Minimally Invasive
Spine Surgery

Minimally Invasive Spine Surgery

Edited by

Alexander R. Vaccaro
Thomas Jefferson University and the Rothman Institute
Philadelphia, Pennsylvania, USA

Christopher M. Bono
Harvard Medical School
Brigham and Women's Hospital
Boston, Massachusetts, USA

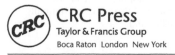

CRC Press
Taylor & Francis Group
Boca Raton London New York

CRC Press is an imprint of the
Taylor & Francis Group, an **informa** business

First published 2007 by Informa Healthcare USA, Inc.

Published 2019 by CRC Press
Taylor & Francis Group
6000 Broken Sound Parkway NW, Suite 300
Boca Raton, FL 33487-2742

© 2007 by Taylor & Francis Group, LLC
CRC Press is an imprint of Taylor & Francis Group, an Informa business

First issued in paperback 2019

No claim to original U.S. Government works

ISBN 13: 978-0-367-45306-0 (pbk)
ISBN 13: 978-0-8493-4029-1 (hbk)

Visit the Taylor & Francis Web site at
http://www.taylorandfrancis.com

and the CRC Press Web site at
http://www.crcpress.com

Library of Congress Cataloging-in-Publication Data

Minimally invasive spine surgery/edited by Alexander R. Vaccaro, Christopher M. Bono.
    p. ; cm. -- (Minimally invasive procedures in orthopedic surgery; 3)
    Includes bibliographical references and index.
    ISBN-13: 978-0-8493-4029-1 (hardcover : alk. paper)
    ISBN-10: 0-8493-4029-2 (hardcover : alk. paper)
    1. Spine--Surgery. 2. Spine--Endoscopic surgery. 3. Microsurgery.
    I. Vaccaro, Alexander R. II. Bono, Christopher M. III. Series.
    [DNLM: 1. Spine--surgery. 2. Surgical Procedures, Minimally
    Invasive--methods. WE 725 M6648 2007]

RD768.M55 2007
617.5'6059--dc22   2007015261

This book is dedicated to my wife, Terri, and my daughter, Alissa Rose, whose love and warmth calm the storms of everyday life, which allows me to focus on such academic endeavors.

Christopher M. Bono

I would like to dedicate this book to my wife, Midge, who plays so many roles in my life, such as friend, personal advisor, and companion.

Alexander R. Vaccaro

Preface

The field of spinal surgery has borne witness to unprecedented advancements in technology. Among the most exciting has been the development of minimally invasive surgery. It has been promoted under numerous descriptors, such as "minimal access" and "less invasive" and utilizes various visualization techniques, such as endoscopy, tubular retractors, and image-guidance.

Minimally invasive spine surgery has sought to achieve the same surgical goals as standard open surgery while minimizing associated morbidity and recovery times. Increasing numbers of reports of "success" at specialized centers by experienced surgeons have spawned interest within the spine surgical community in general. However, the path to "success" must be carefully appreciated. Many minimally invasive techniques have slow learning curves that require substantially more time than their open equivalents, particularly at the outset of a surgeon's experience. As instruments and access systems continually improve, what *is* available today is easier to use than what *was* available yesterday and potentially more difficult to maneuver than what *will* be available tomorrow. Ultimately, these successive improvements will bring minimally invasive surgery to a level that a general spine surgeon can easily learn and use expeditiously to achieve good results.

Minimally Invasive Spine Surgery offers a comprehensive and up-to-date source for surgeons interested in performing minimal access spinal surgery. The text includes detailed descriptions of a wide array of minimally invasive techniques. To better aid the reader in using this timely work, the chapters are divided into comprehensive sections according to the treatment goal: decompression, stabilization and fusion, percutaneous pain-relieving procedures, and non-fusion/motion-sparing techniques. Going beyond a pure technique-oriented book, each of the chapters includes a discussion of indications, imaging, setup, complications, and clinical outcomes of the individual procedures.

The reader will also quickly appreciate the unique organization of *Minimally Invasive Spine Surgery*. The opening section is intended to develop a grounded framework within which these surgical techniques can be better analyzed and understood. Beyond an excellent discussion on anatomical approaches, other chapters discuss an evidence-based review of minimally invasive surgery, classification of minimally invasive spine surgery techniques, appropriate patient selection, and the future direction of these surgical techniques and technology. Whether planning an endoscopic discectomy or percutaneous pedicle screw insertion, spinal surgeons must have a comprehensive understanding of the indications, technical execution, limitations, and bailouts of these minimally invasive procedures. It is the editors' hope to provide this important information for a broad range of conditions and techniques. Thoughtful consideration of these issues can help surgeons safely and effectively adopt minimally invasive spine surgery into their everyday practices.

Christopher M. Bono
Alexander R. Vaccaro

Acknowledgments

For their commitment, evident in the quality of the chapters contained within this book, we would like to thank all of the contributing authors. Their expertise, time, and patience are very much appreciated in light of the difficult question of finding the delicate balance between clinical responsibilities, academic work, and family.

Contents

Contributors

Henry Ahn Division of Orthopedic Surgery, St. Michael's Hospital, University of Toronto, Toronto, Ontario, Canada

Todd J. Albert Department of Orthopedics, Thomas Jefferson University, Philadelphia, Pennsylvania, U.S.A.

D. Greg Anderson Department of Orthopedic Surgery, Thomas Jefferson University, Philadelphia, Pennsylvania, U.S.A.

Paul A. Anderson Department of Orthopedic Surgery and Rehabilitation, University of Wisconsin, Madison, Wisconsin, U.S.A.

Douglas G. Armstrong Division of Pediatric Orthopedics, Rainbow Babies and Children's Hospital, Case Medical Center, Case Western Reserve University, Cleveland, Ohio, U.S.A.

Paul Arnold Department of Neurosurgery, University of Kansas, Kansas City, Kansas, U.S.A.

Ferhan Asghar Department of Orthopedic Surgery, Vanderbilt University Medical Center, Nashville, Tennessee, U.S.A.

Sushil K. Basra Department of Orthopedics, University of Medicine and Dentistry of New Jersey, Newark, New Jersey, U.S.A.

Kathleen S. Beebe Department of Orthopedics, University of Medicine and Dentistry of New Jersey, Newark, New Jersey, U.S.A.

John M. Beiner Department of Orthopedics, Yale University School of Medicine, New Haven, Connecticut, U.S.A.

Carlo Bellabarba Department of Orthopedics and Sports Medicine, and Neurological Surgery, Harborview Medical Center, University of Washington School of Medicine, Seattle, Washington, U.S.A.

Joseph Benevenia Department of Orthopedics, University of Medicine and Dentistry of New Jersey, Newark, New Jersey, U.S.A.

Randal R. Betz Shriners Hospitals for Children, Philadelphia, Pennsylvania, U.S.A.

Christopher M. Bono Department of Orthopedic Surgery, Harvard Medical School, Brigham and Women's Hospital, Boston, Massachusetts, U.S.A.

Darrel S. Brodke Department of Orthopedic Surgery, University of Utah, Salt Lake City, Utah, U.S.A.

T. Desmond Brown Department of Orthopedic Surgery, Boston University School of Medicine, Boston, Massachusetts, U.S.A.

Jens R. Chapman   Department of Orthopedics and Sports Medicine, and Neurological Surgery, Harborview Medical Center, University of Washington School of Medicine, Seattle, Washington, U.S.A.

Yung Chen   Spinal Diagnostics and Treatment Center, Daly City, California, U.S.A.

Bernard A. Coert   Department of Neurosurgery, Stanford University Medical Center, Stanford, California, U.S.A.

Linda Park D'Andrea   Brandywine Institute of Orthopedics, Pottstown, Pennsylvania, U.S.A.

Michael D. Daubs   Department of Orthopedic Surgery, University of Utah, Salt Lake City, Utah, U.S.A.

Rick Davis   Department of Orthopedic Surgery, Vanderbilt University Medical Center, Nashville, Tennessee, U.S.A.

Richard Derby   Spinal Diagnostics and Treatment Center, Daly City, and Division of Physical Medicine and Rehabilitation, Stanford University Medical Center, Stanford, California, U.S.A.

Tom Faciszewski   Department of Orthopedic Spine Surgery, Marshfield Clinic, Marshfield, Wisconsin, U.S.A.

Daniel R. Fassett   Department of Neurosurgery, University of Utah, Salt Lake City, Utah, U.S.A.

Steven R. Garfin   Department of Orthopedic Surgery, University of California, San Diego Medical Center, San Diego, California, U.S.A.

Grigory Goldberg   Thomas Jefferson University, Philadelphia, Pennsylvania, U.S.A.

Jay Govind   Department of Anesthesia and Pain Medicine, The Canberra Hospital and The Australian National University, Canberra, Australian Capital Territory, Australia

Jonathan N. Grauer   Department of Orthopedics and Rehabilitation, Yale University School of Medicine, New Haven, Connecticut, U.S.A.

Troy D. Gust   Department of Neurosurgery, University of Kansas, Kansas City, Kansas, U.S.A.

Qusai M. Hammouri   Department of Orthopedics and Rehabilitation, Yale University School of Medicine, New Haven, Connecticut, U.S.A.

Neal G. Haynes   Department of Neurosurgery, University of Kansas, Kansas City, Kansas, U.S.A.

Harry N. Herkowitz   William Beaumont Hospital, Royal Oak, Michigan, U.S.A.

Alan S. Hilibrand   Department of Orthopedic Surgery, Thomas Jefferson University and the Rothman Institute, Philadelphia, Pennsylvania, U.S.A.

Ken Y. Hsu   Orthopedic Surgery, St. Mary's Spine Center, San Francisco, California, U.S.A.

Mark M. Kayanja   Cleveland Clinic Spine Institute, The Cleveland Clinic Foundation, Cleveland, Ohio, U.S.A.

A. Jay Khanna   Johns Hopkins Orthopedics, Good Samaritan Hospital, Baltimore, Maryland, U.S.A.

Larry T. Khoo   Division of Neurosurgery, Department of Surgery, David Geffen School of Medicine, University of California, Los Angeles Medical Center, Los Angeles, California, U.S.A.

Choll W. Kim   Department of Orthopedic Surgery, University of California, and the San Diego VA Medical Center, San Diego, California, U.S.A.

Daniel H. Kim   Department of Neurosurgery, Baylor College of Medicine, Houston, Texas, U.S.A.

Se-Hoon Kim   Department of Neurosurgery, Korea University Medical Center, Seoul, Republic of Korea

Dimitriy Kondrashov   Orthopedic Surgery, St. Mary's Spine Center, San Francisco, California, U.S.A.

Joon Y. Lee   Department of Orthopedic Surgery, University of Pittsburgh, Pittsburgh, Pennsylvania, U.S.A.

Max C. Lee   Department of Neurosurgery, Milwaukee Neurological Institute, Milwaukee, Wisconsin, U.S.A.

Sang-Heon Lee   Spinal Diagnostics and Treatment Center, Daly City, California, U.S.A.

Isador H. Lieberman   Cleveland Clinic Spine Institute, The Cleveland Clinic Foundation, Cleveland, Ohio, U.S.A.

Moe R. Lim   Department of Orthopedic Surgery, University of North Carolina–Chapel Hill, Chapel Hill, North Carolina, U.S.A.

Sameer Mather   Department of Orthopedic Surgery, University of North Carolina–Chapel Hill, Chapel Hill, North Carolina, U.S.A.

Fergus McKiernan   Center for Bone Diseases, Marshfield Clinic, Marshfield, Wisconsin, U.S.A.

A. A. Mehbod   Department of Orthopedic Surgery, Massachusetts General Hospital, Boston, Massachusetts, U.S.A.

Lance K. Mitsunaga   Department of Orthopedic Surgery, University of California, and the San Diego VA Medical Center, San Diego, California, U.S.A.

Peter O. Newton   Department of Orthopedics, Children's Hospital San Diego, San Diego, California, U.S.A.

Erbil Oguz   Department of Orthopedic Surgery, Gulhane Military Medical Academy, Ankara, Turkey

Michael A. Pahl   Department of Orthopedic Surgery, Thomas Jefferson University, Philadelphia, Pennsylvania, U.S.A.

Chetan K. Patel   Beaumont Comprehensive Spine Center, Royal Oak, Michigan, U.S.A.

Deepan Patel   Department of Orthopedics, Thomas Jefferson University, Philadelphia, Pennsylvania, U.S.A.

Frank M. Phillips   Department of Orthopedic Surgery, Rush Medical Center, Chicago, Illinois, U.S.A.

Thomas J. Puschak   Panorama Orthopedics and Spine Center, Golden, Colorado, U.S.A.

Raja Rampersaud   Division of Orthopedic Surgery and Neurosurgery, Toronto Western Hospital, University of Toronto, Toronto, Ontario, Canada

James Sanfilippo   Department of Orthopedics, Thomas Jefferson University, Philadelphia, Pennsylvania, U.S.A.

Rick C. Sasso   Indiana Spine Group, Indianapolis, Indiana, U.S.A.

Dilip K. Sengupta   Dartmouth-Hitchcock Medical Center, Lebanon, New Hampshire, U.S.A.

Roshan P. Shah   Department of Orthopedics and Rehabilitation, Yale University School of Medicine, New Haven, Connecticut, U.S.A.

Donald C. Shields   Division of Neurosurgery, Department of Surgery, David Geffen School of Medicine, University of California, Los Angeles Medical Center, Los Angeles, California, U.S.A.

Kern Singh   Department of Orthopedic Surgery, Rush University Medical Center, Chicago, Illinois, U.S.A.

William Tally   Department of Orthopedics, Thomas Jefferson University, Philadelphia, Pennsylvania, U.S.A.

Chadi Tannoury   Department of Orthopedic Surgery, Thomas Jefferson University, Philadelphia, Pennsylvania, U.S.A.

George H. Thompson   Division of Pediatric Orthopedics, Rainbow Babies and Children's Hospital, Case Medical Center, Case Western Reserve University, Cleveland, Ohio, U.S.A.

Daisuke Togawa   Cleveland Clinic Spine Institute, The Cleveland Clinic Foundation, Cleveland, Ohio, U.S.A.

Eeric Truumees   Department of Orthopedic Surgery, Beaumont Comprehensive Spine Center, Royal Oak, Michigan, U.S.A.

Vidyadhar V. Upasani   Department of Orthopedic Surgery, University of California, San Diego, California, U.S.A.

Alexander R. Vaccaro   Department of Orthopedic Surgery and Neurosurgery, Thomas Jefferson University and the Rothman Institute, Philadelphia, Pennsylvania, U.S.A.

Michael Vives   Department of Orthopedics, University of Medicine and Dentistry of New Jersey, Newark, New Jersey, U.S.A.

K. B. Wood   Department of Orthopedic Surgery, Massachusetts General Hospital, Boston, Massachusetts, U.S.A.

Anthony T. Yeung   Arizona Institute for Minimally Invasive Spine Care, Phoenix, Arizona, U.S.A.

Christopher A. Yeung   Arizona Institute for Minimally Invasive Spine Care, Phoenix, Arizona, U.S.A.

Jason Young   Department of Orthopedic Surgery, Loyola University Medical Center, Maywood, Illinois, U.S.A.

Paul H. Young   Department of Surgery, St. Louis University School of Medicine, St. Louis, Missouri, U.S.A.

James F. Zucherman   Orthopedic Surgery, St. Mary's Spine Center, San Francisco, California, U.S.A.

1 Anatomical Approaches for Minimally Invasive Spine Surgery

Donald C. Shields and Larry T. Khoo
Division of Neurosurgery, Department of Surgery, David Geffen School of Medicine, University of California, Los Angeles Medical Center, Los Angeles, California, U.S.A.

Grigory Goldberg
Thomas Jefferson University, Philadelphia, Pennsylvania, U.S.A.

Alexander R. Vaccaro
Department of Orthopedic Surgery and Neurosurgery, Thomas Jefferson University and the Rothman Institute, Philadelphia, Pennsylvania, U.S.A.

INTRODUCTION

Traditional open surgical approaches to the spine require disruption of muscular and ligamentous components in order to expose bony structures. Spinal stability supplied by these components is therefore compromised as part of the surgical exposure. Decreased spinal stability and other morbidities associated with open surgical approaches have led to the development of minimally invasive spinal exposure techniques. The text that follows provides a description of anatomical structures and potential complications associated with various minimally invasive approaches to the spine.

ANTERIOR CERVICAL FORAMINOTOMY APPROACH

The anterior cervical foraminotomy exposure was designed to negate the need for bone fusion and immobilization, while maintaining spinal stability following anatomical decompression of the spinal cord. Approximating the skin incision required for the standard anterior cervical spine approach, a 3- to 5-cm transverse incision is made along the anterior neck ipsilateral to the radiculopathy just medial to the sternocleidomastoid muscle. Subcutaneous tissue and platysma muscle are immediately observed and sharply dissected. The loose connective tissue layer deep to the platysma is undermined for greater mobility, and the middle layer of the deep cervical fascia enclosing the omohyoid muscle is incised. The carotid sheath and sternocleidomastoid muscle are retracted laterally, and the strap muscle, trachea and esophagus, medially. An anterior cervical discectomy retractor system exposes the ipsilateral longus colli muscle rather than the midline anterior disc surface (Fig. 1). As the longus colli muscle is reflected to further increase exposure, the lateral dissection is limited by the uncovertebral joints to prevent injury to the vertebral vessels as they pass through the foramen. As the vertebral artery courses anterior to the C7 transverse process and beneath the longus colli, care must be taken not to injure the vertebral artery while removing the medial portion of the longus colli. After the medial portions of the transverse processes of adjacent vertebrae have been identified, the ipsilateral uncovertebral joint between them is visualized. Often the uncovertebral joint interface is directed approximately 30° cephalad from the horizontal plane of the intervertebral disc; spondylotic changes may obscure this anatomy. The uncovertebral joint is drilled between the transverse processes to the level of the posterior longitudinal ligament, leaving a piece of thin cortical bone attached laterally to the ligamentous tissue covering the vertebral artery. This remnant of uncinate process is dissected to expose the vertebral artery. Care is also taken to drill the base of the uncinate process as the exiting nerve root lies just adjacent to it. Posterior osteophytes can now be drilled away by crossing the midline diagonally toward the opposite margin of the spinal cord dura. The posterior longitudinal ligament is incised for decompression of the ipsilateral nerve root and spinal cord.

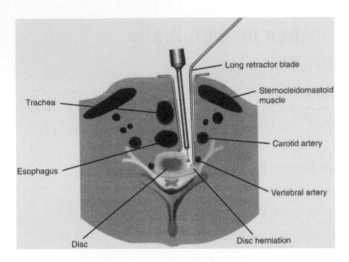

FIGURE 1 Anterior cervical foraminotomy exposure with retraction of the carotid sheath and sternocleidomastoid muscle laterally, and the strap muscle, trachea, and esophagus, medially.

Complications associated with this technique include perforation of the ipsilateral vertebral artery (1–3). Because the vertebral artery occasionally enters the transverse foramen at a level adjacent to C6, the longus colli is incised carefully under the operating microscope. Also, the thin layer of cortical bone left covering the medial portion of this artery helps prevent injury to the vessel. Damage to the recurrent laryngeal nerve upon exposure must also be avoided. A left-sided approach may reduce this risk at lower cervical levels as the nerve runs a more predictable course along the anterior border of the sternocleidomastoid. Care must also be taken to prevent injury of other anterior cervical structures (i.e., esophagus, carotid artery) by using blunt dissection during the exposure.

POSTERIOR CERVICAL APPROACHES
Anatomy and Pertinent Landmarks

The C2, C7, and T1 spinous processes are among the most prominent palpable landmarks in the posterior cervical spine and are easily located even in larger individuals. There is often difficulty in differentiating C7 from T1; therefore, a spinal needle may be placed and a lateral radiograph obtained to determine the proper level. Unfortunately, in larger individuals or in the presence of a short, stocky neck, radiographic visualization may be difficult and may require a "swimmer's view" to visualize down to this level. Also, the C7 spinous process is thicker and not bifid like the cephalad vertebral levels (C3–C6), and has a tubercle at its end.

The ligamentum nuchae is a fibroelastic septum that takes origin from the occiput and inserts into the C7 spinous process (1). It sends septa to each of the cervical spinous processes and serves to longitudinally divide the lateral paracervical muscles. The posterior paracervical muscles of the cervical spine are arranged in three layers. The most superficial layer consists of the trapezius muscle. It originates from all the spinous processes of the cervical spine. The next layer consists of the splenius capitis that originates in the midline and inserts into the occipital bone. The deep layer is composed of three layers. From the most superficial to the deepest, they are the semispinalis capitis, the semispinalis cervices, and the multifidus muscles and short and long rotators.

Posterior Cervical Foraminotomy

Posterior cervical approaches are often employed to address the site of neurological compression while avoiding risk of injury to the anterior neck structures, including the trachea, esophagus, thyroid, thymus, carotid arteries, jugular veins, vagus nerve, recurrent laryngeal nerve, superior laryngeal nerve, ansa cervicalis, and thoracic duct. Minimally invasive posterior foraminotomy exposures are further designed to extend these benefits while avoiding the loss of structural integrity required in open approaches. After incision of the skin and the underlying subcutaneous tissue, the cervical fascia is exposed. Sharp dissection of the fascia allows for easier passage of the sequential dilating cannulas with a minimum force. The underlying posterior neck musculature primarily responsible for neck extension, lateral bending, and rotation is then exposed. These fibers run in a longitudinal or oblique fashion, and placement of sequentially dilating tubes can be accomplished with minimal tissue trauma by muscle splitting and stretching.

The tubular retractor system is then used to perforate the superficial, intermediate, and deep muscle layers (Fig. 2). The superficial layer is composed of the trapezius, splenius capitis, and semispinalis capitis muscles. Deeper to this is the intermediate layer including the levator scapulae, spinalis cervicis, longissimus capitis, and inferior oblique capitis muscles, while the deep layer includes the rotator cervicis brevis, rotator cervicis longus, and interspinalis cervicis muscles. Once the tubular retractor is set in the desired position, a bovie electrocautery with a long tip is used to remove the remaining muscle and soft tissues overlying the lateral mass and facet. It is best to begin this dissection laterally where the bone is clearly felt. The dissection can then be continued medially to expose the laminofacet junction, avoiding compromise of the interlaminar space at this point. Often, the ligamentum flavum is thinned or absent near the lateral edge of the interlaminar space, placing the dura and spinal cord at higher risk. With the bone well-visualized, a small straight endoscopic curette is used to scrape the inferior edge of the superior lamina and the medial edge of the lateral mass-facet complex. This exposure is then continued beneath the lamina and facet with the use of a small angled curette. This curette is used to hook under the lamina and to free the soft tissue from its periosteal attachment. Adequate dissection of the underlying flavum and dura from the bone defines the relevant anatomy and helps to prevent incidental dural tears. After the plane has been defined, a small angled Kerrison rongeur is utilized to begin the foraminotomy. The decompression is carefully continued inferiorly and laterally along the course of the neural foramen.

Potential complications with this procedure include durotomy, vertebral artery perforation, neural element compromise, and spinal cord injury (4,5). Percutaneous K-wire or Steinmann pin placement is a common initial step employed by many practitioners of this technique, followed by subsequent serial dilatation using a tubular retractor system such as the METRx tubes (Medtronic, Sofamor-Danek; Memphis, TN). In the posterior cervical region, the fascia typically encountered is thicker than that found in the thoracodorsal fascia. As a result, excessive force is often needed to persuade the dilators through this dense layer, which can result in inadvertent plunging of the dilators. Thus, the posterior cervical fascia can be sharply incised to avoid injury during serial dilation with the tubes. Direct visualization under lateral fluoroscopy is important to assess the depth of penetration of the K-wire or pin during initial placement. Furthermore, anteroposterior fluoroscopic imaging is helpful to ensure safe docking on the facet complex. Medial migration can lead to durotomy or direct neural injury to the cord, and lateral migration can result in damage to the exiting nerve root or the vertebral artery in the foramen transversarium.

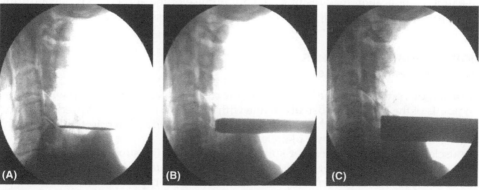

FIGURE 2 Posterior cervical foraminotomy approach following sharp dissection of the fascia for easy passage of dilating cannulas as shown with sequential lateral cervical spine radiographs (**A–C**).

THORACOSCOPIC APPROACHES

Thoracoscopic exposures have been used extensively in thoracic surgery for a variety of pathologies that affect the chest and mediastinum (6–9). This technique decreases the risk of shoulder girdle dysfunction and intercostal neuralgia, and is associated with a lower rate of pulmonary morbidity than open thoracotomy (10–12). Thoracoscopic spinal exposures have thus been developed to approach ventral midline lesions that compress the spinal cord (13).

The location of vascular structures such as the aorta and vena cava is an important consideration in deciding which side to enter. The aorta often has a variable location with respect to the spinal column, while the vena cava location does not vary appreciably. Midline lesions above the level of T9 can often be approached from the right side, allowing more space for manipulation in the absence of the aorta. Although the azygous venous complex is present on the right side, coagulation of these structures is sometimes preferable to aortic retraction. Once the approach trajectory has been established, a 1.5-cm skin incision above the intercostal space along the posterior axillary line allows blunt dissection of the external, middle, and internal intercostal muscles. The segmental nerve and vessels coursing beneath the rib are avoided by incision superior to the rib. The parietal pleura is then opened bluntly after deflating the ipsilateral lung with single-side ventilation. With direct visualization to ensure a path clear of lung or pleural adhesions, an optical 10-mm channel is introduced. By compressing the skin with a finger, the exact entry point of the next two to three portals along the anterior axillary line is identified under internal thoracoscopic visualization. The subsequent trocars can be inserted after blunt dissection of the different layers of the lateral chest wall with small scissors. The cephalo-caudad axis of the camera is oriented to the view of the primary operative surgeon to allow for normal translation of his hand movements to the monitor. The pleura is then dissected from the surface of the spine, and the segmental intercostal vessels are ligated. Of note, with levels from T1 to T10, the head of the rib articulates with the same numbered vertebral body and superior disc space (Fig. 3).

After dissection of the anterior longitudinal ligament, the spinal canal is exposed by removing the rib head and pedicle. Care must be taken at this point to avoid avulsion of the sympathetic trunk and splanchnic nerves anterior to the rib heads. A cavity is drilled in the dorsal vertebral body and disc space to provide enough room to insert tools, to avoid manipulation of the spinal cord, and to expose normal dura rostral and caudal to the herniated disc. The cavity is hemispherically shaped for small- to moderate-sized disc herniations and rectangular for larger herniations. The spinal cord and nerve roots are decompressed microsurgically under direct visualization.

Complications associated with this procedure include ipsilateral radiculopathy if the segmental nerve root is damaged during manipulation. Durotomies with spinal cord compromise can also occur if the pedicle drilling advances too deeply. Additional complications include transient atelectasis and pleural effusions, which often respond adequately to pulmonary physiotherapy and throacentesis, respectively. A postoperative hemothorax is also possible with damage to thoracic intercostal vessels upon removal of chest tubes. Ultimately, however the most devastating complication may result from compromise of the aorta or vena cava during exposure. Appropriate understanding of the thoracic anatomy is essential in avoiding this.

POSTERIOR LUMBAR APPROACHES
Anatomy and Pertinent Landmarks

The posterior spinous processes of the lumbar spine are easily palpable. The line drawn between the highest points of the iliac crest is usually in line with the L4–L5 interspace. A precise method of localizing a spinal level is with the placement of a spinal needle down to the level of the posterior spinal elements followed by a plain lateral X ray.

The muscles of the posterior lumbar spine are made up of the superficial, intermediate, and deep layers. The superficial layer consists of the latissimus dorsi and thoracolumbar fascia. The intermediate layer consists of serratus posterior and the erector spinae muscles (iliocostalis, longissimus, and spinalis, from lateral to medial). The deep layer consists of the multifidus and rotator muscles (2).

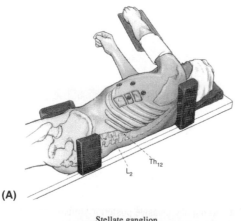

(A)

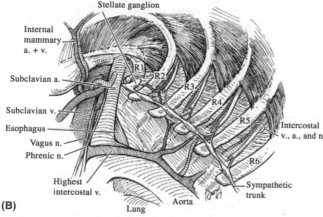

(B)

FIGURE 3 Thoracoscopic approach via the left chest wall is achieved after deflating the ipsilateral lung with single-side ventilation. Common sites for port entry are marked along the anterior and posterior axillary lines (**A**). Medial and posterior chest wall anatomical structures are also depicted as seen through a portal placed along the left anterior axillary line (**B**).

Posterior Foraminotomy

As with posterior foraminotomy exposures of the cervical spine, minimally invasive posterior lumbar approaches are designed to avoid the loss of structural integrity required in open approaches. The skin is incised approximately 1.5-cm lateral to the midline ipsilateral to the site of nerve root compression. A layer of underlying fat and subcutaneous tissue of various thicknesses separates the skin and thoracolumbar fascia. Sharp dissection of this fascia allows for passage of the sequential dilating cannulas with minimum force. Deep to this fascia lies the erector spinae muscle column. The three components of the erector spinae from superficial to deep include the iliocostalis lumborum, longissimus thoracis, and spinalis muscles. Each of these originates inferiorly via a broad tendon attached to the posterior aspect of the iliac crest, sacrum, sacroiliac ligaments, and the sacral spinous processes. The iliocostalis column inserts superiorly into the angles of the ribs while the longissimus attaches to the transverse processes of the vertebra. The spinalis muscle also arises inferiorly from the common origin and attaches superiorly to the spinous processes of the superior lumbar and thoracic vertebra. The erector spinae muscle group extends the vertebral column when acting in unison and laterally flexes the spine if acting unilaterally. Deep to the erector spinae, the surgeon encounters the smaller transversospinalis muscle group, which includes the semispinalis, multifidus, and rotatores, respectively. The muscle fibers in this group attach from the transverse process to the spinous process of the superior adjacent level. The semispinalis muscles extend the cervical and thoracic portions of the vertebral column when acting in unison, and rotate these regions toward the opposite side when acting unilaterally. Similarly, the multifidus and rotatores groups stabilize the spine, flex the trunk laterally, and rotate the superior vertebra to the opposite side. The dilating cannula apparatus is designed to spread these muscles laterally and medially to expose the bony structure below, while avoiding loss of spinal stability afforded by these muscle groups (Fig. 4).

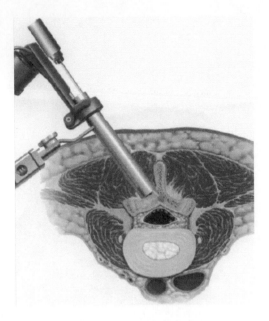

FIGURE 4 Minimally invasive posterior lumbar approaches spread erector spinae muscles laterally and medially to expose the bony structure below. Portions of the lamina, inferior articulating process of the superior vertebra, and the superior articulating process of the inferior vertebra are drilled away. The spinal canal and exiting nerve root are thus exposed for removal of any disc fragments present.

Once the muscular and tendonous components are removed from the underlying lamina and facet joints, a drill is used to remove the inferior articulating process of the superior vertebra and the superior articulating process of the inferior vertebra deep to it. The spinal canal and exiting nerve root is then exposed for removal of any disc fragments present.

Complications associated with this approach include muscle spasm, which may last for several days postoperatively. Muscle relaxants are typically sufficient to address this issue. Durotomy can also occur with the high speed drill or sharp objects inserted near the neural structures. Pyogenic disc space infection and missed free disc fragments have also been reported using this approach (14,15).

EXTREME LATERAL INTERBODY FUSION APPROACH

The extreme lateral interbody fusion (XLIF) approach is designed to utilize a direct lateral, retroperitoneal exposure to visualize the intervertebral disc without significant muscular disruption. It also allows more freedom for the surgeon to change the aperture of the operative corridor according to clinical needs. A retroperitoneal approach enables access to spinal nerve root tumors, lateral free-fragment disc protrusions, ossified posterior longitudinal ligament disease, and spondylolisthesis (with lateral entrapment) without sacrifice of the pedicle, facet joint, or transverse processes.

With this approach, the patient is placed in a lateral decubitus position to allow abdominal organs to fall away from the lumbar spine. The adjustable surgical table is flexed so as to increase the iliac crest–rib cage distance. The disc in question is localized with lateral fluoroscopy, and marked directly lateral to the disc space. A 1- to 2-cm longitudinal skin incision is placed posterior to this mark at the lateral border of the erector spinae muscle. Through this incision, subcutaneous soft-tissue layers are dissected bluntly using the surgeon's finger. Blunt dissection scissors can also aid in spreading the subsequent external oblique, internal oblique, and transversus muscle layers. The paraspinal transverse fat layer can then be visualized. Care must be taken at this point to avoid perforation of the abdominal peritoneum. Inside the retroperitoneal space, the surgeon's finger is again used to push the peritoneum anteriorly. The finger can now palpate the iliopsoas muscle, and sweep anteriorly to confirm the direct lateral incision mark (Fig. 5). The second incision is then made at this mark, and the dilator set is introduced with palpation of the initial dilator tip with the surgeon's finger still in place to avoid peritoneal perforation. As the initial dilator approaches the iliopsoas muscle, its location is verified with fluoroscopy. Iliopsoas fibers are bluntly displaced anteriorly to expose the disc space. Of note,

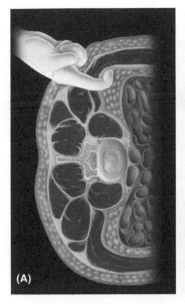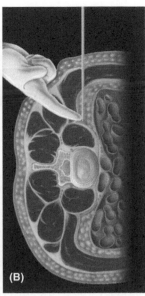

FIGURE 5 The extreme lateral interbody fusion approach is aided by use of the surgeon's finger to confirm the peritoneum is pushed forward to open the retroperitoneal space (**A**). The dilator set can then be introduced with palpation of the initial dilator tip to avoid peritoneal perforation (**B**).

care must be taken to avoid damage to the anterior great vessels and more lateral lumbosacral plexus during this procedure (16). Subsequent dilators are placed for direct visualization of the lateral annulus. A 15- to 20-mm annulotomy is created, and standard disc removal and endplate preparation are performed as necessary (17).

Complications associated with this procedure include perforation of the peritoneal space during exposure. Damage to the ipsilateral renal vascular structures can lead to significant bleeding. This can be prevented with blunt dissection of the initial posterior insertion. The small dilator tube may also perforate the peritoneum during insertion if the surgeon's finger is not used to guide its trajectory. Moreover, exiting nerve roots of the lumbosacral plexus at the level of the iliopsoas muscle can be injured with sharp dissection of the muscle. Also, during removal of the disc fragments, anatomical boundaries must be observed anteriorly to avoid the aorta and spinal canal posteriorly as these structures are poorly visualized from a lateral, retroperitoneal approach.

MINIMALLY INVASIVE ANTERIOR LUMBAR INTERBODY FUSION APPROACH

Anterior approaches to the lumbar spine were designed to provide direct access to ventral pathology, to avoid dissection of lumbar paraspinal musculature, and to place bone grafts in the predominant load-bearing column of the lumbar spine. Minimally invasive anterior lumbar interbody fusion approaches have more recently been developed to achieve these results with minimal distraction of abdominal cavity contents. While the traditional open transperitoneal approach to the lumbar spine is performed through either midline, paramedian, or Pfannensteil incision, minimally invasive techniques employ three or four smaller incisions for placement of laparoscopic channels. An approximately 1- to 3-cm-wide midline incision just above the pubis is utilized for insertion of the interbody components, while small paramedian incisions allow for insertion of working forceps. An umbilical incision is also created for placement of a viewing camera. Midline incisions pierce the linea alba, while paramedian exposures enter the external oblique, internal oblique, and transverse abdominis muscles. Entrance into the abdominal cavity via the transversalis fascia, extraperitoneal fat layer, and peritoneum, respectively, can then be achieved. Abdominal contents can sometimes be mobilized out of the pelvic inlet as the patient is placed into a steep Trendelenburg position. Once bowel segments are moved to allow viewing of the sacral promontory, the posterior portion of the parietal peritoneum can be dissected with electrocautery. In males, a blunt Kittner dissector should be used to avoid injury to the presacral sympathetic plexus, which can result in retrograde ejaculation.

The presacral sympathetic plexus is a continuation of the sympathetic trunk, which enters the abdominal cavity posterior to the medial arcuate ligament. The sympathetic trunk is a direct continuation of the thoracolumbar sympathetic nerves coursing along the anterolateral aspect of the lumbar vertebral bodies with close approximation to the iliopsoas attachments. At the level of the third and fourth lumbar vertebrae, these ramify about the inferior mesenteric artery and the inferior mesenteric ganglion. About 80% of these ramifications occur on the left side of the aorta. Once ramified, these fibers are referred to as the superior hypogastric plexus as they course inferiorly in the retroperitoneal space. They cross the left common iliac artery/vein and lie anterior to the fifth lumbar vertebra within the prevertebral space. These sympathetic fibers control the normal transport of semen and prevent retrograde ejaculation by closing the bladder neck during ejaculation.

One of the initial anatomical structures observed in the midline is the median sacral artery and vein complex. As these vessels do not reliably predict the midline of the vertebral body, the preoperative MRI images should be reviewed for the presence of eccentric anterior osteophytes, which may give the surgeon a false localization of the midline. The great vessels and iliopsoas muscles also aid the surgeon in selecting the proper site for entry into the disc space. Of note, the bifurcation of these vessels is variable and is important for approaches to the L4–5, and L5–S1 disc spaces. The bifurcation of the vena cava occurs inferior to that of the aorta and is usually located above the L5–S1 disc space. The vena cava bifurcation is also to the right of the aorta with the left common iliac vein passing through the aortic bifurcation (Fig. 6). Injury to the left common iliac vein is therefore common during approaches to this area. Superior to this level, the aorta gives off paired segmental vessels, which pass laterally over the middle portion of the lumbar vertebral bodies. The segmentals are attached by soft tissue and can be mobilized and ligated as needed. Care must be taken as the segmentals actually arise from the dorsal surface of the aorta, and ligation too close to the origin may result in retraction behind the aorta. The vessel may then be very difficult to locate as it continues to vigorously bleed. The blood supply to the spinal column is also derived from these segmental vessels, which feed the vertebral bony elements, the paraspinal muscles, and the extradural space. A main dorsal branch emerges as the segmental arteries approach the neural foramina. This branch continues posteriorly below the transverse process and supplies the bone of the posterior elements and the paraspinal muscles. Shortly after its origin, the dorsal branch gives off an intraspinal branch, which feeds the nerve root and dura. At specific levels, separate anterior segmental medullary arteries arise from the dorsal segmental artery and supply the anterior two-thirds of the spinal cord. One such vessel, the artery of Adamkiewicz, occurs commonly at the upper lumbar or lower thoracic levels. As a major feeder to the anterior spinal artery, paraplegia may result if this vessel is ligated. Venous structures in this area are somewhat less predictable than that of the arterial vessels. However, the iliolumbar vein is most often a left-sided venous segmental structure, similar to the other segmental veins that drain into the vena cava at each mid vertebral level. The inferior location and large size of this vessel are important to note. The vein courses

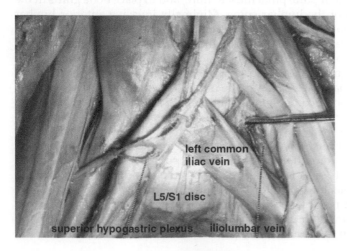

FIGURE 6 The anterior lumbar interbody fusion approach requires consideration of critical vascular and nervous structures. The bifurcations of the aorta and vena cava are typically observed rostral to the L5-S1 disc space. The superior hypogastric plexus is shown anterior to the left common iliac vein in this specimen.

medially deep to the iliopsoas to join the left common iliac vein, and may attach directly to the vena cava.

In addition to vascular structures in this region, the iliopsoas muscles can aid the surgeon in localization of the midline. The iliopsoas muscle lies along the anterolateral aspect of the spine between the transverse processes and the lateral vertebral bodies and discs. It originates from the lumbar transverse processes and lateral bodies of lower thoracic and lumbar vertebra with an insertion onto the lesser trochanter of the femur. The kidney, ureter, and perinephric fat are located anterior to the iliopsoas. Of note, the ureter passes along the iliopsoas muscle and then lies anterior to the iliac vessels. After confirmation of the midline, the disc space can be entered via annulotomy and cleaned. Progressively larger distractors are then tamped into the disc space to appropriately restore the disc height in preparation for implant insertion.

Significant complications can result during this exposure if anatomical relationships are ignored. Due to the high flow of abdominal great vessels, the most devastating complications are related to avulsion of the aorta, vena cava, and iliac arteries/veins. Blunt dissection of soft tissues adjacent to these structures is critical in avoiding this. In males, retrograde ejaculation is a potential risk with lower lumbar exposures as sympathetic fibers course anteriorly to the disc space (18–20). Blunt dissection is thus recommended along the anterior border of the spinal column. Perforation of other abdominal contents (i.e., bowel, ureters) with resulting peritoneal contamination can similarly be avoided if their anatomical relationships are respected by the surgeon.

MINIMALLY INVASIVE TRANSSACRAL APPROACH FOR L5-S1 FUSION

The paracoccygeal approach for L5–S1 fusions was designed to avoid bony dissection, prevent L5–S1 annulus disruption, and minimize dissection of posterior muscular and ligamentous structures. The patient is initially placed in a prone position, and the paracoccygeal notch is palpated. A 1.5-cm incision is made through the skin and levator ani muscle/fascia 20-mm caudal to the notch for entry into the presacral space.

Anatomical borders of this space anteriorly include the visceral fascia covering the posterior aspect of the mesorectum. The parietal fascia lining the sacrum and coccyx bounds the presacral space posteriorly. The anterior (pelvic) surface of the sacrum is shaped in a concave fashion in both transverse and rostrocaudal directions (21). As the sacrum is formed by the fusion of five vertebral bodies, four transverse ridges are noted along this surface with a corresponding anterior neural foramen on each side. The foraminae are oriented in a slightly anterolateral direction allowing passage for exiting anterior divisions of sacral nerves and lateral sacral arteries. Also, three symmetrical muscular attachments are noted on the anterior surface of the sacrum. The piriformis muscle group is found lateral to the ventral foraminae originating from the sacral lateral masses. The iliacus group is attached to the superior lateral aspect of the sacrum, and the coccygeus to the inferior lateral sacrum. Important vascular structures related to this approach include the median sacral artery, as discussed previously (22). This vessel lies posterior to the parietal fascia, and may descend in a variable trajectory over the sacral promontory. The vascular supply to the rectum is likewise outside of the presacral space contained within the visceral fascia covering the posterior mesorectum. Thus, the surgeon is limited to the midline in the coronal plane between the iliac vessels (mean distance of 6.4 cm) and sagittally within the presacral space with an average diameter of 1.2 cm.

With the midline sacral promontory and median sacral artery located, a guide pin introducer is inserted with fluoroscopic confirmation. An axial port is thus placed into the anterior surface of S1 (Fig. 7). Gradual dilation of a trans-osseous working channel within the vertebral column is then formed for L5–S1 discectomy using disc cutters, which debulk the nucleus pulposa and remove disc fragments via suction. After endplate abrasion, the L5 and S1 bodies are fused with inserted bone graft and an axial titanium rod fixation device. Thus, the disc space height can be restored to normal without dissection of the annulus or supporting muscle groups.

Complications associated with this procedure include perforation of the pelvic contents. Injury to the rectum, iliac vessels, and median sacral artery can be avoided if their trajectories are appreciated by the surgeon during exposure. In case of median sacral artery injury, several

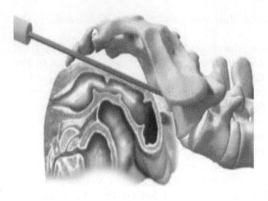

FIGURE 7 The paracoccygeal approach for L5-S1 fusions is achieved via the presacral space. An entry point approximately 20-mm caudal to the paracoccygeal notch allows placement of a guide pin introducer into the midline presacral space toward the anterior surface of S1.

anastomoses to paired lateral sacral arteries may help to preserve blood supply to the sacrum and coccyx, preventing significant vascular compromise. Biplanar fluoroscopy can also be used to avoid complications by ensuring a midline approach through the presacral space.

Thus, while these and other minimally invasive approaches to the spine decrease the disruption of surrounding tissues, they require an accurate understanding of anatomical relationships as the surgeon's view is often more limited than that of traditional open exposures.

REFERENCES

1. Jho HD. Microsurgical anterior cervical foraminotomy for radiculopathy: a new approach to cervical disc herniation. J Neurosurg 1996; 84:155–160.
2. Jho HD. Decompression via microsurgical anterior foraminotomy for cervical spondylytic myelopathy: technical note. J Neurosurg 1997; 86:297–302.
3. Johnson JP, Filler AG, McBride DQ, Batzdorf U. Anterior cervical foraminotomy for unilateral radicular disease. Spine 2000; 25:905–909.
4. Adamson TE. Microendoscopic posterior cervical laminoforaminotomy for unilateral radiculopathy: results of a new technique in 100 cases. J Neurosurg 2001; 95 (suppl 1) :51–57.
5. Khoo LT, Laich DT, Perez-Cruet MJ, Fessler RG. Posterior cervical microendoscopic foraminotomy. In: Perez-Cruet MJ, Fessler RG, eds. Outpatient Spinal Surgery. St. Louis: Quality Medical Publishing Inc., 2002:71–93.
6. Coltharp WH, Arnold JH, Alford WC Jr, et al. Videothoracoscopy: improved technique and expanded indications. Ann Thorac Surg 1992; 53:776–779.
7. Kaiser LR. Video-assisted thoracic surgery. Current state of the art. Ann Surg 1994; 220:720–734.
8. Landreneau RJ, Mack MJ, Hazelrigg SR, et al. Video-assisted thoracic surgery: basic technical concepts and intercostal approach strategies. Ann Thorac Surg 1992; 54:800–807.
9. Mack MJ, Aronoff RJ, Acuff TE, Douthit MB, Bowman RT, Ryan WH. Present role of thoracoscopy in the diagnosis and treatment of diseases of the chest. Ann Thorac Surg 1992; 54:403–409.
10. Ferson PF, Landreneau RJ, Dowling RD, et al. Comparison of open versus thoracoscopic lung biopsy for diffuse infiltrative pulmonary disease. J Thorac Cardiovasc Surg 1993; 106:194–199.
11. Hazelrigg SR, Landreneau RJ, Boley TM, et al. The effect of muscle-sparing versus standard posterolateral thoracotomy on pulmonary function, muscle strength, and postoperative pain. J Thorac Cardiovasc Surg 1991; 101:394–401.
12. Landreneau RJ, Hazelrigg SR, Mack MJ, et al. Postoperative pain-related morbidity: video-assisted thoracic surgery versus thoracotomy. Ann Thorac Surg 1993; 56:1285–1289.
13. Oskouian RJ, Johnson JP, Regan JJ. Thoracoscopic microdiscectomy. Neurosurgery 2002; 50:103–109.
14. Mayer HM. Spine update. Percutaneous lumbar disc surgery. Spine 1994; 23:2719–2723.
15. Luft C. Automated percutaneous lumbar discectomy (APLD)—method and 1-year follow-up. Eur Rad 1992; 2:292.
16. Rohen JW, Yokochi C. Color Atlas of Anatomy. 2nd ed. New York: Igaku-Shoin, 1988.
17. Dezawa A, Yamane T, Mikami H, Miki H. Retroperitoneal laparoscopic lateral approach to the lumbar spine: a new approach, technique, and clinical trial. J Spinal Disorders 2000; 13:138–143.
18. Christensen FB, Bunger CE. Retrograde ejaculation after retroperitoneal lower lumbar interbody fusion. Int Orthop 1997; 21:176–180.

19. Flynn JC, Price CT. Sexual complications of anterior fusion of the lumbar spine. Spine 1984; 9:489–492.
20. Tiusanen H, Seitsalo S, Osterman K, Soini J. Retrograde ejaculation after anterior lumbar interbody fusion. Eur Spine J 1995; 4:339–342.
21. Cheng JS, Song JK. Anatomy of the sacrum. Neurosurg Focus 2003; 15:1–4.
22. Moore KL. Clinically Oriented Anatomy. 3rd ed. Baltimore, MD: Williams and Wilkins, 1992.

2 | Evidence-Based Review: Minimally Invasive Spine Surgery vs. Open Surgery

Ferhan Asghar and Rick Davis
Department of Orthopedic Surgery, Vanderbilt University Medical Center, Nashville, Tennessee, U.S.A.

Christopher M. Bono
Department of Orthopedic Surgery, Harvard Medical School, Brigham and Women's Hospital, Boston, Massachusetts, U.S.A.

INTRODUCTION

Minimally invasive approaches to surgical procedures have gained popularity over the last several decades. The proposed benefits of these approaches include diminished surgical trauma, scarring, preservation of anatomy, earlier patient recovery, improved cosmesis, and potentially better (or at least equivalent) clinical outcomes. In light of skyrocketing costs for medical care, the evidence supporting these proposed benefits becomes increasingly important. Clinical studies reporting the results of minimally invasive surgery would be the basis of evidence, with comparison of less invasive versus traditional open techniques being most useful.

While a multitude of studies documenting the safety and efficacy of various minimally invasive spine surgical procedures exists, there is a relative paucity of comparisons of the two. Surgeons must therefore be cautious when interpreting the results of such procedures and extrapolating their efficacy to their patients. In the current age of evidence-based medicine, spinal surgeons must critically evaluate these new techniques to determine whether they are both minimally invasive and equally effective as their open counterparts. Notwithstanding the deficiencies in the current literature, it is this chapter's purpose to review the existing evidence comparing the results of a variety of minimally invasive techniques to their open counterparts.

CERVICAL SPINE: OPEN VS. MICROENDOSCOPIC POSTERIOR FORAMINOTOMY

Inherent in its approach, anterior cervical surgical techniques, such as discectomy and fusion, might be considered an open yet minimally invasive procedure. Although debate continues whether use of a microscope might improve results, it seems that the one- to two-inch transverse incision required for such an operation is cosmetically appealing, and offers adequate visualization and working space for the surgeon without the need for endoscopic instruments such as tubular retractors.

In contrast, open posterior cervical surgery usually requires a fairly large incision, even for a single-level procedure. In addition, it seems to be associated with a greater degree of postoperative pain, likely from the degree of muscle-stripping and retraction required. With this, interest in developing minimally invasive techniques of posterior cervical spine procedures has been fostered. In order to minimize the incision size and degree of muscle dissection, surgeons have utilized tubular retraction systems that are placed through paramedian incisions, which allow dissection between the fibers of the paraspinal muscle bellies. Currently, the most popular posterior cervical procedure performed using minimally invasive technique is an endoscopic foraminotomy. Indicated for unilateral radiculopathy from degenerative foraminal stenosis or a disc herniation, advocates also boast that it is motion-sparing, unlike the alternative, which is an anterior discectomy and fusion.

Despite its growing popularity, there are only a handful of studies reporting the outcomes of a microendoscopic posterior cervical foraminotomy (1,2). To date, there is only one study that has attempted to compare endoscopic foraminotomy with open surgery. In a nonrandomized, prospective trial, Fessler and Khoo (1) compared the results of 25 patients who underwent a posterior microendoscpic foraminotomy and 26 patients who underwent an open foraminotomy for cervical radiculopathy. They found that patients who underwent the open procedure had nearly twice the blood loss, three times the postoperative inpatient stay, and four times the duration of narcotic pain medication use. Patients who underwent endoscopic surgery had an 87% rate improvement in axial neck pain and a 92% rate of improvement in radicular symptoms. Those who had open surgery had comparable results, reporting an 89% and 88% rate of axial neck pain and radicular symptom resolution, respectively. The authors concluded that endoscopic foraminotomy for cervical radiculopathy is safe and produces equivalent results as an open procedure, though with short-term (perioperative) advantages.

OPEN VS. ENDOSCOPIC ANTERIOR THORACIC DECOMPRESSION

The morbidity of an open thoracotomy is substantial. Rates of intercostal neuralgia and postoperative incisional pain are high. In addition to being less frequent than cervical or lumbar disc herniations, the morbidity of open anterior thoracic surgery can be prohibitive of thoracic discectomy except for the most serious conditions, such as myelopathy from spinal cord compression.

With the lung deflated, the chest cavity is a natural dead space. In distinction to other forms of minimally invasive approaches using laparoscopy or tube retractors, thoracoscopy capitalizes on this working space. With presumed decreased morbidity, spinal surgery using thoracoscopic techniques may have helped broaden the number of potential candidates for thoracic disc excision and/or fusion (3–5). Notwithstanding the number of series reporting acceptable results of thoracoscopic discectomy (3–5), no dedicated comparisons of endoscopic versus open thoracic disc excision could be found in the authors' review of the literature.

Interestingly, there have been two published series comparing thoracoscopic with open treatment of spinal disorders. In a French study, Mangione et al. (6) compared the outcomes of thoracosopic surgery for a variety of spinal disorders in 29 patients versus open surgery in 24 patients. They found that minimally invasive surgery took significantly longer (246 minutes vs. 172 minutes) but had less blood loss (447 ml vs. 837 ml). The rate of complications was not different. Unfortunately, long-term follow-up or clinical outcomes were not reported. Compared with a cohort of patients who underwent an open procedure, Dickman et al. (7) found that patients who underwent a thoracoscopic corpectomy and fusion had less blood loss, lower chest tube output, and shorter intensive care stays.

OPEN VS. MINIMALLY INVASIVE LUMBAR DISCECTOMY

Minimally invasive techniques have a long history in the treatment of lumbar disc pathology. Although they have lost much of their initial popularity, a substantial body of randomized, controlled data concerning chemonucleolysis, percutaneous lumbar discectomy, and percutaneous laser discectomy exists. For example, van Alphen et al. (8) randomized 151 patients with a lumbar herniated disc to either chemonucleolysis or open discectomy. Of the 73 patients who underwent the minimally invasive procedure, 16 experienced an increased radicular pain compared with none in the 78 patients in the open group. After chemonucleolysis, 18 (25%) eventually underwent open surgery compared with only two reoperations in the open group. Perhaps, what is most concerning is that open surgery following failed chemonucleolsis was successful in only 44% of the cases. Mayer and Brock (9) compared the results of percutaneous endoscopic discectomy in 20 patients versus open discectomy in 20 patients in a randomized, controlled trial. Of note, only contained or small uncontained herniations were included. At two years follow-up, radicular pain had been resolved in 80% of the percutaneous group and 65% of the open discectomy group, which was not a statistically significant difference ($P = 0.3$).

Such techniques rely on indirect decompression of the nerve roots through reduction of intradiscal pressure. Thus, they appear to be most effective for contained herniations/ protrusions that do not extend far beyond the posterior annulus (see Chapter 12). So-called arthroscopic discectomy (a misnomer, as it is not an intra-articular procedure) was then developed, allowing direct visualization and excision of extruded or uncontained disc fragments (10,11). In the authors' search, only two randomized controlled studies were found comparing endoscopic with open discectomy.

In a randomized, controlled trial of 60 patients with a single-level lumbar disc herniation, Hermantin et al. (12) found comparable rates of satisfactory outcome following open discectomy (93%) and endoscopic discectomy (97%). While statistical analysis was not reported, the length of time that the patients were out of work was higher in the open group (49 days) than in the endoscopic group (27 days). Importantly, the investigators excluded disc herniations that exceeded one-half of the anteroposterior diameter of the spinal canal and advised that such large fragments should be approached by open methods.

In an interesting study that focused on the systemic response to open versus endoscopic discectomy, Huang et al. (13) found satisfactory outcomes in 90% of patients who underwent the minimally invasive procedure versus 92% who underwent an open disectomy. C-reactive protein and interleukin-6 levels (both indicators of systemic inflammatory response to trauma) were lower in the endoscopic group, leading the authors to suggest that, with comparable clinical results, the lower systemic insult with minimally invasive surgery may justify its use.

Advocates of using a microscope to perform a lumbar discectomy have claimed the ability to work through a smaller incision. However, there are many surgeons who perform a so-called open discectomy using loupe magnification through equivalently sized incisions. Thus, the technical differences between the so-called microscopic discectomy (which implies that the surgeon utilized a microscope for visualization) and standard open lumbar discectomy have become blurred. Regardless, data comparing the two procedures does exist. Henriksen et al. (14) conducted a prospective, randomized study of 39 patients who underwent a microscopic discectomy compared with 40 who underwent a standard discectomy. While the fascial incision was significantly shorter in the microscopic group (31 mm compared with 70 mm in the open group), the skin incision was kept the same length to blind the patients to the type of surgery. There were no differences in outcomes, pain, or length of stay in the hospital, leading the investigators to conclude that there was no immediate benefit to the microscopic procedure. Ultimately, the decision to use a microscope, loupes, or no magnification is primarily determined by surgeon preference, as it does not seem to affect the outcomes.

DECOMPRESSION FOR LUMBAR STENOSIS PROCEDURES

As familiarity with endoscopic techniques has increased, surgeons have attempted to treat other lumbar disorders besides disc herniation. In a nonrandomized study, Khoo and Fessler (15) reported results of 25 patients who underwent microendoscopic laminotomy for lumbar stenosis and compared them with a similar group who underwent open decompression (laminectomy). They found that patients in the open group had a shorter operation (88 minutes vs. 109 minutes), but had more blood loss (193 cc vs. 68 cc), longer inpatient stays (94 hours vs. 42 hours), and used more narcotics postoperatively. Despite these perioperative differences, overall clinical outcomes were similar between the two groups at final follow-up.

OPEN, MINI-OPEN, AND LAPRASCOPIC ANTERIOR LUMBAR INTERBODY FUSIONS

As lumbar fusion became a more popular procedure for the treatment of degenerative disc disease, various minimally invasive techniques for its execution had been developed. While only recently have minimally invasive posterior fusion techniques come about (which will be discussed next), experience has been considerably longer with minimal access anterior lumbar interbody fusion (ALIF). Advancements in laparoscopy for nonspinal surgery were a major driving force toward the development of laparoscopic ALIF. A number of studies over the past decade have compared the results of this procedure with both standard open and so-called mini-open ALIF.

In a nonrandomized, prospective, multicenter study, Regan et al. (16) compared a group of 240 patients who underwent a laparoscopic, transperitoneal ALIF with a group of 591 patients who underwent an open, retroperitoneal ALIF with threaded, stand-alone cages. Of importance, there was a 10% rate of conversion to open surgery, which the investigators felt was probably avoidable with better patient selection. The overall incidence of complications was not found to be statistically significantly different between the two groups (14% in the open vs. 19% in the laparoscopic group), although the rate of retrograde ejaculation was higher in the laparoscopic group. Patients undergoing the laparoscopic procedure sustained less blood loss (142 cc vs. 207 cc), and had a shorter hospital stay (3.3 days vs. 4 days). Operative time was higher in the minimally invasive group (201 minutes vs. 142 minutes), but this difference decreased as surgeons became more experienced. What is glaringly missing from this study, unfortunately, was documentation of the clinical outcomes or fusion rates.

Zdeblick and David (17) performed a prospective, nonrandomized study of 25 patients who underwent a laparoscopic ALIF versus 25 who underwent a mini-open ALIF at L4-5. There was no statistical difference in operative time, blood loss, or length of hospitalization for single-level cases; operative time was higher for two-level laparoscopic compared with open procedures. Importantly, they found a substantially higher overall complication rate in the laparoscopic group (20% vs. 4%). Furthermore, there was more difficulty in gaining adequate exposure with the laparoscopic technique, which resulted in placement of only a single cage in 16% of the cases, whereas two cages were inserted in all patients undergoing mini-open ALIF. No clinical outcomes or fusion rates were reported. In a retrospective study of 98 patients, Kaiser et al. (18) also found longer operative times with laparoscopic versus mini-open ALIF, a difference that was statistically significant for procedures at the L5-S1 level. While the immediate postoperative complication rate was higher with a mini-open ALIF, the rate of retrograde ejaculation was significantly higher in the laparoscopic group (17.6% vs. 4.3%).

Some have had better success with laparoscopic surgery at the L5-S1 level (19,20). Chung et al. (20) prospectively compared 25 patients who underwent laparoscopic ALIF with 22 who underwent a mini-open ALIF at the L5-S1 disc. The clinical outcomes, including pain scores, Oswestry Disability Index scores, and fusion rates were equivalent in both groups. Operative complications occurred in three laparoscopic cases and two open cases. Operative time was statistically higher in the laparoscopic group.

In a retrospective review of 31 transperitoneal laparoscopic versus 14 mini-open L5-S1 ALIFs, Rodriguez et al. (21) surprisingly found shorter operative times for the laparoscopic approach. However, no difference in analgesic requirements, length of hospital stay, or rate of complications was found. Of interest in times of cost containment, laparoscopy cost $1374 more than the mini-open approach.

MINIMALLY INVASIVE POSTERIOR LUMBAR FUSION AND INSTRUMENTATION

Techniques of minimally invasive posterior lumbar fusion and instrumentation have recently been developed. In general, these require specialized retractor systems, paraspinal muscle splitting surgical approaches, and heavy reliance on intraoperative fluoroscopic imaging. Pedicle screws, utilizing cannulated systems, have been devised that allow insertion through minimal incisions (22). Such techniques have seen their most popular use as adjunct stabilization following an ALIF (23). Others have developed methods of crossing the spinal canal to perform a minimally invasive transforaminal interbody fusion (TLIF) (24). Despite the growing popularity of these procedures, as well as development of a plethora of new types of instrumentation and retractors systems, there is minimal clinical data available. In fact, in the authors' review of the literature, there is no available data comparing minimal access posterior fusion or instrumentation with traditional, standard open procedures.

CONCLUSION

It is clear that more comparative trials, preferably randomized, controlled trials, are needed to better evaluate the efficacy and potential advantages of minimally invasive spine surgery. Larger-scale, prospective trials with sufficient follow-up periods will allow the best assessment.

Readers should be wary of favorable findings with minimally invasive techniques in studies with low numbers, as this can be a sign of type I or alpha error. Likewise, small studies that conclude there are no differences between techniques should be scrutinized for adequate power, as they are at risk of committing type II or beta error (25,26). Glaringly missing in the majority of the studies reviewed in this chapter, a power analysis should be considered mandatory when reporting the results of a randomized controlled trial.

While initial results in centers experienced with minimally invasive spinal surgery have been encouraging, the slow learning curve that must be endured is an important consideration when making general recommendations for the less experienced surgeon. It is also prudent to say that patient and pathology selection (as discussed in another chapter in this text) will have a strong influence on the outcomes of such techniques.

REFERENCES

1. Fessler RG, Khoo LT. Minimally invasive cervical microendoscopic foraminotomy: an initial clinical experience. Neurosurgery 2002; 51:36–45.
2. Adamson TE. Microendoscopic posterior cervical laminoforaminotomy for unilateral radiculopthy: results of a new technique in 100 cases. Neurosurgery 2001; 95:51–57.
3. Stillerman CB, Chen TC, Couldwell WT, et al. Experience in the surgical management of 82 symptomatic herniated thoracic discs and review of the literature. J Neurosurg 1998; 88:623–633.
4. Perez-Cruet MJ, Kim BS, Sandhu FA, et al. Thoracic microendoscopic discectomy. J Neurosurg Spine 2004; 1:58–63.
5. Anand N, Regan JJ. Video-assisted thoracoscopic surgery for thoracic disc disease. Classification and outcome study of 100 consecutive cases with minimum 2 year follow-up. Spine 2002; 27:871–879.
6. Mangione P, Vadier F, Senegas J. Thoracoscopy versus thoracotomy in spinal surgery: comparison of two paired series. Rev Chir Orthop 1999; 85:574–580.
7. Dickman CA, Rosenthal D, Karahalios DG, et al. Thoracic vertebrectomy and reconstruction using a microsurgical thoracoscopic approach. Neurosurgery 1996; 38:279–293.
8. van Alphen HA, Braakman R, Berfelo MW, et al. Chemonucleolysis or discectomy? Results of a randomized multicentre trial in patients with a herniated lumbar intervertebral disc (a preliminary report). Acta Neurochir Suppl (Wien) 1988; 43:35–38.
9. Mayer HM, Brock M. Percutaneous endoscopic discectomy: surgical technique and preliminary results compared to microsurgical disectomy. J Neurosurg 1993; 78:216–225.
10. Kambin P, Gellman H. Perctuaneous lateral discectomy of the lumbar spine: a preliminary report. Clin Orthop 1983; 174:127–132.
11. Kambin P, Sampson S. Posterolateral percutaneous suction-excision of herniated lumbar intervertebral discs: report of interim results. Clin Orthop 1986; 207:37–43.
12. Hermantin FU, Peters T, Quartarao L, et al. A prospective, randomized study comparing the results of open discectomy with those of video-assisted arthroscopic microdiscectomy. J Bone Joint Surg Am 1999; 81:958–965.
13. Huang TJ, Hsu RW, Li YY, et al. Less systemic cytokine response in patients following microendoscopic versus open lumbar discectomy. J Orthop Res 2005; 23:406–411.
14. Henriksen L, Schmidt K, Eskesen V, et al. A controlled study of microsurgical versus standard lumbar disectomy. Br J Neuosurg 1996; 10:289–293.
15. Khoo LT, Fessler RG. Microendoscopic decompressive laminotomy for the treatment of lumbar stenosis. Neurosurgery 2002; 51:146–154.
16. Regan JJ, Yuan H, McAfee PC. Laparoscopic fusion of the lumbar spine: minimally invasive spine surgery. A prospective multicenter study evaluating open and laparoscopic lumbar fusion. Spine 1999; 24:402–411.
17. Zdeblick TA, David SM. A prospective comparison of surgical approach for anterior L4-L5 fusion: laparoscopic versus mini anterior lumbar interbody fusion. Spine 2000; 25:2682–2687.
18. Kaiser MG, Haid RW, Subach BR, et al. Comparison of the mini-open versus laparoscopic approach for anterior lumbar interbody fusion: a retrospective review. Neurosurgery 2002; 51:97–103.
19. Zucherman JF, Zdeblick TA, Bailey SA, et al. Instrumented laprascopic spinal fusion. Prelminary results. Spine 1995; 20:2029–2034.
20. Chung SK, Lee SH, Lim SR, et al. Comparative study of laparoscopic L5-S1 fusion versus open mini-ALIF, with a minimum 2-year follow-up. Eur Spine J 2003; 12:613–617.
21. Rodriguez HE, Connoly MM, Dracopoulos H, et al. Anterior access to the lumbar spine: laparoscopic versus open. Am Surg 2002; 68:982–983.
22. Foley KT, Gupta SK. Percutaneous pedicle screw fixation of the lumbar spine: preliminary clinical results. J Neurosurg 2002; 97:7–12.

23. Lee SH, Choic WG, S.R. L, et al. Minimally invasive anterior lumbar interbody fusion followed by percutaneous pedicle screw fusion for isthmic spondylolisthesis. Spine 2004; 30:838–843.
24. Schwender JD, Holly LT, Rouben DP, et al. Minimally invasive transforaminal lumbar interbody fusion (TLIF): technical feasibility and initial results. J Spinal Disord Tech 2005; 18:S1–S6.
25. Bhandari M, Whang W, Kuro JC, et al. The risk of false-positive results in orthopaedic surgical trials. Clin Orthop Rel Res 2003; 413:63–69.
26. Bailey CS, Fisher CG, Dvorak MF. Type II error in the spine surgical literature. Spine 2003; 29:1146–1149.

3 | Definition and Classification of Minimally Invasive Spine Surgery

Erbil Oguz
*Department of Orthopedic Surgery, Gulhane Military Medical Academy,
Ankara, Turkey*

Qusai M. Hammouri and Jonathan N. Grauer
*Department of Orthopedics and Rehabilitation, Yale University School of Medicine,
New Haven, Connecticut, U.S.A.*

Michael A. Pahl
*Department of Orthopedic Surgery, Thomas Jefferson University, Philadelphia,
Pennsylvania, U.S.A.*

Alexander R. Vaccaro
*Department of Orthopedic Surgery and Neurosurgery, Thomas Jefferson University and the
Rothman Institute, Philadelphia, Pennsylvania, U.S.A.*

INTRODUCTION

Prior chapters in this volume have introduced the concept and history of minimally invasive spine surgery (MISS). In this chapter, we attempt to answer two simple yet not completely resolved questions. What is MISS and who is the correct patient for MISS?

As we try to answer the first question, we examine the different procedures that fall under the banner of MISS, define general categories of the procedures, and briefly describe each. The second part of this chapter considers issues that influence the decision to perform MISS. Surgeon and patient considerations are discussed in detail. The last part of this chapter deals with practical considerations of selecting the optimal patient for MISS.

DEFINITION OF MINIMALLY INVASIVE SPINE SURGERY

MISS has been defined in many different ways, but so far no clear definition that everyone agrees upon has emerged. We will define MISS as *any spinal surgery that specifically attempts to minimize tissue damage*. Within this definition, MISS can be categorized based on its therapeutic effect into:

1. Injection procedures
2. Decompression procedures
3. Instrumentation and fusion procedures
4. Vertebral body augmentation and nonfusion procedures.

It can also be divided into four categories based on the technology or approach used to perform these procedures, which include:

1. Percutaneous procedures
2. Thoracoscopic/laparoscopic (endoscopic) procedures
3. Surgery through a tube
4. Minimal incision procedures.

Most of the procedures performed using these approaches can be readily performed through an open method. The lure of MISS is decreasing patient morbidity and recovery time.

However, MISS procedures may be technically demanding and instrument-dependent, have slow learning curves, and have increased operative times. These potential limitations must be balanced against the fact that most of these procedures have not been proven to be superior to their open counterparts.

TECHNOLOGICAL CLASSIFICATION
Percutaneous Procedures

Percutaneous transforaminal and epidural injections are commonly used for diagnostic and therapeutic purposes. A needle is docked at a desired location and anesthetic, with or without steroid medication is delivered. This is generally performed with fluoroscopic guidance. Although many would not include mention of these procedures in a surgical chapter, the anatomy and principles of such techniques are a launching point for many other MISS techniques.

Percutaneous intradiscal procedures were popularized when chymopapain was injected into the disc space to dissolve the nucleus pulposus (chemical discectomy). This technique has since fallen out of favor. However, other techniques such as discography, percutaneous nucleotomy, and intradiscal electrothermy (IDET) have employed a similar approach (1).

In a different class of procedures, percutaneous vertebral augmentation has been introduced as a minimally invasive option for stabilizing vertebral compression fractures (2,3). A needle or needles are placed down the pedicle, or in an extrapedicular manner, and polymethylmethacrylate or similar bone cement-curing agent is injected into the vertebral body.

Finally, percutaneous pedicle screw systems have been developed. With fluoroscopic or computerized image guidance, the pedicle can be cannulated and a screw placed in a percutaneous manner (Fig. 1). The greatest technical limitation with percutaneous systems is the placement of the rod in a way that avoids further soft-tissue disruption. Additionally, as the posterior anatomy is not directly exposed, bone grafting is not possible with this technique, and at this time it is mainly used to mechanically supplement anterior fusion procedures. Mini-open procedures, however, can be used to expose and decorticate the posterior elements in order to deliver a bone-grafting substance for a fusion procedure (Fig. 2).

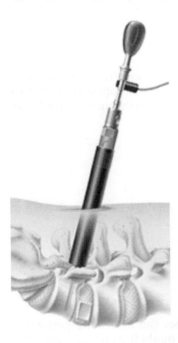

FIGURE 1 SpheRx™ cannulated pedicle screw (NuVasive® Inc., San Diego, CA, U.S.A.).

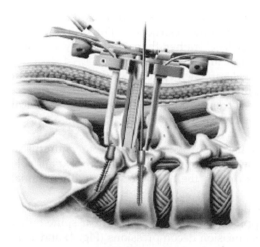

FIGURE 2 SpheRx™ pedicle screws as shown placed through MaXcess® access system (NuVasive® Inc., San Diego, CA, U.S.A.).

Thoracoscopy/Laparoscopy

Laparoscopic lumbar spine surgery was introduced by Obenchain in the early 1990s for anterior discectomy and interbody fusions (4–6). However, identified risks, including sexual dysfunction and visceral and vascular injuries, were encountered more frequently than with open procedures and were more technically challenging to repair (4–6). With these risks and limitations to exposure, laparoscopic spinal procedures have generally fallen out of favor.

A retroperitoneal endoscopic approach with balloon dilatation has also been described. Originally used for urological procedures, this was adapted to access the lumbar spine without the need for gas insufflation or violation of the peritoneal cavity (1). Although this offered potential advantages, it has also fallen out of favor due to its complexity in comparison with the more commonly used mini-open techniques.

As open thoracotomies are associated with significant postoperative discomfort, it was clearly desirable to attempt to approach the thoracic spine with less invasive techniques. Video-assisted spinal thoracoscopy was first accomplished by Mack et al. in 1993 (7). During the procedure, the lung on the exposure side is deflated, and an endoscope is introduced. Other portals are then made for working access. This technique has gradually evolved and has been used to perform a number of different procedures, including decompressions, anterior releases, bone grafting, and anterior instrumentation. With the large potential space of the thoracic cage, this has been much more successful and widely accepted than laparoscopic techniques.

Surgery Through a Tube

With the desire to perform less destructive surgery, posterior techniques have been developed to serially dilate portals of surgical access. Once a path has been dilated, a tube is generally placed down the path and secured to the table, in essence acting as a directed retractor system. There are many versions of this theme that have been developed with varying defining features.

For illumination, many tubular retractors have fiberoptic lighting features. For others, microscopes can be used. For visualization, endoscopes have been used by some systems. More commonly, however, one looks directly down such tubes with loupe or microscope magnification.

The first procedure performed through such tubular systems was a foraminotomy and discectomy. However, with refined tools and growing experience, larger procedures have become more common, including more extensive decompressions, posterior instrumentation, and posterior interbody work.

Minimal Incision Procedures

The greatest limitations of MISS are the technical and instrument demands. Surgical goals are the same; however, some of the techniques have grown greatly in complexity, albeit with varying returns. Consequently, there has been an emphasis to return partially toward traditional open surgical techniques but with less soft-tissue and bony destruction. Thus, the obvious change in terminology to "minimal incision approaches," rather than "minimally invasive surgery," has been adopted to better describe such surgical endeavors.

The "mini-open" anterior lumbar retroperitoneal approach epitomizes this movement in thought. Formal open anterior lumbar approaches often involved extensive soft-tissue dissection. Laparoscopic/endoscopic procedures, as noted, were fraught with significant technical limitations. Now, small para-rectus abdominus incisions are routinely used to grant access to the anterior lumbar spine.

The direct lateral retroperitoneal approach has also been advanced for intradiscal procedures. The extreme lumbar interbody fusion (XLIF) procedure uses an expandable retractor system through a small lateral incision to reach the anterior spine with minimal approach-related morbidity (Fig. 3).

Another classic example of the shift toward less destructive approaches is the recent renewed interest in the Wiltse paraspinal muscle-splitting approach to the posterior lumbar spine rather than the traditional midline open exposure. Minimal incision decompressions (Fig. 4) and TLIF (transforaminal lumbar interbody fusion) procedures can be performed using this exposure corridor, with or without posterior instrumentation (Figs. 5 and 6).

SURGEON CONSIDERATIONS

Although there are many potential advantages to minimally invasive lumbar procedures, the techniques do have limitations and drawbacks. As with any novel surgical technique, a learning curve is associated with the development of proficient technical skills. As one transitions from classic open techniques to minimally invasive techniques, there is generally increased time required for similar procedures. This is true for any new procedure that one learns and, to some degree, the time required gradually decreases as one's familiarity with a procedure increases. A rare exception may be the development of some anterior or lateral minimal procedures that are designed to avoid the need for vessel exposure or mobilization (such as the XLIF). Once experience is gained with these techniques, surgical exposure time may be considerably decreased.

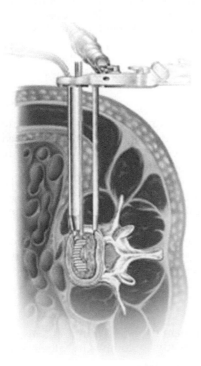

FIGURE 3 Extreme lumbar interbody fusion (XLIF™) approach through MaXcess® access system.

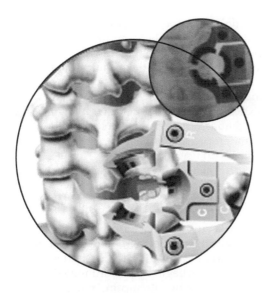

FIGURE 4 Minimally disruptive posterior cervical decompression through MaXcess® microaccess system.

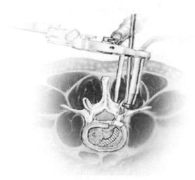

FIGURE 5 Minimally disruptive transforaminal lumbar interbody fusion through MaXcess® access system.

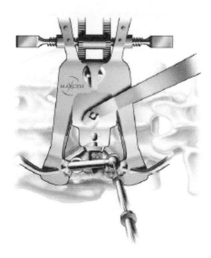

FIGURE 6 Minimally disruptive transforaminal lumbar interbody fusion with SpheRx™ pedicle screw fixation.

Regardless of their allure, newer minimally invasive methods may ultimately prove challenging or impossible to achieve the desired surgical goals. Although a thorough understanding of the three-dimensional anatomy of the spinal pathology in question is a prerequisite for both open and minimally invasive procedures, the surrounding anatomy is often not visualized with minimal incision surgery and may confuse or hinder the safe and timely performance of complex spinal procedures.

Additional equipment is generally needed for minimally open procedures. Instruments are generally longer, frequently bayoneted, and with a lower profile to minimize obscuring visualization. Contrary to tubular systems, mini-open retractor systems can often use conventional instruments and direct illuminated visualization that can reduce the technical challenges and learning curve.

Without direct visualization, the value of image guidance and fluoroscopy cannot be undervalued. This, unfortunately, adds further expense and time to master the imaging modality, as well as the unfortunate consequences of potential radiation exposure. Computerized navigational systems are constantly being evaluated and improved, but have not gained widespread popularity as a result of their cost and difficulties with use and accuracy.

Although minimal incision procedures can be performed adequately using loupe magnification, many surgeons exploit the aid of an operating microscope because of the enhanced illumination. Depending on a surgeon's training and experience, this transition may also be associated with a learning curve of its own.

In general, there are many potential roadblocks to a surgeon mastering new minimally invasive techniques. However, there are often clear bailouts to convert to traditional open techniques if difficulties are encountered or if there is question of achieving the desired surgical goals in a safe and effective manner. To this end, most surgeons begin by performing relatively simple minimally invasive techniques such as a discectomy before attempting more complex surgical endeavors. Additionally, retractors that allow customizable exposure allow the user a gradual transition from larger to smaller exposures as confidence builds.

Surgeons' adoption of minimally invasive techniques has thus been found to progress in parallel with their desire to confront the frustrations associated with the required learning curve and the ability of their institutions to afford the initial expense of this new technology.

REFERENCES

1. Jaikumar S, Kim DH, Kam AC. History of minimally invasive spine surgery. Neurosurgery 2002; 51(5 suppl):S1–S14.
2. Martin JB, Jean B, Sugiu K, et al. Vertebroplasty: clinical experience and follow-up results. Bone 1999; 25(2 suppl):11S–15S.
3. Barr JD, Barr MS, Lemley TJ, et al. Percutaneous vertebroplasty for pain relief and spinal stabilization. Spine 2000; 25(8):923–928.
4. Obenchain TG, Laparoscopic lumbar discectomy: case report. J Laparoendosc Surg 1991; 1(3): 145–149.
5. Zucherman JF, Zdeblick TA, Bailey SA, et al. Instrumented laparoscopic spinal fusion. Preliminary results. Spine 1995; 20(18):2029–2034; discussion 2034–2035.
6. Mathews HH, Evans MT, Molligan HJ, et al. Laparoscopic discectomy with anterior lumbar interbody fusion. A preliminary review. Spine 1995; 20(16):1797–1802.
7. Mack MJ, Regan JJ, Bobechko WP, et al. Application of thoracoscopy for diseases of the spine. Ann Thorac Surg 1993; 56(3):736–738.

4 | Patient Selection for Minimally Invasive Spinal Surgery

D. Greg Anderson and Chadi Tannoury
Department of Orthopedic Surgery, Thomas Jefferson University, Philadelphia, Pennsylvania, U.S.A.

INTRODUCTION

Minimally invasive spinal surgery (MISS) is a developing field of surgery allowing surgeons to perform spinal procedures through smaller incisions. The primary intention of MISS is to limit the collateral damage to the spinal soft-tissue envelope, thus diminishing postoperative pain and allowing earlier recovery and return to activities. It is actually a collection of techniques and operations utilizing specialized retractors, hand instruments, and equipment that make it possible to operate through the limited exposure. The theoretical advantages of the less invasive approach includes decreased soft-tissue disruption, less postoperative pain, less blood loss, less hospitalization, better cosmesis, and faster recovery times (1). Minimally invasive surgical techniques have been described for essentially all areas of the spine over the past few decades (2,3). Although pioneers in the field began to describe small incision spine surgery more than 30 years ago, it has not been until the last few years that advancements in technology have produced a more generalized interest within the spinal community in less invasive approaches to spinal problems.

Examples of technological advances that have played a role in the development of MISS include advanced spinal imaging, microscopes, endoscopes, cannulated screw technology, tubular retraction devices, fiberoptic lighting, and image guidance technology. Using combinations of these technologies, many traditional spinal operations can be performed in a less invasive fashion. However, not all patients or spinal problems are ideal candidates for a less invasive surgical approach. In this chapter, we discuss the considerations that go into the patient selection process for a minimal access spinal procedure.

PRINCIPLES OF LESS INVASIVE SPINAL SURGERY

Although the exact line between a traditional open operation, a mini-open procedure, and a percutaneous procedure is not always easy to define, the applications of the principles of less invasive spinal surgery are much more important than the length of the skin incision. A minimally invasive spinal procedure should always begin with careful analysis of advanced imaging studies (magnetic resonance imaging, computed tomography, and radiographs) to define the exact location of the spinal pathology. This is critical because relevant anatomic regions of the spine much be visualized and treated during the less invasive procedure just as with a traditional open operation. Next, the location of surgical incisions should be localized in the operating room prior to beginning the procedure. This is usually performed using a C-arm fluoroscopy unit and is particularly important because the surgeon must ensure that the small skin incisions will allow access to the relevant region of the spinal column. During the exposure process, the soft tissues (i.e., skin, muscles, fascia, ligaments) should be handled with care to minimize soft-tissue trauma. Often, serial dilators are used to spread rather than cut the fascicles of the paraspinous muscles. Care should be taken to limit prolonged retraction or excessive electrocautary of soft tissues around the spine. The blood and nerve supply to the paraspinal muscles should be meticulously spared.

Specialized retractor systems are often utilized to maintain a working portal between the skin and the spine, and allow direct visualization of the relevant spinal pathology. Visualization during surgery is facilitated by good lighting and magnification, which should be routinely used. Working through a tubular retraction system may require longer instruments, which are

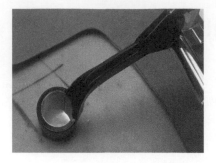

FIGURE 1 Tubular retractor in place for a posterior lumbar exposure. Note the integral light source and table mounted "arm" that secures the retractor during the operative procedure.

often bayoneted to allow the surgeon to keep his/her hand away from the visualization corridor. A long, thin, high-speed burr/drill is often used to remove bone during a decompression procedure or to decorticate the spine for a fusion.

Although less invasive procedures are performed through smaller skin incisions, the same adequate decompression and/or fusion procedure must be performed in order to have results comparable with traditional open surgical approaches. Although the term MISS implies that the procedure is minor, the actual invasiveness of the case is defined by the nature of the spinal condition. However, less exposure-related trauma to the soft-tissue envelope around the spine should be expected when compared with the traditional approach for a given procedure. Complete treatment of the spinal pathology should never be sacrificed in order to perform surgery through a smaller incision.

With experience, discectomies, decompressions, posterolateral fusion, interbody fusion, and spinal instrumentation can be achieved with less invasive techniques in all areas of the spine (cervical, thoracic, and lumbar). Although the same principles can be allied to approaches for both the anterior and posterior region of the spine, it is the posterior region where the greatest benefits of less invasive spinal surgery are seen compared with a traditional approach. This is because the traditional approach to the posterior spine causes substantial stripping and injury to the paraspinous muscles and can be associated with significant postoperative pain. These approach-related problems can be limited by a less invasive approach.

One of the most important skills that must be learned in order to perform less invasive spinal surgery is the technique of operating through a tubular retractor. Tubular retractors are now available in a variety of configurations (Fig. 1). In most cases, the tubular retractor is introduced over a series of soft-tissue dilators (Fig. 2). Tubular retractors are generally attached to a table-mounted retractor holder, allowing the position and angulation of the tubular retractor to be maintained (Fig. 3). Some tubular retractors can open or expand to allow enhanced visualization of the spine. When placing the tubular retractor, each dilator should be advanced and "docked" against bone. In this way, the amount of soft tissue remaining over the spine can be minimized. Once the tubular retractor is in place (and verified by fluoroscopy) surgery through the tube can commence. The surgeon must generally remove a small amount of soft tissue and identify anatomic landmarks as the first step in working through the tubular retractor. Visualization is facilitated by good lighting and magnification. Many surgeons prefer to use a

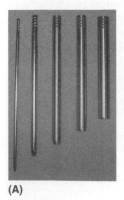
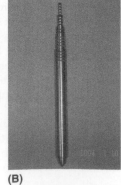

(A)   **(B)**

FIGURE 2 Serial dilators used to spread or dilate the operative corridor for a minimally invasive spinal procedure. (**A**) shows the dilators individually, while (**B**) shows the dilators placed one on top of the other as would be performed when dilating the soft tissue corridor in preparation for the placement of a tubular retractor.

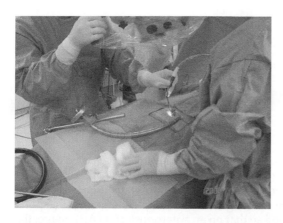

FIGURE 3 Operative microscope in place to view the spine through a tubular retractor. Lighting and illumination are optimized through the use of a high-quality operative microscope.

microscope to visualize the spinal anatomy through the tubular retractor (Fig. 3). Use of the microscope provides optimal magnification and illumination, while providing better depth perception than endoscopic viewing.

"Wanding" allows the surgeon to reach different areas of the spine. This is performed by loosening the table-mounted retractor holder and placing the largest dilator through the tube to act as a handle for manipulation of the tubular retractor. The tubular retractor can then be angled or translated under the skin to reach a different area of the spine such as the contralateral side of the spinal canal or the adjacent spinal level (Fig. 4).

The movement of instruments within a tubular retractor system is dictated (geometrically) by the diameter and length of the tube (Fig. 5). For this reason, the shortest tubular retractor that will reach from the skin to the spine should be chosen. An overly short tubular retractor should be avoided as it will allow muscle tissue to creep into the operative field and obscure the surgeon's visualization of the spine.

When working through a tubular retractor, visualization along the edges of the tube and just beyond the edges of the tube is obscured by soft tissue. Therefore, care must be taken when decompressing the dural sac in this region to avoid an accidental dural tear. Compared with traditional spinal surgery, tactile feedback plays a larger role in minimal access spinal surgery as the surgeon's visual feedback might be diminished. The experienced minimally invasive spinal surgeon will have good palpation skills in referencing spinal anatomy in a tactile fashion. Also, imaging feedback plays a larger role in less invasive spinal procedure and provides localization or confirmation of position and trajectory during a wide variety of procedures. In

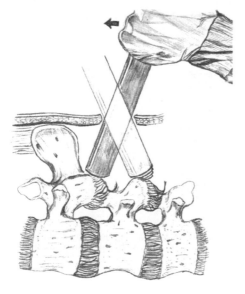

FIGURE 4 Figure shows a wanding maneuver, which allows the surgeon to adjust the position of the tubular retractor to operate on different regions of the spine.

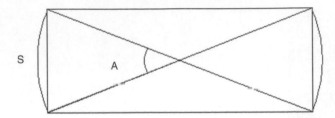

FIGURE 5 This figure illustrates the principle that a shorter or wider tube allows the surgeon better ability to maneuver instruments during the operation. As the length of the tube increases or the width (S) of the tube decreases, the angle (A) that the surgeon may use to operate within the tube decreases.

summary, navigation of the spine during minimal access spinal procedure depends on a combination of direct visualization, tactile feedback, and fluoroscopy.

Minimally invasive spinal surgery is more dependent on fluoroscopy than traditional open surgery. For this reason, it is important to obtain good fluoroscopic images of the spinal region of interest. The vertebrae should be aligned so that on an anteroposterior (AP) image, the spinous process is centered between the pedicles, and the superior endplate is parallel to the fluoroscopy beam (Fig. 6A). On the lateral image, the pedicles should be superimposed and only a single posterior cortex of the vertebral body should be seen (Fig. 6B). Patient with severe osteopenia or obesity may be challenging to image using a C-arm because the bony anatomy may be obscured or difficult to visualize. If adequate fluoroscopic images cannot be obtained, an alternative surgical strategy may be required.

FACTORS THAT AFFECT THE SELECTION PROCESS
Obesity

Although all spinal procedures are more difficult to perform in obese patients, the use of a minimally invasive surgery in this patient population requires special consideration. Because the distance between the patient's skin and spine is greater, the surgeon must ensure that the tubular retractor system and spinal instruments are long enough to reach the patient's spine. In some cases, this can be estimated or measured using preoperative imaging studies such as a computed tomography (CT) scan or magnetic resonance imaging (MRI) if the imaging window is large enough to show both the spine and surrounding soft tissues to the level of the skin. However, only at the time of surgery can the surgeon actually measure the exact depth from the skin to the spine with the patient in the surgical position. This is generally performed with a graduated (calibrated) soft-tissue dilator prior to selection of the optimal length tubular retractor. If the patient's soft-tissue depth is greater than the available retractors and/or hand instruments, an alternative surgical technique must be used. Working through a long tube in an obese patient is more difficult because the instruments cannot be angled as well to adjust to the local spinal anatomy (Fig. 5). Although a minimally invasive approach is more difficult in obese patients, less invasive surgery in this population has the potential to offer even greater benefits than in a thinner patient due to the large open incision that would be required to reach the spine

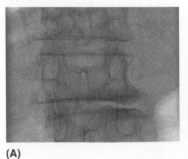

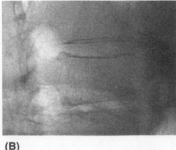

(A)   **(B)**

FIGURE 6 Properly aligned anteroposterior image is shown in (**A**) with the endplate parallel to the X-ray beam and the spinous process midway between the pedicles. Properly aligned lateral view is shown in (**B**) with the endplate and posterior body parallel the X-ray beam and the pedicle superimposed.

with a traditional approach. The minimally invasive surgeon is able to use an incision that is equal to the diameter of the chosen tubular retractor rather than having to increase the size of the incision to visualize the depth of the surgical wound. Thus, when surgery can be carried out in a less invasive manner, the obese patient should benefit significantly.

Revision Surgery

Revision spinal surgery is always more difficult than primary spinal surgery because of scaring of the perispinal tissue. A particularly challenging situation arises when the revision procedure requires a decompression of the spinal canal through an area of severe scaring as might be seen in a case of recurrent disc herniation. The principles of revision surgery call for a wider exposure with identification of the spinal canal structures through an area of unoperated normal anatomy prior to dissecting through a region of dense peridural scar. Sharp curettes are useful in defining the edges of a prior bony decompression and can be used with the sharp "cutting" surface against the bone, while the blunt "spoon" side is placed against the soft tissues and dura to decrease the risk of dural injury. Good mobilization of the dural sac must be achieved prior to retraction of the neural elements. Although this type of case can be achieved in a less invasive fashion, it should be performed only after the surgeon has considerable experience working through a tubular retractor with cases not involving revision surgery. When attempting a revision case in a less invasive fashion, the surgeon should be ready to convert to a wider exposure if needed to safely expose the necessary regions of the spinal canal.

Dural Laceration

Despite careful techniques, an occasional unintentional durotomy is a complication that every spinal surgeon must be ready to address. Dural tears are more common with revision spinal surgery compared with primary cases (4). They are also more common early in the learning curve of both traditional spinal surgery and MISS. The exact treatment of a dural tear depends on many factors, including the location and size of the tear, the quality of the dural tissue, the region of the spine (cervical vs. lumbar) and the health of the patient. When possible, significant dural tears should be directly repaired at the time they are encountered. A variety of adjuvants to dural repair are available, including dural sealants (e.g., fibrin glue) and dural patches. A direct water-tight repair may not always be possible due to the location of the tear and quality of the dural tissues. In such cases, other means such as subarachnoid drains, dural sealants, and flat bed rest may be useful (5). Direct repair of a dural laceration through a small tubular retractor can be difficult. If a direct repair is required (as a result of the nature of the tear) and it is not achievable while working through a tubular retractor, conversion to an open exposure should be performed.

Learning Curve

All medical procedures have a learning curve, meaning that the surgeon becomes better at performing the procedure with experience. Minimally invasive spinal surgery has a well-documented learning curve. The exact number of cases that are required to become proficient at the use of less invasive approaches is dependent on the experience and technical skills of the individual surgeon and the complexity of the specific surgical technique. However, during the early learning curve, the surgeon should expect that more time will be required to perform the procedure and that the number of technical complications encountered will be greater. For this reason, it is a good idea to begin with more simple spinal procedures when embarking on a new or modified surgical procedure. As the surgeon becomes experienced, more difficult cases can be undertaken with a less invasive approach. It is also a good idea to plan for a longer operative time than usually required during the early learning curve of minimally invasive procedures. Simple, primary (first-time) discectomies in thin patients are an example of a good type of case for the surgeon to undertake in the early learning curve of operating through a tubular retractor. As the surgeon becomes adept at performing minimally invasive surgery, more complex cases will be feasible.

Time Efficiency

Depending on the nature of the exact spinal procedure, the experience of the surgeon and various patient variables (i.e., obesity, revision surgery), it may take more time to perform an operation using a minimally invasive approach as compared with the traditional open approach. The added time under anesthesia may be outweighed by the benefits of less blood loss, less postoperative pain, and early mobilization afforded by the less invasive approach. However, the risks of a prolonged anesthesia are patient-dependent and are affected by a variety of factors including patient age and medical comorbidities. In general, small procedures (i.e., disc herniations, single-level decompressions) are fairly quick procedures whether performed with a traditional or a less invasive technique. In contrast, larger and more complex procedures such as a posterior lumbar interbody fusion with instrumentation is a longer procedure, especially early in the learning curve of an individual surgeon (6). It is important that each surgeon be realistic about the added operative time and risk when comparing the options of a traditional versus a less invasive surgical approach for a given patient.

Localized Spinal Pathology

Minimally invasive surgery is best suited to localized spinal problems. In other words, a person with a single, large sequestered disc fragment is generally an excellent candidate for a less invasive surgical approach. In contrast, a problem that is more diffuse (affects a larger area of the spine), such as a person who requires bilateral decompression at three levels, is less well-suited to an efficient MISS approach. In part, this is because of the added time that is required to localize each of the levels individually and to increase the complexity of performing a bilateral decompression at each of the levels. Similarly, a person who requires a long spinal fusion is a less ideal candidate for a minimally invasive approach in most surgeons' hands. However, the potential benefits in performing larger operations with a less invasive approach can be dramatic because the traditional open approach to such problems is relatively morbid. As the instrumentation and techniques evolve, it is likely that surgeons will be able to undertake spinal problems affecting larger regions of the spine with a less invasive approach.

Complexity of the Procedure

The more complex the spinal procedure, the more difficult it is to achieve with a minimally invasive approach. Minimally invasive procedures generally involve more equipments than traditional open procedures. Each piece of equipment and each surgical step that the surgeon must perform adds complexity to the operation. The surgeon must be familiar with the specific technique that is being undertaken and should maintain a variety of surgical options when embarking on a highly complex procedure. In particular, the risks and benefits should be carefully weighed and discussed with the patient when choosing a less invasive surgical approach for a given case.

Fluoroscopy/Radiation Exposure

Fluoroscopy is utilized for almost all less invasive procedures. Some procedures, such as the placement of percutaneous pedicle screws, require a significant amount of fluoroscopy. The additive effects of fluoroscopy during occupational exposure to radiation can be significant for the surgeon and surgical team. For this reason, the surgeon should take steps to limit the effective radiation exposure to operative personnel. Modern, high-efficiency fluoroscopy equipment should be used because the radiation produced by these units is significantly less than that with older fluoroscopy units. Proper protective lead aprons with thyroid shield protection should be worn by the surgeon and staff in the operating room. Leaded glasses should be worn to protect the cornea. Steps should be taken to "cone down" or columnate the radiation beam so that only the necessary anatomy is visualized. Short "snapshots" rather than continuous fluoroscopy should be used when possible. The surgeon should stand when possible so that the radiation beam is directed away. The surgeon should keep his hands away from the fluoroscopy path during imaging. Proper dosimetry badges should be worn on the outside of the surgeon's gown and checked regularly. When possible, the surgeon should step back when using fluoroscopy as the radiation dose drops dramatically as a function of distance from the source.

PATIENT SELECTION FOR SPINAL SURGERY AND MINIMALLY INVASIVE SPINAL SURGERY

Patient selection is generally considered to be the most important issue predicting success of any spinal procedure. Despite this, patient selection has many variables and remains one of the most challenging aspects of spinal practice. Choosing a good candidate for surgery is much more important than the surgical approach (i.e., MISS vs. traditional open surgery) and much has been written about the topic of patient selection. It is crucially important to have an accurate diagnosis or understanding of the cause for the patient's pain prior to considering spinal surgery. Generally, surgery has been much more reliable for degenerative conditions causing neurologic symptoms (e.g., spinal stenosis with neurogenic claudication) than for degenerative conditions causing axial back pain. Surgery is unlikely to be successful if the surgeon is unsure or incorrect as to the cause of the patient's symptoms. Also crucial is the patient education process. Prior to surgery, an adequate discussion should be undertaken as to the symptoms that are likely to be responsive to a surgical solution as opposed to those symptoms that may remain. This will help the patient to understand and anticipate an appropriate clinical response to surgery and will improve the patient's satisfaction that the goals of surgery have been met by the procedure. Finally, the surgeon must be vigilant in identifying barriers to improvement. Examples of barriers to improvement would be psychologic pathology, secondary gain as a result of pending legal or workman's compensation claims, and narcotic or tobacco abuse. Whenever possible, these barriers should be addressed prior to proceeding with surgery to improve the odds of a successful clinical outcome. Most agree that favorable factors with regard to a good clinical outcome from spinal surgery include a high degree of motivation on the part of the patient, a higher level of education, and/or intelligence on the part of the patient, and the personal ownership/responsibility that a patient takes in the recovery process (7,8).

A good candidate for spinal surgery has a good chance of a successful clinical outcome despite the choice of surgical approach (i.e., traditional open vs. less invasive). Thus, the primary impetus for considering a less invasive approach is to lessen the perioperative pain and hasten the recovery process rather than affecting the long-term outcome. Selection of a less invasive approach for a given patient therefore must be based in large part on the nature of the procedure and the experience of the individual surgeon. Simple procedures (i.e., sequestered disc fragments) are generally good candidates for a less invasive operation and present a favorable risk to benefit ratio in the hands of most surgeons. However, a minimally invasive transforaminal lumbar interbody fusion is a complex procedure and would likely present an unfavorable risk to benefit ratio to an inexperienced surgeon, but can be quite reliable in the hands of a highly experienced minimally invasive spinal surgeon.

The risk and benefit ratio approach can be applied to each individual case as the surgeon considers the type of spinal problem, patient characteristics, and his own experience in the field of less invasive spinal surgery to determine whether the minimally invasive approach is a good option. Of particular importance is the discussion of this surgical judgment process with the patient. The surgeon should take the time to educate the patient on the surgical and nonsurgical options and surgical approaches (MISS vs. traditional open) that are available for their problem. It is important to have a frank discussion about the risks and benefits of each type of approach including the risks inherent to a minimal access operation. This discussion should be documented as part of the formal consent for surgery. By involving the patient in the surgical judgment process, the surgeon empowers the patient to be an active participant in their health problem and improves the odds of a good outcome with surgery.

CONCLUSION

Minimally invasive spinal surgery offers many advantages compared with traditional open surgery and, with experience, can be successfully applied to many spinal problems. Patients generally experience less pain and enjoy a quicker recovery with a properly performed minimally invasive approach than with a traditional open approach. However, like all medical therapies, minimally invasive surgery has certain drawbacks, limitations, and risks. In particular, these techniques are dependent on surgeon experience, particularly when performing complex spinal operations in a minimally invasive fashion.

The patient selection process should include a thoughtful consideration of the technical and medical issues that are relevant to the particular case and how these might impact a minimally invasive approach to the spinal problem. These issues should be openly discussed with the patient, using the risk to benefit ratio analogy to guide the decision process. Each patient should understand that if a minimally invasive approach is chosen, there is a chance that the procedure may need to be converted to a larger open incision for a variety of technical reasons. Conversion to a larger open incision should not be viewed as a failure of the minimally invasive approach but rather as the application of sound surgical judgment during the surgical procedure.

Good patient selection remains the cornerstone of a good clinical result following surgery. More important than the approach utilized is the selection of an optimal surgical candidate. A patient who is a poor candidate for a traditional open spinal procedure is also a poor candidate for a minimally invasive spinal operation. By application of these principles, a surgeon can enjoy success and safety as he learns and uses less invasive spinal surgery techniques to the benefit of spinal patients.

REFERENCES

1. Jaikumar S, Kim DH, Kam AC. History of minimally invasive spine surgery. Neurosurgery 2002; 51 (5 suppl):S1–S14.
2. Williams RW. Lumbar disc disease. Microdiscectomy. Neurosurg Clin N Am 1993; 4(1):101–108.
3. Tong HC, Williams JC, Haig AJ, et al. Predicting outcomes of transforaminal epidural injections for sciatica. Spine J 2003; 3(6):430–434.
4. Tafazal SI, Sell PJ. Incidental durotomy in lumbar spine surgery: incidence and management. Eur Spine J 2005; 14(3):287–290; e-pub: Nov 17, 2004.
5. Bosacco SJ, Gardner MJ, Guille JT. Evaluation and treatment of dural tears in lumbar spine surgery: a review. Clin Orthop Relat Res 2001; 389:238–247.
6. Khoo LT, Palmer S, Laich DT, et al. Minimally invasive percutaneous posterior lumbar interbody fusion. Neurosurgery 2002; 51(5 suppl):S166–S171.
7. Moon MS. The outcome of posterolateral fusion in highly selected patients with discogenic low back pain. Spine 1997; 22(12):1419–1420.
8. Parker LM, Murrell SE, Boden SD, et al. The outcome of posterolateral fusion in highly selected patients with discogenic low back pain. Spine 1996; 21(16):1909–1916; discussion: 1916–1917.

5 | The Future Direction of Minimally Invasive Surgery: Is Its Fate Controlled by the Physician, Patient, Industry, or Insurance?

Eeric Truumees
Department of Orthopedic Surgery, Beaumont Comprehensive Spine Center, Royal Oak, Michigan, U.S.A.

Chetan K. Patel
Beaumont Comprehensive Spine Center, Royal Oak, Michigan, U.S.A.

INTRODUCTION

Promising new technologies are presented to spine surgeons daily. One hallmark of a successful practice involves its critical evaluation and adoption of new technologies. A given technology's benefits in terms of operative morbidity and improved outcomes must be weighed against its training requirements and the potential for increased malpractice exposure associated with deviation from the "tried and true." For many surgeons, practice costs are rising rapidly while revenues are declining. These same practitioners may see their ranks swelling as freshly trained orthopedic surgeons and neurosurgeons open practices in their area. Increasingly, these new surgeons are seen less as colleagues and more as competition for a decreasing number of insured patients.

In this frenzied environment, medical decisions are made. For our purposes, the most important decisions are: if and when to perform spine surgery, and, which type of spine surgery to perform. Ideally, the surgeon recommends a course of management based on Class 1 literature proving the superiority of a single approach for a given pathology. The patient decides based on their symptoms and their surgeon's recommendations.

The reality can be wildly different. In spine surgery for degenerative disorders, major controversies remain as to which treatments are most effective. In the absence of clear-cut literature support, the surgeon makes recommendations based on the available literature, experience, anecdote, and, increasingly, influence from other parties. First, some patients come to the physician's office with powerfully entrenched, preconceived notions as to the most appropriate course of treatment. Sadly, these notions are often based on misleading or false information gleaned from disreputable internet sources.

While physicians may respond to this "pressure" from patients, they bring their own internal bias into the decision-making process as well. For some, an important distinction surrounds the definition of minimally invasive surgery (MIS) itself. Some surgeons shave a few centimeters from the length of their open fusion incision and call the procedure "less invasive." For others, MIS means tubular retractors. Most inclusively, MIS refers to a wide variety of percutaneous, endoscopic, and partly open spine procedures.

Given the differences in available definitions, surgeon perceptions of the future of minimally invasive spine surgery (MISS) in general or of individual procedures also vary widely. Some techniques that were described years ago have yet to gain a firm foothold in surgical practice (e.g., percutaneous discectomy); others have rapidly spread across North America (e.g., kyphoplasty). Some procedures enjoyed a brief moment of fame at the lectern of national spine meetings only to be dismissed a few years later (such as transperitoneal endoscopic anterior lumbar interbody fusion). Still others are endangered by refinement of traditional procedures. (Panels of pediatric spinal deformity experts describe sharply lower rates of endoscopic anterior release and fusion for thoracic deformity in favor of an all-posterior, multilevel pedicle screw approach.)

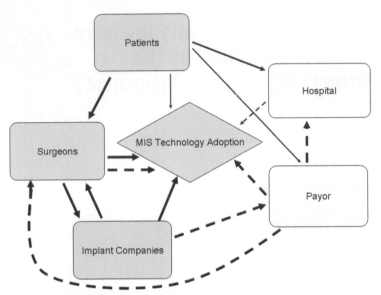

FIGURE 1   The complex web of relationships among the various parties involved in manufacturing, buying, using, and benefitting from MIS technology and their influence on the utilization of these technologies. The directions of the arrows suggest one party exerting influence on the other. The solid arrows represent positive influence (i.e., the first party tends to influence the second in a way that would increase the utilization of MIS implants and technologies. Thinner lines represent more marginal influence. The dashed arrows represent negative influence, wherein the first party tends to influence the second to decrease the use of these technologies. The point of the graphic is to suggest that simple supply and demand economics are not the driving forces here. Also, note that the payer, for example, can exert negative pressure on several parties to decrease the utilization of these technologies, The surgeon may both increase and decrease utilization. *Source*: From Ref. 44.

Overall, while interest in and utilization of MIS principles are gradually increasing, the fate of these techniques is not entirely clear. Outside parties are increasingly affecting the choices that are available to patients and that physicians have available. First, insurance companies limit treatment options by denying coverage for a subset of the available procedures. Then, hospitals, under increasing pressure to control costs, limit physician access to certain, expensive technologies. Finally, the medical device industry seeks to influence physicians' attitudes by a variety of direct and indirect means.

This chapter examines how the challenges of utilization of new medical technology affect MISS. In reality, a vast number of outside parties influence treatment decisions in spine surgery (these include employers, various government agencies, credentialing boards, professional peers, patient's friends, neighbors, residents, and colleagues). For simplicity, a five-element spine community, the patient, the physician, the hospital, the insurance company, and the implant manufacturer is considered. Each subsequent section details how that element affects the others. These relationships are simplified in Figure 1. The goal is to see how each element either drives or retards the implementation of MIS technique through its influence on the other elements. Two caveats must be considered: First, a chapter of this type exaggerates the influence of the forces described; second, the potency of these forces varies significantly by region, hospital type, and patient population.

ROLE OF THE PHYSICIAN

Physicians have a critical role in the acceptance of MIS techniques for spine surgery. Today, that impact can be both positive and negative. For example, some physicians' desire to offer so-called cutting-edge spine care drives the availability of MIS. Others, reluctant to devote the time to learn technically challenging new procedures, "restrain" MIS.

This section emphasizes that the treating surgeon, however, gains patients from referring physicians who may preferentially send patients to either traditional or "less invasive" surgeons.

Similarly, the availability of skilled endoscopists may affect the success of an MIS spine program in a given hospital.

Physician behavior is felt to account for a sixfold variation in the rates of spine surgery across the United States (spinal fusion rates vary 10-fold) (1). That is, rather than differences in rates of spinal pathology per se, the so-called surgical "footprint" including utilization of spinal imaging and nonoperative interval affects, to a large degree, who will get spine surgery and when in the course of their disease (2). These same physician-controlled parameters, no doubt, affect the rate at which MIS techniques are utilized.

This variability stems from both more and less legitimate surgeon reasoning. Unfortunately, surgeon ego and issues of being the first to try a certain technique in their region or be able to complete a given procedure entirely through the scope may stimulate some early MIS adopters. For others, MIS is a larger part of their practice marketing strategy than a rational treatment strategy. Some physicians may use MIS techniques as a justification to inappropriately relax surgical indications, thereby increasing surgical volume.

These considerations hold for a hospital's support for MIS. Large hospital systems market MIS practices. On the other hand, increased up-front costs and operating room (OR) time requirements have tempered enthusiasm in many institutions. For some, "carve-out" payments for expensive technologies allow them to profit above current diagnostic-related group (DRG) levels. When carve-outs are not available, pressures to limit use of similar technologies increase.

Successful implementation of minimally invasive spine principles requires long hours of additional surgeon training. This can incur a cost to the surgeon through the expense of the training courses as well as the lost practice revenue while attending the course (3). Notwithstanding the often long and frustrating learning curve, many surgeons remain skeptical about MIS claims. They cite increased OR time, increased radiation exposure, and poor reimbursement as detracting factors (4,5). A given surgeon's attraction to MIS may be influenced by the availability of competent colleagues for surgical access and the surgeon's desire to collaborate (4).

The malpractice environment in a given state may make surgeons more or less likely to employ new techniques. During the learning curve associated with MIS procedures, the risks to patients are higher (3,6). For some surgeons, this incremental risk, particularly in litigious areas, will keep them from employing these new techniques.

Malpractice issues have other, more subtle effects as well. The highly variable malpractice climate state-to-state significantly affects surgeon migration and decisions to practice in certain states. Younger surgeons who are more likely to have been trained in MIS techniques are less likely to settle in states in "malpractice crisis." For example, a recent survey found that 75% of the physicians in training in Pennsylvania planned to leave the state after residency. Pennsylvania already ranks 41st out of the 50 states in the percentage of physicians under 35 years old (7). In these states, patient access to any spine care physician is limited and that restriction may be more evident for MIS and other subspecialized modalities.

Some community spine surgeons, while interested in MIS, are reticent to begin training in current techniques. They suspect easier procedures will be introduced. That some MIS procedures have gone out of vogue quickly has left early proponents feeling burned (e.g., endoscopic cage placement). Others, such as the prominent neurosurgical spine specialist Edward Benzel, ascribe their reluctance to pursue MIS techniques to an engrained medical conservatism "related to wisdom associated with experience and maturity" (4).

Historically, cost containment has not been a priority for many surgeons. Faced with the perception of high malpractice risk and declining reimbursements, physicians seek to maximize the odds of a good patient outcome with little thought to the cost associated with any, small incremental benefit to the patient. This attitude fosters spiraling procedural costs. Commentators warn that, given this "reckless" spending, physicians will lose decision-making authority. These authors counsel slow, careful incorporation of expensive technologies into common spine practice (8).

ROLE OF THE PATIENT

Patients affect the adoption of new spine technologies in two ways. Most importantly, as healthcare consumers, patients will seek out new, cutting-edge treatments. Second, patient characteristics may influence the surgeon's decision of whether to offer these new techniques to a given patient.

Spinal surgery for degenerative conditions is especially vulnerable to patient influence for two key reasons. First, traditional management strategies are popularly regarded as less than satisfactory. Open, spinal fusion operations in particular have received marked negative publicity in recent years in both the popular media and nonsurgical medical literature (9–11). Given the gradual development of symptomatic spinal degeneration, patients have ample opportunity to discuss their problems with friends, relatives, neighbors, and other specialists. These patients actively explore treatment options as "consumers" of healthcare rather than passive participants (12).

While the surgeon's recommendation may be the most important guide, patients increasingly affect their management by presenting alternatives. Some surgeons describe this influence by labeling some new spine technologies as "patient-driven." The implication is that if the surgeon refuses the patient's request for a given spine procedure to be performed in a specific way, the patient will simply leave and get the procedure performed elsewhere.

The extent to which patient pressures affect physician practice is unknown. Undoubtedly, some patients seek multiple opinions and choose the surgeon offering a less invasive technique. Physicians and hospitals, sensitive to patient preferences, present themselves as "minimally invasive surgery institutes."

The ethical legitimacy of these efforts depends on their underlying impetus. Spine surgery is no different from other healthcare concerns in that patient perceptions may be widely distorted (13). For example, patients assume that MIS is somehow less risky than traditional, open techniques. In fact, for novice technicians, less invasive techniques increase the rates of nerve root injury (3).

In their pursuit of a rapid recovery and a cosmetically more appealing scar, patients rarely understand the differences between the immediate and long-term morbidity of a given surgical approach (12). In some cases, while MIS techniques allow patients to recover more quickly, the long-term outcome are not different (14). The physiologic consequences of spine fusion in terms of a lost motion segment are not diminished by a less invasive approach.

MIS techniques dovetail into wider social imperatives of "new and improved" treatments. Some patients emphasize a technologic solution for their symptoms. These patients demand a rapid "fix" for their problem that does not obligate them to participate in their own recovery. Laparoscopic obesity surgery is a great example of "high-tech" and risky surgery that is applied to a problem with less risky, low-tech solutions (eat less and exercise).

MIS marketing is at its worst when the less invasive nature of the surgical approach is used to justify relaxed surgical indications and decreased patient responsibility in terms of activity modification, exercise, rehabilitation, weight loss, and smoking cessation. An aggressive nonoperative regimen offered early in a patient's treatment course can significantly reduce rates of spinal imaging, surgical consultation, and surgery itself, without affecting patient satisfaction (15). Similarly, completion of formal education programs diminishes utilization of spinal imaging and surgery (1).

While a patient's largest role in driving MIS flows from the choice of a physician and hospital, other patient-centered characteristics substantially affect use of MIS in individual cases. That is, surgeons treat various patient groups differently. For example, spine surgeons have markedly different discussions with the Internet-searching patient than with their more medically naïve neighbor. Moreover, surgeons may be more reluctant to try newer surgical techniques in certain patient groups. For example, MIS techniques may be more readily offered to thin over obese, athletic over sedentary, and younger over older patients (16).

The burgeoning world literature emphasizing inferior surgical outcomes in workers compensation patients affects surgeons' approach to them. Many spine surgeons are more reluctant to operate on these patients, but, if surgery is recommended, a less invasive approach may be more palatable. A recent study described a large number of compensation patients with substantial postoperative disability. These patients were unable to return to work. Of the 1000 patients studied, none had objective deficits precluding activity. Chronic, postoperative pain, theoretically from the surgical approach, among other factors, was blamed (17). Less invasive techniques, with their attendant effects on the psychological aspects of recovery, may improve these outcomes.

Today, some physicians may feel pressure from patients to adopt new techniques in spine surgery because of perceptions, rather than proof, of superiority compared with traditional management. Occasionally, the role of the patient in driving the utilization of MIS is based on individual patient characteristics. In reality, some of these patient characteristics may be valid discriminators of surgical outcome. Hopefully, with time, we will be able to identify specific characteristics that accurately predict outcomes for nonoperative MIS, or traditional open surgical techniques (18).

ROLE OF THE INSURANCE COMPANY

The expense of new spine technologies has created large incentives for insurance companies to influence the rate at which these new technologies are adopted. How much the payer reimburses the hospital and surgeon affects the providers' ability to offer the service in question. Secondarily, the patient's insurance coverage affects how and when he approaches the healthcare system for treatment of a degenerative spine condition.

At $5267 per capita in 2003, the United States spent, by far, more on healthcare than any other nation (Switzerland was next at $3446) (7). From 2001 to 2005, premiums for family health coverage increased 60% (19). "The biggest driver to increased healthcare costs is new medical technology including new drugs, new devices, and new ways to use existing technology" (19).

Despite the explosion in technology costs, most physicians and patients are only partly restricted as to the techniques or modalities they consider. Yet, analysts suggest that payers are increasingly affecting medical decision-making. Most directly, an insurer may decline to cover the costs of a procedure. Most American family budgets cannot accommodate the hospital and professional fees associated with spine surgery. If coverage is declined, in most cases, the surgery will not be performed. Some insurance companies continue to consider certain MIS techniques "investigational," which means that they are not obligated to pay for them.

Payers may also affect surgeons' decision-making in more subtle ways. If a surgeon perceives two operations as similar in their risk, work, and results, but he receives significantly less revenue for one of the operations, he may be more likely to offer the more generously reimbursed procedure to the patient. Simply put, poorly reimbursed procedures are less likely to "catch on." A number of examples of these phenomena exist in spine surgery today and they may be extrapolated to MIS.

Over the past six years, kyphoplasty, for example, has achieved rapid and widespread surgeon and patient acceptance as a means of treating painful vertebral compression fractures. In that this percutaneous procedure may be performed under local anesthesia and some patients can be discharged from the hospital the same day, it certainly meets criteria as a minimally invasive spine technique (6). How kyphoplasty affects payer's costs is more controversial. Compared with standard, operative management, kyphoplasty is much cheaper. Traditionally, however, osteoporotic patients with painful VCF have been treated nonoperatively, often in a brace. Compared with the cost of a brace alone, kyphoplasty is more expensive. In returning nonambulatory, intractable pain patients to more normal function, kyphoplasty decreases the expense of lengthy inpatient and rehabilitation hospital stays (6,20).

Surgeon and facility reimbursement for kyphoplasty, however, remains variable, and on the whole, lower than comparable procedures in other body systems. Anecdotally, more surgeons offer kyphoplasty in states with higher reimbursements. In 2005, one-level procedure reimbursed $327 in Michigan and more than $1000 in other states. Several Michigan spine surgeons reported that, once kyphoplasty reimbursements declined to less than the reimbursement for the easier vertebroplasty procedure, they stopped offering kyphoplasty and began referring patients for vertebroplasty.

Adverse payer decisions also impact hospitals which, in turn, affect medical decision-making. At our institution, kyphoplasty was initially offered in late 1999. After two years, citing the costs of the disposables required, the hospital withdrew support for the procedure. As more outcomes data became available, the procedure was reintroduced in 2003.

Disc replacement fulfills some of the criteria of an MIS procedure in that it attempts to diminish the morbidity associated with its predecessor operations. As with more typical MIS procedures, a disc replacement costs more than previous operations and provides a keen example of how insurance companies can markedly impact the future of a new medical technique.

The payer response to the cost of the DePuy Charité has clearly affected its early adoption. As of this writing in mid-2005, many insurers continue to refuse to pay for this procedure. Some payers approve the procedure, but reimburse the hospital at levels significantly below the estimated $30,000 to $45,000 costs for a single-level arthroplasty (21). These fiscal difficulties may underlie the shortfall of discs implanted, which has been 25% below the manufacturer's projections. One surgeon, Scott Tromanhouser of the Boston Spine Group, has reported that 80% of his patients were denied coverage (21). This same report lists other new MIS spine technologies such as intradiscal electrothermal annuloplasty (IDET) were impeded by insurance companies. The insurance companies claim that no long-term outcome data justify the new technology's additional cost (21).

The economic analyses performed for disc replacement can, to a degree, be extrapolated to other, cutting-edge spine technologies such as MIS. The potential impact of these devices on medical and practice economics and practice patterns is tremendous (11,22,23).

A patient's healthcare coverage also effects how aggressively he pursues care. Insured patients use more health resources because third-party payers are paying most of the cost (19). For elective surgery, patients typically "face only modest co-pays and rarely know how effective individual service might be" (19). By extension, perhaps if patients were asked to pay the difference between standard spine operations that cost less (at least up front), they may choose to forgo the more expensive minimally invasive options presented.

On the opposite side of the spectrum, uninsured patients do not seek care until their problems are far more advanced and more difficult to treat. Moreover, they are more likely to seek care through emergency rooms rather than physicians' offices. These tendencies make it unlikely that uninsured patients will be offered MISS options at the same rate as insured patients (19). Further, fewer physicians practice in communities with large numbers of uninsured patients. This dearth also limits an uninsured patient's access to MISS (19).

For a capitated patient population, providers assume some of the risk and costs of any surgical intervention offered and thereby have an incentive to decrease costs in terms of the numbers and expense of procedures performed (16). How these factors affect the utilization of MIS techniques in health maintenance organization (HMO) patients may depend on how sensitive the formula is to immediate versus mid-term costs. If providers are credited for cost savings for early discharges or reduced physical therapy or pharmaceutical needs, the increased "up-front" costs may be negated. Similarly, with further refinement of surgical technique, MIS dissections may actually save OR time, thereby counterbalancing the increased implant costs, where they exist (24).

Some argue that HMOs and other capitated systems "remove the decision-making authority from both the patients and the practitioner and put it into the hands of those who hold the money—the employers, insurance companies, and the government" (19). Presently, insurance companies and other payers may be seen as a force against the increased implementation of MIS techniques in the spine. Over time, as MIS outcomes and economic data are increasingly available, on the other hand, payers' attitudes may change (25). For example, MIS procedures promise to discharge hospitalized patients earlier and return workers compensation patients to employment more quickly. While these mid-term savings may take longer for payers to grasp, undoubtedly they will encourage payers to support these techniques more actively (26). As more and more corporations decide to cover their own medical costs as part of self-insurance strategies, techniques that offer earlier return to work will likely receive increasing support.

ROLE OF THE HOSPITAL

As with the insurance companies, many hospitals are seen as restraining factors in the rate of spread for MIS spine techniques. In reality, the hospital may be both favorably and unfavorably affected by the current state of MIS. In the current climate, however, financial interests are wielding increasing influence. Simply put, MIS increases case costs while, in some cases, decreasing case revenues.

This issue is best put into perspective by understanding the economic impact of spine surgery on the typical hospital. At the average U.S. hospital, spine surgery is responsible for 21% of inpatient volumes and 25% of orthopedic revenues (22). Expensive new technologies increasingly jeopardize these revenues (Fig. 2). Given the cost of the hospital stay, OR staff, medications, labs, and the like, an ideal procedure's implant costs remain below 20% of the revenue for that procedure. Yet, the current average in spine surgery has risen above 50% (the mean implant costs for a two-level fusion is $10,000). With some newer MIS techniques, especially when bone morphogenic proteins are used with expensive new implant systems, more than 80% of the revenue is consumed by implants alone (27). In others, a three-level kyphoplasty, for example, the implants and disposables outstrip the hospital's entire reimbursement for the procedure (Kyphon, Sunnyvale, California, 2002).

In most cases, MIS procedures cost the hospital more than the traditional procedures they replace. These additional costs come in several forms. First, the hospital typically already has all of the equipment required to perform traditional, open spinal surgery. MIS requires major "up-front" costs such as microscopes, endoscopes, and in some cases, surgical navigation systems. These costs cannot be charged back to individual patients.

On a case-by-case basis, MIS techniques also require greater hospital resources such as OR time, endoscopic staplers, trocars, and light sources (28). MIS cases tend to be coupled with increased utilization of other, expensive technologies such as bone morphogenic proteins. Surgeons argue that the decrease in operative morbidity from a meticulous endoscopic approach is quickly lost if iliac crest bone harvest is required. As a result, they request bone morphogenetic protein (BMP) for these patients.

Where the surgery is to be performed has a marked impact on many aspects of the procedure. The types of OR equipment available and the skill of the OR staff in using that equipment may turn what is a routine procedure in one hospital into a technical fiasco in another. MIS, in theory, allows for faster recovery from surgery both in the short and mid-term. Ideally, these techniques would allow a greater percentage of spine cases to be performed on an outpatient basis, significantly lowering hospital costs (29). The safety, efficacy, and cost advantages of this approach have previously been demonstrated in the lumbar microdiscectomy procedures (30–32).

The advent of techniques requiring only short inpatient stays fostered the development of spine specialty hospitals. These hospitals are often partnerships between local surgeons and venture firms from outside the region. They are financially attractive to surgeons utilizing the centers who earn not only their usual procedure fee, but also a portion of the profit of the enterprise as a whole. The surgeon's incentive to select patients for these less invasive procedures rises as well.

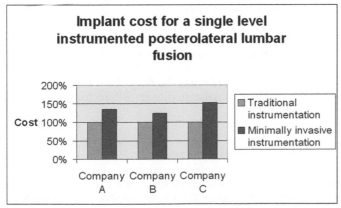

FIGURE 2 MIS technologies are typically more expensive than their traditional counterparts, although the premium for these devices varies among companies. For the companies surveyed here, their MIS offering can range from 20% to a full 50% more than traditional implants for a single level posterolateral fusion procedure. *Source*: From Ref. 44.

The presence of spine specialty hospitals influences regional surgery patterns. A recent Wall Street Journal article summarized the history of Rapid City, North Dakota, Neurosurgeon Larry Tueber's Black Hills Surgery Center. From the founding of its center to 2005, the rate of outpatient spine surgery in Rapid City doubled (33). Presently, Rapid City has one of the highest rates of lumbar surgery in the United States. In other areas, the dominant hospital system attempts to starve out specialty hospital competition by persuading payers to exclude rival facilities from their provider rolls (34). Dr. Tueber took his company public in 2004, earning $9 million for himself and $37.6 million for the other investors, 35 of 37 of whom were surgeons (33).

By increasing case costs, MIS techniques may consume more of the hospital's revenue per procedure. Unfortunately, in some cases, the revenue the hospital receives for the procedure is less than for more traditional spine procedures. MIS procedures may be deemed "experimental" by the insurance companies which often then deny payment to both the physician and the hospital. The physician's uncompensated surgery carries real costs to his practice, but the hospital's stake is much higher in terms of outlay for implants and other hard procedure-related expenses. Even when MIS procedures are covered by the payer, the level of compensation is tagged to payments levels associated with the more traditional surgery that the MIS procedure replaces.

How a given hospital responds to the financial challenges of MIS techniques depends greatly on its financial model. Unlike a community hospital hosting private practice surgeons, a staff model institution will be adversely affected by the utilization of two separate surgical teams in endoscopic spine surgery, for example. Alternatively, in some settings, the presence of allied specialties such as interventional neuroradiology also affects how rapidly percutaneous and other MIS procedures are adopted by orthopedic and neurosurgical spine surgeons (35).

Similarly, different hospital systems have different strategies to recoup capital outlay (27). In general, a hospital receives a flat sum for treating a given patient with a given diagnosis (a DRG) (9). The earliest example in orthopedic surgery came in total joint replacement wherein the Centers for Medicare and Medicaid Services (CMS) would pay a hospital a set fee to provide a total knee replacement, for example. If a more expensive implant was used, the hospital's profit from the procedure declined linearly with the increased expense. Similarly, additional inpatient days, laboratory and radiology costs came out of this bottom line. This funding scheme has led hospital administrators and researchers to closely examine the costs and benefits of the technologies routinely employed in surgery (24,36). The cost-effectiveness and clinical utility of intraoperative red blood cell salvage in routine degenerative spine cases has been questioned (37,38). Moreover, unlike some general hospitals, spine specialty centers strictly limit surgeon access to one brand of implants, for which it negotiates deep discounts (33).

While DRGs have become standard, at least for Medicare patients, some institutions have negotiated "carve-outs" for expensive new medical technologies (39). Here, the hospital receives the usual payment, but has negotiated a special rate, for example cost plus fifteen percent, for the new technology. In spine, these carve-outs have been widely used to finance the use of BMP in routine anterior lumbar interbody fusion procedures (40,41).

Recognizing the role physicians play in choosing expensive medical technologies, some hospitals have sought to induce physicians to utilize lower cost implants and surgical technologies through gainsharing. Currently, costs control factors in physician decision-making but only to a limited degree. In the future, should gainsharing become prevalent, physicians may take a much more aggressive approach in cost management. This may decrease their interest in utilization of the disposables and more expensive implants associated with MIS techniques (42).

ROLE OF INDUSTRY

Historically, spine surgery consisted of simple decompressive procedures. Fusions only rarely required instrumentation. Instrumentation, when used, consisted mainly of stainless steel wire. More recently, the explosion of implant use has resulted in a gargantuan spinal implants market. In 2004, spinal implants represented a full 16% of the entire $22.4 billion dollar musculoskeletal market (which includes casting supplies, wheelchairs, and the like) (22,23). This huge market, $3.5 billion in 2004, gives the device industry both the power and the incentive to influence medical decision-making toward increased utilization of expensive new technologies such as MIS (10,43).

While the spine market overall is growing 15% to 20% per year, niche-oriented hightechnology markets such as disc arthroplasty and MIS are growing by more than 100% annually (22,23). The influence of industry on spine surgery is best demonstrated by the relative utilization of implants or expensive disposables relative to the increase in spine cases overall. Between 1990 and 2000, there was a 20% increase in the number of cases performed, versus population growth during that interval of less than 5% (44). The percentage of this greater number of cases utilizing instrumentation increased by more than 10%. During the same interval, despite a stable average manufacturing cost of $45, the average price charged for a pedicle screw increased from the 1990 range of $135–160 to a range in 2000 of $255–700 (44).

With MISS, even decompression procedures will require expensive, proprietary instruments. The procedures typically require purchase and disposal of items that are reusable in more traditional spine procedures, such as fiberoptic light sources and expandable tubular retractors or their covering sleeves.

When fusion is to be performed through minimal access systems, the systems may mate only with proprietary implants conveniently sold by the manufacturer of the MIS retractor. Of course, these newer implants are significantly more expensive than previous generations of implants (22,45). Further, there is no evidence that these expensive new implants are in any way more effective than their less expensive predecessors. In fact, for many indications, clear evidence supporting instrumentation in fusions for degenerative conditions remains elusive (14,45).

Despite the lack of clear superiority in outcomes data, these technologies have continued to flourish (14). Industry is thrilled by their success and no doubt works tirelessly to support and further this trend in a number of critical ways. The most important avenue of influence is with the physicians who, in most cases, retain the power to decide which implant system is going to be used in a given case. More recently, the medical device manufacturers have increasingly targeted insurance companies, hospitals, and the patients themselves in an effort to increase utilization of their implants.

A number of avenues of influence exist between spine surgeons and the spine implant industry. Advertising to physicians in professional journals is only a small part of this influence (43). Independent observers have long claimed inappropriate interactions between physician and industry at lavish dinners and local meetings (43). Industry supports individual physicians through consulting agreements and by providing promotional material and patient educational materials. More important avenues of industry influence involve financial support of surgeon education and research. As with other areas of medicine, declining practice and hospital revenues and federal support have occurred in a context of increased costs of musculoskeletal research.

Given the relative lack of National Institute of Health (NIH) funding for research, academic spine surgeons have increasingly sought industry funding. As of this writing, more than 70% of spine trials are funded by industry sources (46). A recent study concluded that "while the public benefits immeasurably" from this support, there are a number of areas for potential conflict and bias. Guidelines should be established that delineate the role, if any, of the supporting company in the final statistical analysis and writing of any manuscripts arising from the funded research.

Examples of potential problems within industry sponsored research include the common confidentiality agreements. These agreements seek to block publication of negative results. In September of 2000, a biopharmaceutical company, Immune Response, filed a $7 million lawsuit against the University of California at San Francisco after researchers reported negative findings from a clinical trial about the company's experimental vaccine (46). In other cases, disputes center around industry demands to revise manuscripts written by investigators.

Harsh critics like Augustus Sarmiento ascribe the industry's influence on research and other "scientific" pursuits to the "unrestrained greed and business interests of the healthcare industry (overpowering) the philosophy, values, and ethics of medicine" (47). Academic "publish or perish" timelines for promotion and tenure fly in the face of escalating clinical demands on the academic surgeon and the limited availability of NIH or other federal funding. Some critics feel that the increase in industry-funded research has an innate bias in the type of project selected. That is, industry-funded projects tend to serve industry's aims of selling more implants.

One recent review in *Spine* found that industry-funded papers were significantly more likely to report positive results (48). Sarmiento has argued against the profusion of the so-called throw-away spine journals published at the behest of implant manufacturers and serving their aims, and, he feels, read preferentially to the peer-reviewed journals (47).

Beyond sponsorship of research, industry has long been intimately involved in the process of continuing medical education for practicing physicians. New technologies, such as MIS, require training. While, some physicians are trained in MIS during their residencies and fellowships, the depth and variety of trainee experience with new medical technologies varies widely (49,50). In any event, given the rate of change in the practice of spine surgery today, within four or five years in practice, these young practitioners will be seeking training in the new techniques.

For practical purposes, most current MIS techniques are learned during a surgeon's years of active clinical practice. For those physicians in practice, continuing medical education comes in a number of forms. Ideally, physician interest arises from careful review of Class I data in the peer-reviewed literature. The physician then gets more information on evolving trends at national meetings sponsored by unbiased specialty societies. When new technical skills are required, these are obtained through attendance in cadaver courses sponsored by the same, neutral societies. The surgeon should then visit a site actively utilizing the new techniques to gain more first-hand experience. Ultimately, depending on the complexity of the procedure or the preoperative planning required, mentorship by an experienced practitioner at the surgeon's home institution takes place.

Of course, this scheme is rarely practical. Often, surgeons hear of new techniques and technologies from representatives of the manufacturer, who may spend long hours with the surgeon in the OR each day. As with the population at large, surgeons are tempted by the promise of new techniques. "The stepwise progression of formulation of an idea, preclinical testing, prospective randomized studies, multicenter studies, and registry studies cannot be reconciled with the speed the public demands or to satisfy the hunger for answers to newly developed questions. Before one idea can be tested, what appears to be a better solution for the same problem comes along" (51).

When a surgeon expresses interest in a new technique, a manufacturer's representative may invite the surgeon to learn more at a course hosted by the manufacturer. These courses may be very useful to the surgeon participant, but concerns about how well alternative treatments are presented and the bias inherent in this arrangement remain. It has been alleged that these courses "emphasize their newest, and most expensive implants" (47). Henry Crock has stated that "mastery (of new procedures) is best gained by personal tuition under the guidance of a busy experienced surgeon. The trend toward learning surgical techniques in workshop settings or in short courses organized by manufacturers of surgical equipment … may lead to the triumph of technology over reason" (52).

Even professional society-sponsored educational events do not occur outside the influence of industry. The societies receive large grants to subsidize course costs. In return, the company receives access to the participants in one form or another. In national meetings, the companies will maintain booths where surgeons can be "detailed" on their latest offerings. Meeting hosts will encourage participants to visit these booths and will acknowledge the generosity of the companies sponsoring their meeting (53). At more intimate, society-sponsored cadaver courses, industry representatives, beyond subsidizing the meeting's cost, will often provide bench-side assistance with implants and may answer surgeons' questions about appropriate utilization of their products.

Another aspect of physician education relates to consultancy arrangements between the physicians and industry. When a manufacturer hosts a course on a new spine technology, it typically invites current users of that technology to speak on the subject, giving basic medical information as well their experiences with the implant in question. That surgeon often performs this service as part of a consulting arrangement with the company. Here, the surgeon's time and expertise are compensated by the company. If the surgeon is consistently negative about the product, one would assume that the company would not ask that surgeon to speak at the next meeting (53).

Unfortunately, when misused, these consulting arrangements may have more unsavory aspects as well. Allegations that consulting deals and physician payments were offered in some cases more as a way to reward the surgeon for using that company's products have surfaced for at least one major spine manufacturer (54,55).

In some cases, the surgeon has contributed to the design and development of the implant and receives a royalty for its use. This may affect utilization of certain spine techniques in isolated cases, but does not likely represent a factor in surgical decision-making overall. Allegations that some well-known surgeons have been paid royalties for designs in which they were minimally involved have also arisen (43). Here, manufacturers have been accused of "buying" that surgeon's reputation to associate it with their new product.

Certainly, the "blame" for abuses in these relationships cannot be solely leveled at implant manufacturers. Surgeons have been willing and, occasionally, enthusiastic participants. As with hospital and research interests, declining practice reimbursements in the face of increasing costs such as malpractice tend to encourage physicians to pursue alternative income streams (10,43,55). Ideally, surgeon investigators are primarily interested in increasing knowledge for the improvement in quality of life. Today, commercial motivations are, at the very least, more superficially apparent than in past years. Some spine surgeons have gone so far as to trademark the technical terms they employ to describe their procedures (56).

In 2004, the trade group representing most spine implant manufacturers, Advamed, released strict new guidelines to curb the potential for these abuses (54). Medical specialty societies such as the American Academy of Orthopedic Surgeons (AAOS), while citing patient benefits from the innovation in product safety and efficacy that stems from surgeons working closely with the implant manufacturers, have taken more visible roles in guiding member physicians on appropriate parameters for their relationships with industry (57).

Despite these changes, many if not most spinal academicians serve as consultants for one or more implant manufacturers. This can lead to areas in which there are more experts discussing new technologies than there are investigators studying these devices scientifically (10). Others continue to criticize this system and its effect on dissemination of new information and on the "medical–industrial complex" (55,58).

While the industry–surgeon relationship remains paramount, manufacturers increasingly attempt to influence patients through direct-to-consumer advertising. As this advertising increases, patient demand for new technologies may increase with the increased knowledge of their availability (22). A number of industry Web sites have been created that direct patients as to their options for their spinal pathologies. Critics state that these Web sites focus on operative treatment over nonoperative treatment and utilization of expensive new technologies over more traditional approaches. In addition, the Web site ownership by the medical manufacturer is often at times not apparent.

The manufacturers also strive to convince insurance companies and other payers of the importance of their new technologies in patient care in order to secure physician and hospital reimbursement. Interestingly, the implant manufacturers spend the least amount of effort and money addressing the concerns of the real customers for their products, the hospitals that pay for the implants out of shrinking revenues (22).

CONCLUSIONS

Physicians are taught to make recommendations solely based on what is best for the individual patient. Internal influences such as the surgeon's training affect the array of options from which the ultimate treatment may be chosen (59). Surgical "personality" in terms of an underlying conservatism or aggressiveness of approach also influences the rate at which they adopt new spine technologies. Together, these factors affect the so-called "surgical footprint" that has created wide differences in the rates of spine surgery across North America (2,5) These philosophical differences are also being seen in the informal audience surveys conducted at spine meetings. In four different spine meetings in June and July of 2005, the future of MIS techniques in spine surgery ranged from certain triumph to disdain. One group of surgeons agreed with the statement, "I haven't taken down the midline posterior elements in five years." Another group, pointing to what they felt was an overly slow acceptance rate of MIS techniques beyond vertebroplasty and kyphoplasty, agreed that "tubes are dead."

Increasingly, new influences have entered the decision-making between physicians and patients. First, patients bring additional information and strong opinions into their discussions with their surgeons. Second, insurance companies and hospitals attempt to control costs by limiting the types of treatments on the menu of options. Industry seeks to influence patients and insurers and, to a greater degree, the surgeons themselves. If successful, their influence will serve to further blur the physician's role as, first and foremost, the patient's advocate.

Incumbent upon all physicians, particularly surgeons utilizing expensive new technologies, is to understand the ramifications of their clinical decisions and the wide array of outside influences on those decisions. These influences are unlikely to die away. More likely, they will become stronger. Patients and physicians will be best equipped to make the best decision if they understand the role of these outside parties. As physicians, our first responsibility is to our patients. We should seek to offer them the best option, even if this is not the one they are requesting.

Second, we have a responsibility to the payers and the hospital to contain costs where possible and appropriate. Many expensive new technologies have very little data supporting their additional cost. Indiscriminate use of these technologies will inevitably lead to some outside party controlling even more directly our access to them.

Physicians utilizing new technologies should make themselves and their patients available for data collection. In the future, we will need to justify our expenditures to a far greater degree. Class I data including randomized clinical trials with large numbers of patients will be increasingly seen as necessary before expensive procedures are approved. We will be able to improve patient access to the best of these new technologies by presenting payers with quality of life-year analysis (QALY) and economic data proving that, while up-front costs are higher, long-term costs are lower (40).

In the meanwhile, before recommending any surgery, the physician should ask: Why am I doing this procedure? If I have an economic interest in one of the patient's options, has that been disclosed? Is this really an area where the additional cost is justified?

REFERENCES

1. Lurie, JD, Weinstein JN. Shared decision-making and the orthopaedic workforce. Clin Orthop Relat Res 2001; 385:68–75.
2. Lurie JD, Birkmeyer NJ, Weinstein JN. Rates of advanced spinal imaging and spine surgery. Spine 2003; 28(6):616–620.
3. Truumees E, Lieberman IH, Fessler R, Regan J. Minimally invasive spinal decompression and stabilization techniques. In: Benzel, E, ed. Spine Surgery: Techniques, Complications, Avoidance, and Management. Philadelphia: Elsevier, 2005:1274–1308.
4. Vaccaro A, Benzel E. Foreword and preface. In: Regan J, Lieberman I, eds. Atlas of Minimal Access Spine Surgery. St. Louis: Quality Medical Publishing, 2004:xi–xiii.
5. Thoman D, Phillips E. Training and credentialing. In: Regan J, Lieberman I, eds. Atlas of Minimal Access Spine Surgery. St. Louis: Quality Medical Publishing, 2004:63–65.
6. Truumees E, Hilibrand A, Vaccaro A. Percutaneous vertebral augmentation. Spine 2004; 4(2):218–229.
7. Hasson M. Liability costs not a big factor in high U.S. health care spening. Orthopaedics Today. New Jersey:Thorofare, 2005:47.
8. Herring SA. A plea for professional behavior. North American Spine Society presidential address, Montreal, Canada, 2002. Spine 2003; 3(1):5–9.
9. Faciszewski T. Spine policy. What's in a name? Spine 2001; 1(4):300.
10. McDonnell DE. History of spinal surgery: one neurosurgeon's perspective. Neurosurg Focus 2004; 16(1):E1.
11. Singh K, Vaccaro AR, Albert TJ. Assessing the potential impact of total disc arthroplasty on surgeon practice patterns in North America. Spine 2004; 4 (suppl 6):S195–S201.
12. St. John W. The Irish Patient and Dr. Lawsuit. New York, 2005.
13. Health R. New York Times, 2005.
14. Sasaoka R, Nakamura H, Konishi S, et al. Objective assessment of reduced invasiveness in MED compared with conventional one-level laminotomy. Eur Spine J 2005; S0940–6719.
15. Klein BJ, Radecki RT, Foris MP, et al. Bridging the gap between science and practice in managing low back pain. A comprehensive spine care system in a health maintenance organization setting. Spine 2000; 25(6): 738–740.

16. Brinker MR, O'Connor DP. Utilization of orthopaedic services in a capitated population. J Bone Joint Surg Am 2002; 84-A(11):1926–1932.
17. Berger E. Late postoperative results in 1000 work related lumbar spine conditions. Surg Neurol 2000; 54(2):101–106, discussion 106–108.
18. Karppinen J, Ohinmaa A, Malmivaara A, et al. Cost effectiveness of periradicular infiltration for sciatica: subgroup analysis of a randomized controlled trial. Spine 2001; 26(23):2587–2595.
19. Kelley R. Uninsured in America. The Cost Factors. Orthop Today 2005: 48–49.
20. Lieberman IH, Dudeney S, Reinhardt M-K, Bell G. Initial outcome and efficacy of "Kyphoplasty" in the treatment of painful osteoporotic vertebral compression fractures. Spine 2001; 26(14): 1631–1638.
21. Feder B. When FDA Says Yes, but Insurers Say No. New York Times, 2005.
22. Lieberman IH. Disc bulge bubble: spine economics 101. Spine 2004; 4(6):609–613.
23. Viscogliosi A, Viscogliosi J, Viscogliosi M. The Future of Spine Surgery: Beyond Total Disc. New York: Viscogliosis Bros., LLC, 2004.
24. Castro FP, Jr Holt RT, Majd M, Whitecloud TS. A cost analysis of two anterior cervical fusion procedures. J Spinal Disord 2000; 13(6):511–514.
25. Faro FD, Marks MC, Newton PO, et al. Perioperative changes in pulmonary function after anterior scoliosis instrumentation: thoracoscopic versus open approaches. Spine 2005; 30(9):1058–1063.
26. Fritzell P, Hagg O, Jonsson D, et al. Cost-effectiveness of lumbar fusion and nonsurgical treatment for chronic low back pain in the Swedish Lumbar Spine Study: a multicenter, randomized, controlled trial from the Swedish Lumbar Spine Study Group. Spine 2004; 29(4):421–434, discussion Z3.
27. Mendenhall S. Spine costs: a bigger problem than joints. OR Manager 2005; 21(4): 21–22.
28. Mathias JM. Lessons learned from new spine program. OR Manager 2004; 20(8):14, 16–17.
29. Mikkola H, Hakkinen U. The effects of case-based pricing on length of stay for common surgical procedures. J Health Serv Res Policy 2002; 7(2):90–97.
30. An HS, Simpson JM, Stein R. Outpatient laminotomy and discectomy. J Spinal Disord 1999; 12(3):192–196.
31. Asch HL, Lewis P, Moreland DB, et al. Prospective multiple outcomes study of outpatient lumbar microdiscectomy: should 75 to 80% success rates be the norm? J Neurosurg 2002; 96 (suppl 1):34–44.
32. Singhal A, Bernstein M. Outpatient lumbar microdiscectomy: a prospective study in 122 patients. Can J Neurol Sci 2002; 29(3):249–252.
33. Armstrong D. A surgeon earns riches, enmity by plucking profitable patients. Wall Street Journal, 2005; 40:A1–A7.
34. Romano M. All's fair in healthcare? Heartland Spine & Specialty Hospital alleges HCA Midwest Division conspired with local payers to drive it out of business. Mod Health Care 2005; 35(19): 6–7, 1, 10.
35. Berquist TH, McLeod RA, Unni KK. Postgraduate musculoskeletal fellowship training in the United States: current trends and future direction. Skeletal Radiol 2003; 32(6):337–342.
36. Runy LA. Data Page. Fix the spine and the bottom line. Hosp Health Network 2004; 78(10):22.
37. Chanda A, Smith DR, Nanda A. Autotransfusion by cell saver technique in surgery of lumbar and thoracic spinal fusion with instrumentation. J Neurosurg 2002; 96 (suppl 3):298–303.
38. Reitman CA, Watters WC III, Sassard WR. The cell saver in adult lumbar fusion surgery: a cost-benefit outcomes study. Spine 2004; 29(14):1580–1583, discussion 1584.
39. Becker C. GPOs reserve judgment. New company will finance spinal-implant purchases. Mod Healthc 2005; 35(22):16.
40. Ackerman SJ, Mafilios MS, Polly DW Jr. Economic evaluation of bone morphogenetic protein versus autogenous iliac crest bone graft in single-level anterior lumbar fusion: an evidence-based modeling approach. Spine 2002; 27(16 suppl 1):S94–S99.
41. DeJohn P. Spinal cage contracting: it's a backbreaking chore. Hosp Mater Manage 2002; 27(4):1, 9–10.
42. Reicin G. Will Gainsharing break the back of the orthopaedic device makers? Orthopaedics Today, 2005:1, 68, 70.
43. Reports, B.N.a.R.W. Artificial joint makers probed. USA Today, 2005.
44. Lieberman, I. The economics of disc arthroplasty. Who is going to pay for it? Innovative Techniques in Spine Surgery. MX: Cabo San Lucas, 2005.
45. Lenke L, Anderson G, Bridwell K. Summary statement: fusion technologies. Spine 2003; 28(20): S243–S244.
46. Mello M, Clarridge B, Studdert D. Academic Medicinal Centers' Standards for Clinical Trial Agreements with Industry. NEJM 2005; 352:2202–2210.
47. Sarmiento A. Barebones: a surgeon's tale. The Price of Success in American Medicine. Amherst, New York: Prometheus Books, 2003:379.
48. Shah R, Albert TJ, Bruegel-Sanchez V, et al. Industry support and correlation to study outcome for papers published in Spine. Spine 2005; 30(9):1099–1104.
49. Garfin SR. Editorial on residencies and fellowships. Spine 2000; 25(20):2700–2702.
50. Lee TT, Klose JL. Survey on neurosurgery subspecialty fellowship training. Congress of Neurological Surgeons Education Committee. Surg Neurol 1999; 52(6):641–644, discussion 644–645.

51. Fardon D. Developing and future methods for spine care. In: Fardon D, Garfin S, eds. Orthopaedic Knowledge Update: Spine. Rosemont, IL: American Academy of Orthopaedic Surgeons, 2002:491.
52. Crock H. Foreward. In: Mayer HM, ed. Minimally Invasive Spine Surgery. Heidelberg: Springer Verlag, 2000:247.
53. Kassirer J. Doctors and Drug Companies. Boston Globe, 2005:A15.
54. Feder B. Subpoenas seek data on orthopedics makers' ties to surgeons. New York Times, 2005.
55. Kassirer J. On the Take: How Medicine's Complicity With Big Business Can Endanger Your Health Oxford: Oxford University Press, 2005:272.
56. Yeung A. The evolution of percutaneous spinal endoscopy and discectomy. State of the art. Mt. Sinai J Med 2000; 67(4):327–332.
57. Weinstein S. Orthopedic Firms' Ties With Doctors Scrutinized. Wall Street Journal, 2005.
58. Ausman JI. The death of spine surgery as we know it today. Surg Neurol 2004; 61(4):315.
59. Anderson DG, Silber J, Vaccaro A. Spine training. Spine surgery fellowships: perspectives of the fellows and directors. Spine 2001; 1(3):229–230.

6 | Microscopic Anterior Cervical Discectomy and Foraminotomy

Michael D. Daubs
Department of Orthopedic Surgery, University of Utah, Salt Lake City, Utah, U.S.A.

INTRODUCTION

The use of the anterior approach for cervical decompression and fusion was first described by Robinson and Smith in 1955 (1) and Cloward in 1958 (2). The successful use of the anterior approach for cervical discectomy without fusion has also been reported by several authors (3–5). However, in these studies, despite no interbody bone grafting being performed, a large number of motion segments spontaneously fused. It was evident that in order to preserve motion through the disc space, a less invasive approach was needed. In 1968, Verbiest (6) described an anterolateral approach to the neuroforamen, which involved sectioning of the longus colli muscle, exposure of the transverse process, and mobilization of the vertebral artery. In 1976, Hakuba (7) reported a similar approach that he described as the "trans-unco-discal approach." In this approach, the sternocleidomastoid and longus colli muscles were sectioned and the disc was completely excised. Half of the patients in that series fused despite no interbody graft placement. In 1989, Snyder and Bernhardt (8) reported their results with a fractional interspace decompression, where only the lateral one-third of the disc was excised. They reported minimal disc space collapse and a 4% rate of spontaneous fusion.

In 1996, Jho (9) described a microscopic anterior cervical foraminotomy procedure whereby the transverse process and uncovertebral joint were exposed and the decompression was performed through the gradual removal of the uncinate process. Since the original description by Jho, there have been several modifications to this procedure (10,11). The evolution of the technique has led to less removal of the uncinate process and a direct trajectory to the neuroforamen through the lateral vertebral body (10,11). With these technical modifications, the procedure is now performed with less disc disruption, less bone removal, and less risk of vertebral artery injury.

INDICATIONS

This technique is indicated for unilateral radiculopathy secondary to soft disc herniation or uncovertebral osteophytes at one or two adjacent levels. This technique is not indicated for bilateral or polysegmental radiculopathies, or in patients with documented radiographic instability. Patients with severe neck pain in conjunction with a unilateral radiculopathy may have poor outcomes.

CONSIDERATIONS FOR PREOPERATIVE PLANNING
Physical Exam

This technique is aimed at patients with unilateral cervical radiculopathy. The physical exam should confirm unilateral symptoms. The positioning for this technique is similar to the open anterior cervical discectomy and fusion procedure. A patient must be able to tolerate their neck in slight extension. Patients with a fixed kyphotic deformity may present a problem with positioning.

Imaging

Standard anterior–posterior, lateral, and oblique radiographs allow visualization of the bony anatomy including the uncovertebral joint and foramina. If neck pain is part of the chief complaint, flexion extension radiographs should be considered to rule out instability. Magnetic resonance imaging (MRI) evaluation of the cervical spine is sufficient in most cases. If better bone detail of the foramen is needed, a thin-slice computed tomography (CT) scan should be considered. The pathway of the vertebral arteries should be reviewed on the axial cuts of the MRI to rule out any abnormalities that might hinder the approach. Although rare, a vertebral artery anomaly at the planned operative level is an absolute contraindication due to the increased risk of injury.

SURGICAL TECHNIQUE

The operation is performed with the patient under general anesthesia on a standard operating room table. The patient is positioned supine with the neck in a slight extension and a gel cushion behind the shoulders. Cervical traction is not needed. Taping the shoulders after pulling with longitudinal traction will help visualize the lower cervical segments on lateral radiographs. The approach is similar to that used for a standard open anterior cervical discectomy. The incision is made on the same side as the radiculopathy. It is helpful to use fluoroscopic imaging when marking the incision level. A radio-opaque tool should be used to check the proper trajectory to the symptomatic disc level. If the trajectory is improved with the neck in a neutral position, the shoulder roll should be removed. The neck is prepared and draped in the standard fashion as if performing an open anterior cervical discectomy and fusion.

A 3- to 4-cm transverse skin incision is made on the anterolateral aspect of the neck with two-thirds of the incision medial to the sternocleidomastoid muscle. The platysma is sectioned along the line of the skin incision. Sharp and blunt dissection technique is used to develop the fascial interval between the sternocleidomastoid and the medial strap muscles. The dissection is directed down to the spinal column with the trachea and esophagus retracted medially and the carotid artery and the sternocleidomastoid laterally. The prevertebral fascia is bluntly dissected exposing the anterior cervical body, the intervertebral disc, and the medial border of the longus colli muscle. A lateral radiograph is performed to confirm the correct level. A standard anterior cervical retraction system is used to maintain the exposure.

Next, the medial border of the longus colli muscle is split perpendicularly, retracted or excised to expose the medial aspect of the transverse process of the vertebrae above and below and the lateral border of the of the uncinate process (Fig. 1). The author prefers a retractor to mobilize the longus colli muscle laterally (Fig. 2). If the longus colli muscle is excised, bipolar cautery is used along the excision line. When exposing the C-7 level, care must be taken to avoid injury to the vertebral artery where it runs between the transverse process and the longus colli muscle. In the original description of this procedure by Jho (9), the vertebral artery was deliberately exposed when operating at the C6-C7 level. Saringer (11) recommended avoiding direct exposure of the vertebral artery. Whether it is directly exposed or not, its location should be known and it must be diligently protected to avoid injury.

An operating microscope is now utilized to perform the remaining steps of the procedure. The operative field of view includes the lateral aspect of the intervertebral disc, the lateral portion of the cephalad vertebral body, and the lateral portion of the caudad vertebral body and the uncinate process (Fig. 1). There are two possible approaches into the foramina for decompression. Jho's (9) original description was of a transuncal approach (Fig. 3). In this approach, the uncinate process is drilled with a 2.0-mm high-speed burr to create a void approximately 6 to 8 mm in transverse diameter and 10 mm in height. The drilling continues until a thin posterolateral rim of cortical bone remains (Fig. 3C). Caution should be used while drilling the base of the uncinate process. Lateral to the thin cortical remnant of the uncinate process is the vertebral artery, and posterior to it is the nerve root (Fig. 3F). Once the uncinate process remnant is detached from its base, the thin cortical pieces are removed with a curette and

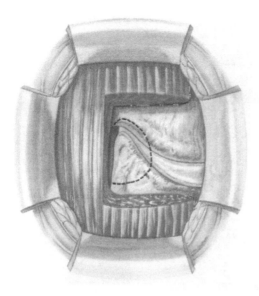

FIGURE 1 Schematic drawing showing the exposure for an anterior cervical microforaminotomy. The medial portion of the longus colli has been excised to expose the uncovertebral joint, the lateral aspect of the cephalad and caudad vertebral bodies. *Source*: Adapted from Ref. 15.

Kerrison rongeur, completing the foraminotomy. The nerve root displaces anteriorly once the final decompression is completed.

At this point in the procedure, the posterior longitudinal ligament covers the vertebral artery and the nerve root. If there is a herniated disc that has ruptured through the posterior longitudinal ligament, the ligament is incised and removed with a 1- or 2-mm Kerrison ronguer. Epidural bleeding can be a problem when removing the posterior longitudinal ligament. Bipolar cautery is used for hemostasis. If a disc has ruptured beyond the posterior longitudinal ligament

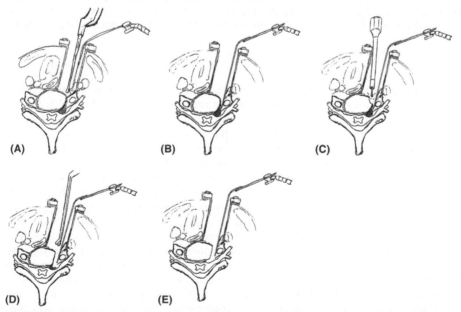

FIGURE 2 Microscopic anterior cervical foraminotomy/discectomy. (**A**) Longus colli muscle is mobilized allowing dissection around the lateral aspect of the vertebral body. (**B**) Placement of a thin (1/4–3/8 inch) malleable retractor between the vertebral body and the vertebral artery. (**C**) The lateral portion of the uncovertebral joint is drilled until a thin posterior rim remains that is removed with curettage and Kerrison ronguer. (**D**) The herniated disc and uncovertebral osteophytes are removed to decompress the exiting nerve root. (**E**) The decompression is completed, and the exiting nerve root is free of compression. *Source*: Adapted from Ref. 14.

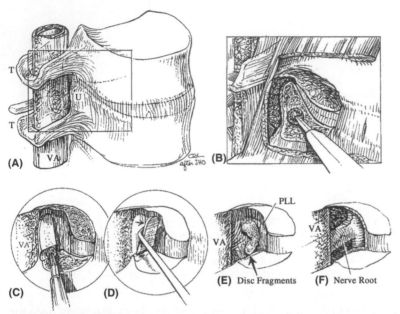

FIGURE 3 Schematic drawings displaying microsurgical foraminotomy. (**A**) An overview of cervical structures seen in the anterior approach. The surgical exposure is outlined by the box and enlarged in subsequent illustrations. (**B**) The medial portion of the longus colli muscle is excised to expose the uncovertebral joint and the medial portion of the upper and lower transverse processes. (**C**) Under an operating microscope, the uncovertebral joint is drilled to the posterior longitudinal ligament. (**D**) A piece of the thin cortical bone (*small arrow*) of the uncinate process covering the vertebral artery is fractured and carefully removed. The vertebral artery can be identified by its pulsation. (**E**) The compressed nerve root is distended forward by bone decompression. A tail of the herniated disc fragment may be visible through a tear in the posterior longitudinal ligament (*large arrow*). (**F**) The posterior longitudinal ligament is removed to confirm decompression of the nerve root. The nerve root is then visible from its origin in the spinal cord to its exit behind the vertebral artery. Removal of the posterior longitudinal ligament may not be necessary if there is no defect. *Abbreviations*: PLL, posterior longitudinal ligament; T, transverse process; VA, vertebral artery; U, uncinate process. *Source*: Adapted from Ref. 9.

(Fig. 3E), a defect in the posterior longitudinal ligament is usually seen along with the attached disc fragment. The posterior longitudinal ligament is not routinely removed if suspicion for a ruptured disc fragment is low. The path of the nerve root is easily visualized through the operating microscope. A small nerve hook is used to check the adequacy of the decompression.

Saringer (11) first described a modification to Jho's (9) original technique (Fig. 4). He described leaving the lateral aspect of the uncinate process for protection of the vertebral artery, and recommended further decompressing the foramen with removal of bone from the cephalad verterbral body endplate (Fig. 4B). Jho (10) also reported several modifications to the original procedure. He termed the new approach as a vertebral transcorporeal approach. In the approach, the starting point for the foraminotomy is the lateral, inferior 5 mm of the cephalad vertebral body, similar to that described by Saringer (11) and shown in Figure 4B. The anterior aspect of the uncinate process is not removed, and instead, the approach extends posteriorly through the most inferior and lateral aspect of the cephalad vertebral body to the posterior portion of the uncinate process. The more cephalad approach to the foramen allows for the cephalad slope of the intervertebral disc in the sagittal plane and provides a direct trajectory to the most compressing aspect of the uncinate process which is the posterior lip. Only the posterior aspect of the uncinate process is then removed. The modifications reported by Saringer (11) and Jho (10) improved the foraminal decompression and reduced the amount of disc disruption during the procedure.

Once the decompression is completed, the closure is performed in the same manner as for an anterior cervical discectomy and fusion. The platysma is closed with 3-0 absorbable suture and the skin with a subcuticular suture. Drains are not routinely used. Patients are placed in a soft collar for comfort only and instructed to begin gentle range of motion exercises

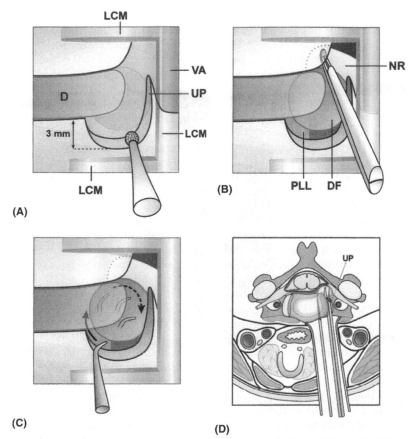

FIGURE 4 Artist drawings depicting microscopic anterior cervical foraminotomy. (**A**) The medial portion of the longus colli muscle (LCM) is excised and the lateral portion of the disc (**D**) and the uncinate process (UP) is exposed. The UP is drilled out. A thin piece of the lateral wall of the UP is left, serving as a landmark and a protective layer for the underlying vertebral artery (VA). Periosteum covers the nerve root, disc fragments, and the lateral portion of the posterior longitudinal ligament (PLL). The intervertebral disc (**D**) is maintained in its form. The VA is not exposed. (**B**) Periosteum, cartilaginous, and degenerative fibrous tissue between the tip of the UP and the cephalad endplate and osteophytes at the posterolateral cephalad endplate are removed using a 1- or 2-mm thin foot Kerrison ronguer. Disc fragments (DF), parts of the nerve root (NR), and lateral parts of the PLL are exposed. (**C,D**) Microscopic and axial depiction of the last step of the operation. Herniated disc fragments are mobilized with a microhook and removed with micropunch accomplishing the decompression of the nerve root. *Source*: Adapted from Ref. 11.

immediately. Activity is advanced as tolerated and return to full activities is allowed at six weeks.

COMPLICATIONS

As with most surgical procedures, many of the complications associated with this procedure can be avoided by an absolute familiarity with the anatomy of this region of the cervical spine. Knowledge of the microanatomy and orientation of the transverse process, the uncinate process, the nerve root, and the vertebral artery are essential. Experience with the use of an operating microscope is also mandatory. Proper illumination and visualization with the operating microscope will aide in reducing complications and improving the success of this procedure.

Pitfalls

Injury to the vertebral artery is a possibility with this procedure. It is most vulnerable to injury at the C6-C7 level where the artery travels between the transverse process of C7 and the longus colli muscle before entering the transverse foramina at C6. The incision of the longus colli muscle should be performed proximal to the transverse process of C6. The dissection should then be directed caudally with identification of the vertebral artery. The vertebral artery also in rare cases enters the transverse foramen at C4, C5, and C7 (12). The MRI should be evaluated to rule out these anomalies. The vertebral artery is also at risk at its location lateral to the uncinate process. By not removing the lateral and anterior aspects of the uncinate process during the approach, the vertebral artery should remain protected.

Nerve root injury can also occurr with this procedure. The nerve root is located posterior and lateral to the uncinate process. The posterior longitudinal ligament lies between the nerve root and the uncinate process. A small lip of bone at the posterior aspect of the uncinate process can be left while drilling with the high-speed burr. This will prevent accidental injury with the drill. The posterior lip can then be carefully removed with 1- or 2-mm Kerrison ronguers.

Horner's syndrome is a possibility if the lateral dissection of the longus colli extends beyond the anterior tubercle of the transverse process. The sympathetic nerves are located along the lateral border of the longus colli muscle. If the dissection and retraction are restricted medial to the anterior tubercle, this complication can be avoided.

Epidural bleeding can occur and cause difficulties with visualization in the relatively small operative field. This most often occurs when taking down the posterior longitudinal ligament. This is best avoided by not taking down the ligament routinely unless there is a high suspicion of an extruded fragment of disc beyond the posterior longitudinal ligament. Bipolar cautery is used to stop the bleeding if it occurs. Surface hemostatic agents are also helpful. Hemostatic agents that have the potential to swell after being placed should not be left upon closing. Bleeding should be completely under control prior to closing to prevent possible neurologic compression or airway compromise.

Another possible complication includes operating on the wrong disc level. Because the operative field and exposure are smaller than with open procedures, this complication is more common with minimally invasive surgeries. A lateral radiograph is absolutely necessary. Even after the radiograph is taken, it is easy to slide up or down one level along the lateral disc area. The uncinate process is located cephalad to the intervertebral disc. When in doubt, a repeat radiograph should be performed, or intraoperative fluoroscopic imaging utilized.

The intent of the minimally invasive approach is to maintain motion, prevent disc injury, and the cascade of disc degeneration and auto-fusion. An aggressive wide exposure that disrupts a large portion of the lateral intervertebral disc will accelerate disc degeneration and lead to either a spontaneous fusion or chronic neck pain.

Bailouts

In the event of a vertebral artery injury, a direct repair should be performed. The approach allows for direct visualization of the vertebral artery. It is more accessible than when performing a standard anterior discectomy and fusion approach. The anterior tubercle of the transverse foramen proximal and distal to the level of injury should be removed with a Kerrison rongeur. This exposes the artery and allows for direct repair. Careful review of the MRI will help identify any anomalies of the vertebral artery and reduce the risk of injury.

Epidural bleeding can be a problem if the posterior longitudinal ligament is excised. The best prevention is to avoid the routine excision of the ligament unless there is an extruded disc fragment. An extrusion is usually visualized as a defect in the posterior longitudinal ligament with a portion of the fragment extending into the foramen (Fig. 3E). If excessive epidural bleeding does occur, the operating table should be placed in reverse Trendelenburg. Temporary application of surface hemostatic agents to the area along with micropatties will stop the bleeding. However, any hemostatic agent that has the potential to swell postoperatively should be removed prior to closure.

As with the standard open anterior cervical discectomy approach, recurrent laryngeal injury can occur. Saringer et al. (11) reported transient injury to the recurrent laryngeal nerve injury in two patients in his series.

If technical difficulties arise with the minimally invasive approach and the decompression cannot be properly performed, the procedure should be converted to a standard open anterior cervical discectomy and fusion.

OUTCOMES

The microscopic anterior cervical foraminotomy has been shown to be effective in relieving unilateral radiculopathy resulting from soft disc herniation and uncovertebral osteophytes. Johnson et al. (12) reported 85% good to excellent results with improvement on a modified Oswestry Pain Scale in 91% of patients. No patient had evidence of instability or loss of disc height on lateral radiographs at three months postoperatively. Saringer et al. (11) reported complete relief of radicular symptoms in 97% of their patients. They reported one recurrent disc herniation. No patient showed signs of instability radiographically. Jho et al. (10) reported results on 104 patients. Seventy-nine patients underwent a one-level operation and 25 had a two-level procedure. Good to excellent results were reported in 99% of the patients. One patient had a fair result. Of the 59 patients who underwent postoperative dynamic radiographs, none of them had evidence of a spontaneous fusion. One patient developed a postoperative discitis and subsequently had disc collapse and spontaneous fusion. Transient Horner's syndrome was reported in two patients. The results in all three studies cited were similar whether the surgery was performed for a soft disc herniation or foraminal stenosis secondary to uncovertebral osteophytes.

SUMMARY

Microscopic anterior cervical discectomy and foraminotomy is a safe, effective, minimally invasive technique for the treatment of unilateral radiculopathy resulting from soft disc herniation or foraminal stenosis due to uncovertebral osteophytes. Experience with microscopic procedures and knowledge of the microscopic anatomy of the region is of utmost importance. As with all minimally invasive procedures, the balance between safety, effectiveness, and the minimal approach must be maintained. Avoiding damage to the disc space is the key to the long-term success of this procedure.

The future trend for this procedure is performing it through an endoscope. There are no long-term reports yet published, but the initial results of the endoscopic approach in a small number of patients has been good with minimal complications (13). If the outcomes are improved, this may become the standard.

Indications

Unilateral cervical radiculopathy secondary to a soft disc herniation or foraminal stenosis secondary to uncovertebral osteophytes.

Outcomes

Good to excellent results reported in 90% of patients with unilateral cervical radiculopathy.

Complications

- Vertebral artery injury
- Nerve root injury
- Horner's syndrome
- Epidural bleeding
- Recurrent laryngeal nerve injury

REFERENCES

1. Robinson RA, Smith GW. Anterolateral cervical disc removal and interbody fusion for cervical disc syndrome (abstract). Bull Johns Hopkins Hosp 1955; 96:223–224.
2. Cloward RB. The anterior approach for removal of ruptured cervical discs. J Neurosurg 1958; 15:602–614.
3. Bertalanffy H, Eggert HR. Clinical long-term results of anterior discectomy without fusion for treatment of cervical radiculopathy and myelopathy. A follow-up of 164 cases. Acta Neurochir 1988; 90:127–135.

4. Hankinson HL, Wilson CB. Use of the operating microscope in anterior cervical discectomy without fusion. J Neurosurg 1973; 43:452–456.
5. Martins AN. Anterior cervical discectomy with and without interbody bone graft. J Neurosurg 1976; 44:290–295.
6. Verbiest H. A lateral approach to the cervical spine: technique and indications. J Neurosurg 1968; 28:191–203.
7. Hakuba A. Trans-unco-discal approach. A combined anterior and lateral approach to cervical discs. J Neurosurg 1976; 45:284–291.
8. Snyder GM, Bernhardt AM. Anterior cervical fractional interspace decompression for treatment of cervical radiculopathy. A review of the first 66 cases. Clin Orthop 1989; 246:92–99.
9. Jho HD. Microsurgical anterior cervical foraminotomy for radiculopathy: a new approach to cervical disc herniation. J Neurosurg 1996; 84:155–160.
10. Jho HD, Kim WK, Kim MH. Anterior microforaminotomy for treatment of cervical radiculopathy: Part 1—Disc-preserving "functional cervical disc surgery." Neurosurgery 2002; 51–52:46–53.
11. Saringer W, Nobauer I, Reddy M, et al. Microsurgical anterior cervical foraminotomy (uncoforaminotomy) for unilateral radiculopathy: clinical results of a new technique. Acta Neurochir 2002; 144:685–694.
12. Daseler DH, Anson BJ. Surgical anatomy of the subclavian artery and its branches. Surg Gynec Obstet 1959; 108:149–174.
13. Saringer WF, Reddy B, Nobauer-Huhmann, et al. Endoscopic anterior cervical foraminotomy for unilateral radiculopathy: anatomical morphometric analysis and preliminary clinical experience. J Neurosurg 2003; 98(2 suppl):171–180.
14. Johnson JP, Filler AG, McBride DQ, Batzdorf U. Anterior cervical foraminotomy for unilateral radicular disease. Spine 2000; 25(8):905–909.
15. Jho HD, Ha HG. Operative techniques in orthopaedics. Operative Techniques in Orthopaedics, 1998; 8(1):46–52.

7 | Microscopic Posterior Foraminotomy/ Laminotomy for Nerve Root Decompression

Troy D. Gust, Neal G. Haynes, and Paul Arnold
Department of Neurosurgery, University of Kansas, Kansas City, Kansas, U.S.A.

INTRODUCTION

In 1943, Semmes and Murphy described a unilateral rupture of the sixth cervical disc resulting in compression of the seventh cervical root in the neural foramen (1). Around the same time, Spurling and Scoville (2,3), as well as Frykholm (4), described the technique of posterior foraminal decompression. Less than 10 years later, anterior cervical discectomy and interbody fusion using autograft was described by Robinson and Smith (5). This procedure was later revised by Cloward in 1958, with the addition of disc excision, removal of compressive structures, and fusion with a bone dowel (6). In 1960, Bailey and Badgley published their method of onlay strut grafting for cervical stabilization (7).

Although an anterior approach with discectomy and fusion seems to be favored by most spine surgeons, the posterior approach via microscopic posterior laminotomy/foraminotomy (laminoforaminotomy) remains a less invasive and effective approach to certain cervical diseases. Over the last 20 years, innovative advances in microscopy, endoscopy, and image guidance systems have led to the development of minimally invasive spine surgery. This concept entails a goal of achieving outcomes that compare favorably with open techniques, thereby minimizing risks to the patient and allowing a more speedy recovery. Most recently, the role for microendoscopic discectomy (8,9) in the cervical spine has challenged the traditional open microsurgical laminoforaminotomy for certain cervical spine disorders.

The following chapter discusses the indications, contraindications, preoperative planning, including physical examination and radiological studies, a brief description of the open surgical technique, complications, and outcomes of the laminoforaminotomy.

INDICATIONS

The current surgical literature supports the posterior froaminotomy/laminotomy approach for several cervical and cervicothoracic disorders. These include posterolateral disc herniation, isolated spondylotic foraminal stenosis, multilevel spondylotic foraminal stenosis without central stenosis, persistent radiculopathy despite previous anterior cervical discectomy and fusion, and cervical disc disease in patients for whom an anterior approach is contraindicated (9). Cervicothoracic disc herniation and radiculopathy are uncommon; however, posterior cervical foraminotomy alone or with a concurrent discectomy may be occasionally indicated, instead of the anterior approach, to avoid potential complications at the caudal cervical spine, including injury to large vascular structures, pharynx, and esophagus (10,11).

The effectiveness of the posterior cervical foraminotomy/laminotomy for decompression of the lateral recess and neural foramen to address unifocal or multifocal radicular complaints as a result of lateral spurs or disc herniation has been well-documented in numerous publications over the last four decades (12–19). In fact, compared with anterior cervical techniques, the posterior approach via a "keyhole" type of osteotomy may provide better exposure for decompression of the exiting root and for removal of lateral osteophytes and discs (9). In an anatomical study, Raynor found that via a posterior decompression, between 3 and 5 mm of the cervical root can be visualized, whereas only 1 to 2 mm can be appreciated through a standard anterior procedure (20). Like all procedures, however, posterior cervical foraminotomy must be used judiciously for primary cases of posterolateral disc herniations, osteophytic compression, focal lateral thickening of the ligamentum flavum, or facet thickening and arthropathy (8).

According to Roh et al. (9), indications for cervical surgery by any approach include unremitting pain despite maximal conservative therapy and/or a progressive neurological deficit, especially weakness.

For cases of myelopathy, central or paracentral stenosis secondary to a soft disc or osteophytic origin, deformity or instability, the laminoforaminotomy technique may not be the ideal procedure (8,15). Spondylosis or ossification of the posterior longitudinal ligament, associated with a kyphotic deformity, regardless of age, should be managed with direct anterior decompression and fusion, posterior laminoplasty (21–24), or both, rather than indirect posterior decompressive procedures. When myelopathy accompanies multifocal radiculopathy, hemilaminectomy, laminectomy, or laminoplasty may be warranted (12,17,25–32). However, in a series reported by Baba, excellent-to-good results were reported in 76% of patients undergoing en bloc open-door laminoplasty, and foraminotomy for selected patients with proven myelopathy and distinct unilateral radicular symptoms (33). The operative choice for lateral or foraminal pathology attributed to soft disc herniation, hypertrophied ligament or ossification of posterior longitudinal ligament (OPLL) degenerative spondylotic changes of the uncovertebral joints, osteophytes arising from the posterior articular facets or root sleeve fibrosis, includes both anterior or posterior approaches, including anterior discectomy with or without fusion or posterior laminoforaminotomy (11,13).

CONSIDERATIONS FOR PREOPERATIVE PLANNING

Preoperative planning should include a detailed history and physical exam, as well as a thorough neurological exam, with affected nerve roots identified by sensory, motor, and reflex abnormality. Specific attention to this detail will help identify which patients will most benefit from nerve root decompression alone as opposed to those who would benefit from more aggressive procedures. The history should include the length of time symptoms have occurred as well as any medications that the patient is taking that can inhibit coagulation, platelet function, or wound healing. Patient selection should exclude patients who have not had at least a trial of nonsurgical therapy, as surgery should be reserved for patients with radicular symptoms that do not improve with conservative management (34,35). Patients with nonsegmental symptoms should also be excluded (18). Preoperative labs should include coagulation studies, as well as platelet count and platelet function studies. Preoperative imaging should include magnetic resonance imaging (MRI) if possible (Fig. 1). A thin slice computed tomography (CT) or myelogram can be especially helpful if MRI is not possible (Figs. 2 and 3), or if the MRI does not show a clear lesion that corresponds to a neurological deficit identified by physical exam (18).

SURGICAL TECHNIQUE

The standard operative procedure for dorsal foraminotomy was first described by Frykholm in 1951 (12). The prone position, sitting position, or Concord position have all demonstrated comparable results. All patients have placement of bilateral sequential compression devices

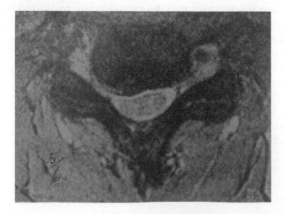

FIGURE 1 Axial T2 weighted magnetic resonance imaging shows right-sided C5-6 herniated disc with foraminal narrowing.

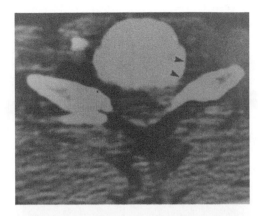

FIGURE 2   Plain axial computed tomography scan shows left-sided herniated disc.

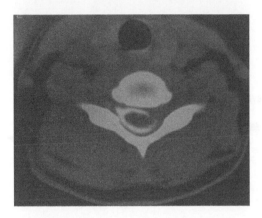

FIGURE 3   Postmyelogram computed tomography shows large herniated disc with nerve root cut-off.

prior to surgery, and prophylactic antibiotics are administered. Routine use of a Foley catheter is not carried out. Continuous intraoperative somatosensory evoked-potential monitoring (SSEP) can be performed during the entire procedure to assess spinal cord function. However, electromyography (EMG) during foraminal nerve root dissection to signal impending motor root damage is not routinely used.

After careful endotracheal intubation is established, the patient's head is placed in a Mayfield three-point pinholder, and the patient is then log-rolled into the prone position and secured to the operating table. The head and neck are mildly flexed with the operating table tilted approximately 30° in the reverse Trendelenburg's position to assure that the cervical spine is parallel to the floor. Intraoperative fluoroscopy or radiography is used to confirm the correct operative level and minimize the skin incision. A 2- to 3-cm incision is marked between the two appropriate spinous processes. A skin incision is made in the posterior midline with the disc space centered on the incision. The paravertebral muscles are then stripped subperiosteally on the symptomatic side from the spinous process and the lamina of the adjacent vertebra (Fig. 4).

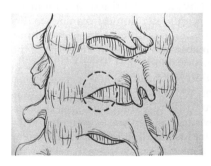

FIGURE 4   The bone to be removed is outlined.

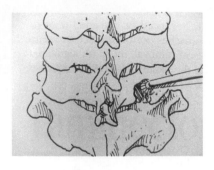

FIGURE 5 A keyhole foraminotomy is performed with a high-speed drill.

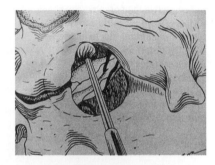

FIGURE 6 A keyhole foraminotomy is performed with a high-speed drill.

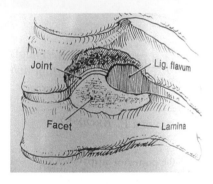

FIGURE 7 The ligamentum flavum is identified.

Hemostasis is achieved by electrocautery. Meticulous care concerning the paraspinous deep veins, as well as the venous structures within the interlaminar space is important to prevent excessive blood loss. The appropriate level is confirmed by radiological studies.

Under microscopic magnification, a high-speed air drill is used to thin bone over the lamina facet junction (Figs. 5 and 6). A small portion of the inferior articular process and the superior articular process may be removed with a small diamond burr. Once thinned to the underlying cortical margin, a small angled curette is used to remove the remaining bone. The amount of facet joint resection should not exceed 50% in order to preserve spinal stability (36). After the laminotomy is completed, the ligamentum flavum is identified and removed with either a knife or 1 to 2 mm Kerrison punches (Fig. 7). Careful attention is taken not to disrupt the venous plexus. The vascular cuff is identified, and intraoperative findings determine the surgeon's decision whether or not to open the cuff (37). Inspection begins in the axilla of the nerve root and, if indicated, the disc is removed using a No. 11 blade and pituitary rongeur, after elevation of the root (Figs. 8 and 9). Thorough exploration is conducted above, below, and medial to the nerve to insure that all fragments have been removed. The decompression is complete when a fine dental probe exits the foramen without difficulty (Fig. 10).

After satisfactory decompression is obtained, the wound is copiously irrigated with antibiotic solution and inspected for sources of bleeding. Hemostasis is achieved with bipolar electrocautery or gelfoam before closing. The muscle and fascia are reapproximated with

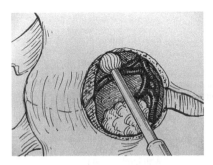

FIGURE 8   The foraminatomy is enlarged, and the disc is identified and removed.

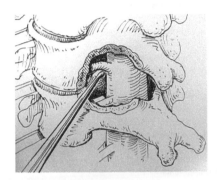

FIGURE 9   The foraminatomy is enlarged, and the disc is identified and removed.

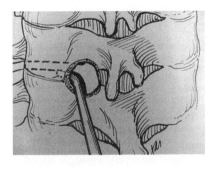

FIGURE 10   The decompressed foramen is probed.

absorbable sutures. The subcutaneous tissue is then approximated with interrupted absorbable sutures. The skin layer is closed with a running subcuticular stitch. A semicompressive dressing is applied to the incision. The patient is log-rolled back to the supine position, the Mayfield headholder is then removed, and all pin sites are carefully inspected for bleeding.

Postoperatively, patients are given postoral or intravenous opioids for pain control. A collar may be used for patient comfort. Diet is advanced as tolerated. Physical therapy services may be utilized to encourage early ambulation. Patient discharge is generally the same day or the next morning.

COMPLICATIONS AND THEIR MANAGEMENT

The complication rate in posterior foraminotomy/laminotomy is quite low in most series (0–10%) (Table 1) (31). They range from simple suture abscess to life-threatening tension pneumocephalus, brain and spinal cord ischemia, and death. Review of the literature notes that the most common neurological complication is transient nerve root paresis, the majority of which are resolved within six days (18). This is most likely because of the concomitant edema associated with revascularization of an ischemic nerve root. As might be expected, the longest nerve roots (C5) are the most commonly affected. Excessive blood loss was noted to be more common in the prone position, especially in obese individuals, while air embolism (32), tension pneumocephalus, and hypotension causing brain and cord ischemia are a risk of operating in the sitting

TABLE 1 Complications

Study	Rate (%)	Complication
Henderson et al. (16)	1.5	Ten wound infections
		Two wound dehiscence
Krupp et al. (17)	5	One spastic tetraparesis (resolved)
		One worsening of pre-existing paresis
		Two durotomy without clinical sequela
		Five postop deep venous therapy without clinical sequela
		Two PE
Aldrich (40)	0	
Fessler and Khoo (8)	6	Two durotomy treated with lumbar drain
		One partial thickness dural tear
Herkowitz et al. (11)	12.5	Two persistent serous drainage
Woertgen et al. (34)	4	Two durotomy without clinical sequela
Silveri et al. (43)	1	One suture abscess
Jodicke et al. (35)	15	Two transiently intensified paresis
		One durotomy without clinical sequela
		Two residual radicular irritation
		One fracture of lateral process of T1
Williams (31)	10	Eight severe muscle spasms—resolved <6 days
		Three worse radiculitis—resolved <6 days
		Five C5 paresis—resolved <6 days
		Two severe paresthesias—resolved <6 days
		One profound numbness—resolved <6 days
		Four prolonged paresis
		One wound infection
Witzman et al. (32)	1.5	One wound dehiscence
Grieve et al. (15)	1	One nerve root damage requiring brachial plexus graft
Kumar et al. (27)	2.2	One superficial wound infection
		One deep wound infection requiring I&D

Abbreviations: I&D, incision and drainage; PE, physical examination.

position. Incidental durotomy with cerebrospinal fluid (CSF) fistula formation was also reported in numerous series, but was no more common with the posterior approach than with anterior procedures. Injury to the vertebral artery is exceedingly rare but potentially one of the more serious complications (10). Nerve root and spinal cord injury was another reported but uncommon complication. In one case, a nerve root was damaged severely enough to later require brachial plexus grafting to regain function (27,33). Recurrence of symptoms at the same level was reported in a small number of cases (11,34), and appears to be more common with longer follow-up (35). It is not clear if this is because of incomplete decompression initially, or hypertrophy and scarring as a result of surgery, though both may ultimately play a role. There was one reported case of recurrent radiculopathy following lateral mass fracture (36). Additionally, instability of the cervical spine may result from overaggressive resection of the facet joint (37). Cadaver studies suggest that instability results only if >50% of the facet is resected (10,15). Bilateral foraminotomies are rarely required at the same level, and it would be unusual to need to resect 50% of the joint on even one side to obtain adequate decompression (10–12,15–17,19,24,27,31,32,34,35,38–44). Wound infection appears to be much lower compared with the most posterior cervical surgeries, most likely because of the smaller size of the incision and less retraction ischemia.

OUTCOMES

The surgical outcomes following posterior cervical foraminotomy are consistent in most of the available large series, with a favorable outcome in >90% of the cases (range 70–100%) (16), though criteria defining good outcome differ markedly. There are numerous studies showing a large series of patients with favorable outcomes, as this is a well-established procedure (Table 2). In the largest study to date, Henderson et al. (16) reported 846 posterior cervical foraminotomies for hard and soft disc disease in 736 patients. They reported a 96% favorable outcome with

TABLE 2　Outcomes

Study	Number of cases/ analyzed	Mean length of follow-up (in months)	Favorable outcome	Recurrence at same level
Henderson et al. (16)	846	21	96%	3.3%
Krupp el al. (17)	230/161	42	98% soft	0%
			84% hard	
			91% mixed	
Aldrich (40)	36	26	100%	0%
Fessler and Khoo (8)	25 MEF	16	92% radiculopathy	NR
	26 Open		87% neck pain	
			88% radiculopathy	NR
			89% neck pain	
Herkowitz et al. (11)	16	50	75%	NR
Woertgen et al. (34)	54/51	12	94%	NR
Silveri et al. (43)	84/60	73	98%	NR
Jodicke et al. (35)	39	33	96% (six weeks)	15%
			85% (long-term)	
Williams (31)	235	NR	100%	2%
Witzman et al. (32)	67	19	93%	NR
Grieve et al. (15)	77/63	40	85%	NR
Kumar et al. (27)	89	8.6	95.5%	6.7%

Abbreviation: NR, not recorded.

regard to pain relief, and a 98% improvement in motor deficit. Krupp et al. reported an excellent or good result with foraminotomy in 98% of the 161 patients analyzed; unfortunately, a large number of these patients in this study were lost to follow-up. They separated outcome by hard, soft, and mixed disc pathology, with favorable outcomes of 98%, 84%, and 91%, respectively (17). Aldrich performed 36 lateral facetectomies for posterolateral soft discs, with 100% favorable outcome (40). Fessler and Khoo performed 25 microendoscopic foraminotomies (MEF) and 26 open laminoforaminotomies for cervical root compression for either foraminal stenosis or disc herniation, with a 92% and 87% favorable outcome for radiculopathy and neck pain, respectively, using MEF, and 88% and 89% favorable outcome for the same two criteria using an open procedure (8). Herkowitz et al. compared anterior cervical fusion (ACF) and laminotomy-foraminotomy, and demonstrated a 75% good or excellent outcome in the 16 patients treated with the posterior approach (11). Woertgen et al. analyzed 51 of 54 patients following foraminotomy at one year with a 94% favorable outcome (74% complete resolution of symptoms and 20% more with some improvement) (34). Silveri et al. retrospectively analyzed 60 of 84 patients with a mean follow-up of 73 months with a 98% good to excellent results (43). Jödicke et al. report a 96% good or excellent outcome at six weeks and a 85% good or excellent outcome at a mean of 33 months following foraminotomy (35). Interestingly, at early follow-up soft discs have a greater ratio of good outcomes in this study than do hard discs; however, at long-term follow-up, there is no statistical difference between the two groups. They also reported a 15% same-level recurrence rate. Williams reported a 100% resolution of radicular pain in 235 patients undergoing foraminotomy over a 10-year period; however, they made no mention of mean follow-up (31). Witzman et al. report a 93% diminution or complete resolution of radicular symptoms at a mean of 19 months after foraminotomy in a series of 67 patients (32). Grieve et al. reported a 25% to 100% improvement in arm pain in 85% of the patients treated with foraminotomy for spondylotic radiculopathy both at one month postop and at the time of the questionnaire with a mean follow-up of 40 months (15). Kumar et al. (27) reported a series of 89 patients followed retrospectivly for a mean of 8.6 months using clinic notes only rather than questionnaires. They reported 95.5% good or excellent results using foraminotomy for treatment of spondylotic radiculopathy.

The most consistently cited variable determining favorable outcome was length of preoperative symptoms; patients with a shorter duration of symptoms tended to have better outcomes. Additionally, patients with far lateral discs had better results than those with central discs, and soft disc patients did better than those with hard discs. There was also a very clear pattern of favorable outcome in patients with symptoms that correlated to dermatomal

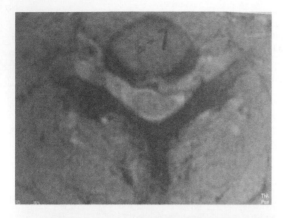

FIGURE 11 The preoperative magnetic resonance imaging shows C6-7 herniated disc.

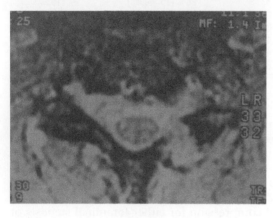

FIGURE 12 The postoperative magnetic resonance imaging shows decompression of the nerve root.

distribution, as opposed to patients with overlapping symptoms with more than one level. This relationship held true even when more than one level was decompressed. Additional poor prognostic factors include pending legal disputes or disability claims. All of these factors were more strongly correlated to outcome than age or gender (Figs. 11 and 12).

SUMMARY

Posterior laminotomy/foraminotomy is historically a very successful surgery with few complications when used to treat appropriately selected patients. Optimally, far lateral soft and hard discs are best treated with foraminotomy/laminotomy, especially if disease exists at one or two levels. The advantages of the minimally invasive foraminotomy over a posterior laminectomy are less pain, blood loss, and fewer wound infections. The advantages of foraminotomy/laminotomy over the anterior approach is better exposure to the nerve root, and avoidance of the structures of the anterior neck, no loss of mobility secondary to fusion, and minimal risk of destabilization of the cervical spine. As instrumentation and techniques continue to get better, the trend for more minimally invasive procedures will continue to grow, and patients will seek out surgeons who are capable of relieving their pain through a smaller incision. Additionally, economic forces dictating shorter hospital stays after spinal procedures will also favor surgeons using minimally invasive techniques. The next logical step in this progression may be surgical robotics for even less invasive spine surgery, as it has already happened in the fields of urology, cardiovascular, and general surgery.

SUMMARY
Indications for Laminotomy/Foraminotomy

- Posterolateral disc herniation
- Isolated spondylotic foraminal stenosis

- Multilevel spondylotic foraminal stenosis without central spinal stenosis
- Persistent radiculopathy despite previous anterior cervical discectomy and fusion (ACDF)
- Isolated patient subgroups with contraindicated anterior approaches.

Outcomes

- Generally greater than 90% reduction in pain
- Generally greater then 90% improvement in motor function
- Rare to have recurrence at the same level
- No evidence of destabilization.

Complications

- Low incidence of transient paresis
- Low incidence of wound infection
- Low incidence of durotomy
- Occasional immediate worsening of symptoms which resolves in less than six days.

REFERENCES

1. Semmes RE, Murphy F. The syndrome of unilateral rupture of the sixth cervical intervertebral disc. JAMA 1943; 121:1209–1214.
2. Scoville WB. Rupture of the lateral cervical disk and its operative technique. Proceedings of the Harvey Cushing meeting, Boston, 1946.
3. Spurling R, Scoville WB. Lateral rupture of the cervical intervertebral discs: a common cause of shoulder and arm pain. Surg Gynae Obst 1944; 78:350–358.
4. Frykholm R. Deformities of dural pouches and strictures of dural sheaths in the cervical region producing nerve root compression. J Neurosurg 1947; 4:403–413.
5. Robinson RA, Smith GW. Anterolateral cervical disk removal and interbody fusion for cervical disc syndrome. Bull John Hopkins Hospital 1955; 96:223–224.
6. Cloward RB. The anterior approach for removal of ruptured cervical disks. J Neurosurg 1958; 15:602–617.
7. Bailey RW, Badgley CE. Stabilization of the cervical spine by anterior fusion. J Bone Joint Surg 1960; 42A:565–594.
8. Fessler RG, Khoo LT. Minimally invasive cervical microendoscopic foraminotomy: an initial clinical experience. Neurosurgery 2002; 51:537–545.
9. Roh SW, Kim DH, Cardoso AC, Fessler RG. Endoscopic foraminotomy using MED system in cadaveric specimens. Spine 2000; 25:260–264.
10. Harrop JS, Silva MT, Sharan AD, Dante SJ, Simeone FA. Cervicothoracic radiculopathy treated using posterior cervical foraminotomy/diskectomy. J Neurosurg (Spine 2) 2003; 98:131–136.
11. Herkowitz HN, Kurz LT, Overholt DP. Surgical management of cervical soft disc herniation. A comparison between the anterior and posterior approach. Spine 1990; 15:1026–1030.
12. Frykholm R. Cervical nerve root compression resulting from disk degeneration and root sleeve fibrosis. Acta Chir Scand 1951; 160:1–149.
13. Epstein NE. Circumferential surgery for the management of cervical ossification of the posterior longitudinal ligament. J Spinal Disord 1998; 11:200–207.
14. Epstein NE. The value of anterior cervical plating in preventing vertebral fracture and graft extrusion after multilevel anterior cervical corpectomy with posterior wiring and fusion: indications, results, and complications. J Spinal Disord 2000; 13:9–15.
15. Grieve JP, Kitchen ND, Moore AJ, Marsh HT. Results of posterior cervical foraminotomy for treatment of cervical spondylitic radiculopathy. Br J Neurosurg 2000; 14:40–43.
16. Henderson CM, Hennessy RG, Shuey HM Jr, Shackleford EG. Posterior lateral foraminotomy as an exclusive operative technique for cervical radiculopathy: a review of 846 consecutively operated cases. Neurosurgery 1983; 13:504–512.
17. Krupp W, Schattke H, Muke R. Clinical results of the foraminotomy as described by Frykholm for the treatment of lateral cervical disc herniation. Acta Neurochir (Wien) 1990; 107:22–29.
18. Zeidman SM, Ducker TB. Posterior cervical laminoforaminatomy for radiculopathy: review of 172 cases. Neurosurgery 1993; 33:356–362.
19. Scoville WB, Whitecomb BB. Lateral rupture of cervical intervertebral disks. Postgrad Med 1966; 39:174–180.
20. Raynor RB. Anterior or posterior approach to the cervical spine: an anatomical and radiographic evaluation and comparison. Neurosurgery 1983; 12:7–13.

21. Epstein NE. Posteior approaches in the management of cervical spondylosis and ossification of the posterior longitudinal ligament. Surg Neurol 2002; 58:194–207.

22. Itoh T, Tsuji H. Technical improvements and results of laminoplasty for compressive myelopathy in the cervical spine. Spine 1985; 10:729–736.

23. Fager CA. Management of cervical disc lesions and spondylosis by posterior approaches. Clin Neurosurg 1977; 24:488–507.

24. Scoville WB, Dohrmann GJ, Corkill G. Late results of cervical disc surgery. J Neurosurg 1976; 45:203–210.

25. Baba H, Chen Q, Vohidak, Imura S, Morikawa S, Tomita K. Laminoplasty with foraminotomy for coexisting cervical myelopathy and unilateral radiculopathy. A preliminary report. Spine 1996; 21:196–202.

26. Chen BH, Natarajan RN, An HS, Anderson GBJ. Comparison of biomechanical response to surgical procedures used for cervical radiculopathy: posterior keyhole foraminotomy versus anterior foraminotomy and discectomy versus anterior discectomy with fusion. J Spinal Disord 2001; 14:17–20.

27. Kumar GR, Maurice-Williams RS, Bradford R. Cervical foraminotomy: an effective treatment for cervical spondylotic radiculopathy. Br J Neurosurg 1998; 12:563–568.

28. Epstein JA, Lavine LS, Aronson HA, Epstein BS. Cervical spondylotic radiculopathy. The syndrome of foraminal construction treated by foraminotomy and the removal of osteophytes. Clin Orthop Rel Res 1965; 40:113–122.

29. Fager CA. Posterolateral approach to ruptured median and paramedian cervical disk. Surg Neurol 1983; 20:443–452.

30. Scoville WB. Classification and surgical approaches to lesions of the cervical disks. J Neurochirurgie 1964; 10:561–563.

31. Williams RW. Microcervical foraminotomy. A surgical alternative for intractable radicular pain. Spine 1983; 8:708–716.

32. Witzmann A, Hejazi N, Krasznai L. Posterior cervical foraminotomy. A follow-up study of 67 surgically treated patients with compressive radiculopathy. Neurosurg Rev 2000; 23:213–217.

33. Scoville WB. Cervical spondylosis treated by bilateral facetectomy and laminectomy. J Neurosurg 1961; 18:423–426.

34. Woertgen C, Holzschuh M, Rotboerl RD, Hueusler E, Brawanski A. Prognostic factors of posterior cervical disc surgery: a prospective consecutive study of 54 patients. Neurosurgery 1997; 40:724–728.

35. Jodicke A, Daentzer D, Kastner S, Asamoto S, Boker D-K. Risk factors for outcome and complications of dorsal foraminotomy in cervical disc herniation. Surg Neurol 2003; 60:124–129.

36. Grundy PL, Germon TJ, Gili SS. Transpedicular approaches to cervical uncovertebral osteophytes causing radiculopathy. J Neurosurg (Spine) 2000; 93:21–27.

37. Zdeblick TA, Zou D, Warden KE, McCabe R, Kunz D, Vanderby R. Cervical stability after foraminotomy. A biomechanical in vitro analysis. JBJS 1992; 74A:22–27.

38. Chestnut, RM, Abitbol JJ, Garfin SR. Surgical management of cervical radiculopathy. Indications, techniques, and results. Orthop Clin N Am 1992; 23:461–474.

39. Rock JP, Ausman JJ. The use of the operating microscope for cervical foraminotomy. Spine 1991; 16:1381–1383.

40. Aldrich F. Posterolateral microdiscectomy for cervical monoradiculopathy caused by posterolateral soft cervical disc sequestration. J Neurosurg 1990; 72:370–377.

41. Kubo S, Goel VK, Yang S-J, Tajima N. The biomechanical effects of multilevel posterior foraminotomy and foraminotomy with double-door laminoplasty. J Spinal Disord Tech 2002; 15:477–485.

42. Casotto A, Buoncristiani P. Posterior approach in cervical spondylotic myeloradiculopathy. Acta Neurochir (Wien) 1981; 57:275–285.

43. Silveri CP, Simpson JM, Simeone FA, Balderston RA. Cervical disc disease and the keyhole foraminotomy: proven efficacy at extended long-term follow-up. Orthopedics 1997; 20:687–692.

44. Snow RB, Weiner H. Cervical laminectomy and foraminotomy as surgical treatment of cervical spondylosis: a follow-up study with analysis of failures. J Spinal Disord 1993; 6:245–250.

8 | Endoscopic Laminotomy/Foraminotomy for Herniated Cervical Disc

Thomas J. Puschak
Panorama Orthopedics and Spine Center, Golden, Colorado, U.S.A.

Rick C. Sasso
Indiana Spine Group, Indianapolis, Indiana, U.S.A.

William Tally and Deepan Patel
Department of Orthopedics, Thomas Jefferson University, Philadelphia, Pennsylvania, U.S.A.

Alexander R. Vaccaro
Department of Orthopedic Surgery and Neurosurgery, Thomas Jefferson University and the Rothman Institute, Philadelphia, Pennsylvania, U.S.A.

INTRODUCTION

Recent advances in techniques that improve intraoperative visualization such as digital fluoroscopy, image navigation systems, and high-resolution endoscopy are being applied to all areas of spinal surgery. These techniques allow surgeries to be performed through smaller incisions with less iatrogenic tissue damage and blood loss. Paraspinal muscle damage associated with surgical dissection and retraction in open procedures contributes to postoperative pain and may be a factor in chronic pain as well. Kawaguchi et al. (1) showed that in the lumbar spine, retractor blade pressure and duration of retraction directly correlated with paraspinal muscle damage. The main goal of minimally invasive procedures is to minimize surgical dissection and paraspinal muscle retraction to theoretically decrease blood loss, minimize postoperative pain, and lead to shorter hospital stays and faster return to full function.

Anterior approaches to the cervical spine avoid the need for muscular division or retraction, which has been traditionally required for posterior access procedures. However, an anterior cervical decompression is not without its shortcomings. In the vast majority of cases, a fusion procedure is performed which may be associated with bone graft donor site discomfort if an autologous source is used and the potential for junctional degeneration may be increased over posterior decompressive procedures. In addition, much less common complications may also be experienced with anterior cervical approaches such as injury to the recurrent laryngeal nerve, esophagus, great vessels, trachea, and the subjective complaint of swallowing difficulty or dysphagia. As a result of these potential problems, disc or foraminal problems that require surgical intervention and that may be equally served by an anterior or posterior procedure, often are managed by the approach associated with the least amount of morbidity.

The simplest and least dangerous approach to the cervical neuroforamen is via a direct posterior exposure. Posterior foraminotomy also has the benefit of avoiding the need for fusion. Unfortunately, this approach requires a defined amount of subperiosteal muscular release and elevation in order to provide adequate visualization of the laterally situated facet joints. The resulting postoperative morbidity including muscular pain, spasms, and stiffness has always been a potential problem for patients and surgeons.

With the effectiveness of posterior cervical laminoforaminotomy for decompression of the lateral recess and neuroforamen (2–4), attempts in performing the procedure through minimally invasive approaches have been made. The "keyhole"-type foraminotomy provides excellent exposure for decompression of the exiting nerve root while avoiding the need for fusion. Posterior and anterolateral osteophytes, as well as soft lateral herniated disc fragments can be easily addressed through this procedure. Because of the depth of the wound, significant muscle dissection is often required during the open procedure, which is associated with increased postoperative neck pain, spasm, and recovery time.

Several minimally invasive posterior cervical retractor systems are now available. Tubular access systems combined with endoscopic visualization similar to those used in the lumbar spine can be used for microendosopic laminoforaminotomy in the posterior cervical spine. A mini-open technique similar to microlumbar discectomy can also be performed using special retractor systems with fiberoptic illuminated blades combined with a surgical microscope for improved visualization. The application of these minimally invasive techniques can help to minimize postoperative pain and disability. This chapter reviews the indications, work-up, and surgical technique of endoscopic posterior cervical foraminotomy. Avoidance and management of complications is also discussed.

INDICATIONS/CONTRAINDICATIONS

The most common indication for posterior foraminotomy is a unilateral single- or multiple-root cervical radiculopathy without instability, significant kyphosis, or severe axial neck pain. The most common etiologies are foraminal stenosis from uncovertebral joint hypertrophy and facet degeneration or acute lateral soft disc herniations. Anterior fusion should be considered in patients with bilateral radiculopathy at the same level to avoid potentially destabilizing the segment. Large central soft disc herniations are more safely and effectively addressed from an anterior approach. Also patients with hard midline disc protrusions may need to be addressed anteriorly. Anterior decompression and fusion should be considered in patients who have more axial neck pain than radicular pain or significant kyphotic deformity. Patients with myelopathy are not adequately decompressed through foraminotomy and either anterior decompression and fusion or posterior decompression through laminectomy or laminoplasty should be performed.

CONSIDERATIONS FOR PREOPERATIVE PLANNING

The diagnosis of cervical radiculopathy is rather specific with patients presenting with predominantly arm pain, weakness, and/or numbness. Symptoms can be quite severe with burning pain and significant weakness. A thorough neurological exam must be performed, both to localize the radiculopathy as well as identify pathology which would require a different surgical treatment. Sensory symptoms traditionally follow dermatomal patterns on exam, while motor deficits are usually specific to muscle groups innervated by the involved root levels. Diminished deep tendon reflexes are often noted and can be helpful in diagnosing the involved root level. Positive nerve root compression signs such as the Spurling's maneuver are often present.

Radiographic examination often involves plain radiographs. Plain films will frequently be normal or show various stages of spondylosis. Plain radiographs are more useful in identifying instability and kyphotic deformity than in identifying the involved stenotic level. Magnetic resonance imaging (MRI) is very helpful in diagnosing foraminal stenosis from spondylosis and acute disc herniations. Cervical computed tomography (CT) scan with myelogram is also helpful in diagnosing foraminal stenosis and nerve root compression in patients unable to obtain an MRI scan. Electrodiagnostic studies such as electromyogram (EMG) are helpful in ruling out peripheral compressive or systemic neuropathies. Cervical selective nerve root blocks can also be used diagnostically for confirmation as well as be a therapeutic treatment tool.

Most patients respond with conservative treatment including rest, observation, oral steroids, nonsteroidal anti-inflammatory drugs (NSAIDs), physical therapy, and epidural or selective nerve root injections. When conservative modalities fail to alleviate pain or if neurologic deficits persist or progress, surgical decompression is indicated.

SURGICAL TECHNIQUE

Posterior approaches to the cervical spine might be performed with the patient in a sitting or prone position. The sitting position has the advantage of minimizing blood loss as a result of collapse of epidural vessels; however, it also has a higher risk of air embolus than the prone position. Placement of the knees higher than the heart and use of compression stockings can help reduce the risk of air embolus. Intraoperative Swan-Ganz catheter placement is helpful in monitoring for air in the venous system.

TABLE 1   Indications for Microendoscopic Posterior Cervical Foraminotomy

Unilateral radiculopathy
  Degenerative/spondylitic
    Uncovertebral osteophytes
    Facet hypertrophy
  Acute disc herniation
    Foraminal soft disc herniation

We prefer prone positioning with the head slightly flexed and held with Mayfield pin-holder headrest or a well-padded horseshoe-shaped headrest. The Mayfield pin-holder headrest offers more rigid control of the head position and completely alleviates potential pressure points on the face of the patient. Mayfield tongs are applied and the patient is proned minimizing manipulation of the head and neck. The patient's chest and iliac crests are supported on gel rolls and the abdomen is allowed to fall free. The arms are positioned anatomically at the patient's side and bony prominences are padded. The face is inspected to make sure that it is not in contact with the frame and that the chin is clear of the end of the table.

The posterior neck is sterilely prepared and draped. The appropriate level for access tube placement is determined using fluoroscopy and a stab incision is made 1 cm lateral to the spinous process. Extending the stab incision through the fascia, which is thick and tenacious at this level, aids in passing the dilators and tubular retraction system. A K-wire or Steinman pin is advanced to the facet under anteroposterior and lateral fluoroscopic guidance. Serial dilators are used to widen the port and the tubular retractor is ultimately docked on the facet complex (Fig. 1). Loupe, microscopic, or endoscopic magnification is utilized based on surgeon preference. The METRx (Medtronic Sofamor Danek, Memphis, Tennessee U.S.A.) tubular retractor system has been the most widely used minimally invasive retractor. It has an excellent light source and special bayoneted instruments that aid in working in the confined space of a tube.

The main difficulty with tubular retractor systems has been the challenge of working in the confined space of a long tube in a plane co-axial with the line of sight. In an attempt to improve the working space and line of sight, minimally invasive expandable retractor systems have developed. These systems are placed unexpanded over the serial dilators and expanded once docked on the facet complex. The Maxcess system (Stryker Spine, New Jersey U.S.A.), one such expandable retractor, can be mounted to the operating table and has illuminated blades.

Once the access has been obtained, the keyhole foraminotomy technique is the same as described in open procedures. A 4-0 curved curette is used to strip the ligamentum flavum from the cranial and caudal lamina edges. A circular lateral laminotomy is made with 1- and 2-mm Kerrison rongeurs to identify the lateral edge of the dural tube and the takeoff of the nerve root (Figs. 2 and 3). A nerve hook or dental instrument is useful to palpate the medial border of the pedicle to identify the lateral edge of the spinal canal and to feel out into the foramen and

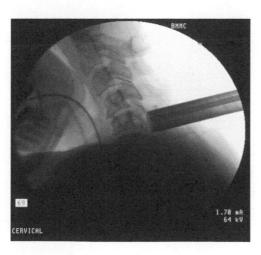

FIGURE 1   Lateral radiograph showing retractor tube docked at C5-6 joint.

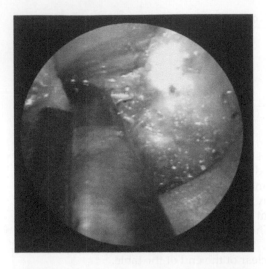

FIGURE 2 Kerrison rongeur biting the inferior C5 lamina creating a keyhole laminotomy.

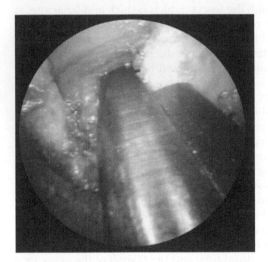

FIGURE 3 Kerrison rongeur biting the superior C6 lamina creating a keyhole laminotomy.

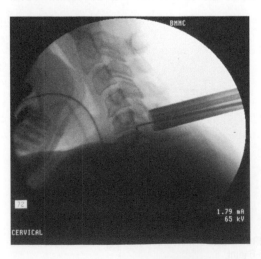

FIGURE 4 Lateral radiograph showing a nerve hook used the palpate the foramen.

TABLE 2 Techniques to Avoid Complications During Endoscopic Posterior Cervical Foraminotomy

Preoperative
  Assure there is no segmental instability at the operative level (flex-ext films)
  Assure there is no significant kyphotic deformity
  Do not perform bilateral radiculopathy
  Do not attempt to decompress a central herniation through this technique
  Avoid if axial neck pain is far greater than radicular symptoms
  Not indicated for myelopathy
Positioning
  Make sure operative level is adequately visualized on fluoroscopy
Intraoperative
  Incise fascia to avoid plunging with dilators
  Use fluoroscopy to make sure retractor is positioned properly over the facet

identify the direction and course of the exiting nerve (Fig. 4). A 3-mm high-speed drill is used to thin the bone over the nerve root. As the root exits between the laminae, the drilling must involve both the superior and inferior portions of the medial facet. The craniocaudal extent of drilling is from pedicle to pedicle. Drilling is performed from medial to lateral and care is taken not to remove more than 50% of the facet to avoid creating iatrogenic instability (5). Irrigation is used to avoid thermal injury to the nerve root. After drilling, the thin remaining cortical rim of bone over the nerve is removed with a curved curette or Kerrison rongeur (Figs. 5–7).

For most spondylotic uncovertebral spurs and smaller soft disc herniations, dorsal decompression of the nerve root is sufficient. With large soft disc herniations, removal of the disc fragments in addition to the bony decompression may be required.

After decompression, the wound is irrigated and closed in layers. A drain is usually not required. Injection of local anesthetic into the muscles and subcutaneous tissues can aid in immediate postoperative pain control. We place the patient in a soft cervical collar for comfort so that the patient is able to discontinue at their discretion.

COMPLICATIONS AND THEIR MANAGEMENT

Inability to appreciate depth and accidental hand movements can lead to durotomy early in the learning curve with this technique as the surgeon learns to work within more limited visual and spatial dimensions. Incidental durotomy with endoscopic posterior cervical foraminotomy has been reported to be 8% early in the learning curve (6,7). Khoo et al. (7) reported an 8% durotomy rate in their first 25 patients; however, after that study they went on to perform over 200 endoscopic foraminotomies with a durotomy rate less than 3%. Minor durotomies can

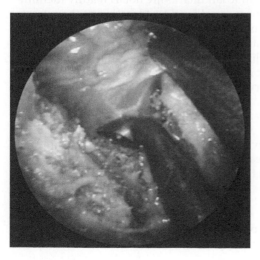

FIGURE 5 A 4-0 curette is used to remove the thinned bone overlying the root in the foramen.

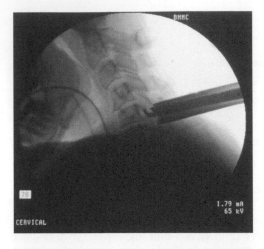

FIGURE 6   Lateral radiograph showing a Kerrison rongeur in the C5-6 foramen.

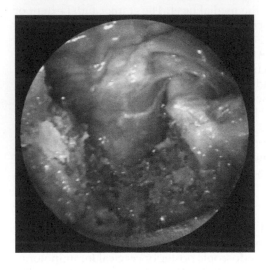

FIGURE 7   Endoscopic view of the keyhole foraminotomy.

usually be managed with gelfoam tamponade. Persistent symptomatic leaks can also be managed with a lumbar drain.

As surgical exposure is very limited and anatomic landmarks are not as readily identified as in open procedures, fluoroscopic confirmation of surgical level and location of the retractor is imperative. After positioning, fluoroscopy should be used to ensure that the appropriate surgical level is easily identified in lateral and anteroposterior projections prior to the sterile preparation and draping. Poor radiographic visualization during the case can lead to improper location of the tubular retractor. Medial placement can lead to durotomy or direct injury of the spinal cord while lateral placement can lead to nerve root injury or inadvertent disarticulation of the facet leading to iatrogenic instability.

Placement of the retractor usually involves percutaneous docking of a K-wire or Steinman pin on the facet followed by sequential dilation with a tubular retractor. The fascia in the posterior cervical spine is quite thick and if excessive force is used to drive the dilators through, inadvertent plunging may occur, which could lead to durotomy or neurologic injury. This complication is easily avoided by directly incising the thick cervical fascia.

OUTCOMES

Adamson and Khoo have both separately reported on their experience with over 125 endoscopic posterior foraminotomies (6,7). These procedures were performed in either a sitting or prone position with a muscle-splitting tubular retractor system and endoscopic visual guidance. Both studies reported less blood loss, shorter hospital stays, lower operative times, and decreased postoperative narcotic pain medicine requirements than in the open procedures. In Khoo's study, resolution of axial and radicular symptoms approached 90% for both the endoscopic and open procedures with no statistical difference noted between the two groups (7).

CONCLUSION

Interest in minimally invasive technologies is growing because of the desire to minimize surgical approach-related morbidity. The goals of minimally invasive surgery are to provide excellent surgical exposure while minimizing injury to soft tissues dissected in the approach. To be widely accepted, these techniques must prove to be safe, efficacious, and reproducible with an acceptable learning curve. They must also prove to decrease postoperative morbidity and allow quicker functional recovery. Early studies of endoscopic posterior cervical foraminotomies are promising in that they have shown equivalent clinical outcomes to open procedures with decreased hospital stays and decreased postoperative analgesic requirements.

REFERENCES

1. Kawaguchi Y, Matsui H, Tsuji H. Back muscle injury after posterior lumbar spine surgery. Part 2. Histologic and histochemical analyses in humans. Spine 1994; 19:2598–2602.
2. Frykholm R. Cervical nerve root compression resulting from disk degeneration and root sleeve fibrosis. Acta Chir Scand 1951; 160:1–149.
3. Henderson CM, Hennessy RG, Shuey HJ, et al. Posterior-lateral foraminotomy as an exclusiove operative technique for cervical radiculopathy: a review of 846 consecutively operated cases. Neurosurgery 1983; 13:504–521.
4. Simpson JM, Silveri CP, Simeone FA, et al. Cervical disk disease and the keyhole foraminotomy: proven efficacy at extended long-term follow up. Orthopedics 1997; 20:687–692.
5. Zdeblick TA, Zou D, Warden KE, et al. Cervical stability after foraminotomy. J Bone Joint Surg 1992; 74(A):22–27.
6. Adamson TE. Microendoscopic posterior cervical laminoforaminotomy for unilateral radiculopathy: results of a new technique in 100 cases. J Neurosurg 2001; 95 (suppl):51–57.
7. Khoo LT, Laich DT, Perez-Cruet MJ, et al. Posterior cervical microendoscopic foraminotomy. In: Perez-Cruet MJ, Fessler RG, eds. Outpatient Spinal Surgery. St. Louis: Quality Medical Publishing Inc., 2002:71–93.

9 Thoracoscopic Excision of Thoracic Herniated Disc

Roshan P. Shah and Jonathan N. Grauer
Department of Orthopedics and Rehabilitation, Yale University School of Medicine, New Haven, Connecticut, U.S.A.

INTRODUCTION

The incidence of clinically significant thoracic disc herniation is approximately one patient per million individuals, or 0.25% to 0.75% of all symptomatic disc herniations (1). The prevalence of thoracic disc herniation has been estimated to be between 11% and 15%, based on magnetic resonance imaging (MRI) and computed tomography (CT)-myelography studies (1). An estimated 80% of thoracic disc herniations occur between the third and fifth decades of life (2). Most herniations occur in the lower thoracic spine, with 26% to 50% of thoracic herniations occurring in the T11–T12 interspace (3).

The vast majority of thoracic disc herniations are managed nonoperatively. Most surgeons, therefore, have significantly less experience with thoracic discectomies than analogous procedures in the cervical and lumbar spine. Indications for surgery include thoracic myelopathy and debilitating pain in a radicular pattern resistant to nonoperative management.

Several surgical techniques have been described to perform a thoracic discectomy based on posterior or anterior approaches. There are certainly advantages and disadvantages to both; however, anterior procedures have been shown in a number of studies to yield a more reproducible decompression in a safe and efficient manner (2,4–6). The most limiting factor for this approach has been the morbidity associated with an open thoracotomy. This has led to the interest in thoracoscopic approaches to symptomatic thoracic disc herniations. Thoracic surgeons first began using video-assisted techniques for surgery in the thoracic cavity in the early 1990s. Spine surgeons adopted thoracoscopy shortly thereafter and have advanced the technology for applications to the thoracic spine (7). In 1993, Mack and Regan reported the use of thoracoscopy to treat symptomatic thoracic disc herniations (8). Advances in minimally invasive techniques and increased interest in these technologies have increased the popularity of thoracoscopic discectomy, particularly among recently trained surgeons.

INDICATIONS

Myelopathy is the most straightforward indication for thoracic discectomy. This may occur in the setting of cord compression secondary to disc herniation. Among this population, acute onset myelopathy is the most clear-cut diagnosis and is associated with the best chance of neurologic recovery following surgical intervention (9–11).

Radiculopathy is a relative indication for thoracic discectomy. This may occur when a disc herniation compresses and/or irritates a nerve root. Classically, thoracic radicular pain begins with axial pain that then radiates unilaterally or bilaterally around the chest wall in a dermatomal distribution. Other symptoms include dermatomal parasthesias or dysesthesias (3). These symptoms may occur with or without concurrent myelopathy. Most patients with radiculopathy will improve with nonsurgical management including nonsteroidal anti-inflammatories, rest followed by physical therapy, and possibly epidural and/or oral steroids, or a hyperextension brace (3). One retrospective review reported that 77% of patients treated conservatively returned to their prior level of functional activity (12). Failed conservative treatment of a thoracic disc herniation may be considered an indication for discectomy.

Axial back pain is the most controversial indication for thoracic discectomy and fusion. Clearly, nonoperative management of this population of patients is the mainstay of treatment.

If surgical intervention is considered, specialized studies have been advocated to correlate the disc pathology with pain. These include anesthetic blocks and discography (1,13). As mentioned before, there is a large prevalence of asymptomatic thoracic disc herniations seen by MRI studies; thus, it is challenging to differentiate the clinically significant thoracic disc herniations from the incidental ones.

If surgical intervention is determined appropriate, one must consider the numerous surgical techniques that have been described. Posterior approaches are appealing based on the familiar anatomy of the posterior dissection. However, these approaches afford limited access and visualization of the anterolateral thecal sac because of inability to manipulate the spinal cord. This might be appropriate for the more laterally based soft disc herniation, but becomes progressively less efficient for more central and calcified disc herniations. Certainly, a larger exposure can be achieved by removing more spinal anatomy; however, there are clear limitations due to the potential for postoperative instability if not coupled with fusion.

Alternatively, anterior approaches allow for optimal access and decompression of central and posterolateral thoracic disc herniations, calcified discs, large herniations, and broad-based discs that span the spinal canal (2). Although many will couple this with an anterior fusion, a recent study suggests that this may not be necessary (14). Unfortunately, these approaches are limited by the morbidity of an anterior thoracotomy.

The indications for thoracoscopic excision of thoracic disc herniations are essentially the same as for open thoracotomy with the difference touted to be reduced approach-related morbidity. Nonetheless, open thoracotomy remains the standard anterior approach and must be carefully weighed against thoracoscopic discectomy. To that end, open thoracotomy remains the preferred option for complex cases such as patients with multilevel lesions, foreseeable anatomic abnormalities, or ossification of the posterior longitudinal ligament. Additionally, adhesions from a previous thoracotomy, migrated disc fragments, hypercoagulability, inability to tolerate single-lung ventilation, or severe cardiac or pulmonary disease may be considered relative contraindications for thoracoscopy.

Thoracoscopy, however, is increasingly recommended for treatment of one- and two-level thoracic lesions at the hands of experienced and practiced surgeons (15). Thoracoscopy is associated with a reduced incidence of post-thoracotomy pain, intercostal neuralgia, pulmonary dysfunction, and scapular dysfunction, as well as shorter length of hospital stay, and fewer complications than thoracotomy (16–22). These advantages may be most noted for discectomies at the uppermost and lowest thoracic levels where open approaches are more challenging (17).

IMAGING

Plain radiographs provide information regarding the overall degenerative status and sagittal and coronal contour of the thoracic spine. They are, however, not helpful in defining compression of the neural elements. For this, MRI is the primary imaging modality, yielding information about disc herniations and surrounding structures of surgical significance such as vascular structures.

One of the very challenging aspects of thoracic imaging is confirming the level of interest on preoperative imaging and correlating with landmarks that can be assessed intraoperatively. In order to allow counting of levels, imaging should be correlated to findings from the upper cervical spine or lumbosacral junction. The importance of this cannot be overstated.

CT scans might be utilized to assess the extent of calcification of a disc herniation. CT-myelography can provide precise definition of the spinal cord and spinal nerves in relation to the bony anatomy. Further, this may be necessary in the patient who cannot have an MRI. MRI combined with CT-myelography provides the maximum preoperative diagnostic information available.

OPERATING ROOM SETUP AND EQUIPMENT

Thoracoscopic discectomy requires general anesthesia and endotracheal intubation with a double-lumen tube for selective ventilation of the contralateral lung. This is generally performed with fiberoptic guidance. The patient is then placed in a lateral decubitus position with the side of the pathology facing up. The patient may be secured with a beanbag or analogous patient-positioning device and an axillary roll is placed. The operating table is flexed to open the intercostal spaces on the side of interest.

The patient should be prepped for a thoracotomy to allow for intraoperative conversion to open thoracotomy if necessary. Neuromonitoring including somatosensory and motor-evoked are often used for this procedure.

The operating room can be set up in a variety of orientations, but these configurations generally allow the surgeons to stand anterior to the patient who is in the lateral position. The scrub assistant can stand at the patient's foot. This allows the video monitors to be easily viewed from their position behind the patient. Additional surgical assistants can stand opposite to the primary surgeon. This requires an additional monitor to be placed in direct view from this position.

Standard minimally invasive surgery equipment includes imaging and video equipment, lighting, and monitors. Traditional endoscopic kits are readily found in hospitals offering laparoscopic procedures. Endoscopes (5–10 mm in diameter) with 0°, 30°, and 45° angles should be used. Surgical drills are similar to those used in open procedures, but have a longer shaft of 8 to 10 inches. Either a diamond or cutting burr can be used. Kerrison rongeurs, straight and angled curettes, pituitary graspers, nerve hooks, and Penfield number 4 dissectors and possibly endoscopic Cobb elevators should be available (each with a long shaft to allow thoracoscopic use). Additional equipments include suction/irrigators, hemostatic tools/agents, bone wax, and cotton-tipped dissectors.

OPERATIVE APPROACH

As with any endoscopic procedure, the placement of portals is crucial to the success of this procedure. Typically, three or four portals are used after the ipsilateral lung is collapsed. These are placed in a triangular formation with the apex portal directly perpendicular to the target disc in the posterior axillary line (Fig. 1). Before placing the first port, a finger is inserted into the port site and swept circumferentially within the chest cavity to check for lung adhesions. After the apex portal is placed, a 30° rigid endoscope is inserted to visualize the placement of the two base ports. The base ports are placed on the anterior axillary line. A fourth optional port can be placed on either the anterior or the posterior axillary line. Soft, flexible ports should be used to reduce the likelihood of intercostal nerve injury.

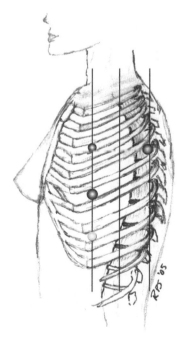

FIGURE 1 Portals are placed in a triangular formation with the apex perpendicular to the target disc level. An optional fourth portal is shown inferiorly on the anterior axillary line. Anterior-, mid-, and posterior-axillary lines are shown.

The spine is then visualized. Important anatomical relationships must be thoroughly understood. The surface contours of the spine provide important information to the surgeon. The middle of each thoracic vertebral body is slightly concave, whereas the disc spaces and end plates form a slightly convex surface. The segmental arteries and veins course over the middle of the vertebral bodies, in the concave contour. The pedicles connect the vertebral bodies with the remainder of the posterior arch. The neural foramen is formed by the boundaries of two adjacent pedicles and contains the exiting nerve roots. The neural foramen also contains foraminal ligaments, epidural fat, epidural venous plexus, and radiculomedullary veins and arteries.

The rib heads articulate with the transverse processes and the pedicles. The costotransverse and costovertebral ligaments are dense, thick, and inelastic. The rib heads above T11 articulate with the base of the pedicle and the vertebral body caudal to or at the level of the disc space. At the T11 and T12 levels, the rib heads articulate with the vertebral bodies caudal to the pedicle and the disc spaces, and thus the rib heads at these levels may be spared. The neurovascular bundle courses on the inferior surface of the ribs, with the vein most adjacent to the ribs, then artery and then nerve.

Upon visualization of the spine, the proper spinal levels should be confirmed relative to levels cited prior to portal placement. This process deserves significant attention with counting from known landmarks. This is generally best accomplished by placing a needle into the presumptive disc space and taking an anteroposterior radiograph. The surgeon should not rely solely on endoscopic rib counting because this is prone to error and the patient may have an anomalous number of ribs.

The deflated lung should be displaced out of the way as needed with endoscopic retractors. This can be facilitated by tilting the operating table anteriorly, allowing the lung to fall further away from the spinal column.

SURGICAL TECHNIQUE

The procedure begins with resection of the parietal pleura covering the medial 2 cm of the rib head and adjacent disc space. This is performed sharply or with electrocautery. The edge of the pleura is grasped and pulled away from the operative field with the aid of a pleural dissector.

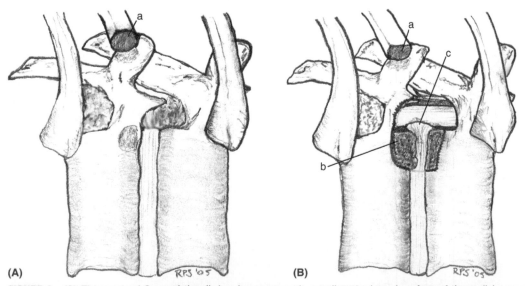

(A)   **(B)**

FIGURE 2   **(A)** The proximal 2 cm of the rib has been removed, revealing the lateral surface of the pedicle, neural foramen, and underlying disc. (a) Resected rib edge. **(B)** The pedicle has been resected and a cavity has been created in the proximal vertebral bodies, revealing the thecal sac and herniated disc. (a) Resected rib edge; (b) resected pedicle and cavity in the proximal vertebral bodies; (c) herniated disc.

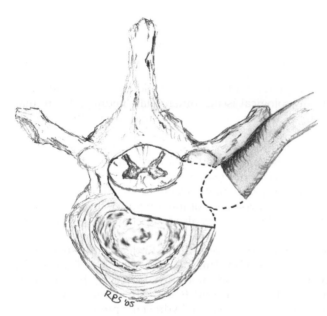

FIGURE 3 Axial view showing the cavity that is created in the vertebral body. The cavity exposes the ventral wall of the spinal canal and extends to the contralateral pedicle. The ventral wall of the spinal canal is cracked back into the space, allowing decompression of the spinal cord.

The segmental vessels located in the middle portion of the vertebral body usually do not have to be sacrificed. If necessary, however, they can be mobilized and divided. The neurovascular bundle coursing along the inferior costal surface should be preserved. Any bleeding can be controlled with a bipolar cauterization.

Once free of the neurovascular bundle, the medial 2 cm of the rib is removed using a burr to expose the lateral surface of the pedicle, neural foramen, and underlying disc (Fig. 2A). Alternatively, the rib can be removed as a single piece by cutting the rib and associated ligamentous attachments. This bone is saved for use as graft material, if needed.

The borders of the pedicle are then defined and the pedicle is resected with a Kerrison rongeur, which exposes the lateral aspect of the thecal sac. Following removal of the pedicle, an empty cavity is drilled in the dorsal disc space and adjacent vertebral bodies (Fig. 2B). This space is exploited when delivering the compressive disc material away from the epidural space. The cavity should be deep enough to expose the ventral dura of the spinal cord to the contralateral pedicle (Fig. 3). There is potential for injuring the exiting nerve root or spinal cord during this step, which can be minimized by maintaining the posterior vertebral wall/annular layers until this is complete. The depth of dissection can be verified by measurement or with fluoroscopy.

The wall is then cracked back into the defect created to relieve pressure on the neural elements. This can be accomplished with curettes or a Kerrison rongeur. Disc material can then be removed.

CLOSURE AND POSTOPERATIVE MANAGEMENT

The thoracic cavity should be irrigated with antibiotic solution and cleared of blood and debris. The thoracic cavity should be thoracoscopically examined for injury and bleeding. Hemostasis must be obtained. Once complete, a chest tube is placed in the posterior portal for drainage. The lung is then reinflated.

The instrument portals should be removed under visualization and the portal sites should be examined internally. Hemostasis of the portal sites can be achieved either internally or externally. Local anesthetic can be injected into the subcutaneous tissue adjacent to the portal incisions. The portal incisions are closed in anatomic layers.

Chest tubes should remain until their output is less than 100 mL/day. Chest radiograph should be obtained to confirm lung reinflation. Postoperative management includes aggressive pulmonary toilet and narcotics as needed for pain.

COMPLICATIONS

Thoracoscopy complication rates vary by series, but the types of complications are similar to those of open thoracotomy. The most serious complications include iatrogenic neurologic deficit, pulmonary embolus, and infection (23). Other types of complications include those related to anesthesia and patient positioning, pulmonary issues (pleuritic pain, pleural effusion, pneumothorax, atelectasis, pneumonia), neurological issues (intercostals neuralgia), vascular injuries (excessive blood loss, chylothorax), and other surgical complications (ileus, dural breach, and incomplete resection of disc fragment) (1,15).

Certainly for specific complications, thoracoscopy is associated with lower rates of problems than is thoracotomy. For example, Rosenthal and Dickman compared 55 patients receiving thoracoscopy with 18 receiving thoracotomy (24). Thoracoscopy resulted in lower rates of intercostal neuralgia (16% vs. 50%). This presumably related to less dissection around the ribs and can be further minimized by careful avoidance of intraoperative levering against the patient's ribs and use of soft plastic trocars. Thoracoscopy also resulted in a lower incidence of atelectasis (7% vs. 33%).

Other complications may be more common or more difficult to deal with when using thoracoscopy. An example of this is the injury to the dura. This may be corrected endoscopically or openly with sutures and/or sealed with fibrin glue and/or a patch. However, the chest tube must be carefully managed to prevent a cerebrospinal fluid (CSF) fistula from developing. In fact, a lumbar drain may be considered to reduce intraspinal hydrostatic pressure.

Certain conditions may increase the likelihood of conversion to open thoracotomy, including extensive lung adhesions, prior thoracic procedure with resultant scar formation, and severely distorted spinal anatomy. When such complications arise, conversion to open thoracotomy should be considered a safe surgical practice. As discussed, the patient should be prepped for possible conversion to thoracotomy and all instruments for thoracotomy should be available. Further, for such circumstances, a long sponge stick should be accessible in order to tampanade bleeding while the chest is opened should it be necessary.

OUTCOMES

Several cohort studies have evaluated thoracoscopic discectomy outcomes (1,15,22,24–27). In one long-term follow-up study, 73% (63/86) of patients had at least a 20% improvement in Oswestry score two years after thoracoscopic discectomy (1).

Good outcomes have been reported with thoracoscopic discectomy when treating patients with myelopathy. In one series, Anand and Regan reported at least a 20% improvement in Oswestry score for 100% (7/7) of patients after two years (1). Han et al. reported an improvement or resolution of myelopathy symptoms in 89% (39/44) and a stabilization of symptoms in 9% (4/44) (25). Symptoms worsened in 2% of the patients (1/44). Oskouian and Johnson reported an average improvement of two Frankel grades for 39% (18/46) of patients with myelopathy and unchanged symptoms in 59% (27/46) (15). Symptoms worsened in one patient (2%) who had had myelopathy for 30 years. Combining these data, 66% of patients with myelopathy improved after thoracoscopic discectomy.

Outcomes for treating radiculopathy symptoms have been similarly optimistic. Han et al. reported an improvement or resolution of symptoms in 84% (27/32) and unchanged symptoms in 16% (5/32) (25). Symptoms did not worsen in any patients. Oskouian and Johnson reported an average of 75% improvement in Oswestry score for patients with thoracic radicular pain (15). Further, all 21 patients experienced some improvement in radicular symptoms. Anand and Regan reported two-year outcomes on a patients with radiculopathy, either alone or with axial and leg pain (1). Of these patients, 72% (37/54) had at least a 20% improvement in Oswestry score. Combining these data, 79% of patients with radiculopathy improved after thoracoscopic discectomy.

Rosenthal and Dickman compared the results of thoracic discectomies performed with thoracoscopy as opposed to open thoracotomy (24). This study found decreased average operating time (205 min vs. 268 min), blood loss (327 mL vs. 683 mL), duration of chest tube usage (1.5 days vs. 3.5 days), narcotic pain medication usage (3.7 days vs. 20.4 days), and hospital stay (6.5 days vs. 16.2 days) in those patients treated with thoracoscopy. Similar results were reported by four other studies (15,22,25,26).

However, there are clearly limitations of thoracoscopy as compared with open techniques. Rosenthal and Dickman's study suggest a higher rate of incomplete resection of disc fragments reporting a 4% incidence of retained disc fragments in the thoracoscopy group compared with 0% in the thoracotomy group. In a later study, the authors reported that three of the 15 patients requiring reoperation secondary to retained disc fragments had undergone thoracoscopy. Only one had undergone open thoracotomy (27). With its better visualization and access, open thoracotomy can be expected to result in more complete disc resection than thoracoscopy. The possibility of incomplete resection must be weighed when deciding between operative approaches.

The learning curve in performing thoracoscopic discectomy is steep. Outcomes are generally less successful when thoracoscopic discectomy is performed by inexperienced surgeons. Several series report poorer outcomes for early cases as compared with later ones (1,15,26). It is important that surgeons train sufficiently and perform the technique frequently to maintain technical skills.

SUMMARY

Overall, thoracoscopic discectomy is a promising technique when compared with more traditional open thoracotomy techniques. This technically challenging procedure requires the correct instrumentation, set up, training, and experience. However, with the correct set up, encouraging outcomes have been reported.

General advancements in the field of minimally invasive technologies continue to change the surgical landscape. Although the incidence of surgically treated thoracic discs may be low, this technique does build off of related minimally invasive techniques that continue to gain a clinical foothold.

Brief Indications

- Myelopathy
- Radiculopathy
- Axial pain (severe, intractable).

Outcomes

- Improvement of myelopathy in 66% of patients.
- Improvement of radiculopathy in 79% of patients.
- Decreased operating time, blood loss, duration of chest tube use, narcotic use, and length of hospital stay as compared with thoracotomy.

Complications

- Pulmonary
  - pleuritic pain
  - pleural effusion
  - pneumothorax
  - atelectasis
  - pneumonia
- Neurological
  - intercostal neuralgia
  - ileus
- Vascular
  - excessive blood loss
  - chylothorax
- Surgical
  - dural breach
  - incomplete resection.

REFERENCES

1. Anand N, Regan JJ. Video-assisted thoracoscopic surgery for thoracic disc disease: classification and outcome study of 100 consecutive cases with a 2-year minimum follow-up period. Spine 2002; 27(8):871–879.
2. Vollmer DG, Simmons NE. Transthoracic approaches to thoracic disc herniations. Neurosurg Focus 2000; 9(4):Article 8, 1–6.
3. O'Connor RC, Andary MT, Russo RB, et al. Thoracic radiculopathy. Phys Med Rehabil Clin N Am 2002; 13(3):623–644.
4. Mulier S, Debois V. Thoracic disc herniations: transthoracic, lateral or posterolateral approach? A review. Surg Neurol 1998; 49(6):599–606.
5. Stillerman CB, Chen TC, Couldwell WT, et al. Experience in the surgical management of 82 symptomatic herniated thoracic discs and review of the literature. J Neurosurg 1998; 88:623–633.
6. Bohlman HH, Zdeblick TA. Anterior excision of herniated thoracic discs. J Bone Joint Surg (Am) 1988; 70(7):1038–1047.
7. Perez-Cruet MJ, Fessler RG, Perin NI. Review: complications of minimally invasive spinal surgery. Neurosurgery 2002; 51(suppl 2):26–36.
8. Mack MJ, Regan JJ, Bobechko WP, et al. Application of thoracoscopy for diseases of the spine. Ann Thorac Surg 1993; 56:736–738.
9. Yonenobu K. Cervical radiculopathy and myelopathy: when and what can surgery contribute to treatment? Eur Spine J 2000; 9:1–7.
10. Fujiwara K, Yonenobu K, Ebara S, et al. The prognosis of surgery for cervical compression myelopathy: an analysis of the factors involved. J Bone Joint Surg Br 1989; 71:393–398.
11. Koyanagi T, Hirabayashi K, Satomi K, et al. Predictability of operative results of cervical compression myelopathy based on preoperative computed tomographic myelography. Spine 1983; 14: 1958–1963.
12. Brown CW, Deffer PA Jr, Akmakjian J, et al. The natural history of thoracic disc herniation. Spine 1992; 17(suppl 6):S97–S102.
13. Johnson JP, Rogers CD. Thoracoscopic discectomy. In: Kim DH, Fessler RG, Regan JJ, eds. Endoscopic Spine Surgery and Instrumentation. New York: Thieme, 2005:111–124.
14. Krauss WE, Edwards DA, Cohen-Gadol AA. Transthoracic discectomy without interbody fusion. Surg Neurol 2005; 63(5):403–409.
15. Oskouian RJ, Johnson JP. Endoscopic thoracic microdiscectomy. Neurosurg Focus 2005; 18(3):E11, 1–8.
16. Rosenthal D, Dickman CA. Thoracoscopic microsurgical excision of herniated thoracic discs. Neurosurg Focus 1999; 6(5):4.
17. Huntington CF, Murrell WD, Betz RR, et al. Comparison of thoracoscopic and open thoracic discectomy in a live ovine model for anterior spinal fusion. Spine 1998; 23(15):1699–1702.
18. Dickman CA, Mican CA. Multilevel anterior thoracic discectomies and anterior interbody fusion using a microsurgical thoracoscopic approach: case report. J Neurosurg 1996; 84:104–109.
19. Horowitz MB, Moossy JJ, Julian T, et al. Thoracic discectomy using video assisted thoracoscopy. Spine 1994; 19:1082–1086.
20. Rosenthal D, Rosenthal R, de Simone A. Removal of a protruded thoracic disc using microsurgical endoscopy. Spine 1994; 19:1087–1091.
21. Landreneau RJ, Hazelrigg SR, Mack MJ, et al. Postoperative pain-related morbidity: video-assisted thoracic surgery versus thoracotomy. Ann Thorac Surg 1993; 56:1285–1289.
22. Regan JJ, Mack MJ, Picetti GD III, et al. A comparison of video-assisted thoracoscopic surgery (VATS) with open thoracotomy in thoracic spinal surgery. Today Ther Trends 1994; 11:203–218.
23. Fessler RG, Sturgill M. Review: complications of surgery for thoracic disc disease. Surg Neurol 1998; 49(6):609–618.
24. Rosenthal D, Dickman CA. Thoracoscopic microsurgical excision of herniated thoracic disc. J Neurosurg 1998; 89:224–235.
25. Han PP, Kenny K, Dickman CA. Thoracoscopic approaches to the thoracic spine: experience with 241 surgical procedures. Neurosurgery 2002; 51(suppl 2):88–95.
26. Johnson JP, Filler AG, McBride DQ. Endoscopic thoracic discectomy. Neurosurg Focus 2000; 9(4): Article 11, 1–8.
27. Dickman CA, Rosenthal D, Regan JJ. Reoperation for herniated thoracic discs. J Neurosurg 1999; 91:157–162.

10 | Thoracoscopic Corpectomy

Lance K. Mitsunaga and Choll W. Kim
Department of Orthopedic Surgery, University of California, and the San Diego VA Medical Center, San Diego, California, U.S.A.

INTRODUCTION

The anterior approach to the thoracic and thoracolumbar spine is a well-established procedure for spinal cord decompression, vertebral body reconstruction, and stabilization via internal fixation for the treatment of trauma, tumor, infection, spondylosis, or deformity. However, traditional anterior approaches to the thoracic and thoracolumbar spine require open thoracotomies or thoracoabdominal approaches that are associated with significant morbidity and extended postoperative rehabilitation. The advancement of video-assisted thoracoscopic surgery (VATS) and its application to disorders of the spine have provided an alternative, minimally invasive approach for many procedures requiring access to the thoracic or thoracolumbar spine. Thoracoscopic surgery has been successfully used to perform discectomy for herniation, anterior release for spinal deformity, fusion, drainage of intervertebral disc space abscesses, and corpectomy (1,2). This chapter addresses key issues relevant to performing a thoracoscopic corpectomy for the treatment of fractures, tumors, and infections. Thoracoscopic spinal instrumentation is discussed in Chapter 21.

ADVANTAGES OF THORACOSCOPY VS. THORACOTOMY FOR CORPECTOMY

There are several advantages of thoracoscopic corpectomy compared with conventional procedures that require open thoracotomy. When compared with open thoracotomy procedures, thoracoscopic approaches are associated with lower incidences of post-thoracotomy pain syndrome, pulmonary impairment, and shoulder dysfunction (3–6). Furthermore, patients who undergo thoracoscopic procedures experience reduced postoperative pain, shorter recovery times, less incisional pain, better cosmetic outcomes, and earlier mobilization compared with patients treated with open procedures (3–8). In addition, thoracoscopic procedures require less pain medication, shorter hospital stays, and reduced operative times compared with open procedures, once the surgeon has gained experience and attained expertise in the thoracoscopic approach (2,9,10). Thoracoscopy affords complete direct visualization and exposure of the anterior aspects of the spine and spinal cord (7,9,11,12). Improved visualization of the anterior surface of the dura during thoracoscopic corpectomy is a potential advantage compared with open thoracotomy. Visual access to and magnification of the targeted spine segment is superior via the thoracoscopic approach (12,13). Also, surgical assistants are better able to visualize the operative field and, thus, can provide more effective assistance to the primary surgeon (13).

Thoracoscopy permits visual access to and exposure of the spine from the T4-T5 disc space to the T12–L1 disc space. In addition, a thoracoscopic transdiaphragmatic approach to the thoracolumbar junction has been demonstrated to allow access to the entire thoracolumbar junction down to L3 (11,12,14).

DISADVANTAGES OF THORACOSCOPY VS. THORACOTOMY FOR CORPECTOMY

While thoracoscopic approaches may prove effective for resection of vertebral body tumors, intradural tumors require open posterior or posterolateral procedures because closure of the dura is extremely difficult via thoracoscopy (15). More importantly, the main disadvantage of thoracoscopic surgery is the fact that there is a substantial learning curve associated with this procedure, such that initial attempts at thoracoscopic procedures may result in more intraoperative complications, longer operative times, and higher morbidity rates than expected

(1,3,5,12,16,17). Significant time, experience, and commitment is required for a surgeon to become acclimated in performing thoracoscopic surgery without the benefit of direct, binocular, three-dimensional visualization or the tactile stimuli available in traditional open approaches. Surgeons need extensive training in didactic sessions, surgical laboratories, workshops, and clinical settings to acquire the knowledge, psychomotor skills, and technical expertise necessary to perform thoracoscopic surgery of the spine. It may be difficult for surgeons to adapt to the modifications made to surgical instruments designed for thoracoscopic procedures. For example, the longer arms needed for thoracoscopic instruments can be difficult to control. Many surgical techniques, such as distraction, are especially difficult via the thoracoscopic approach. In addition, thoracoscopic surgery has been associated with higher costs compared with open thoracotomy procedures (16). The cost of specialized technology, equipment, and instrumentation required for thoracoscopy thus represents another obstacle to the implementation of thoracoscopic procedures.

INDICATIONS AND CONTRAINDICATIONS FOR THORACOSCOPIC CORPECTOMY

Thoracoscopic corpectomy for neural decompression and spinal reconstruction is indicated in cases of trauma or other pathology from T5 to L2. Thoracoscopic corpectomy can be performed to treat vertebral lesions, vertebral osteomyelitis, unstable pathologic and traumatic fractures, kyphotic deformity, ankylosing spondylitis, infections, epidural abscesses, and herniated thoracic discs (5,9,13,18–21).

Because thoracoscopic corpectomy, as with any transthoracic procedure, requires collapse of the ipsilateral lung and single-lung ventilation of the contralateral lung, thoracoscopic corpectomy is contraindicated in patients who are unable to withstand one-lung ventilation or continuous high airway pressures with positive pressure ventilation (22–24). Relative contraindications include emphysema, previous chest tube placement, previous thoracotomy, hemostatic disorders, and concurrent anticoagulant therapy (22–24).

Patients should be informed of the possibility that conversion to an open thoracotomy procedure may be required, along with the risks involved with both general and thoracoscopic surgery, such as injury to viscera or major blood vessels, nerve damage, sympathectomy syndromes, loss of blood, instrumentation failure, pneumothorax, pseudoarthrosis, malunion, infection, pulmonary complications, diaphragmatic herniation, and paralysis (4,11,12,14,20,25,26).

ANESTHESIA

Thoracoscopic corpectomies are performed under general endotracheal anesthesia. Insufflation of carbon dioxide into the thorax is not necessary because sufficient visualization and exposure of the affected spine region and adequate surgical space is afforded by the fixed environment enclosed by the thoracic cavity and collapse and retraction of the ipsilateral lung. A double-lumen endotracheal one-lung ventilation is utilized. Placement of the double-lumen endotracheal tube can be guided by bronchoscopic visualization.

EQUIPMENT AND INSTRUMENTATION REQUIREMENTS

Thoracoscopic corpectomy procedures require surgical equipment specially designed for video-assisted thoracic surgery. Modifications to standard instruments for use in thoracoscopic surgery may include increased lengths, angled tips to provide for an unobstructed view of the instrument tip intraoperatively, and shafts that are calibrated with depth indexes so that instrument depth can be assessed. In addition, successful thoracoscopic corpectomy requires a harmonic scalpel, endoscopic fan retractors, and a combined suction-irrigation apparatus (Fig. 1).

PATIENT POSITIONING AND OPERATING ROOM SETUP

The patient should be positioned in a lateral decubitus position on a radiolucent table with the operative, affected half of the patient's body on top and the patient's back perpendicular to the floor. If trauma or pathology does not suggest a left- or right-sided approach, then a right-sided

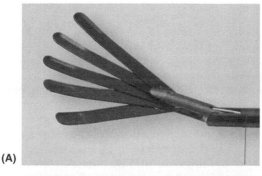

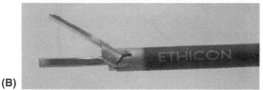

(A)

(B)

FIGURE 1 Special equipment. (**A**) Articulating fan retractor. Fan closes to allow passage through the ports. It is used to retract the lung and diaphragm. (**B**) Curved-tip grasping harmonic scalpel used for pleural incision, coagulation of segmental vessels, and subperiosteal dissection of the vertebral body.

approach is preferred for access to spinal segments T5–T8 because the left hemithoracic region in this area is often obscured by the heart and aorta. For access to the thoracolumbar junction from T9 to L2, on the other hand, a left-sided approach is recommended. A left-sided approach for thoracoscopic procedures of the thoracolumbar spine aids caudal displacement and retraction of the diaphragm, which is lower on the left, due to the presence of the liver below the right diaphragm.

The patient is secured with supports at the sacrum, pubic symphysis, and scapula. The patient's top arm is placed at 90° with respect to the coronal plane of the patient's body by resting it on an arm rest in order to prevent its interference with the operative area (Fig. 2). Confirm proper positioning, free tilt, and arc of the C-arm. The patient should then be draped anteriorly from the sternum, posteriorly from below the spinous processes, rostrally from the axilla, and inferiorly from 8 cm below the iliac crest (11,12,27).

With the patient properly positioned and draped, the surgeon and the surgical assistant operating the camera should be located posterior to the patient. The C-arm head is also positioned posterior to the patient, between the surgeon and the assistant operating the camera. Another surgical assistant and a video monitor are located anterior to the patient. This allows visual access for both the primary surgeon and the assistants. The table is adjusted so that the patient is in the true lateral position. This provides an additional degree of orientation by allowing the surgeon to use three-dimensional spatial cues to align instruments.

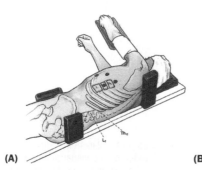
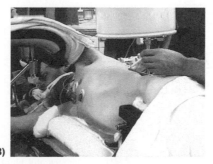

(A)   (B)

FIGURE 2 Illustration and photograph of patient in the lateral decubitus position. A right-sided approach is recommended for the upper thoracic spine and a left-sided approach for the thoracolumbar junction. *Source*: From Ref. 12.

PORTAL PLACEMENT

A true lateral projection of the fractured or pathologic vertebra is visualized with an X-ray image amplifier. The anterior–posterior and end-plate borders of the injured or pathologic vertebra are drawn on the patient's skin with a marking pen (Fig. 2). The first adjacent, healthy vertebrae superior and inferior to the injured spinal segment should also be projected and indicated on the skin with a marking pen. At this point, localization of the 10-mm working port is possible. Its position should be drawn directly over the target vertebra (Fig. 3). Placement of the 10-mm scope portal for insertion of the endoscope depends on which segment of the spine is targeted. Scope ports should be marked two or three intercostal spaces above the working port for thoracoscopic corpectomies performed on T9–L2, or two or three intercostal spaces *below* the working port for fractures or pathology of the upper or middle thoracic spine. The 5-mm port for suction and rinsing should be marked 5 to 10 cm anterior and rostral to the working port, while the 10-mm port for diaphragm or lung retraction should be marked as anterior to the working port as possible. Figure 3 illustrates the recommended portal configuration to perform a thoracoscopic corpectomy of the thoracolumbar spine.

Caution should be taken to avoid misplacement of the suction/rinsing port too far from the working port, which would not allow for suction and irrigation of the entire operative region (14). Also, the fan retractor port should be positioned as anterior as possible to ensure that the retractor does not interfere with the surgical area (14). Once the port positions have been indicated with a marking pen, the patient should be prepped, disinfected, and draped in a fashion that would allow for conversion to an open procedure, if necessary. All scope portals are preinjected with bupivacaine and dilute epinephrine.

The first portal to be placed should be the portal positioned most rostrally, which helps minimize the risk of injury to the lungs, diaphragm, and spleen by allowing the remaining portals to be placed under thoracoscopic guidance. A skin incision of 1.5-cm long is made overlying the intercostal space. The muscles of the chest wall can be dissected in a zigzag direction according to the orientation of the muscle fibers and a blunt dissection technique opens up the intercostal space. Once ventilation to the ipsilateral lung is stopped it can collapse, and the pleura can be opened by performing a blunt puncture under direct visualization. Direct visualization allows the surgeon to verify the presence of an entrance to the thoracic cavity unobstructed by lung or pleural adhesions, allowing for insertion of a 10-mm trocar. If necessary, finger dissection can be used to release the lung from the chest wall. The endoscope angled at 30°, previously prepared with an antifog solution, should be inserted into the first port and directed toward the next trocar to be introduced. Under endoscopic visual guidance, compression of the patient's skin with the surgeon's finger allows the insertion site for the other trocars to be visualized within the thorax. The remaining trocars and instruments can be introduced once blunt dissection of the thoracic wall muscles is performed.

Once all the trocars and instruments have been placed, rotate the endoscope such that a standard surgical orientation is displayed on the video monitor, in which the spine is parallel to the bottom of the video monitor, and the rostral–caudal orientation of the spine on the video

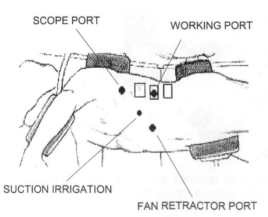

SCOPE PORT

WORKING PORT

SUCTION IRRIGATION

FAN RETRACTOR PORT

FIGURE 3   Recommended portal placement. The cephalad port is made first under direct visualization using careful blunt dissection. The remaining ports are made under direct visualization with the thoracoscope. Portals can be individualized to patient and disease as necessary. *Source*: From Ref. 27.

monitor corresponds to that of the patient from the point of view of the surgeon. The standard surgical orientation, combined with a true lateral position of the patient in relation to the floor, facilitates the surgeon's ability to orient his actual hand movements to those displayed on the video screen.

SPINAL EXPOSURE OF THE THORACOLUMBAR JUNCTION (T11–L2)

Open anterior approaches to the thoracolumbar spine below the T12–L1 intervertebral disc space are complicated by the presence of the diaphragm. A thoracoscopic transdiaphragmatic approach to the thoracolumbar junction has been described in detail in several reports (11,12,14). This technique obviates the need for complete detachment of the diaphragmatic insertion, as required in open procedures. The most caudal diaphragmatic attachment to the spine, found at the costadiaphragmatic recess, inserts perpendicularly onto the spine just above the L2 body. The L2 body can be exposed by creating a limited 5- to 6-cm opening in the diaphragm at this attachment site. An ultrasonic knife is used to make a semicircular incision that courses along the spine and ribs. Using blunt dissection and a fan retractor, this technique provides exposure to L2 and occasionally L3. If necessary, the psoas muscle can be detached in a subperiosteal fashion to expose the vertebral body. The incision should run parallel to and 1 to 2 cm away from the diaphragmatic insertion. This remaining diaphragmatic strip is used to close the diaphragm.

CORPECTOMY AND DECOMPRESSION

Under both fluoroscopic and thoracoscopic visualization, the intervertebral discs of the injured spine segment can be seen. The disc spaces adjacent to the affected vertebra are marked with an ultrasonic scalpel to indicate the boundaries of the corpectomy. The pleura is incised longitudinally and the segmental vessels are exposed using the harmonic scalpel with a grasping tip. This step requires significant care as brisk bleeding may occur. Once the segmental vessels are exposed, the harmonic scalpel is used to coagulate the vessels by using a gentle brushing technique longitudinally along the vessels. If bleeding is encountered, tamponading with long, endoscopic sponges allows continued coagulation until bleeding is controlled.

The rib heads overlying the disc spaces are exposed (Fig. 4A). These rib heads are excised to gain access to the posterior aspect of the disc and the entire neuroforamen. Fluoroscopic guidance with the image at the cross-table position provides an anteroposterior view of the spine. In this view, osteotomes and elevators can be used to separate the disc from the endplate completely to the contralateral side. Long pituitary rongeurs, curettes, and endplate scrapers are then used to complete the discectomies.

The vertebral body is then exposed in a subperiosteal fashion. This dissection is carried out posteriorly to the neuroforamen. A long probe is used to identify the posterior vertebral body wall through the neuroforamen. An osteotome that is equipped with modifications for a

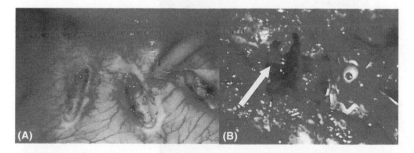

FIGURE 4 Thoracoscopic view. (**A**) Initial view from endoscope. Harmonic scalpel is used to identify and mark the rib heads of the levels of interest. The spine runs longitudinally along the top of the figure. Lateral fluoroscopic image aids in identifying the correct levels. The instrument shown is a combined suction-irrigation system. (**B**) View after corpectomy. *Arrow* shows exposed dural tube after decompression. A titanium mesh cage containing bone graft is also shown at right. See Figure 5 for corresponding imaging studies.

thoracoscopic approach, such as calibrations on the arm of the instrument indicating instrument depth, is used to fragment the bone. Cross-table fluoroscopic imaging may be used during this step. The thoracoscopic corpectomy procedure then proceeds similar to the traditional open approach. Rongeurs are used to resect fragmented segments of the vertebral body and high-speed drills are used to resect bone in the spinal canal region. High-speed drilling should be employed as little as possible because the long shafts of the specialized drills employed in the thoracoscopic approach can be difficult to control.

Having created a large corpectomy cavity in the vertebral body, the remaining rim of the posterior cortex can be resected to complete decompression of the spinal canal. A long probe is used to localize the neuroforamen and inferior edge of the pedicle. A flat, blunt probe, such as a long Penfield 4 elevator, is then used to free the dural tube from the posterior longitudinal ligament by way of the neuroforamen. The thickness of the remaining posterior wall can be assessed. If necessary, the bone can be thinned with curettes or a high-speed drill. Curettes, pituitary rongeurs, and Kerrison rongeurs are used to resect the posterior vertebral body wall and posterior longitudinal ligament. The blunt elevator is used to ensure that the dural tube is not adherent to the tissue to be resected. The corpectomy cavity can now be prepared to receive a bone graft or cage for spinal reconstruction (Fig. 4B).

VERTEBRAL RECONSTRUCTION

The structural graft or cage can be wrapped in an antifriction plastic bag to avoid injury to the surrounding tissue during transport through the thoracic cavity. The working portal is now removed to allow the graft to be placed into the defect. The corpectomy defect can be opened to accept the graft by imparting an antikyphotic moment on the spine. This is most readily accomplished by gently applying posterior pressure manually to the patient's back or by utilizing distractible cages. Alternatively, an anterior plating system can be used to distract the corpectomy site (described in Chapter 21). Final reconstruction can be performed with an anterior plate or posterior instrumentation (Fig. 5).

POSTOPERATIVE MANAGEMENT

Extubation of the patient can often follow immediately after the surgical procedure. However, elderly patients and patients with respiratory or cardiovascular conditions may require

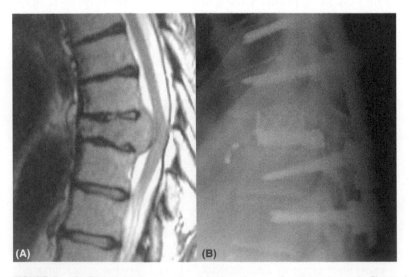

FIGURE 5 (**A**) T2-weighted magnetic resonance image of patient shown in Figure 4. T9 pathologic fracture as a result of multiple myeloma. (**B**) Postoperative radiograph after anterior corpectomy and strut fusion with a titanium mesh cage.

mechanical ventilation for 24 to 28 hours. Anterior–posterior and lateral chest X rays are obtained. X rays should be used to verify normal lung expansion. The chest tube should not be removed until air leakage ceases or until drainage is less than 150 mL per 24 hours (28). Chest tubes can usually be safely removed at one day postsurgery.

The standard postoperative schedule usually involves respiratory exercises on the first postoperative day. Physical therapy is started on the first or second postoperative day. The patient may return back to work at 12 to 16 weeks postsurgery (11,27). X rays should be obtained two days, six weeks, three months, six months, and one year postoperatively. Patients are transitioned to oral medications in preparation for discharge. The need for bracing is similar to open surgeries.

COMPLICATIONS

The potential complications associated with the thoracoscopic corpectomy procedure are similar to those that can also occur with open anterior thoracotomy, although the rate of incidence for each complication may vary between thoracoscopic and open approaches. For thoracoscopic surgery, heightened vigilance is needed against laceration of the lungs with the fan retractor. If lung puncture does occur, endoscopic lung staples can be used to close the leak. Injury to the liver or spleen (secondary to diaphragmatic puncture) can potentially occur during portal insertion. However, these complications can be avoided by placing all portals under direct visualization outside the thoracic cavity and, except for the first portal, under thoracoscopic guidance inside the thoracic cavity. The risk of diaphragmatic injury can be minimized by placing the first portal at the sixth or seventh intercostal space, while injury to the subclavian artery and vein is best avoided by refraining from placing portals in the first or second intercostal space (20,23,29,30).

The risk of intercostal neuralgia in thoracoscopic spine surgery is reported to be relatively low. In one prospective study assessing complications in 78 patients who underwent various thoracoscopic spine procedures, intercostal neuralgia was experienced by six patients (7.7%) (20). This complication was transient in all cases, resolving within six weeks postoperatively. In another series of 371 patients treated thoracoscopically for thoracic and thoracolumbar fractures, only 5.4% of the patients experienced any complication related to endoscopic access, including intercostal neuralgia (12,14). The risk of intercostal neuralgia can be minimized by using thoracic trocars that are flexible and as small as possible (not larger than 12 mm) (20,23,26,29–31). In addition, risk of intercostal neuralgia can be minimized by using 1% marcaine with epinephrine to perform a local block of the intercostal nerve, and by ensuring that ports are inserted near the surface of the superior rib to prevent injury to the neurovascular bundle (29). Although intercostal neuralgia as a result of thoracoscopic spine surgery is usually transient, if this complication persists, intercostal nerve block (with agents such as carbamezapine) and radiofrequency rhizotomy have been shown to be effective treatments (31,32).

Neurologic injury to the spinal cord or nerve roots is commonly because of poor identification of the dura during decompression. Thus, it is important to identify the neuroforamen and the base of the pedicle prior to removing any material impinging on the spinal cord. Neurophysiologic monitoring is used in nearly all cases

OUTCOMES

A large study by Beisse et al. reported their experience with a thoracoscopic procedure to treat thoracic and thoracolumbar fractures from T3 to L3 (12,14). Three hundred and seventy-one patients underwent thoracoscopic surgery involving anterior reconstruction using iliac crest grafts or titanium cages with anterior instrumentation. Sixty-five percent of the patients had injuries requiring posterior internal fixation before anterior thoracoscopic surgery, while 35% of the patients underwent only the anterior thoracoscopic procedure. With surgical experience and improvements in endoscopic instrumentation, mean operative times were reduced from about six hours in the initial cases to approximately 2.5 to 3 hours for cases later in the series of 371 patients. Blood loss averaged 650 mL for the 150 patients undergoing monosegmental corpectomy later in the series. The Z-plate, an anterior internal fixation system not specifically designed for thoracoscopic use, was employed in the first 197 patients. This fixation system was associated with a one-year fusion rate of 86%, five cases of partial implant loosening, and one complication. The MACS-TL implant, specially designed for endoscopic placement, was later introduced and employed in 150 patients. This fixation system was associated with a one-year fusion rate of 91%. Two cases of partial implant loosening were reported with the MACS-TL system, but these complications were likely because of osteoporotic bone and not implant failure.

Of the 371 patients included in this study, conversion to an open procedure was required in four patients, occurring at a rate of 1.2%. However, two of these patients requiring open conversion were among the first five patients treated. Complications related to endoscopic access, including intercostal neuralgia, pleural effusion, and pneumothorax were observed at a rate of 5.4%. Complications not related to endoscopic access were seen in 4.3% of patients. One incident was reported for each of the following complications: transient compressive neuropraxia, splenic injury, and Frankel grade worsening from D to B. In addition, one deep wound infection, five superficial wound infections, and one diaphragmatic splitting-related complication (transient L1 sensory deficit) were observed.

Dickman et al. (9) compared the clinical outcomes of 17 patients who underwent thoracoscopic corpectomy with those of the seven patients who underwent thoracotomy for corpectomy. There were no observed differences between the two cohorts of patients in terms of the degree of decompression, vertebral reconstruction, or stabilization with instrumentation that was performed. Nor were there any demonstrated differences in mean operative times between patients who underwent thoracoscopy versus thoracotomy for corpectomy. However, in the group treated thoracoscopically, blood loss, chest tube drainage, duration of administration of analgesics, and length of intensive care unit and hospital stays were reduced compared with patients undergoing the open procedure.

SUMMARY

Thoracoscopic corpectomy is a safe and effective procedure to treat injury or pathology affecting T5–L2, including metastic disease of the spine, vertebral osteomyelitis, and vertebral body fracture (33–38). The major challenge presented by the thoracosopic corpectomy procedure is the significant learning curve and technical demands associated with this surgery. Promising outcomes have been reported for the thoracoscopic corpectomy procedure by several groups. This operation is associated with decreased blood loss, less postoperative pain, and shorter hospital stays than conventional open approaches. Thoracoscopic procedures provide an alternative, minimally invasive approach to the thoracic and thoracolumbar spine.

REFERENCES

1. Regan JJ, Mack MJ, Picetti GD 3rd. A technical report on video-assisted thoracoscopy in thoracic spinal surgery: preliminary description. Spine 1995; 20(7):831–837.
2. Mack MJ, Regan JJ, McAfee PC, et al. Video-assisted thoracic surgery for the anterior approach to the thoracic spine. Ann Thorac Surg 1995; 59(5):1100–1106.
3. Visocchi M, Masferrer R, Sonntag VK, et al. Thoracoscopic approaches to the thoracic spine. Acta Neurochir (Wien) 1998; 140(8):737–743; discussion 743–744.
4. Kaiser D, Ennker IC, Hartz C. Video-assisted thoracoscopic surgery – indications, results, complications, and contraindications. Thorac Cardiovasc Surg 1993; 41(6):330–334.
5. Han PP, Kenny K, Dickman CA. Thoracoscopic approaches to the thoracic spine: experience with 241 surgical procedures. Neurosurgery 2002; 51(5 suppl):S88–S95.
6. Landreneau RJ, Hazelrigg SR, Mack MJ, et al. Postoperative pain-related morbidity: video-assisted thoracic surgery versus thoracotomy. Ann Thorac Surg 1993; 56(6):1285–1289.
7. Dickman CA, Karahalios DG. Thoracoscopic spinal surgery. Clin Neurosurg 1996; 43:392–422.
8. Burgos J, Rapariz JM, Gonzalez-Herranz P. Anterior endoscopic approach to the thoracolumbar spine. Spine 1998; 23(22):2427–2431.
9. Dickman CA, Rosenthal D, Karahalios DG, et al. Thoracic vertebrectomy and reconstruction using a microsurgical thoracoscopic approach. Neurosurgery 1996; 38(2):279–293.
10. Ferson PF, Landreneau RJ, Dowling RD, et al. Comparison of open versus thoracoscopic lung biopsy for diffuse infiltrative pulmonary disease. J Thorac Cardiovasc Surg 1993; 106(2):194–199.

11. Kim DH, Jahng TA, Balabhadra RS, et al. Thoracoscopic transdiaphragmatic approach to thoracolumbar junction fractures. Spine J 2004; 4(3):317–328.

12. Khoo LT, Beisse R, Potulski M. Thoracoscopic-assisted treatment of thoracic and lumbar fractures: a series of 371 consecutive cases. Neurosurgery 2002; 51(5 suppl):S104–S117.

13. McAfee PC, Regan JR, Fedder IL, et al. Anterior thoracic corpectomy for spinal cord decompression performed endoscopically. Surg Laparosc Endosc 1995; 5(5):339–348.

14. Beisse R, Potulski M, Buhren V. Endoscopic techniques for the management of spinal trauma. Eur J Trauma 2001; 27:275–291.

15. Dickman CA, Apfelbaum RI. Thoracoscopic microsurgical excision of a thoracic schwannoma: case report. J Neurosurg 1998; 88(5):898–902.

16. Newton PO, Wenger DR, Mubarak SJ, et al. Anterior release and fusion in pediatric spinal deformity: a comparison of early outcome and cost of thoracoscopic and open thoracotomy approaches. Spine 1997; 22(12):1398–1406.

17. Cunningham BW, Kotani Y, McNulty PS, et al. Video-assisted thoracoscopic surgery versus open thoracotomy for anterior thoracic spinal fusion: a comparative radiographic, biomechanical, and histologic analysis in a sheep model. Spine 1998; 23(12):1333–1340.

18. Huang TJ, Hsu RW, Liu HP, et al. Video-assisted thoracoscopic treatment of spinal lesions in the thoracolumbar junction. Surg Endosc 1997; 11(12):1189–1193.

19. Rosenthal D, Marquardt G, Lorenz R, et al. Anterior decompression and stabilization using a microsurgical endoscopic technique for metastatic tumors of the thoracic spine. J Neurosurg 1996; 84(4):565–572.

20. McAfee PC, Regan JR, Zdeblick T, et al. The incidence of complications in endoscopic anterior thoracolumbar spinal reconstructive surgery: a prospective multicenter study comprising the first 100 consecutive cases. Spine 1995; 20(14):1624–1632.

21. Dickman CA, Rosenthal DJ. Thoracoscopic corpectomy. In: Dickman CA, Rosenthal DJ, Perin NI, eds. Thoracoscopic Spine Surgery. New York: Thieme Medical Publishers, Inc., 1999: 271–291.

22. Dieter RA Jr, Kuzycz GB. Complications and contraindications of thoracoscopy. IntSurg 1997; 82(3):232–239.

23. Goldstein JA, McAfee PC. Minimally invasive endoscopic approach to the spine. In: Cueto-Garcia J, Jacobs M, Gagner M, eds. Laparoscopic Surgery. New York: McGraw-Hill, 2003:609–614.

24. Regan JJ. Endoscopic spinal surgery: anterior approaches. In: Frymoyer JW, ed. The Adult Spine: Principles and Practice. Vol. 2. 2nd ed. Philadelphia: Lippincott-Raven Publishers, 1997:1665–1684.

25. Huang TJ, Hsu RW, Sum CW, et al. Complications in thoracoscopic spinal surgery: a study of 90 consecutive patients. Surg Endosc 1999; 13(4):346–350.

26. Perez-Cruet MJ, Fessler RG, Perin NI. Review: complications of minimally invasive spinal surgery. Neurosurgery 2002; 51(5 suppl):S26–S36.

27. Balabhadra RS, Kim DH, Potulski M, et al. Thoracoscopic decompression and fixation (MACS-TL). In: Kim DH, Fessler RG, Regan JJ, eds. Endoscopic Spine Surgery and Instrumentation: Percutaneous Procedures. New York: Thieme Medical Publishers, Inc., 2005:180–198.

28. Brau SA. Video endoscopic approach to the thoracic spine. In: Watkins RG, ed. Surgical Approaches to the Spine. 2nd ed. New York: Springer, 2003:360–366.

29. Perin NI, Dickman CA, Papadopoulos SM, et al. Perioperative management for thoracoscopic spine surgery. In: Dickman CA, Rosenthal DJ, Perin NI, eds. Thoracoscopic Spine Surgery. New York: Thieme Medical Publishers, Inc., 1999:87–93.

30. Isaacs RE, Perez-Cruet MJ, Fessler RG. Complications in the treatment of L1 burst fractures. Tech Neurosurg 2003; 8(2):130–139.

31. Oskouian RJ, Johnson JP. Endoscopic thoracic microdiscectomy. Neurosurg Focus 2005; 18(3):e11.

32. Buscher HC, Jansen JB, van Dongen R, et al. Long-term results of bilateral thoracoscopic splanchnicectomy in patients with chronic pancreatitis. Br J Surg 2002; 89(2):158–162.

33. Landreneau RJ, Mack MJ, Hazelrigg SR, et al. Video-assisted thoracic surgery: basic technical concepts and intercostal approach strategies. Ann Thorac Surg 1992; 54(4):800–807.

34. McAfee PC. Thoracolumbar spinal corpectomy. In: Regan JJ, McAfee PC, Mack MJ, eds. Atlas of Endoscopic Spine Surgery. St. Louis: Quality Medical Publishing, Inc., 1995:189–197.

35. Liu PC, Yuan HA. Anterior thoracic and lumbar approaches. In: Bono CM, Garfin SR, eds. Spine. Philadelphia: Lippincott Williams & Wilkins, 2004:221–230.

36. Regan JJ, McAfee PC. Thoracoscopy and laparoscopy of the spine. In: Bridwell KH, DeWald RL, eds. The Textbook of Spinal Surgery. Vol. 2. 2nd ed. Philadelphia: Lippincott-Raven Publishers, 1997:2313–2331.

37. Blum MG, Sundaresan SR. Video-assisted thoracoscopic surgery. In: Jones DB, Wu JS, Soper NJ, eds. Laparoscopic Surgery: Principles and Procedures. 2nd ed. New York: Marcel Dekker, Inc., 2004:527–537.

38. Bolesta MJ. Minimally invasive orthopedic and spinal surgery: a brief overview. In: Jones DB, Wu JS, Soper NJ, eds. Laparoscopic Surgery: Principles and Procedures. 2nd ed. New York: Marcel Dekker, Inc., 2004:569–573.

11 Endoscopic Laminotomy, Foraminotomy, and Discectomy for Herniated Lumbar Disc

Anthony T. Yeung and Christopher A. Yeung
Arizona Institute for Minimally Invasive Spine Care, Phoenix, Arizona, U.S.A.

HISTORY AND EVOLUTION OF THE TECHNIQUE

Minimal access surgery for lumbar disc herniation was first independently reported by Kambin et al. (1) and Hijikata (2) in 1973. The technique utilized a posterolateral approach to the foraminal zone of the disc bordered by the superior facet dorsally, the exiting nerve ventrally, and the endplate of the inferior vertebra caudally. The goal was to decompress nerve roots secondary to lumbar disc herniation by the "inside–out technique" of central and posterior nuclectomy and fragmentectomy. Advances in technique and instrumentation since Kambin, however, has allowed the surgeon to also enlarge the medial or lateral foramen by decompression of the lateral and ventral portions of the facet joint complex to reach the dorsal 25% of the disc and the epidural space. Thus, the full spectrum of disc herniations is feasible with advanced endoscopic instrumentation and techniques that can either target the extruded fragment in the epidural space directly or with a combination of the "inside–out technique" (3).

The early efforts were limited to a nonvisualized central discectomy to achieve an indirect decompression of the nerve roots (1,2,4), but improvements in surgical equipment and technique evolved gradually over the next 30 years. In the last seven years, the important and major equipment improvements include: (*i*) various angled high-resolution rod lens operating endoscopes, (*ii*) variable sized of working channels (2.0–4.2 mm), (*iii*) beveled and slotted cannulas, (*iv*) flexible shavers and pituitary forceps, (*v*) various sized hinged pituitary forceps, (*vi*) a bipolar flexible high-frequency/low-temperature radiofrequency (RF) electrode, (*vii*) multidirectional Holmium Yttrium-Aluminum-Garnet lasers, (*viii*) high-speed diamond and endoscopic motorized burrs enlarge the lateral and subarticular foramen (3). An improved fluoroscopically guided approach method introduced by Yeung and reported by Tsou (5,6) outlined a consistent technique for entry into all lumbar posterior disc spaces including the L5–S1 level. These refinements, including adapting the use of more extreme lateral and posterior trajectories plus the more routine use of biportal approaches, have enhanced the capabilities of foraminal endoscopic discectomy to deliver surgical results similar to the results obtainable by traditional transcanal approaches for treating common lumbar disc herniations (6–9).

New operating tools have also expanded operative capabilities that allow the surgeon to inspect many painful conditions in a degenerative lumbar spine.

INDICATIONS

Indications for surgical intervention are similar to indications for traditional transcanal discectomy. However, endoscopic access to the spine does not have the same paradoxical effects of surgery through the transcanal approach and does not have to invade the sensitive spinal canal. The capability of visualizing and probing patho-anatomy in a unanesthetized patient provides the endoscopic surgeon a technique that will allow him to study discogenic axial and neuropathic spinal pain, and consider treatment alternatives of foraminal decompression and tissue modulation that is not in the armamentarium of traditional approach surgeons (9). The full spectra of conditions causing back pain and sciatica from degenerative conditions of the lumbar spine are therefore potential indications for the accomplished and experienced endoscopist.

Ideal indications are for upper lumbar and contained disc herniations, far-lateral disc herniations, discogenic pain from annular tears elicited by low pressure, low-volume evocative discography™, and discitis. Extruded disc herniations accessible from the axial plane of the disc are possible for the experienced endoscopic surgeon. Upper lumbar herniations are especially better accessed through the foraminal approach, as the traditional transcanal approach may require extensive laminectomy and facetectomy that might destabilize the spine.

The Learning Curve

Due to the steep learning curve, there are currently only a handful of endoscopic spine surgeons who practice posterolateral lumbar endoscopy as a major part of their practice. The obvious benefits for the patient, however, keep interest in the technique high. The learning curve for spinal endoscopy is steeper than the traditional microscopically assisted open procedures with or without the use of tubular retractors. As long as the pathoanatomy can be reached, there are no contraindications to the technique; there are only relative contraindications dictated by the skill of the surgeon in accessing the targeted pathology safely. Some sequestered and migrated herniations are inaccessible in the spinal canal via the transforaminal approach and the more direct posterior approach is preferred. Surgeon-performed interventional injection techniques of foraminal epidurography, therapeutic steroid injections, discography, and adjunctive therapy are helpful to determine if such a herniation is accessible or not. Mastering these injection techniques is thus important to help the surgeon in evaluating appropriate candidates for the posterolateral technique. The more experienced the endoscopic surgeon, the more he will prefer the transforaminal portal.

CONSIDERATIONS FOR PREOPERATIVE PLANNING
The Preoperative Physical Exam

The examination is similar to that for traditional surgery. Findings of radiculopathy causing reflex change, sensory change, or focal muscle weakness that are indications for microdiscectomy are also indications for endoscopic discectomy. For endoscopic discectomy, however, when back pain and sciatica is exacerbated with active or passive extension, this is a good physical sign that foraminal decompression of the disc will provide pain relief. When there is more back pain than leg pain from central disc herniations that do not lateralize to the spinal nerves, excellent results are obtained for central disc herniations (10).

Preoperative Imaging, Diagnostics, and Therapeutic Injections

Standard magnetic resonance imaging (MRI) with or without gadolinium that demonstrates mechanical elevation or deformity of the spinal nerves also provides confirmation of the findings on physical examination. Positional MRIs (standing or sitting) in the position causing greatest pain may provide dynamic information on the size and extent of the protrusion not seen in a recumbent MRI. Preoperative discography by the operating surgeon is emphasized for the endoscopic surgeon. Surgeon-performed discography provides useful information for patient selection as it gives as much information for avoidance of surgery as it does for surgical indication. When the endoscopic surgeon performs his own discography, the process provides him additional clinical information on his patient, which is lost to the variability of discography reports. In the preoperative setting, discography provides information on the internal architecture of the nucleus and the competency of the annulus (9). If discography elicits concordant pain, the technical aspect of the discography and the patient's response to the procedure itself provides invaluable information that can only be appreciated by the surgeon who uses the same approach to the patho-anatomy (9). A foraminal epidural gram and therapeutic foraminal injection using the same skin entry portal will serve to provide information useful to the surgeon that cannot be easily obtained by an independent discographer. The provision of a therapeutic injection in conjunction with the evocative injection may also provide some temporary relief of back pain and sciatica when the pain is mediated by the inflammatory response. Surgeons who do their own discography are able to better select patients for endoscopic discectomy as they soon learn to correlate discography results with the visualized patho-anatomy at surgery. In an experienced surgeon-discographer's hands, there will be far less false positive discograms than if an evocative discogram is done by an independent discographer. A "false-positive" discogram will therefore only be a false interpretation of a positive discogram, as the endoscopic surgeon learns to correlate the visualized pathoanatomy at surgery. The most common finding is inflamed granulation tissue in the annular tear. The epidural gram, needle placement, and skin portal approach is almost exactly the same as with the surgical skin portal. The technique is different than the approach used by interventional pain specialists and radiologists. When it is particularly difficult to correlate the patient's sciatic pain, electromyogram (EMG) and conductions studies with special attention to H reflex and F wave changes may help localize the spinal nerve involved.

Surgical Technique

The first learning barrier is the percutaneous approach itself. The posterolateral or transforaminal approach to the disc through Kambin's triangle is not routinely taught in most spine surgery training programs. Precise needle placement and subsequent cannula and endoscope placement between the exiting and traversing nerve roots is needed to avoid patient discomfort and nerve injury in the awake patient. Eliciting a painful response from the patient can be intimidating to the spine surgeon not accustomed to operating on an awake patient. Patients will not tolerate multiple misguided needle passes and this may frustrate the surgeon as well. With practice, spine surgeons can become accomplished to accessing the disc via the posterolateral approach. Yeung has developed a standardized method for optimal needle placement that should lower the initial learning curve.

The second learning barrier is becoming comfortable with the anatomic relationships within the foramen. All spine surgeons are trained in the posterior approach to the spine and are familiar with the anatomic relationships when viewed from this posterior approach. They are not accustomed to looking at the anatomy from the posterolateral or foraminal portal, and area of the "hidden zone" rarely visualized by traditional surgeons. The clear visualization provided by the newer rod lens endoscopes and a new understanding of the patho-anatomy and anatomic relationships help overcome preconceived rigid concepts that affect traditional surgical indications.

Another learning barrier is the ability to recognize anatomy on the video screen. Most neurosurgeons do not have much if any experience using endoscopes. Most orthopedic spine surgeons have used scopes for knee and shoulder surgery and are accustomed to looking at the two-dimensional video screen. The ability to move the scope and view structures from many vantage points rather than simply magnifying the same view, help overcome this two-dimensional viewpoint. Dedication to learning the technique and utilizing it are important in establishing and maintaining skill recognizing endoscopically viewed anatomy.

Once these learning barriers are overcome, surgeons competent with the technique will prefer posterolateral endoscopic spine surgery to the traditional posterior approach for most disc herniations.

Surgical Equipment

The most widely available system for posterolateral endoscopic discectomy is the Yeung Endoscopic Spine Surgery System (YESS) by Richard Wolf. The YESS system consists of the following instruments.

- Multichannel, 20° oval spinal endoscope with 2.7-mm working channel and integrated continuous irrigation (inflow and outflow) ports (Fig. 1)
- Multichannel, 70° oval spinal endoscope
- 7-mm working cannulas with various open-slotted, beveled, and tapered ends
- Two-channel tissue dilator/obturator
- Specialized single- and double-action endoscopic rongeurs for visualized fragmentectomy
- Larger straight and hinged rongeurs for discectomy and targeted fragmentectomy
- Trephines for annulotomy and foraminoplasty
- Micro rasps, curettes, and penfield probes

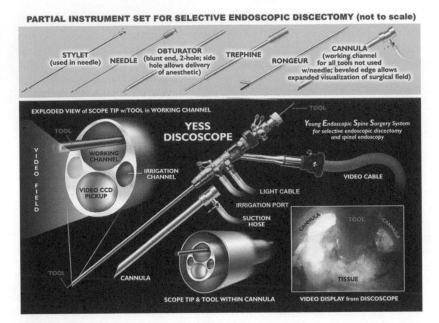

FIGURE 1 Partial instrument set for selective endoscopic discectomy.

- Annulotomy knife
- Flexible bipolar radiofrequency probe for hemostasis, thermal contraction of the annular collagen, and thermal ablation of the annular nociceptors (Ellman trigger-flex bipolar probe).

Second-Generation Scopes and Equipment

Second-generation foraminal scopes have larger operating channels (3.1 and 4.2 mm) that allow for larger forceps and motorized equipments such as high-speed burrs to aid in foraminal decompression. These new endoscopes can be used for lateral and central stenosis, treatment of failed back surgery syndrome (FBSS) caused by stenosis, and dorsal laminotomy if the scope is used fully endoscopically in the dorsal approach. The dorsal approach is especially useful for extruded fragments at L5–S1.

Adjunctive Equipment

- Straight and flexible suction-irrigation shavers for discectomy [Endius microdiscectomy system (MDS)]
- Side-firing Holmium-YAG laser (Trimedyne)
- Direct-firing Holmium-YAG laser (Lisa)
- High-speed diamond burrs
- Fluid pump for continuous irrigation
- Video endoscopy tower
- VHS, DVD and computer equipment for surgical documentation.

Operating Room Setup

Proper operation room setup requires a radiolucent table with a hyperkyphotic frame, one C-arm, and a tower with the usual monitor for endoscopic viewing. Foot pedals controlling the radiofrequency probe, shaver, suction, C-arm, and laser should be ergonomically arranged. Required personnel include the anesthesiologist, scrub tech, circulator, C-arm technician, and a surgical assistant if a biportal approach is planned.

Patient Positioning

The patient is placed prone on the radiolucent hyperkyphotic frame (Kambin frame, U.S. Surgical) with the arms away from the side of the body. Care is taken to line up the patient with the C-arm to ensure a perfect posterior-anterior and lateral view on the fluoroscopy. The spinous processes should be centered between the pedicles on the posterior–anterior (PA) view and the endplates parallel on the lateral view. The surgical level must be centered to avoid parallax

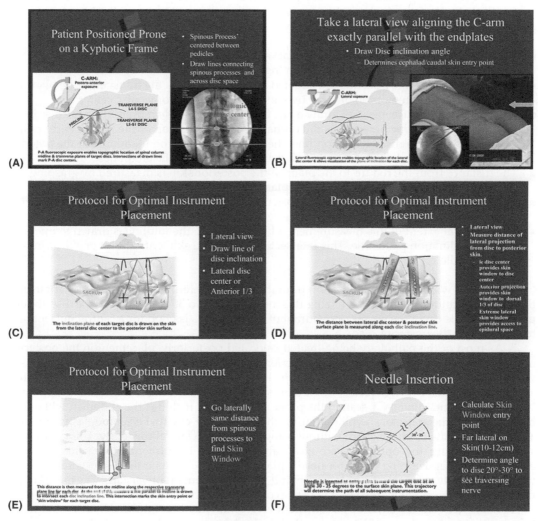

FIGURE 2 **(A–E)** The procedure is carried out in an operating room, under aseptic conditions, using only local anesthesia and conscious sedation. Do not use propofol! Free hand C-arm biplane guidance method is used. Two basic C-arm projected images are utilized, posteroanterior and lateral projections. Both views require parallelism of the X-ray beam to the target endplates. When the intervertebral disc is not perpendicular to the floor, the C-arm tube is tilted until the beam (*dotted line*) is parallel to the disc endplates (Ferguson view). The skin window is estimated by measuring the distance from the anterior disc to the skin or placing the skin window as far lateral on the back as possible before the skin window goes anteriorly. **(F)** Axial view needle trajectory. From the skin window aim the approach needle toward the disc at 20° to 30° in the frontal plane. The path is medial to quadratus lumborum. This avoids inadvertent visceral penetration. The trajectory places the posterior one-third of the disc and the epidural space within reach of the operating tools. Use more vertical angle if epidural procedure is not needed. Enter the disc through the annular window and place the needle tip in midline. In the lateral projection, the needle tip need not pass the midpoint of the disc. Provocation contrast/blue dye discography is performed in this position.

error. Anesthesia consists of a half percent of local lidocaine infiltration, supplemented by versed and fentanyl for conscious sedation. The sedation is kept light enough to allow patient feedback if they experience any painful nerve root irritation.

OPERATIVE APPROACH
Protocol for Optimal Central Needle Placement (Fig. 2A–F)

Utilizing a thin metal rod as a radio-opaque marker and ruler, lines are drawn on the skin to mark surface topography for guidance in free hand biplane C-arm needle placement. These surface markings help identify three key landmarks for needle placement: the anatomic disc center, the annular foraminal window (centered within the medial and lateral borders of the pedicles), and the skin window (needle entry point).

- Utilizing a metal rod as radio-opaque marker and ruler, draw a longitudinal line over the spinous processes to mark the midline on the PA view.
- Draw a transverse line bisecting the targeted disc space to mark the transverse disc plane on the PA view. The intersection of these two lines marks the anatomic disc center.
- On the lateral fluoroscopic view draw a line on the patient's side representing the disc inclination plane. This line determines the cephalad/caudal position of the needle entry point. When drawing this disc inclination line, the tip of the metal rod should be at the anterior aspect of the disc and the rod should bisect and be parallel to the endplates.
- The distance from the rod tip to the plane of the posterior skin is measured by grasping the rod at the point where the posterior skin plane intersects it.
- This distance is then measured on the posterior skin from the midline along the transverse plane line.
- At the lateral extent of this measurement a line parallel to the midline is drawn to intersect the disc inclination plane line. This intersection marks the skin entry point or skin window for the needle.

The skin window's lateral location from the midline determines the trajectory angle into the foraminal annular window. Utilizing this method, a 20° to 30° trajectory to the disc should place the needle tip in the posterior quadrant of the disc. This is good for a central nucleotomy to decompress the posterior disc.

As most of the pathology being treated is located posteriorly, placement in the posterior one-third of the disc is optimal. With experience, the surgeon may want to move the skin window more laterally for the optimal needle placement into the posterior one-third of the disc and epidural space with a trajectory angle of less than 20 degrees. If an extreme lateral approach is considered, obtaining a CT scan in the prone position that includes the abdomen will determine whether the trajectory avoids injuring the abdominal cavity. Foraminoplasty will also allow access to the epidural space without using the extreme lateral trajectory. This coordinate system of finding the optimal anatomical landmarks for instrument placement will help decrease the steep learning curve for needle placement and eliminate the less accurate "down the tunnel" method favored by radiologists and pain management physicians. The more lateral the skin entry, the surgeon must be aware to avoid entering the abdominal cavity by the needle or cannula. To avoid too anterior placement, it is recommended that the needle entry point not be more lateral than the most lateral aspect of the back before it curves anteriorly.

The positive disc inclination plane of the L5–S1 disc is noteworthy. A steep positive inclination line (lordosis) will position the optimal skin window more cephalad from the transverse plane line, avoiding the "high iliac crest." A flatly inclined L5–S1 disc will position the optimal skin window with the iliac crest obstructing the trajectory of the needle. The skin window will have to start more medial to avoid the iliac crest, and sometimes the lateral one-quarter of the facet joint complex must be resected to allow for posterior needle placement in the disc.

The first neutrally aligned disc inclination plane is usually at L4–L5 or L3–L4. A neutrally aligned disc inclination plane is in the same plane as the transverse plane line, thus the skin window is in line with the transverse plane line. A negatively inclined disc, often at L1–L2 and L2–L3, places the skin window caudal to the transverse plane line.

Needle Placement

Infiltrate the skin window and subcutaneous tissue with one half percent lidocaine. Insert a six-inch long, 18-gauge needle from the skin window at a 20° to 30° angle from the coronal plane anteromedially toward the anatomic disc center. Infiltrate the needle tract with one half percent lidocaine as you are advancing the needle. The superficial portion of the needle trajectory is usually outside of the C-arm viewing perimeter on the PA view. Once the needle tip is visible within C-arm viewing perimeter, tilt the C-arm beam parallel to the disc inclination plane, the Ferguson view. This allows one to visualize the advancing needle in the true disc inclination plane. Advance the needle toward the target foraminal annular window. If minor directional adjustments are necessary, use the plane of the needle bevel and hub pressure to navigate (i.e., if the needle bevel is facing dorsal, the needle will tend to move ventral when advancing it). At the first bony resistance or before the needle tip is advanced medial to the pedicle; turn the C-arm to the lateral projection. Do not advance the needle tip medial to the pedicle during the initial approach. Doing so risks inadvertent traversing nerve root and dural puncture.

Most frequently, the first bony resistance encountered is the lateral facet. Increase the trajectory angle to aim ventral to the facet and continue the approach toward the foraminal annular window. Turning the needle bevel to face dorsal helps the needle tip skive off the undersurface of the facet. The C-arm lateral projection should confirm the needle tip's correct annular location. In the lateral view, the correct needle tip position should be just touching the posterior annulus surface. In the posteroanterior view, the needle tip should be on the medial border of the facet. These two views of the C-arm confirm that the needle tip has engaged, the safe zone, within the foraminal annular widow.

While monitoring the posteroanterior view, advance the needle tip through the annulus to the midline (anatomic disc center). Then check the lateral view. If the needle tip is in the center of the disc on the lateral view you have a central needle placement, which is good for a central nucleotomy. Ideally the needle tip will be in the posterior one-third of the disc indicating posterior needle placement. This is ideal for accessing most herniations.

Evocative Chromo-Discography™

Perform confirmatory contrast discography at this time. The following contrast mixture is used: 9 cc of Isovue 300 with 1 cc of indigo carmine dye. This combination of contrast ratio gives readily visible radio-opacity on the discography images, and intraoperative light blue chromatization of pathologic nucleus and annular fissures which help guide the targeted endoscopic fragmentectomy.

Chromodiscography is an integral part of posterolateral selective endoscopic discectomy. The indigo carmine preferentially stains the acidic degenerated nucleus pulposus. This helps orient the surgeon to the endoscopic anatomy and selectively remove the herniated and unstable nucleus pulposus. The surgeon can follow the blue stained tissue to the annular tears and the herniation tract.

The ability of discography to evoke a concordant painful response is also helpful to confirm the disc as a pain generator. The literature on discography is currently considered controversial. It is controversial partly because of the high inter-observer variability by discographers in reporting the patient's subjective pain as well as the ailing patient's inability to give a clear response, especially if pain response is altered by the use of analgesics or sedation during the procedure. The surgeon who is accomplished in endoscopic spine surgery should do the discography himself in order to decrease the interobserver variability in interpreting the patient's response and thus better select for appropriate patients. One of the main uses of discography is to exclude patients who are overly pain sensitive and thus poor surgical candidates.

Instrument Placement

Insert a long thin guide wire through the 18-gauge needle channel and into the disc. Remove the needle and slide the bluntly tapered tissue dilating obturator over the guide wire until the tip of the obturator is firmly engaged in the annular window. An eccentric parallel channel in the obturator allows for four quadrant annular infiltration using small incremental volumes of one-half percent of lidocaine in each quadrant, enough to anesthetize the annulus, but not the nerve roots. Hold the obturator firmly against the annular window surface and remove the guide wire. Infiltrate the full thickness of the annulus through the obturator's center channel using lidocaine.

The next step is the through-and-through fenestration of the annular window by advancing the bluntly tapered obturator manually or with a mallet. Annular fenestration is the most painful step of the entire procedure. Advise the anesthesiologist to heighten the sedation level just prior to annular fenestration. Advance the obturator tip deep into the annulus and confirm on the C-arm views. Now slide the beveled access cannula over the obturator toward the disc. Advance the cannula until the beveled tip is deep in the annular window. Remove the obturator and insert the endoscope to get a view of the disc nucleus and annulus. If there is leg pain during the insertion of the cannula, the leg pain can be avoided by rotating the cannula with the open end toward the exiting nerve. This will allow the cannula to get past the nerve while it is advanced past the nerve. The cannula is then rotated to protect the nerve while it is advanced further.

Alternatively, if you are worried about further extruding a large disc herniation or if you want to inspect the outer annular fibers before fenestrating the annulus, the surgeon can engage the outer annulus with the blunt obturator. Then the beveled cannula is advanced over the obturator to the annulus. The obturator is removed and the endoscope is inserted. The outer annular fibers can be inspected to ensure that no neural structures are in the path of the cannula prior to the annulotomy. Then an annulotome or a cutting trephine can be used for the annular fenestration under direct vision. Prominent disc tissue can be removed prior to entering the disc with the cannula.

The foraminal annular window is an easily identifiable intraoperative anatomic landmark; it is the starting location for endoscopic disc excision. Through the endoscope, the surgeon may see various amounts of blue-stained nucleus pulposus. The general purpose access cannula has a bevel hypotenuse of 12 mm and outside diameter of 7 mm. When the cannula is slightly retracted to the midstraddle position in relationship with the annular wall, the wide angle scope visualizes the epidural space, annular wall, and the intradiscal space in the same field.

DESCRIPTION OF THE PROCEDURE
Performing the Discectomy (Fig. 3A–C)

The basic endoscopic method to excise a noncontained paramedian extruded lumbar herniated disc via a uniportal technique is described here. First enlarge the annulotomy medially to the base of the herniation with a cutting forcep. The side-firing Holmium-YAG laser can also be utilized to enlarge and widen the annulotomy. This is performed to release the annular fibers at the herniation site that may pinch off or prevent the extruded portion of the herniation from being extracted. Directly under the herniation apex a large amount of blue-stained nucleus is usually present, likened to the submerged portion of an iceberg. The nucleus here represents migrated and unstable nucleus. The endoscopic rongeurs are used to extract the blue-stained nucleus pulposus under direct visualization. The larger straight and hinged rongeurs are used directly through the cannula after the endoscope is removed. Fluoroscopy and surgeon feel guides this step. By grabbing the base of the herniated fragment, one can usually extract the extruded portion of the herniation. Initial medialization and widening of the annulotomy reduce the prospect of breaking off the apex of the herniation. The traversing nerve root is readily visualized after removal of the extruded herniation (Fig. 4A–G).

Next, perform a bulk decompression by using a straight and flexible suction-irrigation shaver (Endius MDS). This step requires shaver head C-arm localization before power is activated to avoid nerve/dura injury and anterior annular penetration. The cavity thus created is called the working cavity. The debulking process serves two functions. First it decompresses the disc, removing the unstable nucleus material to prevent future reherniation. Second, it creates a working space to visualize the inner layers of the posterior annulus, annular clefts/tears, the herniation tract, and any residual herniated nucleus pulposus.

Inspect the working cavity. If a noncontained extruded disc fragment is still present by finding blue-stained nucleus material posteriorly, then these fragments are teased into the

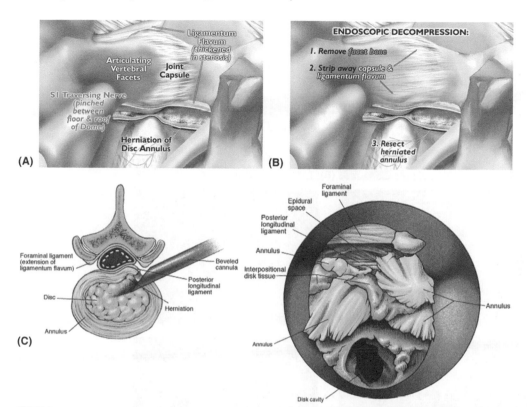

FIGURE 3 (**A**) Degenerative conditions from annular tears to spinal stenosis are visible through the foramen. In severe cases, the ligamentum flavum is pushed against the exiting nerve, causing the normal perineural fat in the foramen to be absent, then causing ischemic inflammation of the nerve. The absence of perineural fat and pulsation of the exiting nerve is an indirect, but more accurate confirmation of lateral stenosis than computed tomography-myelogram and magnetic resonance imaging. (**B**) Endoscopic surgery can address these conditions by decompressing the disc, and by enlarging the foramen accomplished by resecting the undersurface of the superior facet, a portion of the pedicle, and the ligamentum flavum through the foramen, thus decompressing the exiting nerve, the traversing nerve, and the dorsal root ganglion. (**C**) The endoscopic approach for decompressing herniated discs. For decompressing and removing herniated discs, a beveled or slotted cannula is placed in the foramen at the base of the herniation. One-half of the beveled or slotted cannula is in the disc and the dorsal one-half of the cannula is positioned to view the epidural space lateral to the traversing nerve. Rotating and repositioning the open end of the cannula laterally will expose the facet, epidural space containing the traversing nerve, and the exiting nerve while protecting anatomy at the same time. Multiple cannula configurations designed to accommodate variable foramenal anatomy helps the endoscopic surgeon with surgical exposure.

working cavity with the endoscopic rongeurs and the flexible radio-frequency trigger-flex bipolar probe (Ellman) and removed. Creation of the working cavity allows the herniated disc tissue to follow the path of least resistance into the cavity. The flexible radiofrequency bipolar probe is used to ablate any ingrown granulation tissue and contract and thicken the annular collagen at the herniation site. It is also used for hemostasis throughout the case.

The vast majority of herniations can be treated via the uniportal technique. Sometimes for large central herniations the disc needs to be approached from both sides by incorporating a biportal technique.

Closure and Postoperative Management

The incision is closed with steristrips. Sutures are not necessary. Most patients will have dramatic immediate relief of their back and leg pain postoperatively. Some with large herniations will report that their leg pain is gone intraoperatively. No sutures are needed. If there is some bleeding from the incision, it will always stop with a little pressure on the skin. A small abdominal binder may give the patient postoperative comfort and security.

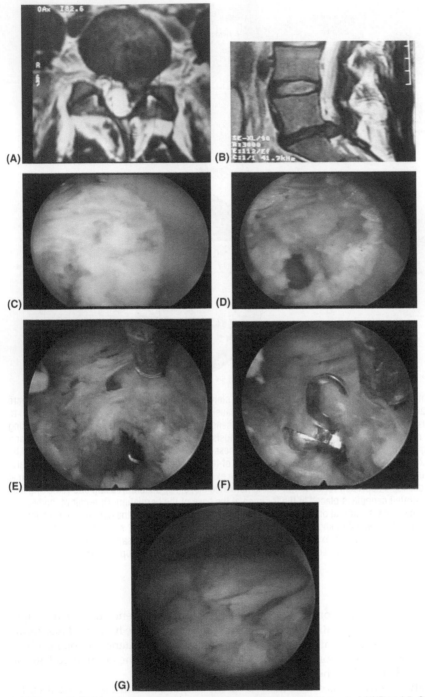

FIGURE 4 (**A,B**) Magnetic resonance imaging of a classic large paracentral HNP at L5–S1 causing back pain and radiculopathy. Lack of containment suspected due to the size of HNP. (**C**) Endoscopic view of the base of herniation from the ipsilateral portal. The indigo-carmine dye and Iso-vue discogram also stains the annulus. (**D**) A collagenous sequestered subligamentous fragment under the traversing nerve caused the decision to establish a biportal approach to probe the nerve and extract the fragment under direct visualization. (**E**) Probing sequestered subligamentous fragment from ipsilateral portal. Note presence of contralateral access cannula at 5 o'clock. (**F**) Biportal manipulation technique with Ellman bipolar triggerflex® probe and endius flexible pituitary rongeur for visualized manipulation of the traversing nerve and removal of sequestered HNP fragment. (**G**) After herniation removal, the traversing nerve pulsates freely in the epidural space confirming complete decompression of the nerve. *Abbreviation*: HNP, herniated nucleus pulposus.

Complications and Their Management

The usual risks of infection, nerve injury, dural tears, bleeding, and scar tissue formation are always present as with any surgery. Dural tears do not require surgical repair. Because we are operating in a closed space, bleeding from the operative site will usually serve as blood patch in small tears. With larger tears, where there is displacement of the nerve rootlets, increasing the flow and pressure of the irrigation fluid will push the rootlets back into the thecal sac. Injection of a sealant such as Flowseal® will help. The postoperative use of a compressive dressing and a brace will help provide compression long enough for the tear to seal enough to avoid spinal fluid leakage and spinal headache. Dysesthesia, the most common postoperative complaint, occurs approximately 5% to 15% of the time, and is almost always transient. It cannot be completely eliminated when operating in the foraminal zone. Its cause remains incompletely understood and may be related to nerve recovery, operating adjacent to the dorsal root ganglion of the exiting nerve, or a small hematoma adjacent to the ganglion of the exiting nerve, as it can occur days or even weeks after surgery (11). If the patient is bothered by the dysesthesia, it can be resolved quickly by a foraminal epidural block and/or a lumbar sympathetic block. The injection of 80 mg of depomedrol mixed with 1 or 2 cc of one-quarter percent of marcaine into the foramen before removing the surgical cannula will decrease postoperative dysesthesia to less than 5%. The incidence of dysesthesia may not be related to any mechanical irritation of the spinal nerves as it can occur with out any irritative response on continous EMG monitioring and can occur days or weeks later. The symptoms are sometimes so minimal that most surgeons do not report it as a "complication." The more severe dysesthetic symptoms are similar to a variant of complex regional pain syndrome, but usually less severe, and without the skin changes. The use of small doses of gabapentin (Neurontin®, Pfizer, Inc., New York, U.S.A.), usually 300 mg t.i.d. will mitigate the discomfort of dysesthesia. Gabapentin is FDA-approved for postherpetic neuralgia, but effective in treatment of neuropathic pain. The off-label use of gabapentin can be titrated to as much as 1800 to 3200 mg/day in case of severe dysesthesia. Postoperative neuropraxia has happened without apparent injury during the operative procedure. The presence of furcal nerves and autonomic nerves in the perineural fat have been documented, and interruption, ablation, or mechanical manipulation of these nerves can cause dysesthesia and neuropathy. This may also be an unavoidable sequella of the foraminal approach, as it is necessary to retract or bluntly traverse the foramen to access the disc. The patient may experience numbness and weakness immediately after the procedure. This is usually temporary and transient since local anesthesia is used routinely. Bowel injury or large vessel injury is extremely rare, but possible if needle, stylette or surgical instruments penetrates the contralateral annulus from an incompetent annulus or from a defect left after removing a disc herniation that has extruded through the annular wall. If this happens, refrain from reflexly pulling the needle or instrument back into the disc. Assess the position of the instrument and monitor the patient intraoperatively and in the recovery room. When the patient is receiving conscious sedation, this type of monitoring is almost always sufficient, but how aggressively the surgeon chooses to observe and manage this type complication cannot be a didactic exercise in surgical judgment. In over 3,000 cases, only one major neuropraxia and bowel injury was encountered. Careful intraoperative fluoroscopic localization and "feeling" the contralateral annulus with the instrument prior to activating it will help prevent the surgical instruments from advancing past the contralateral annular wall.

Avoidance of complications is enhanced by the ability to visualize normal and patho-anatomy clearly, and use of local anesthesia and conscious sedation rather than general or spinal anesthesia. The entire procedure is usually accomplished with the patient remaining comfortable during the entire procedure, and should be done without the patient feeling severe pain except when expected—such as during discography, annular fenestration, or when instruments are manipulated past the exiting nerve. Local anesthesia using one-half percent lidocaine permits generous use of this dilute anesthetic for pain control yet allows the patient to feel pain when the nerve root is manipulated. If the patient is uncomfortable or has pain during the procedure, unless the surgeon expects the pain, such as the extraction of a disc fragment adherent to a nerve, it is best to abort the procedure rather than to further sedate the patient or resort to general or spinal anesthesia. The surgeon is still operating in the "hidden zone" where anomalous nerve structures reside. The overall complication rate, including dural tears, thrombophlebitis, discitis, postoperative radiculopathy, and one isolated case of bowel injury is 4%. Based on an analysis of 100 consecutive patients undergoing intraoperative neuromonitoring compared with a matched sample of 100 consecutive patients without neuromonitoring, it is not possible to eliminate dysesthesia completely, but the unanesthesized patient is the best method in avoiding complications (12).

OUTCOMES

The literature on endoscopic discectomy must be reviewed according to the types of herniations reported and the surgical equipment utilized. Because the endoscopes, endoscopic equipment, and endoscopic methods are in a state of rapid evolution, the current literature must take into account the technique utilized and consider patient selection for the type of herniations studied. In earlier reports, such as with automated percutaneous lumbar discectomy (APLD) or percutaneous laser disc decompression (PLDD), only small contained disc herniations were appropriate for the technique, so comparisons with microdiscectomy literature for extruded disc herniations were not comparing similar patient populations. To provide a more accurate comparison, Tsou reviewed Yeung's endoscopic technique on a subgroup of patients who had objective evidence of radiculopathy secondary to extruded noncontained disc herniations. Ninety-one percent of the patients were satisfied with their results and would opt to undergo the procedure again if they had the same diagnosis and symptoms. A 5% to 10% technical failure rate was salvaged by a second surgery by the transcanal technique. This study can be used to better compare the endoscopic technique with the traditional transcanal microdiscectomy technique. Yeung and Tsou also reported their initial results using the YESS™ system in their first 307 patients with disc herniations who were candidates for transcanal microdiscectomy (5). This study, which included contained nonsequestered intracanal and extracanal herniations produced similar results. Central disc herniations and extraforaminal herniations, when stratified against the transcanal technique identified clear advantages for the foraminal endoscopic approach.

These initial results showed that endoscopic surgery could provide equivalent results to reported results of open microdiscectomy, even with noncontained herniations. Just avoidance of the dorsal muscle column of the spinal canal resulted in less overall surgical morbidity.

SUMMARY

Posterolateral lumbar endoscopy and discectomy introduces a visualized method for minimal access to the disc space as an alternative to the traditional surgical management of lumbar disc herniations. The technique has close overlapping capability with the traditional posterior transcanal open methods. The foraminal approach has advantages over the transcanal approach in upper lumbar herniations and extraforaminal herniations, especially at L5–S1. The foraminal approach allows for the visualization of foraminal pathology in the "hidden zone" of MacNab. It also provides a technique to treat painful annular tears by performing selective nuclectomy and annuloplasty as a new method in treating chronic lumbar discogenic pain (13). The future direction of the technique will become more apparent when a complete nuclectomy is needed for nucleus replacement. It will be recognized that discectomy is not equivalent to nuclectomy, and younger surgeons will have no problem in learning the new technique when it is gradually adopted by current academic training programs.

REFERENCES

1. Kambin P, Gellman H. Percutaneous lateral discectomy of the lumbar spine: a preliminary report. CORR 1983; 174:127–132.
2. Hijikata S, Yamagishi M, Nakayma T. Percutaneous discectomy: a new treatment method for lumbar disc herniation. J Tokyo Den-Ryoku Hosp 1975; 5:39–44.
3. Yeung AT, Yeung CA. Advances in endoscopic disc and spine surgery: foraminal approach. Surg Tech Intern 2003; XI:253–261.

4. Onik G, Helm CA, Ginsbery L, Morris J. Percutaneous lumbar discectomy using a new aspiration probe. AJR 1985; 144:1137–1140.
5. Yeung AT, Tsou, PM. Posterolateral endoscopic excision for lumbar disc herniation: surgical technique, outcome, and complications in 307 consecutive cases. Spine 2002; 27:722–731.
6. Tsou PM, Yeung AT. Transforaminal endoscopic decompression for radiculopathy secondary to intra-canal non-contained lumbar disc herniations: outcome and technique. Spine J 2002; 2:41–48.
7. Schaffer JL, Kambin P. Percutaneous posterolateral lumbar discectomy and decompression with a 6.9 millimeter cannula. Analysis of operative failures and complications. JBJS 1991; 73A:822–831.
8. Hermantin FU, Peters T, Quartararo L, Kambin P. A prospective, randomized study comparing the results of open discectomy with those of video-assisted arthroscopic microdiscectomy. JBJS 1999; 81A:958–965.
9. Yeung AT, Yeung CA. In vivo endoscopic visualization of the patho-anatomy of degenerative conditions of the lumbar spine. Surgical Technology International XV. Tom Laszlo: Universal Medical, 2006:243–256.
10. Seferlis T, Yeung AT. Selective endoscopic discectomy and thermal annuloplasty: a new technique for central disc herniations. J Minim Invas Spinal Tech 2003; 3(1):13–16.
11. Yeung AT, Savitz M. Complications of percutaneous spinal surgery. In: Vacarro, ed. Complications in Adult and Pediatric Spine Surgery. New York: Marcel Dekker, 2005:547–571.
12. Poster exhibit: A prospective study of intraoperative neuromonitoring during selective endoscopic discectomy™ compared to a matched patient sample without neuromonitoring. Spine Arthroplasty Society Global symposium on Motion Preservation Technology, May 4–7, 2005, New York.
13. Tsou PM, Yeung CA, Yeung AT. Selective endoscopic discectomy™ and thermal annuloplasty for chronic lumbar discogenic pain: a minimal access visualized intradiscal procedure. Spine J 2004; 2:563–574.

12 | Unilateral Hemi-Laminotomy for Bilateral Lumbar Decompression (Segmental Sublaminoplasty)

Moe R. Lim
Department of Orthopedic Surgery, University of North Carolina–Chapel Hill, Chapel Hill, North Carolina, U.S.A.

Jason Young
Department of Orthopedic Surgery, Loyola University Medical Center, Maywood, Illinois, U.S.A.

Paul H. Young
Department of Surgery, St. Louis University School of Medicine, St. Louis, Missouri, U.S.A.

Joon Y. Lee
Department of Orthopedic Surgery, University of Pittsburgh, Pittsburgh, Pennsylvania, U.S.A.

Alan S. Hilibrand
Department of Orthopedic Surgery, Thomas Jefferson University and the Rothman Institute, Philadelphia, Pennsylvania, U.S.A.

INTRODUCTION

The gold standard of treatment for symptomatic lumbar spinal stenosis is a wide decompression via a bilateral paraspinal muscle stripping exposure. Although this traditional technique allows maximal neural decompression, there is morbidity related to stripping the paraspinal muscles and resection of stabilizing interspinous/supraspinous ligaments. An alternative is a less invasive microsurgical technique of unilateral hemi-laminotomy for bilateral decompression. Commonly known as lumbar segmental sublaminoplasty, the technique was developed by John A. McCulloch and Paul H. Young over 20 years ago. This technique enables bilateral central and foraminal neural decompression of one or two levels while limiting muscle stripping to one side and preserving the stabilizing midline ligamentous structures.

Lumbar segmental sublaminoplasty compares favorably with other minimally invasive microsurgical decompression techniques such as bilateral hemi-laminotomies (1,2) and interlaminar decompression (3). With bilateral hemi-laminotomies, subarticular stenosis can be addressed while preserving the midline ligaments and bone. However, bilateral muscle stripping is still required and central and foraminal stenosis may not be adequately addressed. With an interlaminar decompression, the cephalad portion of the cephalad lamina and the caudal aspect of the caudal lamina are preserved. Central, subarticular, and foraminal stenosis can be easily addressed. However, bilateral muscle stripping is still required and the midline ligaments and a portion of the spinous processes must be excised to undercut the laminae. Other techniques involve spinous process osteotomies (4) or modified "port-hole" laminotomies (5). In comparison with these techniques, McCulloch and Young's sublaminoplasty may allow the greatest amount of decompression via the least invasive approach.

The technique of segmental sublaminoplasty described in this chapter should not be confused with the other more recently described lumbar laminoplasties such as inverse laminoplasty (6), expansive laminoplasty (7), and restorative laminoplasty (8). These techniques involve hinging open the laminae, as with expansive laminoplasty (7), removing the entire laminae and replanting it after reversing its caudocranial position, as with inverse laminoplasty (6), or shaving the inner compressive elements, as with restorative laminoplasty (8). These novel techniques are not minimally invasive and represent a distant departure from microsurgical decompression methods.

INDICATIONS

The indications for lumbar segmental sublaminoplasty are similar to that of standard lumbar decompression. Patients with degenerative lumbar spinal stenosis and predominant leg pain who have failed conservative therapy are potential surgical candidates. The ideal candidate for sublaminoplasty is a thin patient with unilateral leg pain and radiographic evidence of severe single-level central canal stenosis and unilateral subarticular and/or foraminal stenosis. Notably, subarticular and foraminal decompression is more easily accomplished contralateral to the hemi-laminotomy; thus, the exposure is performed on the side opposite of the patient's radiculopathy. Foraminal decompression of the ipsilateral side often requires an intertransverse process approach, which is more challenging.

Grade I degenerative spondylolisthesis is not a contraindication to sublaminoplasty decompression, although we generally recommend fusion in this setting. In some patients with minimal segmental motion with a collapsed disc and who may be unsuitable for the additional morbidity of a fusion, sublaminoplasty may offer a unique option. Preservation of the stabilizing ligaments and minimal bony resection may help prevent postoperative iatrogenic progression of the spondylolisthesis (9,10).

Patients with a grade II or higher spondylolisthesis are more suitable for a standard wide decompression and fusion, as they are not candidates for sublaminoplasty. Patients with a significant component of congenital spinal stenosis are also poor candidates for sublaminoplasty. In congenital stenosis, neural compression is continuous in the spinal canal and multilevel laminectomies are usually required.

CONSIDERATIONS FOR PREOPERATIVE PLANNING

To maximize neural decompression while minimizing unnecessary bony and soft tissue resection, a thorough understanding of the exact locations of neural impingement is necessary. Although there are many systems which classify the areas of neural compression in lumbar spinal stenosis (11,12), we prefer the precise anatomic descriptions of McCulloch and Young (13,14). They described areas in successive axial cuts as "floors" while areas in successive sagittal cuts were called "zones." Moving caudal to cranial, each segment can be divided into three "floors." The first floor is at the disc level, the most significantly affected with degenerative spinal stenosis. The second floor is at the level of the foramina, which extends from the inferior endplate to the inferior aspect of the pedicle. The most third and most cephalad floor is at the level of the pedicle, which extends from the inferior aspect of the pedicle to the superior endplate. Moving medial to lateral via sagittal cuts, the spinal canal can be divided into two zones. The central zone extends from the medial aspect of the left facet joint to the medial aspect of the right facet joint and spans the entire length of the spine. The lateral zone is further subdivided into the subarticular, foraminal, and extraforaminal zones. The subarticular zone, also known as the lateral recess, extends from the medial aspect of the facet joint to the medial aspect of the ipsilateral pedicle. The subarticular zone spans the pedicle and disc floors. The foraminal zone extends from the medial aspect of the pedicle to the lateral aspect of the same pedicle. It spans the disc and foraminal floors from the inferior aspect of the cephalad pedicle to the superior aspect of the caudal pedicle. Finally, the extraforaminal zone extends lateral to the lateral aspect of the pedicle (Fig. 1).

The primary imaging modality to localize neural compression in lumbar spinal stenosis is magnetic resonance imaging (MRI). The T2-weighted MRI images are useful because of its myelogram effect. The T2 axial cuts are best to evaluate the central and lateral zones for the relative contributions of the disc, congenitally short pedicles, ligamentum flavum, and facet joints to the stenosis. A midline T2-weighted sagittal cut is best to localize the most affected floor(s). Paramedian T1-weighted images are best to evaluate foraminal stenosis, as seen by the obliteration of the normal fat signal surrounding the exiting nerve root and impingement by the caudal superior facet. If MRI is contraindicated, computed tomographic (CT) myelography with sagittal and coronal reconstructions is the modality of choice.

During preoperative planning, the exact locations of neural compression detected on these studies are carefully translated to the bony landmarks seen on the plain films to create a

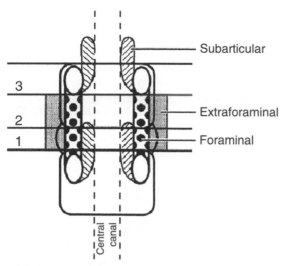

FIGURE 1 Areas of neural compression in lumbar spinal stenosis as described by McCulloch and Young. Areas in successive axial cuts are called "floors" while areas in successive sagittal cuts were called "zones." Moving caudal to via axial cuts, the spine can be divided into three "floors" per segment. The *first* floor is the disc, the most significantly compressed level in degenerative spinal stenosis. The next (*second*) floor is the foraminal level, which extends from the inferior endplate to the inferior aspect of the pedicle. The most cephalad (*third*) floor is the pedicle level with extends from the inferior aspect of the pedicle to the superior endplate. Moving medial to lateral via sagittal cuts, the spinal canal can be divided into the central zone and lateral zone. The central zone extends from the medial aspect of the left facet joint to the medial aspect of the right facet joint, and spans the entire length of the spine. The lateral zone is further subdivided into the subarticular, foraminal, and extraforaminal zones. The subarticular zone (also known as the lateral recess), extends from the medial aspect of the facet joint to the medial aspect of the ipsilateral pedicle. The subarticular zone spans the pedicle and disc floors. The foraminal zone extends from the medial aspect of the pedicle to the lateral aspect of the same pedicle, and spans from the inferior aspect of the cephalad pedicle to the superior aspect of the caudal pedicle (the disc and foraminal floors). Lastly, the extraforaminal zone extends lateral to the lateral aspect of the pedicle. *Source*: From Ref. 14.

so-called surgical roadmap. On the anteroposterior (AP) radiograph, the widths of the interlaminar spaces at the level(s) of the pathology are noted. On the AP and lateral radiographs, the relationships between the posterior elements and disc spaces are studied. In particular, the relationship of the inferior border of the laminae to the floors of pathology is noted to determine the necessary amount of lamina resection.

During the preoperative office visit, the patient's primary symptom and any relevant medical or surgical history are written on the plain radiographs. In addition, the surgical roadmap for the areas of necessary bony resection is drawn out on the radiographs. This strategy allows for a quick final review of the patient's history, location of pathology, and surgical plan in the operating room prior to the start of the procedure.

SURGICAL TECHNIQUE
Patient Position

After intubation, the patient is placed prone on an Andrews frame or table. With the Andrews frame, the hips and knees remain flexed just beyond 90° and the abdomen hangs free. This position reduces the normal lumbar lordosis to widen the interlaminar spaces and allows easier entry into the spinal canal for microsurgical access. In addition, the freely hanging abdomen serves to decompress the epidural vessels to decrease bleeding, which is crucial for this procedure. In positioning the upper extremities, the shoulders should not be abducted beyond 90° to avoid traction on the brachial plexus. The elbows are flexed 90°. After final positioning, the breasts and genitalia are checked to ensure that there are no areas of excessive pressure. We generally ask the anesthesiologist to avoid the use of neuromuscular paralytics during the procedure. This allows the surgeon to see twitching in case of excessive nerve root retraction.

Level Localization

The lateral iliac crest provides the best superficial landmark to help localize the lower lumbar levels. Generally, the bony lateral iliac crest is in the same level as the L4–5 interspace. This provides a convenient landmark as L4–5 is the most commonly involved level. The exact relationship of the L4–5 interspace to the lateral iliac crest can also be confirmed by examining the AP and lateral radiographs. To identify the correct level, we use localizing needles with a preincision lateral radiograph. First, a preliminary skin prep is performed prior to draping. For the L4–5 level, two 18-gauge spinal needles are then inserted obliquely off the midline and onto the lateral spinous processes of L4 and L5. A lateral radiograph is then obtained. Two needles are used to increase the probability that the needle will identify the correct level and will allow the distance between the two needles to be used as a reference length on the magnified radiograph. Once the correct level is confirmed, the level of the correct needle is marked on the skin and 0.5 cc of indigo carmine is slowly injected into the soft tissue as the needle is withdrawn. Once the skin is incised, this dye is followed to bone to direct the surgeon to the correct surgical level. The skin is then reprepped for the procedure. Of note, the indigo carmine may cause the patient's urine to temporarily turn light blue or green.

Surgeon's Position

The operating position of the surgeon depends on the location of the pathology. For central stenosis alone (a rare situation), the surgeon stands on the side of the greater pathology and the hemi-laminotomy is performed on that side. For lateral zone stenosis, the surgeon stands contralateral to the lateral pathology and the hemi-laminotomy is performed on the side contralateral to the pathology. In case of bilateral symptoms, a left-sided approach is generally preferred for a right-handed surgeon.

Placement of Skin Incision

Multiple anatomic and radiographic clues are used to precisely place the skin incision. First, the relationship of our localizing needle to the bony landmarks on the lateral radiograph can help place the incision. Second, the incision is placed in relation to the palpable interspinous process spaces, depending on the desired level of operation. For example, at L5–S1, the disc space is usually directly beneath the palpable L5–S1 interspinous process space. As we proceed cephalad, the disc space is progressively more cephalad in relation to the interspinous process space. The primary location of stenosis is usually at the level of the disc. Therefore, for L5–S1, the incision is centered between the spinous processes of L5 and S1. For L4–5, the incision is shifted slightly cephalad, from the cephalad aspect of the L4 spinous process to the middle of the L4–5 interspinous process space.

Exposure

A 2.5-cm midline incision is usually sufficient for a single-level decompression. Subcutaneous hemostasis is achieved with bipolar coagulation and a small self-retaining Weitlander retractor is placed. A curvilinear incision is then made in the thoracolumbar fascia approximately 1 cm off the midline. If necessary, the fascial incision can extend approximately 1 cm cephalad or caudal to the skin incision. The small flap of deep fascia is reflected upward and serves to preserve and protect the interspinous and supraspinous ligaments and also facilitates fascial reapproximation during closure. The paraspinal musculature is then subperiosteally dissected off the bone using a Cobb elevator and electrocautery. A gauze sponge and Cobb elevator is then used to clean off the bone while exposing the ligamentum flavum at the interspace. The blunt dissection is then carried laterally to the mid-portion of the facet joint, taking care to avoid violating the facet capsule. A McCulloch retractor is placed by positioning the sharp hook ventral and opposite the interspinous ligaments. Care should be taken to ensure that the hook does not impinge on the spinous process as this will hinder the medial and contralateral views. The blade portion of the retractor is then used to retract the paraspinal muscles over the facet joint. The cephalad and caudal pars, half of the caudal and cephalad laminae, the inferior aspect of the interspinous ligament medially, and the middle of the facet joint laterally should be easily visible after the exposure.

The operating microscope is brought in at this stage. The microscope provides greater magnification and anatomic detail. Most importantly, the use of the microscope is essential to maintain three-dimensional visualization through a small incision in a deep wound. The optics of the operating microscope compresses the necessary interocular distance to approximately 25 mm. Therefore, no matter how deep the wound is, as long as a wound diameter of 25 mm is present, three-dimensional visualization is possible. In contrast, three-dimensional visualization with the use of loupe magnifying glasses requires at least a 65-mm wound diameter (the average adult interocular distance) (15).

Ipsilateral Central Decompression (Hemi-Laminotomy)

For an L4–5 decompression, we begin by taking the lower half of the leading lamina (L4) using a side-cutting high-speed burr (Midas Rex M8). Begin medially near the base of the L4 spinous process and proceed laterally toward the ipsilateral side as far as the base of the inferior articular facet (Fig. 2). Note that the lamina bone is thicker laterally than medially and that the ligamentum flavum attachment is more cephalad laterally on the lamina. Care is taken to preserve 5 to 10 mm of the pars interarticularis to prevent postoperative instability. The lamina resection is successively extended cephalad to the origin of the underlying ligamentum flavum. As the resection gets to approximately half of the L4 lamina, the protective ligamentum flavum thins out and terminates, allowing visualization of the epidural fat and dura. At L4–5, approximately half of the leading L4 lamina needs to be resected to adequately decompress the disc "floor." In more cephalad levels (such as L3–4), relatively more of the leading lamina needs to be resected. Also in severe disease or patients with excessive lordosis, shingling of the laminae may necessitate greater bony resection to allow a 2 to 3-cm interlaminar window.

A similar laminotomy is then performed at the cephalad edge of the trailing L5 lamina. The attachment of the ligamentum flavum on the cephalad aspect of the lamina is different from its attachment at the caudal aspect of the lamina (Fig. 3). On the caudal aspect of the lamina, the ligamentum flavum attaches ventrally, serving as a protective layer over the dura while the lamina is being burred. In contrast, on the cephalad aspect of the lamina, the ligamentum flavum attaches only at the edge and dorsal aspect of the lamina. Therefore, there is no underlying ligamentum flavum to protect the dura. Because of this different anatomy, we prefer to use a large #2 curette to detach the ligamentum flavum off the cephalad edge of the trailing lamina. A Kerrison rongeur is then used to perform the laminotomy. Alternatively, a high-speed burr

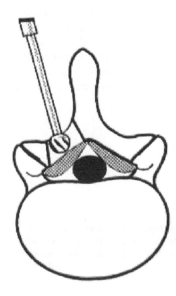

FIGURE 2 Ipsilateral central decompression (hemi-laminotomy). The ipsilateral central decompression is begun by resecting the lower half of the leading lamina using a side-cutting high-speed burr. Begin medially near the base of the L4 spinous process and proceed laterally toward the ipsilateral side as far as the base of the inferior articular facet. *Source*: From Ref. 14.

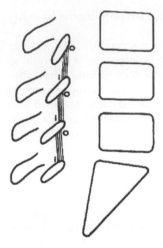

FIGURE 3   The attachments of the ligamentum flavum. On the caudal aspect of the leading lamina, the ligamentum flavum attaches ventrally, serving as a protective layer over the dura while the lamina is being burred. In contrast, on the cephalad aspect of the lamina, the ligamentum flavum attaches only at the edge and dorsal aspect of the lamina. Therefore, there is no underlying ligamentum flavum to protect the dura. *Source*: From Ref. 14.

can be used for the laminotomy. However, a dural tear can occur at this stage if one is not cognizant of the ligamentum flavum attachment.

At this point after the ipsilateral central decompression, further lateral ipsilateral decompression into the subarticular zone is halted. Because of the potential for epidural bleeding laterally, the ipsilateral subarticular stenosis is addressed only after the contralateral decompression is complete.

Contralateral Central Decompression

To safely perform the contralateral central decompression, the line of vision must extend underneath the interspinous ligament and across the midline. Visualization is achieved by aiming the microscope laterally and tilting the table away from the operating surgeon. First, a dural separator is used to free the dura from the overlying ligamentum flavum. The contralateral caudal and cephalad lamina is then undercut with a high-speed burr, beginning at the base of the spinous processes and proceeding laterally within the canal (Fig. 4). In a stepwise fashion, the contralateral cephalad and caudal laminae are burred away, followed by resection of the intervening ligamentum flavum. The ligamentum flavum is resected after the bone to serve as a protective layer over the dura (Fig. 5). This successive resection is carried laterally until the contralateral L5 pedicle is visualized, indicating that the L5 lamina has been adequately resected (Fig. 6). For the L4 lamina, adequate resection is realized when the attachment of the ligamentum flavum is no longer visible. While protecting the dura, the deep portions of the laminae is then burred further to resculpture the central canal and create visible space for the thecal sac. A Murphy probe or dural separator is passed cephalad and caudal in the central canal to confirm adequate decompression. If contralateral visualization remains poor after an adequate central decompression, the deepest portions of the interspinous ligaments can be resected to clear the line of sight to the contralateral side.

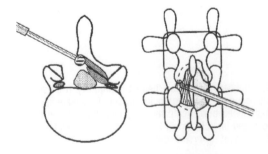

FIGURE 4   Contralateral central decompression. The contralateral caudal and cephalad lamina is then undercut with a high-speed burr and Kerrison, beginning at the base of the spinous processes and proceeding laterally within the canal. *Source*: From Ref. 14.

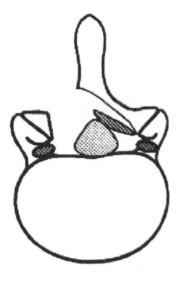

FIGURE 5 Contralateral central decompression. In a stepwise fashion, the contralateral cephalad and caudal laminae are burred away, followed by resection of the intervening ligamentum flavum. The ligamentum flavum is resected after the bone to serve as a protective layer over the dura. *Source*: From Ref. 14.

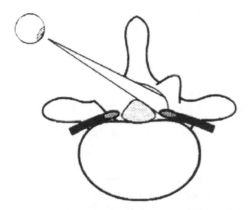

FIGURE 6 Contralateral central decompression. The successive contralateral central decompression is carried laterally until the contralateral trailing pedicle is visualized (L5 pedicle for an L4–5 decompression), indicating that the trailing lamina has been adequately resected. *Source*: From Ref. 14.

Contralateral Subarticular Decompression

Contralateral subarticular decompression begins with visualization of the contralateral caudal L5 pedicle. This pedicle serves as a landmark to define the positions of the disc space and traversing and exiting nerve roots. The lateral attachments of the ligamentum flavum to the medial facet joint capsule can be compressive and are resected using a Kerrison. The traversing nerve root is gently retracted away from the medial border of the pedicle and the medial shelf of the superior articular process is resected with a Kerrison. To complete the subarticular zone decompression, a burr is used to resculpture the remaining bone in a trumpeted fashion to maximize preservation of the facets and pars, and to create a smooth transition between the lamina and L5 pedicle. Adequate contralateral subarticular decompression is achieved when the traversing nerve root is freed from any compression as it courses medial to the L5 pedicle and is easily mobilized.

Contralateral Foraminal Decompression

After adequate decompression of the contralateral central and subarticular zones, a surprisingly good view of the traversing root foramen can be achieved. The bone and soft tissue impinging on the traversing L5 root can be inspected and resected with a curved Kerrison rongeur as the root passes from medial to lateral along the inferior aspect of the pedicle. Decompression of the exiting L4 root is more challenging. Portions of the cephalad lamina and inferior facet may need to be resected further to visualize the inferior aspect of the exiting nerve within the foramen and

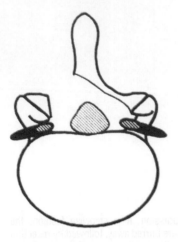

FIGURE 7 Contralateral foraminal decompression. After adequate decompression of the contralateral central and subarticular zones, a surprisingly good view of the traversing nerve root can be achieved. The bone and soft tissue impinging on the traversing root can be inspected and resected with a curved Kerrison rongeur. The exiting root is decompressed by successively resecting the cephalad lamina and inferior facet until the inferior aspect of the exiting nerve is visualized within the foramen and the L4 pedicle can be palpated. *Source*: From Ref. 14.

allow palpation of the L4 pedicle (Fig. 7). As the decompression progresses laterally, visualization may become limited by epidural veins, which become more prominent farther out into the neural foramen. At the conclusion of the contralateral foraminal decompression, a dural separator should be able to follow the exiting and traversing nerve roots all the way out into the extra-foraminal zone without obstruction in all directions.

Ipsilateral Subarticular Decompression

When the contralateral decompression is complete, attention is returned to the ipsilateral pathology. Visualization can be facilitated by redirecting the microscope and tilting the operating table toward the surgeon. Ipsilateral subarticular decompression is begun by removing the medial aspect of the hypertrophied inferior articular process with a burr, Kerrison, or osteotome (Fig. 8). Laterally, following the resected cephalad edge of the caudal trailing L5 lamina should reveal the medial border of the L5 pedicle. From here, the L5 nerve root can be identified and the hypertrophic medial shelf of the superior facet can be safely resected by progressing cephalad along the medial edge of the pedicle. The partial medial facetectomy is performed in a trumpeted fashion such that greater amounts of deep bone are removed than superficial bone (to maximize decompression while minimizing facet resection). Care is taken to preserve at least half of the facet joint to maintain stability. Adequate ipsilateral subarticular

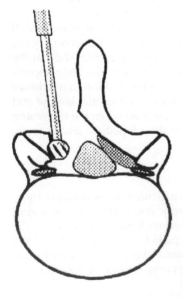

FIGURE 8 Ipsilateral subarticular decompression. Ipsilateral subarticular decompression is achieved by removing the medial aspect of the hypertrophied inferior articular process with a burr, Kerrison, or osteotome. *Source*: From Ref. 14.

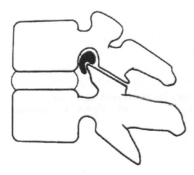

FIGURE 9 Ipsilateral foraminal decompression. The most common cause of foraminal compression is the cephalad tip of the superior facet. Through the intertransverse window, the capsule of the caudal facet joint is opened laterally and the tip of the superior facet is resected. *Source:* From Ref. 14.

decompression is achieved when the facet is flush with the ipsilateral pedicle and the traversing nerve root passes freely toward its foramen.

Ipsilateral Foraminal Decompression

When necessary, ipsilateral foraminal decompression is performed from outside–in using the intertransverse interval. We generally do not perform an ipsilateral foraminal decompression with a laminoplasty unless the patient has bilateral leg pain and radiographic evidence of severe bilateral foraminal stenosis. Also, as the L5 pars is wider than the other levels, an adequate foraminotomy from inside the canal can often be achieved while preserving enough of the pars. Therefore, an ipsilateral foraminotomy is rarely performed for L5.

First, the paraspinal muscles are stripped further laterally to the tips of the transverse processes. The pars and the caudal facet joint are clearly identified. The most common source of foraminal compression is the cephalad tip of the superior facet. Therefore, the capsule of the caudal facet joint is opened laterally and the tip of the superior facet is resected (Fig. 9). The intertransverse membrane is then detached medially using bipolar cautery. The flap of the intertransverse membrane is started inside the facet joint and carried cephalad. The foraminotomy is then continued from lateral to the pars into the canal. A blunt probe placed in the foramen from inside the canal can serve to protect the nerve root. After adequate decompression, a probe should readily pass from inside the canal into the extraforaminal zone and the tip of the probe can be visualized from the intertransverse interval.

Closure and Postoperative Management

Prior to closure, the decompression is reassessed to ensure that the exiting and traversing nerve roots are mobile and pass freely into their respective foramina. The resected bony surfaces are also inspected to ensure that no sharp edges or oozing surfaces exist. Hemostasis is achieved by coating the raw bony surfaces with bone wax and temporarily filling the epidural dead space with gelfoam. The paraspinal muscles are injected with 0.5% Marcaine® for postoperative analgesia and to allow the muscles to oppose the bone. The wound is irrigated with antibiotic solution and routinely closed in layers. A postoperative AP radiograph is obtained in the recovery room to ensure that the correct level has been treated. Patients may be discharged same day with activity as tolerated, provided there have been no intraoperative complications.

COMPLICATIONS AND MANAGEMENT
Complications

The most common complication during lumbar segmental sublaminoplasty is inadvertent dural tear. When encountered, a watertight repair should be performed. There was one dural tear in the two published series totaling 59 patients. In the same studies, there was one wound infection, which was successfully treated with oral antibiotics. Other potential complications include excessive pars resection with postoperative fracture, epidural hematoma, and neurologic injury. However, these complications have not been reported with the sublaminoplasty.

Pitfalls

Neurologic injury can be prevented by careful attention to the anatomic location of the nerve roots at all times during the procedure. Prior to aggressive bone/soft tissue resection, the nerve root should be clearly identified based on its relationship to the pedicle. In mild disease, the nerve roots appear round with its cuff of vasculature and can be readily distinguished from the other tissues. However, in severe disease, the nerve roots may be flattened and can be mistaken for protruding annulus or ligamentum flavum. In addition, using the Kerrison rongeur parallel to the nerve roots can avoid inadvertently biting the nerve roots.

Generally, little epidural bleeding is encountered during central canal decompression. However, epidural venous bleeding is common in the lateral zone. To avoid loss of visualization by bleeding, bilateral central decompression is completed prior to any lateral decompression. When bleeding is encountered, it should be tamponaded with a small strip of gelfoam and Cottonoid®. Attention may be directed to another area of decompression while waiting for hemostasis.

Bailouts

Conversion of a sublaminoplasty to a conventional laminectomy may be necessary in case of dense adhesions in the midline dura or in the event of an inadvertent dural tear. Conversion to a standard bilateral exposure may also be necessary in patients with significant lordosis or obesity where contralateral visualization is poor.

OUTCOMES

The effectiveness of lumbar segmental sublaminoplasty in enlarging the cross-sectional areas of the spinal canal and foramen has been confirmed in cadaveric and clinical studies using postoperative CT (16–18). Clinical outcomes following lumbar sublaminoplasty have been published in two small studies. Weiner and McCulloch (19) prospectively followed a cohort of 30 patients who underwent lumbar sublaminoplasty for symptomatic spinal stenosis without spondylolisthesis. At nine months follow-up, 87% of the patients rated the surgery as very or fairly successful. Average Neurogenic Claudication Outcome Scores (NCOS) were approximately doubled. There were no intraoperative complications. Spetzger et al. (18) retrospectively reviewed a similar cohort of 29 patients. At average 18 months follow-up, 93% of the patients demonstrated marked improvement in walking distance. Eighty-eight percent of the patients reported good or excellent results. One patient had a dural tear and another required reoperation to decompress an additional level.

SUMMARY

Unilateral hemi-laminotomy for bilateral lumbar decompression is a minimally invasive procedure that allows maximal neural decompression. All compressive elements can be adequately visualized and addressed while limiting paraspinal muscle stripping to one side and preserving the stabilizing ligaments.

Brief Indications

Symptomatic degenerative lumbar spinal stenosis without significant associated instability (spondylolisthesis or scoliosis) which has failed conservative therapy.

Outcome

Good to excellent in over 85% of the patients.

Complications

- Dural tear
- Infection

- Pars fracture
- Epidural hematoma
- Neurologic injury.

REFERENCES

1. Thomas NW, Rea GL, Pikul BK, Mervis LJ, Irsik R, McGregor JM. Quantitative outcome and radiographic comparisons between laminectomy and laminotomy in the treatment of acquired lumbar stenosis. Neurosurgery 1997; 41:567–574, discussion 574–575.
2. Tsai RY, Yang RS, Bray RS Jr. Microscopic laminotomies for degenerative lumbar spinal stenosis. J Spinal Disord 1998; 11:389–394.
3. Patond KR, Kakodia SC. Interlaminar decompression in lumbar canal stenosis. Neurol India 1999; 47:286–289.
4. Weiner BK, Fraser RD, Peterson M. Spinous process osteotomies to facilitate lumbar decompressive surgery. Spine 1999; 24:62–66.
5. Kleeman TJ, Hiscoe AC, Berg EE. Patient outcomes after minimally destabilizing lumbar stenosis decompression: the "Port-Hole" technique. Spine 2000; 25:865–870.
6. Yucesoy K, Ozer E. Inverse laminoplasty for the treatment of lumbar spinal stenosis. Spine 2002; 27:E316–E320.
7. Kawaguchi Y, Kanamori M, Ishihara H, et al. Clinical and radiographic results of expansive lumbar laminoplasty in patients with spinal stenosis. J Bone Joint Surg Am 2004; 86-A:1698–1703.
8. Adachi K, Futami T, Ebihara A, et al. Spinal canal enlargement procedure by restorative laminoplasty for the treatment of lumbar canal stenosis. Spine J 2003; 3:471–478.
9. Postacchini F, Cinotti G, Perugia D, Gumina S. The surgical treatment of central lumbar stenosis. Multiple laminotomy compared with total laminectomy. J Bone Joint Surg Br 1993; 75:386–392.
10. Matsudaira K, Yamazaki T, Seichi A, et al. Spinal stenosis in grade I degenerative lumbar spondylolisthesis: a comparative study of outcomes following laminoplasty and laminectomy with instrumented spinal fusion. J Orthop Sci 2005; 10:270–276.
11. Arnoldi CC, Brodsky AE, Cauchoix J, et al. Lumbar spinal stenosis and nerve root entrapment syndromes. Definition and classification. Clin Orthop Relat Res 1976; 115:4–5.
12. Lee CK, Rauschning W, Glenn W. Lateral lumbar spinal canal stenosis: classification, pathologic anatomy and surgical decompression. Spine 1988; 13:313–320.
13. Wiltse LL, Berger PE, McCulloch JA. A system for reporting the size and location of lesions in the spine. Spine 1997; 22:1534–1537.
14. McCulloch JA, Young PH. Essentials of Spinal Microsurgery. Philadelphia, Pennsylvania: Lippincott-Raven, 1998.
15. McCulloch JA, Snook D, Kruse CF. Advantages of the operating microscope in lumbar spine surgery. Instr Course Lect 2002; 51:243–245.
16. Poletti CE. Central lumbar stenosis caused by ligamentum flavum: unilateral laminotomy for bilateral ligamentectomy: preliminary report of two cases. Neurosurgery 1995; 37:343–347.
17. Spetzger U, Bertalanffy H, Reinges MH, Gilsbach JM. Unilateral laminotomy for bilateral decompression of lumbar spinal stenosis. Part II: Clinical experiences. Acta Neurochir (Wien) 1997; 139:397–403.
18. Spetzger U, Bertalanffy H, Naujokat C, von Keyserlingk DG, Gilsbach JM. Unilateral laminotomy for bilateral decompression of lumbar spinal stenosis. Part I: Anatomical and surgical considerations. Acta Neurochir (Wien) 1997; 139:392–396.
19. Weiner BK, Walker M, Brower RS, McCulloch JA. Microdecompression for lumbar spinal canal stenosis. Spine 1999; 24:2268–2272.

13 | Percutaneous Automated Lumbar Discectomy

Sushil K. Basra and Michael Vives
Department of Orthopedics, University of Medicine and Dentistry of New Jersey, Newark, New Jersey, U.S.A.

INTRODUCTION

Low back pain and sciatica are major causes of morbidity in the United States. In many cases, this may be caused by a herniated lumbar disc. As the disc material bulges, it can impinge on a nerve root and cause symptoms. The goal of treatment for this condition is a reduction or elimination of associated symptoms with the least risk and morbidity. Initially, a course of conservative therapy is prescribed to the patient, which includes analgesics and physical therapy. If this fails, surgery is an option. Traditionally, surgery for a herniated disc involves an open procedure, whereby the displaced material and the pressure on the nerve root is removed. While the results in selected patients are predictable, morbidity and complications associated with open discectomy have been described (1,2). As a result, various less invasive, percutaneous techniques have been developed. These include chemonucleolysis, automated percutaneous lumbar discectomy (APLD), laser discectomy, and arthroscopic microdiscectomy. Of these, automated APLD has had the most cases worldwide (more than 125,000), most articles published, and has a remarkable safety record with no reports of permanent nerve injury or great vessel injury in over 50 series in the literature (3). The basic concept of APLD involves a decrease in the disc volume, which leads to a decreased disc pressure and decreased nerve impingement. The purpose of this chapter is to review the development, techniques, patient selection, outcomes, and complications associated with APLD.

HISTORY AND DEVELOPMENT OF AUTOMATED PERCUTANEOUS LUMBAR DISCECTOMY

Open discectomy has been a very effective method for treating patients who have failed physical therapy. However, it is not without its morbidity and complications. A number of large studies have demonstrated these complications. Ramirez et al. detailed the incidence of acute, major complications in a population of 28,395 patients who underwent open lumbar discectomy for radiculopathy in the United States in a community setting (1). Their incidence of a major complication was 1 in 64 patients. The incidence of a major neurological deficit was 29 per 10,000, 10.7 per 10,000 for a pulmonary embolus, and 5.6 per 10,000 for myocardial infarction. The overall incidence of death was 5.9 per 10,000. Of note, there was no difference in complication rates between orthopedic surgeons and neurosurgeons. Stolke et al. demonstrated a complication rate of 13.7% in a prospective study of 481 lumbar discectomies performed by neurosurgeons (2). This included a 1% rate of discitis, one death and three nerve injuries. These complications have lead to the search of less invasive and less morbid procedures such as APLD.

Hijikata et al. were the first to introduce a percutaneous technique for the treatment of herniated discs in 1975 (4). Their technique involved the use of a posterolateral approach to the spine, guide pipes, cannulas, an annulus cutter, discography, forceps, and graspers. Other authors including Kambin et al. and Hoppenfeld introduced variations of this manual technique based on the same concept (5,6). Their method involved percutaneously gaining access to the disc space and then manually removing some of the disc material with graspers to relieve pressure on the nerve roots. Their studies have shown good results with these techniques. However,

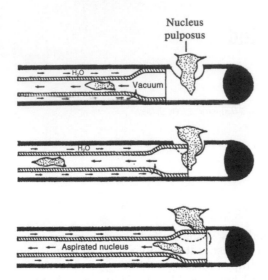

Nucleus
pulposus

FIGURE 1 Drawing of nucleotome illustrating suction through the central bore. The inner cutting sleeve is pneumatically driven across the side port where the disc material is cut. The disc material is then aspirated away, suspended in saline.

there were complications reported such as vascular injuries (iliolumbar artery, venous) and discitis. These may have been related to the multiple entries into the disc space required.

APLD was first introduced in 1984 by Onik et al. (7). The procedure utilizes the nucleotome aspiration probe (Clarus Medical, LLC, Minneapolis, Minnesota, U.S.A.). The probe functions by aspirating nucleus pulposus material through a side port by a sucking and cutting action. There is a 2-mm reciprocating suction cutter. This takes advantage of an inner cutting sleeve, which is pneumatically driven across the side port. The disc material is cut and carried away in a saline solution, suspended between the wall of the nucleotome and the inner cutting sleeve, as seen in Figure 1. This is a relatively safe procedure because the nucleus material is cut and sucked out but the annulus is left intact (except for the entry site). Onik et al. have developed smaller instruments to be used. This, in theory, decreases the chance of nerve or vascular injury. Furthermore, once the probe enters the central portion of the disc it remains there until all the aspiration is completed without having to be removed and replaced multiple times. This reduces the chance of contamination and discitis by one-fifth of the rate with open procedures (8). Currently, the method introduced by Onik et al. is the most widely used method of percutaneous discectomy.

PATIENT SELECTION

Proper patient selection is necessary for predictable results. Patients with leg symptoms greater than back pain are better candidates than those with primarily axial symptoms. In addition, a minimum six-week course of nonoperative treatment should be attempted. This includes anti-inflammatory medications, active (functional-based) physical therapy, and modalities. It is not atypical for patients to have up to six months of physical therapy prior to an APLD. Most studies exclude patients with discogenic disease from being a candidate for APLD. However, a large study by Bonaldi of 1047 patients, evaluated a subgroup of 188 patients with purely discogenic pain. He demonstrated an excellent or good result in 79% of these patients undergoing APLD (9). Other relative clinical contraindications for APLD are workers compensation and previous open surgery at the same level.

There are certain radiographic criteria used to select patients for APLD. All disc herniations should be of the protrusion variation. These, by definition, are contained by either the annulus fibrosis or the posterior longitudinal ligament. Failed procedures will likely result if APLD is performed on patients with free fragments or extruded discs (10). In addition, those patients with disc herniations compromising greater than 50% of the thecal sac should not be treated by APLD as the literature demonstrates that 90% of these have a free fragment (11).

Other radiographic contraindications to APLD include spinal stenosis, lateral recess stenosis, and calcified disc herniations.

Most patients diagnosed with herniated discs are imaged with magnetic resonance imaging (MRI). The MRI will help determine the type of disc herniation (i.e., protrusion, extrusion, sequestered). In addition, MRI will help identify spinal stenosis, arthropathy, and degenerative disc disease. As mentioned previously, the size of the herniation may influence outcome, and this can be evaluated by MRI. Finally, the shape of the herniation, as seen on MRI, may be helpful. Extruded fragments are represented by irregular herniations, that is, they have sharp angles to the annulus. Protruded (contained) herniated discs typically have smooth, regular margins. Some authors advocate a preoperative localization computed tomography (CT) scan (8,10). The CT establishes the exact entry point and pathway for the procedure. More importantly, it excludes the possibility of bowel being in the path of the probe.

A number of practitioners are performing discography routinely prior to APLD. Discography can distinguish between a contained disc and an extruded one. Contrast material contained within the disc space and not flowing to the epidural space is indicative of a protruding/contained disc and suggests appropriate candidacy for APLD.

TECHNIQUE FOR L1–L5 LEVELS

Prior to beginning this procedure, a number of resources will be required. In addition to the physician/surgeon, an anesthetist, a scrub nurse, a circulating nurse and a radiology technician (C-arm operator) will need to be present. The required equipment necessary for the procedure includes the nucleotome console, portable fluoroscopy (C-arm), a radiolucent operating table, a compressed air tank, local anesthesia, and the usual anesthetic-monitoring devices.

Patient positioning and equipment placement are crucial. The patient is typically positioned in the lateral decubitus position with the most symptomatic side facing up toward the ceiling. The patient should be flexed to decrease lumbar lordosis and the hips and shoulders need to be stabilized to prevent any rotation. Care is taken to pad all bony prominences. Some physicians prefer to place the patient in a prone position. In this position, the patient also needs to be flexed to open the disc spaces posteriorly. Regardless of the patient position, the surgical technique and concepts remain the same. With the patient in the lateral position the equipment is next placed in the appropriate location. The physician will stand posterior to the patient, facing his or her back. The anesthetist will be at the head of the operating table. The C-arm is placed on the opposite side of the table from the physician so it is anterior to the patient. The C-arm monitor is placed between the C-arm and the anesthetist, toward the patient's head. The APLD equipment is placed at the foot of the table and a sterile table is placed behind the surgeon or a Mayo stand is placed adjacent to the surgeon. Appropriate anteroposterior (AP) and lateral views of the desired level must be obtainable prior to beginning the procedure. On the AP view, the spinous processes must be midway between the pedicles. On the lateral view, the vertebral endplates should be clearly visualized, as well as the appropriate disc space.

The preoperative CT is reviewed to identify the correct entry point and ensure no bowel or organs are in the trajectory of the probe. At this point, the field is prepped and draped, and the C-arm is also draped. Appropriate perioperative antibiotics are given. A posterolateral entry point, seen in Figure 2, is used which is usually 8 to 12 cm from the midline, staying both parallel to the disc space and midway between the desired endplates. A guide needle is used to

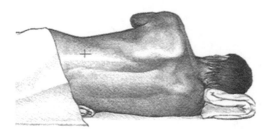

FIGURE 2 Approximate starting point on the skin in the lateral position.

verify, fluoroscopically, the level of the disc space and the midline of the disc. A mark on the skin is placed and local anesthesia is applied to the skin and along the proposed path of the procedure with a long spinal needle. General anesthesia is contraindicated in APLD to decrease the possibility of nerve root injury during the passage of instruments.

A small skin incision is made at the proposed entry site and the guide needle is inserted slowly through the low back musculature. The insertion is visualized fluoroscopically on the lateral view. The needle must be parallel to and midway between the appropriate endplates. The goal of this posterolateral approach is to reach the center of the disc via a trajectory in which the instruments pass posterior to the nerve root and anterior to the superior articular facet (8). Evaluation of certain radiographic landmarks prevents injury to vital structures. On the lateral, an imaginary line along the posterior vertebral bodies is visualized. Anterior to this line lie the nerves, bowel, and great vessels. The tip of the guide needle must reach this point. At the same time, on the AP view, a line is visualized along the medial margins of the pedicles. The thecal sac is presumed to lie medial to this line. The tip of the needle must also be at, but not yet beyond, this point. These positions are demonstrated in Figures 3A and B. Once at these points, a gritty sensation representing the annulus may be felt. If during the insertion of the guide needle the patient experiences any radicular pain, the needle is to be withdrawn and slightly redirected. The radicular symptoms imply that the nerve root has been touched.

Once the needle is identified to be in the correct position, it is inserted into the center of the disc. This central intradiscal position is verified by fluoroscopy. At this point, the knob attached to the guide needle is removed. The straight cannula with a tapered dilator is passed over the guide needle and inserted down to the level of the annulus. This position is verified fluoroscopically in both the AP and lateral views. It is important to monitor the patient for any radicular symptoms during the insertion of the cannula. If radicular symptoms are encountered, the cannula should be angled slightly more posterior to avoid the anterior traversing nerve root. In addition, the guide needle should be monitored to ensure that it has not advanced any further with the insertion of the cannula and dilator. Once this step has been accomplished, the dilator is removed over the guide needle and the cannula is left in place. The dilator extends 2 mm beyond the tip of the cannula. Therefore, the cannula may need to be slightly advanced to ensure it is against the annulus. Once the cannula is against the annulus, the cannula stop (which is a circular device attached to the cannula) can be lowered down against the skin.

The trephine (used to incise the annulus) is placed over the guide wire, through the cannula. This trephine is placed down to the level of the annulus (as verified on fluoroscopy). The trephine is rotated in a clockwise direction with slight pressure to incise the annulus. After

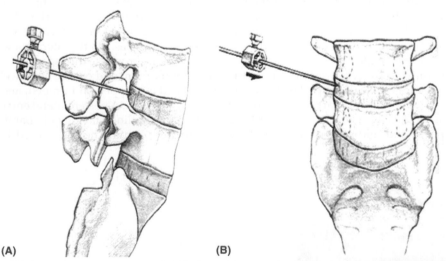

(A)   **(B)**

FIGURE 3   (**A**) Lateral view demonstrating the position of the guide needle on the posterior aspect of the L4–L5 disc, along the posterior vertebral line. (**B**) Anteroposterior view demonstrating the position of the guide needle on the lateral aspect of the L4–L5 disc, lateral to the medial margins of the pedicles.

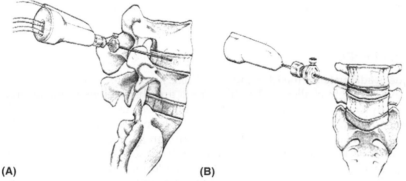

(A)   **(B)**

FIGURE 4   (**A**) Lateral view demonstrating the correct position of the probe in the L4–L5 disc. (**B**) Anteroposterior view demonstrating the correct position of the probe in the L4–L5 disc.

the annulus has been incised, the cannula stop is loosened and the cannula and the trephine are advance until the distal ends are about 5mm into the disc. The cannula stop is repositioned against the skin. The trephine is removed from the cannula followed by removal of the guide needle. Gentle forward pressure is held on the cannula while the guide needle is removed to prevent improper positioning.

The nucleotome probe, with the cannula seal nut, is placed through the cannula. The diameter of the probe is 2 mm, with options available for 2.5- and 3.5-mm diameter probes. The seal nut secures to the cannula stop. There should be a smooth placement of the probe through the cannula. If the probe does not slide easily through the cannula, an obstruction needs to be ruled out. The correct positioning is verified fluoroscopically. The correct positioning of the probe is shown in Figures 4A and B. The probe has an etched mark on its shaft. When this mark is at the level of the seal nut, the cutting port of the probe is 8 mm beyond the tip of the cannula. Figure 5 demonstrates that the ridge on the probe handle faces in the same direction as the cutting port of the probe. Initially, the cutting port should be facing the direction of the herniation. The probe is started via a foot control. At first, the cutting rate of the probe should be placed at the maximum level. This minimizes the chance of clogging the ports. There are three tubes coming off the probe handle. One connects to the suction canister, one connects to irrigation, and one to the air pressure/vacuum. The aspiration process should be bloodless as the nucleus is avascular. There may be slight bleeding from the skin site. If bleeding is encountered during the aspiration, the correct position of the probe should be verified. The angulation of the probe is slightly adjusted in the plane of the disc. Excessive force is never placed on the probe handle. The tip of the probe can break or be damaged against the vertebral endplates. This process is finished once no further disc material is obtained. This usually lasts 20 to 30 minutes. Once this has been completed, the cutting action of the probe is stopped. The probe is withdrawn into the

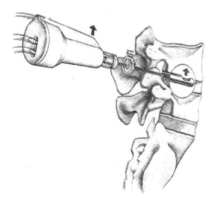

FIGURE 5   The ridge on the probe handle faces the same direction of the cutting side port.

cannula and both the probe and cannula are simultaneously removed. A suture is placed on the skin with a small sterile dressing.

TECHNIQUE FOR L5–S1 LEVEL

The preceding technique is adequate for the L1–L2 to L4–L5 disc levels. However, reaching the L5–S1 disc space may pose a slight challenge. The iliac crests are obstructions to the desired path. This was addressed by a modified technique by Onik et al. in 1989 using a curved cannula (12). The same equipment and patient positioning are needed. The patient can be either in the prone or lateral position. To obtain the entry point on the skin, an AP view is obtained. The sacro-iliac joint is identified on the affected side. A guide needle can be used as fluoroscopic marker and is placed parallel on the sacro-iliac joint. This should extend superiorly until it intersects the top of the iliac crest. A mark is made along this line on the skin. Next, the guide needle is placed parallel to the top of the iliac crest and extended medially toward the line delineating the sacro-iliac joint. The intersection of these lines will be the approximate entry point for the approach. These lines are seen in Figure 6.

Under fluoroscopic guidance in the lateral view, a long spinal needle is used to give local anesthesia and advance in the trajectory of the L5–S1 disc. The trajectory to the disc is verified with this step and adjustments are made as necessary. Once again, general anesthesia is contraindicated for the same reasons stated for the L1–L5 levels. Next, the guide needle is placed along this trajectory. The same anatomic landmarks are observed while placing the guide needle. The tip of the needle should be at the posterior vertebral body line on the lateral view, as seen in Figure 7, and lateral to the medial aspect of the pedicles in the AP view. At this level, the other structures that are at risk for injury are the iliac vessels. As long as the previous landmarks are observed, injury is unlikely. A gritty sensation is felt once the needle is against the annulus and this is verified on fluoroscopy. Sometimes, the straight cannula and dilators can be used to gain access to the L5–S1 disc space if the iliac crests are lower. However, the curved cannula and dilator are often used at this step. They are placed over the guide needle down to the level of the annulus. There is a guide on this curved cannula to aid in its rotation and to keep track of the direction of the curve. It may be difficult to dilate through the tough lumbar fascia with the curved dilator. Therefore, the straight cannula may be used first, followed by the curved dilator. The ensuing steps are the same. A trephine is used to incise the annulus. The cannula and guide needle are advanced into the disc. The guide needle is carefully removed and the nucleotome is placed through the cannula. The probe is straight but flexible enough to be bent around the curve of the cannula. The correct positioning for the curved cannula is shown in Figures 8A and B. Once the disc material is removed, the probe and the cannula are carefully removed. The skin is sutured and a small sterile dressing is applied.

The postoperative protocol is essentially the same as one for a microdiscectomy. The patient is prohibited from any heavy lifting or excessive bending/twisting for six weeks.

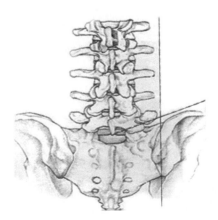

FIGURE 6 Posterior view demonstrating the approximate positioning and intersection of lines to determine the starting point to gain access to the L5–S1 disc.

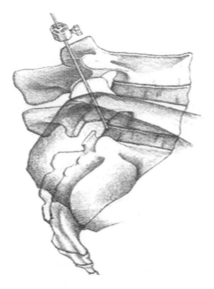

FIGURE 7 Lateral view demonstrating the trajectory of a guide needle to the L5–S1 disc. Note the acute angulation needed to clear the iliac crest.

Patients who have less physically demanding jobs can usually return to work in two to three days. The decision to send patients for physical therapy is based on the individual patient. Most physicians do send the patient for therapy to promote functional recovery.

OUTCOMES OF AUTOMATED PERCUTANEOUS LUMBAR DISCECTOMY

There are a number of studies published in peer-reviewed journals that have reported the outcomes of APLD. While the majority of studies report favorable outcomes, they also highlight that appropriate patient selection is crucial. In addition, experience with the procedure plays a factor.

Onik et al., in a prospective multi-institutional study, evaluated 327 patients who met the strict criteria previously stated (13). The overall success rate was 246 (75.2%) of 327 patients. Success was defined as improvement in radicular pain, no longer taking narcotics, improved functional status, and patient satisfaction. Forty-one of the patients went on to an open surgery.

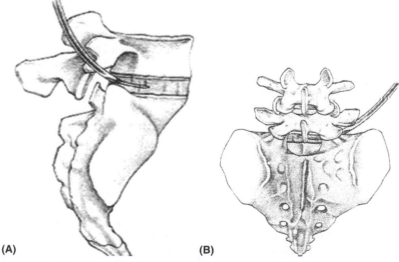

(A)   **(B)**

FIGURE 8 **(A)** Lateral view demonstrating the correct position of the curved cannula and probe in the L5–S1 disc. **(B)** Anteroposterior view demonstrating the correct position of the curved cannula and probe in the L5–S1 disc.

There were two complications, one of which was a psoas hematoma treated with observation and one case of discitis treated with antibiotics.

Davis et al. prospectively evaluated 518 patients who were at least one year post-APLD (14). They showed a total of 439 (85%) of 518 patients having success. Success was defined as improvement in pain, no further use of narcotics, return to preinjury functional status, and patient satisfaction. Seventy percent of 36 patients older than 60 years of age were successfully treated. In addition, 40 of 44 patients who had previous spinal surgery were successfully treated. They concluded that previous surgery at the same or adjacent level should not deter one from performing APLD. This remains a debatable issue among authors. Of the 439 patients successfully treated, 70% returned to work in less than two weeks. There were no reported complications.

Bonaldi evaluated 1047 patients six months after having APLD (9). He used the very strict inclusion and exclusion criteria mentioned previously in this text. The results were excellent or good in 67.5% of the 1047 patients. In addition, he showed excellent or good results in 66 (79.5%) of 83 patients aged 70 or more and in 149 (79%) of 188 patients with purely discogenic back pain. Bonaldi reported two cases (0.17%) of discitis and one acute hematoma of the iliopsoas muscle. Of the 1047 patients, 125 (12%) eventually underwent an open surgery for their symptoms.

Onik presented the summation of 11 papers at the International Percutaneous Meeting in 1989 (15). Of the 3088 patients included in all the studies he quoted there was an overall success rate of 77%. The range varied from 61% to 82% success rates. There were only a total of 12 (0.004%) complications. There were no reported deaths, vascular, or nerve injuries. Another interesting finding reported by Onik was that the average amount of disc material recovered from the procedures was 3.2 g.

Teng et al. in a study from China, conducted a prospective, multi-institutional study as well (16). They evaluated 1474 patients available for follow-up after one year. This study showed an excellent or good result in 82% of the patients. This was defined as either complete resolution of the symptoms or near complete resolution. Interestingly, 79% of patients who had symptoms for greater than two years had an excellent or good result, while 85% of those who had symptoms less than two years had an excellent or good result. This difference was statistically significant. In addition, patients younger than 60 had an 84% rate of excellent or good result, while those older than 60 had a 76% success rate. This difference was also significant. There were nine complications. All of these complications were discitis, eventually treated by antibiotics.

Chatterjee et al. conducted the only randomized prospective study comparing APLD with microdiscectomy (17). This study had a total of 71 patients. Of the 31 randomized to the APLD group, nine (29%) achieved a successful outcome of good or excellent. Of the 40 patients assigned to the microdiscectomy group, 32 (80%) had successful outcomes. This study was designed to recruit more patients but was stopped because of the large discrepancy between the two groups. Chatterjee et al. do mention that a discogram was not routinely obtained in their study and this may have effected their categorization of the type of disc herniation.

Overall, the outcomes of patients, who are carefully selected by the criteria mentioned earlier, are favorable. The majority of patients showed improvement in function, pain, and satisfaction. Those patients who did not report improvement after APLD, were still able to benefit from an open surgery or decided against all further intervention.

COMPLICATIONS OF AUTOMATED PERCUTANEOUS LUMBAR DISCECTOMY

The literature clearly shows that the complication rate from APLD is relatively low (9,13,15,16). The overall rate appears to be around 1%. Among the various studies, discitis (0.2%) and hematoma formation are the most likely complications (8). There have been no reports of any major neurologic or vascular injuries related to APLD. There are a number of theoretical reasons why the complication rate is low. First, its performance under local anesthesia decreases the chance for nerve injury and avoids the risks of general anesthesia. Second, the spinal canal is not entered so the chance for epidural fibrosis is minimal. Third, there is no bone or ligament removal. Therefore, there is no chance of developing postoperative instability. Finally, the disc is entered only once with the probe thereby decreasing the chances of infection as compared with an open procedure.

CONCLUSIONS

Automated percutaneous lumbar discectomy has been shown to be effective and safe in the management of patients with contained herniated lumbar discs. Numerous procedures have been described to treat herniated discs in a minimally invasive technique. Of these procedures, APLD has the most reported cases and has been the most widely studied. The outcomes reported with APLD are favorable. However, careful patient selection is imperative in determining the outcome. Knowledge of the anatomy and technique are important in preventing complications. The complication rate with APLD is low making this a relatively safe procedure. Finally, if APLD is deemed unsuccessful in a patient, or there is a reherniation, the option for an open procedure is still available.

Acknowledgment
The figures and supporting material have been provided by Clarus Medical, LLC, Minneapolis, Minnesota, U.S.A. We gratefully acknowledge their contribution to this chapter.

REFERENCES

1. Ramirez LF, Thisted R. Complications and demographic characteristics of patients undergoing lumbar diskectomy in community hospitals. Neurosurgery 1989; 58:226–231.
2. Stolke D, Sollman WP, Seifert V. Intra and postoperative complications in lumbar disk surgery. Spine 1989; 14:56–58.
3. Onik GM, Kambin P, Chang MK. Minimally invasive disc surgery: nucleotomy versus fragmentectomy. Spine 1997; 22(7):827–830.
4. Hijakata S. Percutaneous nucleotomy: a new concept technique and 12 years experience. Clin Orthop 1989; 238:9–23.
5. Hoppenfeld S. Percutaneous removal of herniated lumbar discs: 50 cases with 10 year follow up periods. Clin Orthop 1989; 238:92–106.
6. Kambin P, Schaffer JL. Percutaneous lumbar discectomy: review of 100 patients and current practice. Clin Orthop 1989; 289:24–34.
7. Onik GM, Helms CA, Ginsburg L, et al. Percutaneous lumbar discectomy using an aspiration arobe. AJNR 1985; 6:290–293.
8. Onik G, Helms CA. Automated percutaneous lumbar discectomy. AJR 1991; 156:531–538.
9. Bonaldi G. Automated percutaneous lumbar discectomy: technique, indications and clinical follow up in over 1000 patients. Neuroradiology 2003; 45:735–743.
10. Maroon JC, Onik G, Sternau L. Percutaneous automated discectomy: a new approach to the lumbar spine. Clin Orthop 1989; 238:64–70.
11. Fries JW, Ahodeely DA, Vijungco JG, et al. CT of herniated and extruded nucleus pulposus. J Comput Assist Tomogr 1982; 6(5):874–887.
12. Onik G, Maroon J, Davis GW. Automated percutaneous discectomy at the L5–S1 level. Clin Orthop 1989; 238:71–76.
13. Onik G, Mooney V, Maroon J, et al. Automated percutaneous discectomy: a prospective multi-institutional study. Neurosurgery 1990; 26:228–233.
14. Davis G, Onik G, Helms C. Automated percutaneous discectomy. Spine 1991; 16:359–363.
15. Onik G. Summation of APLD clinical experience, Paper Thirty Eight, presented at the International Percutaneous Meeting, 1989, Spain.
16. Teng GJ, Jeffery RF, Guo JH, et al. Automated percutaneous lumbar discectomy: a prospective multi-institutional study. J Vasc Interv Radiol 1997; 8(3):457–463
17. Chatterjee S, Roy PF, Findley GF. Report of a controlled clinical trial comparing APLD and lumbar discectomy in the treatment of contained lumbar disc herniation. Spine 1995; 20(9):734–738.

14 | Chemical Dissolution of a Herniated Lumbar Disc: A Review

Henry Ahn
Division of Orthopedic Surgery, St. Michael's Hospital, University of Toronto, Toronto, Ontario, Canada

Raja Rampersaud
Division of Orthopedic Surgery and Neurosurgery, Toronto Western Hospital, University of Toronto, Toronto, Ontario, Canada

INTRODUCTION

Chemical dissolution or chemonucleolysis of a lumbar disc herniation involves the intradiscal injection of an enzyme, such as chymopapain or purified collagenase. The most common form of enzymatic intradiscal therapy is chymopapain, which was isolated from the latex of the *Carica* papaya fruit (1). Chymopapain catalyzes the hydrolytic cleavage of the noncollagen protein connections of proteoglycan aggregates within the disc (2), thereby reducing the water-binding capacity of the nucleus pulposus, which lowers the intradiscal pressure and reduces the magnitude of the disc protrusion compressing the nerve root (3,4). Smith first reported the use of chymopapain in patients with sciatica in 1964 (5). It was not until 1975, when trials began in the United States and Canada. The initial results from a double-blind study conducted at the Walter Reed Army Medical Center showed no statistical difference between good and excellent results for chymopapain (58%) and placebo (49%) (6). However, it was later determined that the study had numerous faults. Further large double-blind trials provided statistical evidence showing the benefit of chymopapain and was granted Food and Drug Administration's (FDA) approval for clinical use in 1982 (7–9).

Collagenase is another enzyme used for intradiscal therapy that splits type 2 collagen fibers found in the nucleus pulposis (10). There have been no reports of anaphylaxis or allergic reactions, but adjacent level endplate erosions have been reported (11). It has not been studied as thoroughly as chymopapain (2). However, the indications and injection technique is similar to chymopapain.

INDICATIONS

Chymopapain is only indicated in the treatment of *clinically significant* sciatica as a result of herniated lumbar nucleus pulposus that has not responded to nonoperative measures such as physiotherapy, nonsteroidal anti-inflammatories, and nerve root blocks, for at least six-week period (2,7). The radiologic level of the disc herniation must match the physical signs and symptoms of the lumbar radiculopathy, and should ideally be a single level. A successful intervention depends on the presence of a contained "soft disc herniation" of nucleus pulposis, rather than a calcified disc as determined by computed tomography (CT) scan (12). Age can be a factor, with better outcomes in patients younger than 30 years of age compared with patients older than 50 who have less mucoprotein to be hydrolyzed and more potential for osseous compression as the cause of the radiculopathy (7,12).

The technique should not be used in patients with back dominant pain, cauda equina syndrome, progressive neurologic deficits, sequestered disc herniations, root compression because of osseous structures such as that in spinal stenosis, arachnoiditis, discitis, spondylolisthesis, recurrent disc herniation after surgery at the same level, or if there is a known allergy to chymopapain or papaya (Table 1) (7,13). Repeat chemonucleolysis is not approved by the FDA. Intradiscal therapy should not be used in pregnant women, as there have been no studies looking

TABLE 1 List of Absolute and Relative Contraindications to Chemonucleolysis with Chymopapain

Contraindications to chemonucleolysis
Absolute contraindications
Allergic sensitivity to chymopapain or papaya
Absence of a disc herniation
Sequestered disc herniation or calcified disc herniation
Spinal stenosis or spondylolisthesis
Cauda equina or progressive neurologic deficits
Pregnant patient
Arachnoiditis
Previous chemonucleolysis with chymopapain
Recurrent disc herniation after surgery at the same level
Relative contraindications
Back dominant or nonradicular pain
History of discitis
Diabetes mellitus

at effect on fetal development. Furthermore, the technique requires fluoroscopy for localization of the needle. Patients with diabetes mellitus, especially with diabetic neuropathy, may not have improvement of their pain following chemonucleolysis and have poorer clinical outcomes (2).

Standard open microdiscectomy is indicated in situations where there is disc sequestration, cauda equina syndrome, progressive neurologic deficits, if the disc is calcified, if there is osseous nerve root compression, or if the patient is allergic to the enzyme. Chemonucleolysis has a time-dependent effect and will not provide the immediate decompression required in urgent cases such as cauda equina syndrome and progressive neurologic deficits.

CONSIDERATIONS FOR PREOPERATIVE PLANNING

As with all interventions careful judgment needs to be utilized in selecting patients for chemonucleolysis. A routine, spine-specific, physical exam should be performed and includes a thorough neurologic assessment. A screening assessment to rule out upper motor neuron abnormalities should be performed. Lumbar radiculopathy and the clinical level are confirmed through a careful assessment of the dermatomes, myotomes, and deep tendon reflexes. Nerve root tension assessment, straight leg raise (with or without bowstring or ankle dorsiflexion reinforcement) or femoral stretch test, should be carried out and considered positive if the patient's radicular symptoms are reproduced (7,12). The presence of a positive straight leg raise test has been shown to correlate with improved good and excellent outcomes following chemonucleolysis (90%) compared with patients with an absent or mild straight leg raise (60%) (12).

If there is any concern about allergies to papaya or chymopapain, patients can be sent for skin testing or blood measurement of immunoglobulin E (IgE) antibodies with tests such as ChymoFast and radio-absorbent tests (RAST). Anaphylactic shock has occurred in studies at a rate of 0.26% to 1.1% (14,15). Skin testing, if performed, should be done in a location capable of resuscitating patients as there have been reports of anaphylactic shock triggered by epidermal injection (16).

Preoperative imaging studies should include upright plain anteroposterior (AP) and lateral radiographs of the lumbar spine to determine the number of lumbar vertebrae and to rule out any structural abnormalities such as a spondylolisthesis. A magnetic resonance imaging (MRI) should be obtained to confirm the presence of a disc herniation and to rule out a sequestered disc fragment. The ideal patient will only have single-level involvement (15). A CT scan should then be used to rule out osseous compression as a result of stenosis or calcification within the disc herniation. The side and level of the herniation based on the CT and MRI should correlate with the patient's symptoms and physical findings.

SURGICAL TECHNIQUE

Chemonucleolysis requires a radiolucent table and C-arm fluoroscope or bi-planar fluoroscopy. The patient's vital signs should be monitored throughout the case. Intravenous lines should be started. Oxygen should also be administered. The patient is positioned in a lateral decubitus position with appropriate padding of bony prominences, and should be securely fastened to prevent movement from the lateral position. The lateral and AP views on the fluoroscope should be assessed to confirm that the appropriate level is visible and centered on the image. The patient should be given preoperative H1 and H2 antihistamines (diphenhydramine and ranitidine) and hydrocortisone to prevent or minimize the risk of an allergic reaction, including anaphylaxis, to chymopapain (2,17). A preoperative dose of antibiotics should be administered to minimize the risk of infection. The injection site should be prepared and draped using sterile technique. The midline is identified using the spinous processes. A mark is then made in line with the intervertebral disc, 8 to 10 cm lateral to the midline. Local infiltrative anaesthetic, such as lidocaine is injected. Ensure that the correct spinal level is clearly identified. A six-inch 18-gauge needle is then inserted directed toward the center of the disc utilizing both AP and lateral fluoroscopic images. The needle tip should be aimed at the triangular safe zone (so-called "Kambin's triangle") of the disc space (18). This area is bordered proximally by the exiting nerve root, inferiorly by the superior endplate of the caudal vertebra, posteriorly by the superior articular process of the caudal vertebra, and medially by the traversing nerve root and the dura. The needle tip should be advanced to the disc space and stopped at an imaginary line connecting the posterior vertebral bodies on the true lateral image (Fig. 1A) and between imaginary lines at the medial and lateral borders of the pedicles on the AP image (Fig. 1B). Once this position is confirmed, the needle tip can be safely advanced and the surgeon should feel a firm "piercing" sensation when going through the annulus. If this sensation is not felt, then the needle may be lateral to the disc. In this situation, the needle should be withdrawn beyond the dorsal thoracolumbar fascia and redirected. Once confident that the needle is in the disc space it is advanced to the center on the disc on both the AP and lateral fluoroscopic images. It is imperative that the needle tip does not enter the subarachnoid space at any time. If this occurs, then the procedure is aborted and can be reattempted in several weeks unless symptoms of a cerebrospinal fluid (CSF) leak are present.

In certain situations, a large L5 transverse process can obstruct proper entry into the L5–S1 disc space. A two-needle entry technique can be utilized in this situation (12). An 18-gauge is inserted either just distal to the L5 vertebral body or caudally just above the S1 endplate by dropping the hand more cephalad. A 22-gauge needle with a curved distal end is inserted through the 18-gauge needle (Figs. 2A and B). If the 18-gauge needle is just distal to the L5 body, the 22-gauge needle bevel should be directed cephalad and the concavity of the curve directed caudal in order to reach the center of the L5–S1 disc space. If the 18-gauge needle is just above the S1 endplate, the 22-gauge needle bevel should be open caudal with the concavity of the curvature directed cephalad.

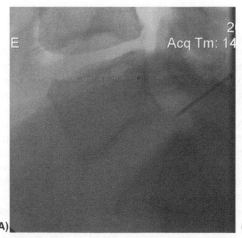 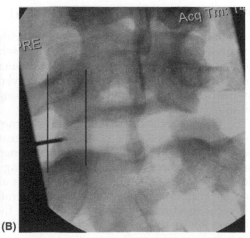

(A) (B)

FIGURE 1 (A) Needle tip should be advanced to the disc space and stopped at an imaginary line connecting the posterior vertebral bodies on the true lateral image. (B) On the anteroposterior image, the needle tip should be between imaginary lines at the medial and lateral borders of the pedicles.

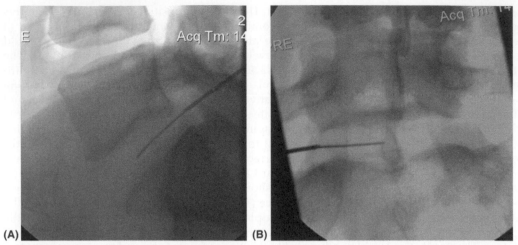

FIGURE 2   (**A**) Two needle technique at L5–S1 with the 22-gauge inner needle bent with the concavity directed caudal and the bevel cranial in order to reach the center of the disc. (**B**) Anteroposterior image of the two-needle technique used to reach the center of the disc at L5–S1.

After central needle placement is verified, the disc integrity and confirmation that there is no communication with the subarachnoid space is then assessed. Two to 2.5 mL of water-soluble contrast medium is injected and resistance of the flow is assessed, along with the pattern of dye flow on fluoroscopy (7). Resistance to flow is high in a normal disc, compared with no resistance in a severely degenerative disc and moderate resistance in a disc with a disc herniation. Patients with severe epidural flow of dye should be excluded as it suggests that the annulus fibrosis and the posterior longitudinal ligament is not intact and that injection of chymopapain will not be contained in the area of disc herniation (12). However, patients with flow out of the disc, only into the subligamentous region can still be treated with chemonucleolysis as the posterior longitudinal ligament is intact, serving as a barrier to the enzyme (7,12).

The amount of chymopapain injected ranges from 2000 to 4000 U. Injection should be given slowly. Some groups advocate a lower dose as 10% of the patients experience back spasm after chemonucleolysis (13). It is not certain whether this side-effect is dose-related. The patient should be closely monitored after the injection for signs of anaphylaxis or allergic response for several hours, along with administration of analgesics for back spasm.

COMPLICATIONS AND THEIR MANAGEMENT

Chymopapain is a known immunogen. The incidence of anaphylaxis is estimated at 0.35% to 0.5% of patients who are not prescreened for sensitivity to chymopapain. African American women, however, have an increased risk of anaphylaxis at 2% (7). Sensitivity testing can prevent or minimize the occurrence of anaphylaxis. Should anaphylaxis occur, epinephrine and hydrocortisone should be administered along with fluids, oxygen, and close monitoring of vital signs.

The safety profile of chymopapain is summarized by 121 "serious" and "unexpected" adverse events reported to the FDA, following treatment of 135,000 patients in the United States between 1982 and 1991 (19). Seven cases of fatal anaphylaxis were reported, along with 24 patients with infection, 32 cases of hemorrhage (including subarachnoid and cerebrovascular), 32 neurologic events such as paraplegia, hemiparesis and foot drop, and 15 miscellaneous events (cardiac and respiratory). The overall mortality rate was 0.019% (19). Of concern were six cases of transverse myelitis. However, follow-up of these reports showed that the typical hyperreflexia and spasticity did not develop and that the actual diagnosis was because of other pathology in four cases such as multiple sclerosis, diabetic neuropathy, and viral infection (13). However, if there is a technical error, and chymopapain enters the cerebrospinal fluid (CSF), an immunogenic response can possibly occur, and this can lead to either an acute or delayed onset of transverse myelitis (2).

Overall, the complication rates of laminectomy/discectomy compared with chemonucleolysis using chymopapain is significantly higher with 17 times more infections, six times more neurologic and vascular complications, and a mortality rate three times greater (19).

OUTCOMES

Five double-blinded randomized trials compared chemonuclelysis with placebo (6,8,9,20,21). Ninety-seven percent of 446 patients were assessed. The meta-analysis by Gibson et al. showed that chymopapain was more effective than placebo in obtaining a successful outcome whether assessed by surgeon or patient (odds ratio, OR: 4.14; 95% confidence interval, CI: 2.04, 8.42). Fewer patients required surgical discectomy after chymopapain treatment as compared with placebo (22).

Five other randomized trials compared chymopapain versus surgical discectomy (23–27). All five trials showed worse results at the one-year mark for chymopapain compared with surgical discectomy. Patients treated with chemonucleolysis were more likely to require a secondary procedure compared with patients treated with surgical discectomy. Thirty percent of patients treated with chymopapain required disc surgery within two years. There were also suggestions that surgical discectomy after failed chemonucleolysis has poorer outcomes than primary discectomy (22).

Chymopapain has also been compared with collagenase in randomized controlled trials (2,28,29). Hedtmann et al. showed no statistical difference between collagenase and chymopapain. However, Wittenberg et al. showed a 72% rate of good and excellent results for the chymopapain group compared with 52% for the collagenase group at the five-year mark. Twenty-eight percent of the collagenase group required microdiscectomy compared with 18% of the chymopapain group.

Most surgeons worldwide have abandoned chymopapain therapy. Chymopapain is no longer manufactured or available in most parts of the world including Canada and Europe. Chemonucleolysis is not as effective as discectomy and has potentially disastrous side-effects including neurologic complications such as subarachnoid hemorrhage, cauda equina syndrome, and transverse myelitis. Furthermore, contemporary microdiscectomy techniques are now routinely performed on an outpatient basis and are associated with reduced morbidity compared with conventional open discectomies. For these reasons, the authors do not perform chymopapain injections.

SUMMARY

Chemonucleolysis is a minimally invasive (percutaneous) treatment option for symptomatic lumbar disc herniations. It is an intermediate option between nonoperative measures and surgical microdiscectomy for soft contained lumbar disc herniations. Chymopapain is the most commonly used form of chemonucleolysis. Results from several randomized controlled trials suggest that chymopapain chemonucleolysis results in poorer outcomes than microdiscectomy, and has a higher likelihood of requiring a second procedure whose outcomes are potentially worse than primary microdiscectomy. With the exception of anaphylaxis, which is unique to chymopapain therapy, complication rates of chymopapain therapy are lower than that following laminectomy/microdiscectomy. As a result of limited anatomic selection criteria, poor overall efficacy, and the potential for disastrous complication the use of chymopapain therapy or other forms of chemonucleolysis have largely been abandoned in Canada and the United States.

Future directions for chemonucleolysis include the development of new intradiscal dissolution substances, which prove to be safer and more efficacious than the current formulations, and may reinitiate greater interest in this form of therapy. However, clear efficacy compared with a contemporary microdiscectomy would have to be shown through rigorous scientific assessment (i.e., well-done large randomized controlled trials).

Indications

- Lumbar radiculopathy unresponsive to nonoperative therapies for at least six weeks.
- Soft, contained disc herniation.
- Radiologic imaging correlates with physical findings and symptoms.

Outcomes

- Chymopapain is more etffective than placebo.
- Chymopapain is less effective than surgical discectomy and has a higher likelihood of requiring a second procedure.

Discectomy after chymopapain therapy may have poorer results than after a primary discectomy.

Complications

- Anaphylaxis (fatal and nonfatal) is estimated at 0.5%.
- Premeditation of patient with H1 and H2 blockers along with hydrocortisone may minimize allergic reactions and anaphylaxis.
- Intrathecal injection can cause paraplegia.
- Epidural injection can lead to epidural hemorrhage.

REFERENCES

1. Jansen EF, Balls AK. Chymopapain: a new crystalline proteinase from papaya latex. J Biol Chem 1941; 137:459.
2. Wittenberg RH, Oppel S, Rubenthaler FA, et al. Five-year results from chemonucleolysis with chymopapain or collagenase: a prospective randomized study. Spine 2001; 26:1835–1841.
3. Suguro T, Degema JR, Bradford DS. The effects of chymopapain on prolapsed human intervertebral disc. Clin Orthop 1986; 213:223–231.
4. Stern IJ. Biochemistry of chymopapain. Clin Orthop 1969; 67:42–46.
5. Smith L. Enzyme dissolution of the nucleus pulposus in humans. JAMA 1964; 187:137–140.
6. Schwetschenau R, Ramirez A, Johnston J, et al. Double-blind evaluation of intradiscal chymopapain for herniated lumbar discs. Early results. J Neurosurg 1976; 45:622–627.
7. Simmons JW, Nordby EJ, Hadjipaviou AG. Chemonucleolysis: the state of the art. Eur Spine J 2001; 10:192–202.
8. Dabezies EJ, Langford K, Morris J, et al. Safety and efficacy of chymopapain (discase) in the treatment of sciatica due to a herniated nucleus pulposus. Results of a randomized, doubleblind study. Spine 1988; 13:561–565.
9. Fraser RD. Chymopapain for the treatment of intervertebral disc herniation. A preliminary report of a double-blind study. Spine 1982; 7:608–612.
10. Sussman BJ, Mann M. Experimental intervertebral discolysis with collagenase. J Neurosurg 1969; 31:628.
11. Brown MD, Tompkins JS. Chemonucleolysis (discolysis) with collagenase. Spine 1986; 11:123–130.
12. Kim YS, Chin DK, Yoon DH, et al. Predictors of successful outcome for lumbar chemonucleolysis: analysis of 3000 cases during the past 14 years. Neurosurgery 2002; 51:S123–S128.
13. Nordby EJ FR, Javid MJ. Chemonucleolysis. Spine 1996; 21:1102–1105.
14. McDermott DJ, Agre K, Brin M, et al. Chymodiactin in patients with herniated lumbar intervertebral discs. An open-label, multicenter study. Spine 1985; 10:242–249.
15. Simmons JW, Stavinoha WB, Knodel LC. Update and review of chemonucleolysis. Clin Orthop 1984; 183:51.
16. Lockey RF, Benedict LM, Turkeltaud PC. Fatalities from immunotherapy (IT) and skin testing (ST). J Allergy Clin Immunol 1987; 79:660.
17. Nordby EJ, Javid MJ. Continuing experience with chemonucleolysis. Mt Sinai J Med 2000; 67:311–313.
18. Kambin P, O'Brien E, Zhou L, et al. Arthroscopic microdiscectomy and selective fragmentectomy. Clin Orthop 1998; 347:150–167.
19. Nordby EJ, Wright PH, Schofield SR. Safety of chemonucleolysis. Adverse effects reported in the United States, 1982–1991. Clin Orthop 1993; 293:122–134.
20. Javid MJ, Nordby EJ, Ford LT, et al. Safety and efcacy of chymopapain (chymodiactin) in herniated nucleus pulposus with sciatica. JAMA 1983; 249:2489–2494.

21. Feldman J, Menkes CJ, Pallardy G, et al. [Double-blind study of the treatment of disc lumbosciatica by chemonucleolysis] Etude en double-aveugle du traitement de la lombosciatique discale par chimionucleolyse. Rev Rhum Mal Osteoartic 1986; 53:147–152.
22. Gibson JNA, Grant IC, Waddell G. Surgery for lumbar disc prolapse. Coch Database Syst Rev 2000.
23. van Alphen HA, Braakman R, Bezemer PD, et al. Chemonucleolysis versus discectomy: a randomized multicenter trial. J Neurosurg 1989; 70:869–875.
24. Muralikuttan KP, Hamilton A, Kernohan WG, et al. A prospective randomized trial of chemonucleolysis and conventional disc surgery in single level lumbar disc herniation. Spine 1992; 17:381–387.
25. Lavignolle B, Vital JM, Baulny D, et al. [Comparative study of surgery and chemonucleolysis in the treatment of sciatica caused by a herniated disk]. Etudes comparees de la chirurgie et de la chimionucleolyse dans le traitement de la sciatique par hernie discale. Acta Orthop Belg 1987; 53:244–249.
26. Ejeskar A, Nachemson A, Herberts P, et al. Surgery versus chemonucleolysis for herniated lumbar discs. A prospective study with random assignment. Clin Orthop 1983; 174:236–242.
27. Crawshaw C, Frazer AM, Merriam WF, et al. A comparison of surgery and chemonucleolysis in the treatment of sciatica. A prospective randomized trial. Spine 1984; 9:195–198.
28. Hedtmann A, Fett H, Steffen R, et al. [Chemonucleolysis using chymopapain and collagenase: 3-year results of a prospective randomized study] Chemonukleolyse mit Chymopapain und Kollagenase. 3-Jahres-Ergebnisse einer prospektiv-randomisierten Studie. Z Orthop Ihre Grenzgeb 1992; 130:36–44.
29. Gibson JNA, Grant IC, Waddell G. The cochrane review of surgery for lumbar disc prolapse and degenerative lumbar spondylosis. Spine 1999; 24:1820–1832.

15 | Odontoid Screw Insertion

Carlo Bellabarba and Jens R. Chapman

Department of Orthopedics and Sports Medicine, and Neurological Surgery, Harborview Medical Center, University of Washington School of Medicine, Seattle, Washington, U.S.A.

INTRODUCTION

Introduced in the early 1980s by Bohler (1) and Nakinishi (2), anterior odontoid screw fixation represents one of only two indications for direct fracture repair in the cervical spine, the other being interfragmentary screw fixation of type II Hangman's fractures. Noncomminuted type II odontoid fractures in patients with favorable bone quality and appropriate body habitus are ideal for anterior odontoid screw fixation. The advantages of anterior odontoid screw fixation over other methods for stabilization of odontoid fractures are supine positioning, minimal soft tissue dissection within existing anatomic planes, and preservation of atlantoaxial motion (3).

INDICATIONS

Overall, the issue of surgical versus nonsurgical treatment of odontoid fractures remains controversial, with a trend toward a gradually decreasing threshold for surgical intervention. The preponderance of evidence suggests that surgical stabilization is appropriate for Anderson and D'Alonzo (4) type II and "shallow" or "high" type III fractures that cannot be maintained in a reduced position using closed means, fractures with distractive patterns of displacement (Fig. 1) (5,6), or fractures with associated spinal cord injury. Relative indications include multiply injured patients, associated closed head injury, initial displacement of 4 mm or more, angulation of 10° or more (5,7–9), delayed presentation (more than two weeks), multiple risk factors for nonunion (10–13), the inability to treat with a halo as a result of advanced age or medical comorbidities (14,15), associated cranial or thoraco-abdominal injury or other medical factors, and the presence of associated upper cervical fractures.

Within these broader surgical indications, the specific indications for anterior odontoid screw fixation are also controversial, and include a fairly narrow spectrum of odontoid fractures. The ideal candidates for anterior odontoid screw fixation are patients with good bone quality who present with acute, isolated (i.e., without associated upper cervical fractures), reducible, noncomminuted type II or "shallow" type III odontoid fractures (3) with either a transverse or anterosuperior to posteroinferior oblique orientation (1,2,16). Beyond this, several controversies remain regarding appropriate relative indications for primary odontoid screw fixation.

Fracture Displacement

As the extent of displacement has been repeatedly correlated with failure of nonoperative care, it is generally agreed that operative fixation of fractures displaced more than 4 mm is indicated, although the exact displacement threshold for operative fixation may vary among surgeons. However, because of concerns regarding the morbidity associated with nonoperative treatment of even less displaced injuries (15–22), fixation of nondisplaced or minimally displaced type II and shallow type III odontoid fractures has also been advocated as a means of achieving more reliable fracture healing, avoiding halo-related complications, and allowing for more rapid return to regular activities (23).

Fracture Acuity

The success of odontoid screw fixation has been reported to be compromised in patients treated six months or more after injury (23). Given the arbitrary method with which this time frame was established, the precise delay after which odontoid screw fixation is no longer a suitable treatment option remains unclear; it might be considerably shorter (1) and most likely varies according to patient-related factors such as comorbidities and nutritional status.

Bone Quality

Compromised bone quality has been reported as a risk for failure of odontoid screw fixation (24), although some studies have shown no correlation between patient age and propensity for fixation failure (16,23). The usual mechanism of failure appears to involve toggling of the screw(s) within the caudal fracture fragment despite maintaining fixation at the odontoid tip, thus allowing for translation of the rostral relative to the caudal fragment. Displacement of the screw shaft through the anterior cortex of the caudal fragment is also a common mechanism of failure, and may be related to technical factors such as a starting point that is not sufficiently posterior. Whereas it is the opinion of some authors that odontoid screw fixation is contraindicated in elderly patients (24), this is clearly not a universal opinion (16,23) and the threshold for defining an elderly patient is often unclear.

Type of Fracture

Type III odontoid fractures treated with anterior screw fixation have been identified as having a higher propensity for fixation failure than type II fractures (23). However, given the fairly broad fracture types that constitute type III injuries, it would be unrealistic to consider all variants at equivalent risk for failure of fixation. It is likely that more rostral or "shallow" type III fractures, which behave similar to type II fractures with regard to displacement patterns, limited surface area for bony healing, and potential disruption of the blood supply to the odontoid tip, leave sufficient bone caudal to the fracture to allow for reliable screw purchase in the caudal fragment and can be reasonably treated with anterior odontoid screw fixation, assuming the presence of other appropriate fracture characteristics (16).

CONTRAINDICATIONS

With the aforementioned caveats in mind, contraindications to odontoid screw fixation include the presence of segmental comminution (13,24) (Hadley Type IIA fracture), oblique fracture orientation from anterior–inferior to posterior–superior, associated upper cervical fracture or ligamentous injury (e.g., distractive fracture pattern, Fig. 1), patients with poor bone quality as a result of osteoporosis or other metabolic bone disorder, low type III odontoid fracture with inferior fracture margin approaching the usual odontoid screw starting point, delayed fracture treatment (more than three to six months), or established pseudarthrosis (1,23).

Technical considerations that may preclude the use of odontoid screw fixation involve the inability to obtain an appropriately cephalad screw trajectory along the sagittal longitudinal axis of the odontoid. This problem may occur when the patient's neck must be excessively flexed to maintain acceptable fracture reduction (Fig. 2), or when the patient is excessively obese or barrel-chested. As discussed next, prior to making the incision for odontoid screw fixation, a radio-opaque/metallic marker placed externally along the intended screw trajectory, as verified by lateral fluoroscopy, can confirm whether the desired trajectory will be achievable.

CONSIDERATIONS FOR PREOPERATIVE PLANNING
Preoperative Physical Examination

Preoperative evaluation of patients being considered for anterior odontoid screw fixation should focus on whether the patient's body habitus might preclude the use of this technique, and whether the patient has had a previous anterior cervical approach and may therefore require additional evaluation for possible pre-existing recurrent laryngeal nerve palsy. In patients who have had a previous anterior cervical approach and have an obvious recurrent laryngeal nerve palsy, any subsequent anterior cervical procedure must be performed ipsilateral to the previous approach in order to avoid the possibility of bilateral recurrent laryngeal

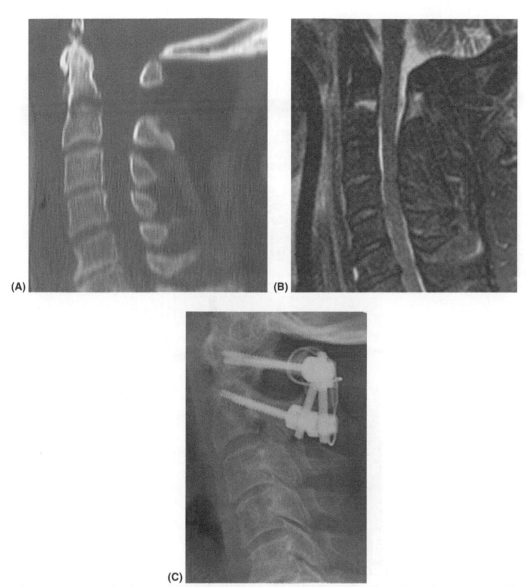

FIGURE 1 Type III odontoid fracture with craniocervical distraction. The presence of associated ligamentous injuries in this injury pattern should raise concern about the suitability of anterior odontoid screw fixation, despite a fracture location and architecture that may seem amenable to anterior screw fixation. (**A**) Sagittal CT and (**B**) MRI images show a type III odontoid fracture with 3 mm of distraction at the fracture site (white *arrow*). This atlantoaxial distractive injury is associated with extensive ligamentous disruption, as illustrated by the posterior element widening and increased signal intensity between C1 and C2 on MRI. Because of the extensive associated ligamentous injury, the odontoid fracture was treated with a posterior approach. (**C**) A lateral radiograph six months after posterior instrumented atlantoaxial arthrodesis shows that anatomic craniocervical alignment has been maintained.

nerve palsies. In patients without clinically obvious recurrent laryngeal nerve palsy, laryngo-scopic evaluation must exclude the presence of subclinical recurrent laryngeal nerve palsy if a contralateral approach is being considered.

All patients should undergo careful neurological evaluation to establish the presence or absence of spinal cord injury, and to establish the appropriate baseline for subsequent serial pre- and postoperative neurological exams. We advocate the use of the American Spinal Injury Association (ASIA) motor score to obtain as objective and reproducible a neurological evaluation as possible.

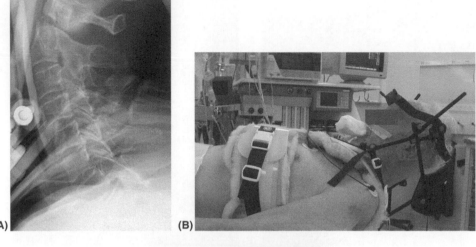

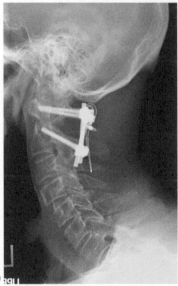

FIGURE 2   Potential impediments to anterior odontoid screw fixation. (**A**) Lateral cervical spine radiograph shows a displaced type II odontoid fracture. External immobilization with a halo vest was not sufficient to stabilize the fracture, which shows 100% posterior displacement of the odontoid tip. Fracture configuration and bone quality appear amenable to odontoid screw fixation. (**B**) However, in part due to the patient's pronounced cervicothoracic kyphosis, the head and neck position needed to maintain odontoid fracture alignment, as shown in this preoperative image, clearly does not allow for the desired odontoid screw trajectory. (**C**) A posterior atlantoaxial arthrodesis was therefore performed, as shown on this lateral radiograph done six months postoperatively. It is essential that contingency plans be made preoperatively in the event that factors arise which may prevent the ability to perform odontoid screw fixation.

Preoperative Imaging
Plain Films

The primary imaging method for identifying odontoid fractures depends on the mechanism of injury and the degree of displacement. Displaced odontoid fractures can easily be identified on lateral cervical spine radiographs (Fig. 3). Associated coronal plane displacement can be seen on open-mouth anteroposterior views. Standard anteroposterior cervical spine radiographs are rarely useful in identifying odontoid fractures, but may shed some light on associated subaxial injuries (25).

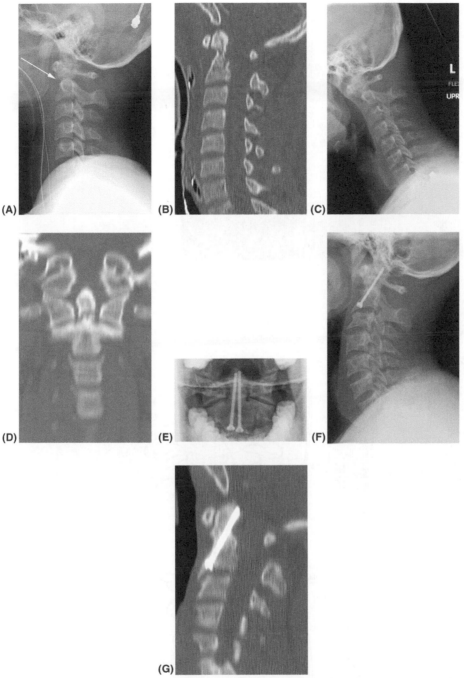

FIGURE 3 Odontoid screw fixation of delayed union of the odontoid. (**A**) Lateral cervical spine radiograph and (**B**) sagittal CT image show a type II odontoid fracture with anterior displacement (white *arrow*). The patient was treated with halo-vest immobilization (**C**) Flexion view of the cervical spine four months after injury shows anterior displacement of the odontoid, manifested as a widened anterior atlanto-dens interval. (**D**) Absence of bony union was confirmed on CT scan, as shown on this coronal CT image through the odontoid. Osteosynthesis of the odontoid was performed using two 2.7 millimeter interfragmentary screws. The smaller 2.7 mm screws were used in lieu of typical small-fragment screws due to the patient's small stature. The presence of fibrous tissue and callus prevented the ability to completely reduce the fracture, but acceptable reduction and interfragmentary compression was achieved, with only slight residual anterior displacement. (**E**) Anteroposterior radiograph, (**F**) lateral radiograph, and (**G**) sagittal CT image two years postoperatively show uneventful fracture healing. Note that formation of an osteophyte at the anterior aspect of the C2-3 disc space (Fig. F, G) is a common but seemingly asymptomatic occurrence after odontoid screw fixation.

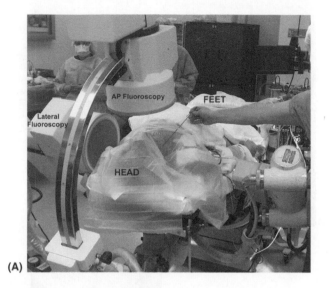

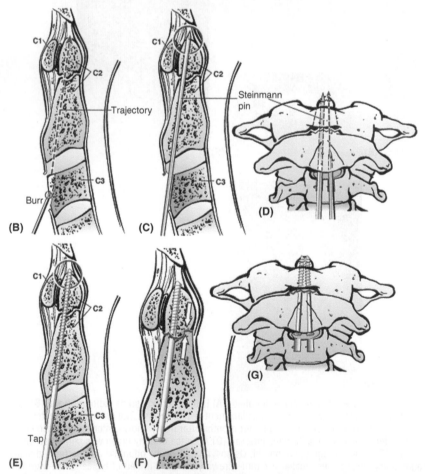

FIGURE 4 Technique of Odontoid Screw Osteosynthesis. (**A**) Biplanar fluoroscopy with two C-arms greatly facilitates odontoid screw fixation procedures. A metallic marker can be used with lateral fluoroscopy to gauge whether the position of the neck will allow for the appropriate screw trajectory, without being impeded by the patient's chest. (**B**) The C2-3 disc space is reached with blunt dissection in the prevertebral plane after performing a Smith-Robinson approach

With low-energy injuries, plain radiographs are often the primary images used for diagnosing odontoid fractures. However, in patients at high risk for odontoid fractures and in whom plain radiographs may be difficult to interpret because of osteoporosis or advanced degenerative changes, a computed tomography (CT) scan should be considered even in the absence of a high-energy mechanism (14). Patients with high-energy mechanisms should have routine CT-imaging, which is increasingly being used as the primary cervical spine screening method in this high-risk patient population (26).

Advanced Imaging

CT scan of the cervical spine is mandatory in patients who have odontoid fractures identified with plain radiographs, and in patients with high-energy mechanisms regardless of whether a fracture has been previously identified on plain radiographs. A CT scan should be strongly considered in elderly patients with low-energy injuries, who are at high risk for odontoid fracture and in whom visualization of the upper cervical spine on plain radiographs can be difficult. Sagittal and coronal CT reformations are essential as transversely oriented fractures may not be apparent on the axial views. A CT scan with coronal and sagittal reformations may also be helpful in identifying segmental comminution, which we generally consider to be a contraindication to odontoid screw fixation (16,24).

We reserve magnetic resonance image (MRI) scanning for patients who have associated neurologic deficits or in whom an associated ligamentous injury, such as a distractive injury pattern (Fig. 1) or rupture of the transverse atlantal ligament is suspected from the appearance of the plain radiographs or CT. Associated ligamentous instability is considered a contraindication to anterior odontoid screw fixation (27).

SURGICAL TECHNIQUE
Operating Room Setup and Equipment

Anterior odontoid screw fixation is carried out with the patient supine on a radiolucent table and the head secured by a fixed cranial holding device, such as Mayfield tongs (Fig. 4). Endotracheal intubation is performed by fiberoptically guided technique. Bite blocks are placed adjacent to the endotracheal tube to enhance visualization on anteroposterior fluoroscopic views. Baseline somatosensory-evoked potentials are established prior to positioning the patient. As this procedure is entirely dependent on radiographic visualization and the ability to achieve acceptable alignment, the most critical and time-consuming parts of this procedure take place before the incision is made. The ability to obtain adequate lateral and open-mouth odontoid views is best achieved with two-image intensifiers. Achieving and maintaining an anatomic, closed reduction of the odontoid fracture with a head and neck position that is amenable to the required screw trajectory requires careful manipulation. If an anatomic reduction cannot be achieved by closed means, if an overly flexed position of the neck is required to maintain an acceptable reduction, or if acceptable fluoroscopic visualization cannot be achieved, posterior atlantoaxial arthrodesis should be considered rather than proceeding with anterior odontoid screw fixation.

FIGURE 4 (*Continued*) through a transverse incision centered over C5. The anterior annulus of C2-3 must be excised and the anterior superior C3 vertebral body and endplate must be partially resected to allow for a sufficiently posterior starting point and sufficiently rostral screw trajectory. (**C**) The appropriate starting point and drill trajectory are demonstrated on the lateral view. The drill trajectory is angled slightly posterior to the anterior cortex of the dens, with the goal of penetrating the tip of the dens just posterior to its apex. (**D**) When placing two screws, the starting point for each screw is approximately 3 mm lateral to the midline, and the drill trajectory on the anteroposterior view follows a slightly medial trajectory. If placing a single screw, the starting point is in the midline on the anteroposterior view. (**E**) Tapping of the far cortex at the tip of the dens is recommended. (**F**) Use of small-fragment partially threaded cancellous screws allows for interfragmentary compression at the fracture site. Achieving screw purchase in the cortex of the odontoid tip is essential to decrease the likelihood of fixation failure. In addition, screw threads should not span the fracture, and should be present only in the rostral fracture fragment in order to achieve interfragmentary compression. (**G**) The desired screw positioning and fracture alignment are demonstrated on the anteroposterior view. *Source*: From Ref. 45.

Another potential obstacle is interference of the chest with the inclination angle required for this instrumentation technique. Large, barrel-chested patients or patients with excessive fixed cervical or cervicothoracic kyphosis may therefore be unsuitable for this technique. Fine adjustment of the patient's head position under fluoroscopy by extending the neck gently without displacing the fracture can aid in attaining the desired trajectory. The presence of sufficient torso clearance to allow for the required odontoid screw trajectory is verified with a metallic object held externally against the patient's chest along the intended screw trajectory as confirmed with lateral fluoroscopy. Because of the possibility that odontoid screw fixation cannot be carried out, contingency plans for alternative fixation methods should always be made.

Operative Approach

A conventional right- or left-sided anterior approach is performed, with the incision usually centered over C5. Correct placement of the incision is important to minimize technical difficulties with odontoid screw fixation. Upon reaching the prevertebral fascia, the dissection is carried rostrally to the C2–3 disc space, which is exposed by reflecting the longus colli muscles laterally. At the C3 level, the superior thyroid artery and vein may cross the operative field and require ligation.

Insertion Technique

A curved, radiolucent submandibular retractor is placed on the anterior vertebral body of C2. Alternatively, by placing this retractor in front of the anterior arch of C1, residual anterior fracture displacement can be corrected by applying posteriorly directed pressure across this retractor. The anterior annulus of the C2–3 disc is excised along with a small wedge of the anterosuperior C3 vertebral body in order to expose the anteroinferior lip of C2. This cortical lip is removed with a high-speed burr to prepare a smooth bony surface for screw placement, which minimizes the risk of compromising the anterior cortex at the base of the axis, a detail that is essential for preserving acceptable fixation of the caudal fragment (Fig. 4). It is critical to the success of this procedure that the starting point is within the inferior endplate rather than the anterior cortex of C2.

An odontoid screw should allow for fracture compression by the use of either terminally threaded screws or by overdrilling the caudal fragment if using fully threaded screws. Although we generally prefer using two screws, fixation can be performed with either one or two screws as single interfragmentary screws have been reported to provide adequate stability in both clinical and biomechanical testing (23,28,29). Two well-placed screws have the advantage of minimizing rotational displacement, but are considered to be technically more challenging. Our preference has been the placement of two 3.5- or 4.0-mm screws, if possible, and to use two 2.7-mm screws if larger screws cannot be accommodated (Fig. 3).

The key elements of screw placement include establishing a starting point that is sufficiently posterior within the inferior endplate of C2, being co-linear to the longitudinal axis of the odontoid, achieving screw thread purchase rostral to the fracture only, and engaging the posterior cortex of the odontoid tip with the terminal screw threads. The specific technique (single or dual, cannulated or solid screws) is a matter of surgeon preference. If noncannulated screws are used, we prefer the use of a Steinman pin rather than a drill bit due to a lower risk of breakage and the absence of bone removal. The first Steinmann pin is left in place after being advanced across the fracture site into the apical cortex under biplanar fluoroscopic guidance. The second Steinmann pin is then used to drill the second channel under biplanar fluoroscopy, followed by determination of screw length with a depth gauge, and subsequent interfragmentary screw placement on the second side. The first Steinmann pin is then removed and replaced with the appropriately sized interfragmentary screw.

Closure and Postoperative Management

After confirming hemostasis, closure of the platysma with interrupted 3-0 absorbable suture is followed by subcuticular closure with nonbraided 4-0 suture. The patient is immobilized postoperatively in a Miami J collar for 12 weeks and is allowed to ambulate as tolerated, to the extent permitted by associated injuries.

COMPLICATIONS AND THEIR MANAGEMENT
Pitfalls

Odontoid fractures, whether treated operatively or nonoperatively, continue to be associated with significant morbidity and even mortality. Fracture nonunion and missed injuries are the most common causes of complications (30). Primary neurologic injury or secondary deterioration are rarely encountered (31,32), and pseudarthrosis of a type II odontoid fracture is a leading cause of secondary neurologic deterioration (31). A pseudarthrosis of the odontoid has been defined as the absence of fracture site bridging after four months of treatment (33).

Major complication rates of up to 28% have been reported with odontoid screw fixation (1,23,34–36), consisting mainly of hardware-related complications (10% to 15%) and superficial wound infections (2%) (23). An associated major pitfall of this procedure is the need for anatomic fracture reduction. Residual fracture displacement is likely to result in either ineffective interfragmentary compression with compromised fracture stability or less than ideal screw position, thus predisposing to failure.

Of the hardware-related complications in one large series (23), one-half were screw disengagements from the C2 body in patients with type III odontoid fractures, putting into question whether this technique is appropriate for odontoid fractures that extend into the inferior C2 body. A second commonly seen hardware-related complication is loosening of the odontoid screw, which occurs primarily when the screw tip has not engaged the apical cortex of the odontoid. Failure of screw fixation may have catastrophic consequences, as demonstrated by reports of quadriplegia and death resulting from fracture displacement after loss of fixation (23,37). A third commonly noted hardware-related complication pertains to screw malposition. A fourth technical error is associated with an excessively anterior starting point, which can leave a thin anterior bony shell along the anterior axis, which either is unable to contain the screw shaft or mandates a screw trajectory that is too posteriorly oriented. If a cannulated screw system is used, care should be taken to avoid advancement of a guide wire rostral to the tip of the odontoid. Although rare, intraoperative spinal cord and cranial nerve injury have been described (34–36). It is apparent from the literature that a considerable learning curve exists with this complex procedure (7,34).

Although fracture union has been reported to be unaffected by delay in surgery of up to six months, long-standing odontoid pseudarthrosis responds poorly to anterior screw fixation, as demonstrated by a mere 25% healing rate in a series of 18 patients who were operated for pseudarthrosis between 18 and 48 months postinjury (23). The 25% hardware-related complication rate in this group of patients, consisting mainly of screw fracture was consistent with previously reported experiences with odontoid screw fixation of pseudarthroses (34). We therefore do not recommend anterior screw fixation as the preferred method for the delayed treatment of injuries.

Complications that have been recognized with the use of the Smith-Robinson approach for other conditions, such as dysphagia, dysphonia, pharyngeal edema, and esophageal or neurovascular injury, have been reported to occur when placing anterior odontoid screws (23,34,37,38).

As previously mentioned, technical considerations that may preclude the use of odontoid screw fixation pertain primarily to physical characteristics that do not allow for acceptable screw trajectory, such as prominent upper thoracic or cervicothoracic kyphosis, barrel chest, and fracture characteristics that require a flexed position to maintain an acceptable reduction (Fig. 2).

Bailouts

In most cases, where odontoid screw fixation either cannot be achieved or has failed to result in fracture healing, posterior C1–2 arthrodesis is the appropriate salvage procedure (Fig. 1). Nonunion rates of 4% or less have been reported using transarticular screw and wired structural bone-graft constructs (7,39,40). Other C1–C2 screw and rod constructs provide additional options for posterior fixation (41). Surgical stabilization of low type III odontoid fractures, if necessary, should generally be in the form of posterior atlantoaxial fixation, because of their high reported failure rates (55%) with odontoid screw fixation (23). Posterior C1–C2 arthrodesis techniques are discussed in greater detail in Chapter 16.

OUTCOMES

Results of anterior odontoid screw fixation have varied in the literature. Although some series have shown excellent success rates, with healing rates approaching 90% in patients treated within six months of injury regardless of patient age and bone quality (16,23,38,42), other series have shown higher complication rates, particularly loss of fixation, in patients with osteoporosis (24). As discussed in greater detail before, failure of type II odontoid fracture healing after odontoid screw fixation has been reported in 10% to 15% of patients, with an overall perioperative complication rate approaching 30% (34,36). In addition to bone quality, sagittal plane fracture obliquity direction similar to that of intended screw placement (i.e., from anterior–inferior to posterior–superior), appears to be associated with lower (75%) healing rates (23). In general, patients with anteriorly displaced odontoid fractures pose a greater challenge to odontoid screw fixation, compared to those with posteriorly displaced fractures. Lack of an anatomic reduction or inability to achieve interfragmentary compression across the fracture can greatly impair the efficacy of odontoid screw fixation. Also, despite the fact that preservation of atlantoaxial motion has been one of the primary advantages cited for anterior odontoid screw fixation over posterior C1–C2 fixation techniques, atlantoaxial motion appears to be compromised, in part, even after odontoid screw fixation (3).

With regard to type III odontoid fractures, the data for type II fractures can reasonably be extrapolated to more rostral type III fractures because they behave similarly. Although operative stabilization is not commonly required in type III injuries that extend more caudally into the C2 body, when surgical intervention is indicated, posterior C1–C2 arthrodesis should be considered the method of choice because of the high reported failure rate of anterior odontoid screw fixation in these injury types (23). Use of newer, more versatile odontoid fracture classification systems (43,44) may help facilitate the distinction between different type III odontoid fracture variants and identify more clearly which ones would be amenable to odontoid screw fixation.

SUMMARY

Anterior odontoid screw fixation is advocated for the treatment of noncomminuted odontoid fractures with intact vertebral body of the axis (1,23,36). Prudent patient selection and meticulous technical execution are necessary to avoid perioperative complications and high failure rates (1,34–36). Failure of odontoid screw fixation has been described in 10% to 15% of patients, with an overall perioperative complication rate of up to 28% (34,36). Vertebral body fracture of the axis, comminution of the odontoid and the presence of osteoporosis offer a poor prognosis for successful fixation. Treatment of odontoid nonunions with anterior fixation alone is generally not recommended, although success has been reported in the treatment of nonunions up to six months postinjury (23). In patients with extensive fracture comminution, compromised bone quality, or in whom achieving the necessary odontoid screw trajectory cannot be accomplished because of unfavorable body habitus or the need for a flexed neck position to maintain reduction, posterior atlantoaxial arthrodesis using either transarticular screw fixation or segmental C1–2 fixation is indicated (chap. 16) (39,41). Posterior atlantoaxial arthrodesis is the recommended treatment for type IIA dens fractures, which are inherently unstable because of a zone of segmental comminution at the odontoid base (13), and fractures in which the fracture line parallels the typical odontoid screw trajectory, in which attempted interfragmentary compression would result in loss of reduction and inadequate fixation (23,34). Rigidly instrumented posterior C1–2 arthrodesis is expected to have the most predictably favorable result in the management of injuries that are not amenable to anterior odontoid screw fixation, and in the salvage of failed anterior odontoid screw fixation (17,34,39).

Brief Indications

- Acute, noncomminuted type II or high type III odontoid fractures
- Transverse or posterior oblique fracture orientation
- Acceptable bone quality

- Absence of associated upper cervical injury
- Absence of ligamentous injury or distractive instability pattern.

Outcomes

- Fracture healing in approximately 90% of the patients
- Preservation of partial atlantoaxial motion.

Complications

- Approximately 30% complication rate
- Ten to 15 percent reported failure of fixation
  - Excessively anterior starting point
  - Failure to gain screw purchase into the odontoid tip
  - Insufficiently cephalad trajectory
  - Screw malposition
  - Fracture obliquity in same orientation as screw trajectory
  - Low type III odontoid fractures
  - Poor bone quality
  - Segmental comminution
  - Remote fracture/established pseudarthrosis
- Failure to achieve anatomic fracture reduction
- Anatomic obstructions to screw placement
  - Prominent chest
  - Upper thoracic/cervicothoracic kyphosis
  - Overly flexed neck position required to maintain reduction.

REFERENCES

1. Bohler J. Anterior stabilization for acute fractures and non-unions of the dens. J Bone Joint Surg Am 1982; 64:18–27.
2. Nakanishi T, Sasaki, T,Tokita, N, Hirabayashi, K. Internal fixation of the odontoid fracture. Orthop Trans 1982; 6:176.
3. Jeanneret B, Vernet O, Frei S, et al. Atlantoaxial mobility after screw fixation of the odontoid: A computed tomographic study. J Spinal Disord 1991; 4:203–211.
4. Anderson LD, D'Alonzo RT. Fractures of the odontoid process of the axis. J Bone Joint Surg Am 1974; 56:1663–1674.
5. Ryan MD, Taylor TK. Odontoid fractures. A rational approach to treatment. J Bone Joint Surg Br 1982; 64:416–421.
6. Graziano G, Colon G, Hensinger R. Complete atlanto-axial dislocation associated with type ii odontoid fracture: a report of two cases. J Spinal Disord 1994; 7:518–521.
7. Clark CR, White AA, III. Fractures of the dens. A multicenter study. J Bone Joint Surg Am 1985; 67:1340–1348.
8. Apuzzo ML, Heiden JS, Weiss MH, et al. Acute fractures of the odontoid process. An analysis of 45 cases. J Neurosurg 1978; 48:85–91.
9. Hadley MN, Dickman CA, Browner CM, et al. Acute axis fractures: a review of 229 cases. J Neurosurg 1989; 71:642–647.
10. Dickson H, Engel S, Blum P, et al. Odontoid fractures, systemic disease and conservative care. Aust N Z J Surg 1984; 54:243–247.
11. Dunn ME, Seljeskog EL. Experience in the management of odontoid process injuries: an analysis of 128 cases. Neurosurgery 1986; 18:306–310.
12. Roy-Camille R, Saillant G, Judet T, et al. Factors of severity in the fractures of the odontoid process (author's translation). Rev Chir Orthop Reparatrice Appar Mot 1980; 66:183–186.
13. Hadley MN, Browner CM, Liu SS, et al. New subtype of acute odontoid fractures (type IIa). Neurosurgery 1988; 22:67–71.

14. Pepin JW, Bourne RB, Hawkins RJ. Odontoid fractures, with special reference to the elderly patient. Clin Orthop 1985; 193:178–183.

15. Bednar DA, Parikh J, Hummel J. Management of type II odontoid process fractures in geriatric patients; a prospective study of sequential cohorts with attention to survivorship. J Spinal Disord 1995; 8:166–169.

16. Founts KN, Kapsalaki EZ, Karampelas I, et al. Results of long-term follow-up in patients undergoing anterior screw fixation for type II and rostral type III odontoid fractures. Spine 2005; 30:661–669.

17. Lind B, Nordwall A, Sihlbom H. Odontoid fractures treated with halo-vest. Spine 1987; 12:173–177.

18. Mirza SK, Moquin RR, Anderson PA, et al. Stabilizing properties of the halo apparatus. Spine 1997; 22:727–733.

19. Bucci MN, Dauser RC, Maynard FA, et al. Management of post-traumatic cervical spine instability: operative fusion versus halo vest immobilization. Analysis of 49 cases. J Trauma 1988; 28:1001–1006.

20. Garfin SR, Botte MJ, Waters RL, et al. Complications in the use of the halo fixation device. J Bone Joint Surg Am 1986; 68:320–325.

21. Glaser JA, Whitehill R, Stamp WG, et al. Complications associated with the halo-vest. A review of 245 cases. J Neurosurg 1986; 65:762–769.

22. Schweigel JF. Halo-thoracic brace management of odontoid fractures. Spine 1979; 4:192–194.

23. Apfelbaum RI, Lonser RR, Veres R, et al. Direct anterior screw fixation for recent and remote odontoid fractures. J Neurosurg 2000; 93:227–236.

24. Andersson S, Rodrigues M, Olerud C. Odontoid fractures: high complication rate associated with anterior screw fixation in the elderly. Eur Spine J 2000; 9:56–59, discussion 60.

25. Ehara S, el-Khoury GY, Clark CR. Radiologic evaluation of dens fracture. Role of plain radiography and tomography. Spine 1992; 17:475–479.

26. Mann FA, Cohen WA, Linnau KF, Hallam DK, Blackmore CC. Evidence-based approach to using CT in spinal trauma. Eur J Radiol 2003; 48:39–48.

27. Dickman CA, Hadley MN, Browner C, et al. Neurosurgical management of acute atlas-axis combination fractures. A review of 25 cases. J Neurosurg 1989; 70:45–49.

28. Sasso R, Doherty BJ, Crawford MJ, et al. Biomechanics of odontoid fracture fixation. Comparison of the one- and two-screw technique. Spine 1993; 18:1950–1953.

29. Graziano G, Jaggers C, Lee M, et al. A comparative study of fixation techniques for type II fractures of the odontoid process. Spine 1993; 18:2383–2387.

30. Geisler FH, Cheng C, Poka A, et al. Anterior screw fixation of posteriorly displaced type II odontoid fractures. Neurosurgery 1989; 25:30–37, discussion 37–38.

31. Fairholm D, Lee ST, Lui TN. Fractured odontoid: the management of delayed neurological symptoms. Neurosurgery 1996; 38:38–43.

32. Crockard HA, Heilman AE, Stevens JM. Progressive myelopathy secondary to odontoid fractures: clinical, radiological, and surgical features. J Neurosurg 1993; 78:579–586.

33. Schatzker J, Rorabeck CH, Waddell JP. Fractures of the dens (odontoid process). An analysis of thirty-seven cases. J Bone Joint Surg Br 1971; 53:392–405.

34. Aebi M, Etter C, Coscia M. Fractures of the odontoid process. Treatment with anterior screw fixation. Spine 1989; 14:1065–1070.

35. Montesano PX, Anderson PA, Schlehr F, et al. Odontoid fractures treated by anterior odontoid screw fixation. Spine 1991; 16:S33–S37.

36. Etter C, Coscia M, Jaberg H, et al. Direct anterior fixation of dens fractures with a cannulated screw system. Spine 1991; 16:S25–S32.

37. Henry AD, Bohly J, Grosse A. Fixation of odontoid fractures by an anterior screw. J Bone Joint Surg Br 1999; 81:472–477.

38. Daentzer D, Deinsberger W, Boker DK. Vertebral artery complications in anterior approaches to the cervical spine: report of two cases and review of literature. Surg Neurol 2003; 59:300–309, discussion 309.

39. Jeanneret B, Magerl F. Primary posterior fusion c1/2 in odontoid fractures: Indications, technique, and results of transarticular screw fixation. J Spinal Disord 1992; 5:464–475.

40. Haid RW, Jr., Subach BR, McLaughlin MR, et al. C1-c2 transarticular screw fixation for atlantoaxial instability: a 6-year experience. Neurosurgery 2001; 49:65–68, discussion 69–70.

41. Harms J, Melcher RP. Posterior c1–c2 fusion with polyaxial screw and rod fixation. Spine 2001; 26:2467–2471.

42. Borm W, Kast E, Richter HP, et al. Anterior screw fixation in type II odontoid fractures: is there a difference in outcome between age groups? Neurosurgery 2003; 52:1089–1092, discussion 1092–1084.

43. Chutkan NB, King AG, Harris MB. Odontoid fractures: evaluation and management. J Am Acad Orthop Surg 1997; 5:199–204.

44. Grauer JN, Shafi B, Hilibrand AS, et al. Proposal of a modified, treatment-oriented classification of odontoid fractures. Spine J 2005; 5:123–129.

45. Bellabarba C, Mirza SK, Chapman JR. Injuries to the craniocervical junction. In: Bucholz RW, Heckman JD, Court-Brown CM, eds. Rockwood & Green, Fractures in Adults, 6 ed. Philadelphia, PA: Lippincott Williams & Wilkins, 2006:1482–1483.

16 | C1–C2 Transarticular Screw Technique

Thomas J. Puschak
Panorama Orthopedics and Spine Center, Golden, Colorado, U.S.A.

Paul A. Anderson
Department of Orthopedic Surgery and Rehabilitation, University of Wisconsin, Madison, Wisconsin, U.S.A.

INTRODUCTION

A variety of techniques for posterior C1–C2 fusion have been described, ranging from in situ to wire to those with rigid internal fixation. Until recently, wiring methods were the most popular including the Gallie and Brooks techniques (1,2). In these techniques, wedged or H-shaped corticocancellous structural bone grafts are keyed into the posterior elements of C1 and C2 and held in place with wires. Postoperative immobilization in halo vests or Minerva braces is usually required and pseudarthrosis rates as high as 10% to 15% have been reported (3). Also, iatrogenic neurologic injury can occur during wire placement. The Halifax clamp which compresses the two adjacent laminae has also been used for atlantoaxial fixation (4). This device has poor rotational stability due to the differences in slopes between the arch of C1 and the lamina of C2 which can lead to clamp dislodgement.

In 1979, Magerl and Seeman described the placement of transarticular screws in conjunction with traditional posterior wiring and bone grafting (5). This construct is biomechanically superior to wiring and clamp techniques (6–10). The increased rigidity of the transarticular screw constructs decreases postoperative external immobilization and lowers pseudarthrosis rates (3). Currently, this technique is considered to be the standard by many spine surgeons for posterior C1–2 fixation (3,11,12). The screws are placed at a low angle relative to the spine starting through the skin quite opposite to T1. In the original description the spine was completely exposed from C1 to T1, but current practice in the majority of cases allows percutaneous placement of screws with open exposure only of C1 and C2.

This chapter describes the surgical technique of arthrodesis using transarticular C1–2 screws. Surgical anatomy, indications, and preoperative assessment will be discussed. We will also identify potential pitfalls to screw placement, discuss how to avoid them, and how to deal with them if encountered.

INDICATIONS

The primary indication for posterior fusion of the atlantoaxial joint is instability from traumatic or inflammatory processes (Table 1). Congenital conditions, such as Down's syndrome or several forms of dwarphism, are also associated with atlantoaxial instability. Regardless of the etiology, atlantoaxial instability can lead to axial neck pain, radiculopathy, and myelopathy. The goals of surgery are to decompress the spinal cord, reduce the C1–2 joint, and stabilize the segment.

Traumatic C1–2 instability occurs from rupture of the transverse atlantal ligament, fracture of the odontoid processes or, less commonly, by complex atlantal injuries. Except in young children, patients with traumatic injuries of the transverse and alar ligaments are candidates for arthrodesis. Displaced and comminuted fractures through the base of the dens (type II) heal poorly nonoperatively and may be stabilized by posterior C1–2 arthrodesis (13). Furthermore, C1–2 arthrodesis may be indicated in elderly otherwise active patients with type II odontoid fractures. A few authors recommend C1–2 for unstable Jefferson fractures (14). Transarticular screw stabilization can also be incorporated into occipitocervical constructs if stability of the occipitocervical articulation is also compromised.

TABLE 1   Indications for C1–2 Arthrodesis

C1–2 instability
Traumatic
Transverse atlantal ligament rupture
Comminuted type II dens fracture
Congenital/developmental
Down's syndrome
Odontoid hypoplasia
Os odontoideum
Occipitalization of C1 with C1–2 instability
Inflammatory
Rheumatoid arthritis
C1–2 osteoarthritis

Chronic post-traumatic insufficiency may present insidiously and diagnosis may be delayed years after the index injury. Initially, the diagnosis can be missed if a patient is neurologically normal and local pain and spasm limit the amount of displacement on imaging. Careful follow-up and repeat flexion–extension radiographs after acute symptoms have helped to avoid missing these injuries.

Congenital insufficiency of C1–2 is seen in several disorders including Down's syndrome and Morquio's syndrome. The incidence of atlantoaxial instability in patients with Down's syndrome may be as high as 20% (15). The instability is because of congenital absence or laxity of the transverse ligament. Often this instability is asymptomatic, although patients may experience symptoms from pain to torticollis and even myelopathy. Patients with instability may need to be restricted from activities that put the head and neck at risk. The topic of prophylactic fusion is controversial, but traditionally fusion is recommended in those with an anterior atlantal dens interval (ADI) greater than 7 mm. Additional assessment of stability of the occipitoatlantal articulations is needed as many patients will have combined sites of instability.

A relatively common etiology of instability is hypoplasia or aplasia of the odontoid and os odontoidium. Some patients present with local mechanical irritation that causes axial pain, headaches, or torticollis, while others develop neurologic symptoms. Neurologic symptoms may be transient after an acute injury or more insidious and chronic in nature. Patients with purely mechanical symptoms usually respond to supportive measures such as rest, immobilization, and physical therapy. They should be followed to ensure that the instability does not progress. Those with progressive neurologic symptoms, significant instability (ADI >10 mm), or significant canal stenosis (space available for the spinal cord <13 mm on axial MRI scan) should undergo posterior C1–2 arthrodesis and decompression if necessary.

Atlantoaxial instability is commonly encountered in rheumatoid arthritis and other inflammatory and some degenerative conditions. Traditionally, observation has been recommended in neurologically stable patients as long as the ADI is less than 9 mm. Measurement of the ADI in patients with rheumatoid arthritis can be misleading as it may not represent the true space available for the spinal cord secondary to the presence of synovial pannus. Boden recommends following the posterior atlantal dens interval (PADI) in patients with rheumatoid arthritis (16). The PADI is the distance between the posterior margin of the dens and the anterior edge of the posterior C1 arch measured on lateral radiographs. Patients with a PADI greater than 14 mm who are neurologically stable should be observed. If the PADI is less than 14 mm, a magnetic resonance imaging (MRI) should be performed and C1–2 fusion (with decompression if necessary) is recommended if the cervicomedullary angle is less than 135°, the cord diameter in flexion is less than 6 mm, or the space available for the spinal cord is less than 13 mm (16). Chronic instability can develop in cases of occipitalization of the atlas or congenital fusion of C2–3 (Klippel-Feil). The increased stress on the adjacent C1–2 segment can lead to attenuation of the transverse ligament over time. Symptoms usually present themselves late because of the gradual development of laxity.

Another less common indication for atlantoaxial fusion is degenerative osteoarthrosis of the C1–2 articulations. This surgery is highly effective in patients with suboccipital neck pain with severe degeneration of the C1–2 articulations (17).

PREOPERATIVE PLANNING

The close proximity of the vertebral arteries, carotid arteries, brain stem, spinal cord, and cranial nerves demand careful assessment to avoid iatrogenic injury prior to and during placement of transarticular screws. A checklist is presented in Table 2 of essential steps to minimize the chance of inadvertent injury.

Surgical Anatomy

The vertebral artery can be divided into four parts: cervical, vertebral, suboccipital, and intracranial (Fig. 1). The vertebral arteries originate from the respective subclavian artery and ascend anterior to the longus coli at C7 and T1. The artery enters the spinal column at C6 and courses cranially in the transverse foramina from C6 to C3. At C2, the artery turns first laterally and then again cranially so that it occupies a far more lateral position in the C1 transverse foramen. This position relatively lengthens, or creates redundancy, of the artery which allows for large excursions of C1–2 rotation without injury or obstruction of blood flow. In C1, the vertebral arteries pass through the transverse foramen and then turn 90° medial and posterior, to lie in a groove on the superior aspect of the posterior arch of the atlas. Approximately 1.5 cm from the midline they turn cranial and anterior, perforating the atlanto-occipital membrane. They ascend first lateral to the medulla, then join anteriorly forming the basilar artery.

Other important structures are the first and second cervical spinal nerves. The first cervical spinal nerve lies in the groove with the vertebral artery which is situated posterior to the lateral mass of the atlas, lateral to the spinal canal, and anterior to the atlanto-occipital membrane. The second spinal nerve lies just dorsal to the C1–2 articulation between the posterior arches. Large epidural venous sinuses are located around the C2 nerve and bleeding from these sites can be difficult to control.

The hypoglossal nerve (CN XII) exits the skull base through the jugular foramen just anterior and lateral to the occipital condyle. It then passes anterior to the lateral part of the C1 lateral mass and C1–2 joint and can be injured if a very long screw is placed. Ebraheim reports that the optimal screw length for the transarticular technique is 38 mm; however, this number may vary depending on the individual's anatomy (18). In order to avoid risking injury to the hypoglossal nerve, care must be taken not to past-point with the drill and the surgeon must select an appropriate length screw based on the individual patient's anatomy.

The internal carotid artery passes anterior to the lateral half of the C1 lateral on its way to the carotid foramen in the base of the skull. Currier has shown in an anatomic study that the distance between the internal carotid artery and the anterior cortex of the center of the C1 lateral mass is 2 to 4 mm with the head and neck in neutral rotation (19).

TABLE 2 Safety Techniques to Avoid Iatrogenic Injury During C1–2 Transarticular Screws

Preoperative
    Assure that stenosis is not present in the position achieved during surgery
    Determine course of vertebral arteries by computed tomography and/or magnetic
        resonance imaging
    Discuss airway management with anesthesia team
Positioning
    Control head position during positioning using Mayfield or a turning table
    Obtain radiographs to assess alignment
    Reduce all misalignments before skin incision
Intraoperative
    Avoid dissection on superior surface of C1 lamina greater than 1.5 mm from the midline
    Avoid screws when vertebral anomalies are present
    Use biplanar fluoroscopy
    Position screws in center of the C1 lateral mass on both anteroposterior views and lateral
        images
    Do not locate screws farther anterior than the posterior margin of the C1 anterior arch
    If an artery is injured, do not place a screw on the opposite side
    Avoid sublaminar wires when stenosis is present

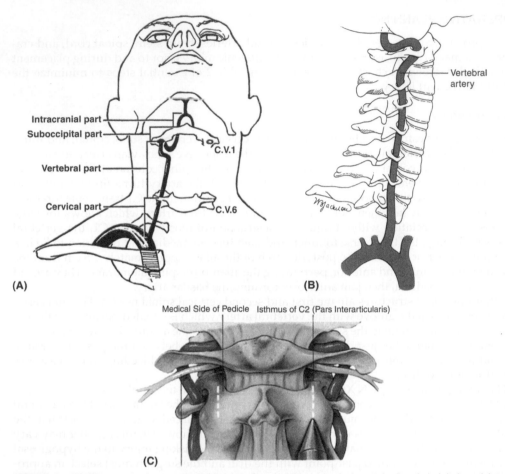

FIGURE 1 (**A**) The vertebral artery is divided into four sections: cervical, vertebral, suboccipital, and intracranial. (**B**) Side view showing the course of vertebral artery entering the spine at C6 and ascending in the foramina transversarium. At C1, the artery turns posterior before piercing the occipito-atlantal membrane entering the foramen magnum. (**C**) Dorsal view of suboccipital spine. At C2, the artery makes two turns, first laterally and then cranial to enter the C1 foramina transversarium that is located in a more lateral position.

During exposure of the laminar arches, one should take care not to injure the vertebral artery. Ebraheim has reported that the medial edge of the vertebral artery groove ranges from 8 to 18 mm from the midline on the superior surface of the C1 lamina (20). Exposure on the superior aspect of the posterior arch of the atlas should not be carried further than 15 mm lateral to midline. In 1% to 2% of cases, the vertebral artery lies in a tunnel, the arcuate foramen, on the superior aspect of the posterior atlantal arch formed by a thin bony arch, the postis ponticulous (21).

Transarticular screws enter the lateral mass of C2, traverse the C2 isthmus and the posterior portion of the C1–2 articulation, and are seated in the lateral mass of the atlas. Knowledge of the vertebral artery path within the axis in each patient is necessary for safe screw placement.

The C2 pedicle lies anterior to the inferior articular process of the axis and is often confused with the isthmus of the pars interarticularis. Reports in the literature indicate that placement of a transarticular screw is not anatomically possible in 10% to 18% of the population because of vertebral artery anomalies (22–25). Mandel reports that when the C2 isthmus measures less than 5 mm in height or width on computed tomography (CT) scan, the placement of a 3.5-mm transarticular screw increases the risk of penetration of the vertebral artery (22).

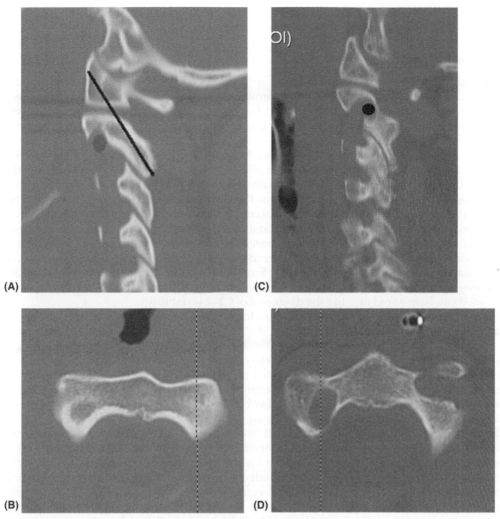

FIGURE 2 (**A**) Sagittal and axial computed tomography (CT). These views are helpful to plan screw course and determine if a transarticular screw is feasible and safe. (**B**) CT axial reconstruction of normal anatomy. (**C**) Axial CT showing a medial course of right vertebral artery making transarticular screw placement unsafe. (**D**) Same patient's sagittal CT showing insufficient bone to safely place a transarticular screw.

Preoperative CT scans with sagittal reconstruction or high-quality sagittal MRI images should be used to evaluate the vertebral artery and C2 isthmus to ensure that safe screw placement is possible (Fig. 2). If there is any question of the ability to safely place a transarticular screw on these images, screw placement should not be attempted. Satisfactory results have been achieved with unilateral screws and supplemental wire fixation (24).

Preoperative Assessment

A thorough history and physical exam is performed. Patients may present with symptoms ranging from mechanical complaints such as axial neck pain, neck spasm, torticollis, and headaches to myelopathy from spinal cord compression. Symptoms are usually worsened with neck flexion. The neurologic exam can range from normal to transient quadriparesis. Complete spinal cord injuries are rare as they are usually fatal at this level. Neurologic complaints may present late. In cases of severe atlantoaxial instability, patients may present with brain stem symptoms such as vertigo, syncope, respiratory distress, and stroke secondary to vertebrobasilar insufficiency from vertebral artery occlusion. Body habitus is important to assess when planning a C1–2 posterior arthrodesis. Excessive thoracic kyphosis or obesity may preclude correct screw trajectory for the C1–2 transarticular approach.

Preoperative Imaging

Standard radiographic assessment includes an open-mouth odontoid view and lateral cervical spine radiograph centered at C2. The bony elements are assessed on these films to identify fractures, various anomalies such as odontoid hypoplasia and os odontoideum, and severe erosive changes which may be because of various inflammatory, neoplastic, or infectious etiologies.

On the lateral view, the ADI is the distance between the posterior aspect of the anterior C1 arch and the anterior aspect of the dens. The ADI serves as a radiographic assessment of the integrity of the transverse ligament. It is normally less than 3 mm in adults and 5 mm in children, and should not change significantly from flexion to extension. Atlantal-dens intervals greater than 5 mm may be associated with spinal cord compression. The lateral radiograph may be misleading if it is taken in the supine position as the C1–2 joint may be reduced as the head falls back in extension. If the patient is alert, conscious, cooperative, and neurologically intact, lateral flexion–extension radiographs can better identify abnormal motion at C1–2. In cases of acute trauma, muscular pain and splinting may limit motion on flexion–extension films leading to a false-negative reading. Repeat flexion–extension radiographs once the acute phase spasms have resided can help avoid missing the diagnosis of C1–2 instability.

All patients who are considered candidates for C1–2 transarticular screw fixation should have a CT scan with sagittal reconstruction or MRI with high-quality sagittal images to assess the course of the vertebral arteries. Although rare, there have been reports of cerebellar infarction and death following iatrogenic vertebral artery injury (26). The size of the C2 isthmus and location of the vertebral artery can be determined on sagittal CT and MRI images. If anatomic constraints suggest that a transarticular screw cannot be safely placed, an alternate method of fixation must be performed. If a unilateral screw can be placed safely, we recommend placement of that screw combined with posterior wiring (27).

In patients with neurologic findings, MRI evaluation should be performed to assess the spinal canal. In patients with rheumatoid arthritis, MRI also provides an assessment of the degree of synovial pannus, the space available for the cord, and the cervicomedullary angle. Signal changes within the cord representing edema or myelomalacia can give information regarding the general physiologic state of the cervical cord. Posterior sublaminar wires should not be passed in the face of canal stenosis. If reduction of the C1–2 joint will not alleviate the stenosis, decompression of the cervical cord should be accomplished by posterior C1 arch laminectomy, possibly with posterior occiput decompression and/or C2 laminotomy.

SURGICAL TECHNIQUE
Anesthesia and Positioning

General endotracheal intubation is traditionally performed, although the degree of instability and neurologic status may necessitate the rise of fiberoptic intubation. After intubation, a neurologic check is performed and then the patient is given a general anesthetic. A bite-block, gauze roll, or wine cork placed between the incisors will optimize the intraoperative visualization of the C1–2 joints on anteroposterior fluoroscopy. We recommend spinal cord monitoring with motor-evoked potentials and/or somatosensory-evoked potentials in cases of significant instability or high-grade stenosis.

Mayfield tongs are placed and the patient is proned minimizing manipulation of the head and neck (Fig. 3). The patient's chest and iliac crests are supported on gel rolls and the abdomen is allowed to fall free. The arms are positioned anatomically at the patient's side and bony prominences are padded. The C1–2 joint is reduced with gentle extension and traction of the neck while mildly rotating the chin caudally. The Mayfield is tightened and secured to the bed on a "U-frame," which allows unobstructed anteroposterior and lateral fluoroscopic views during surgery. After positioning, the reduction is confirmed by fluoroscopy. The shoulders are gently taped without excessive tension to avoid brachial plexus traction. Alternatively, the

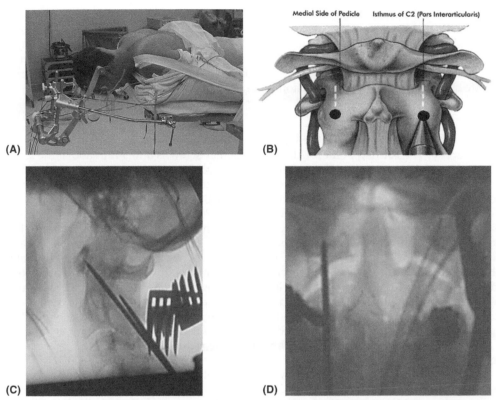

Medial Side of Pedicle   Isthmus of C2 (Pars Interarticularis)

FIGURE 3 (**A**) Intraoperative positioning on open-mouth radiograph. The Mayfield device is attached to the top of the U-shaped outrigger bar. (**B**) In line with C2 isthmus and 3 to 5 mm above the C2–3 facet joint, 3-mm drill holes are placed that identify the starting point for screw insertion. (**C**) Positioning of two 2.5-mm K-wires on lateral radiographs. The K-wires are directed toward the center of the anterior arch of C1. (**D**) First guide pin seen on open mouth is positioned in the center of the C1 lateral mass.

patient can be positioned prone on the Jackson table with the head held in the Mayfield device attached to the table with a special clamp.

Exposure

The posterior scalp is shaved and the neck and posterior iliac crest are prepared and draped in a sterile manner. A midline incision is made from just caudal to the external occipital protuberance to approximately C3. Dissection is carried sharply down to the spinous processes in the ligamentum nuchae to minimize bleeding. The posterior elements are stripped subperiosteally to the lateral margins of the C2 facet and C3 lateral mass so that the C2 3 facet joint is well visualized. The posterior arch of C1 is exposed taking care not to carry the dissection further than 15 mm lateral on the posterior arch to avoid injuring the vertebral artery. In our experience, gentle blunt dissection with a Cobb elevator on the posterior arch of C1 is effective in minimizing bleeding from the venous plexus that is found between C1 and C2 laterally. If bleeding is encountered, it is best controlled by packing with gel foam–thrombin and compression.

Adjunctive Wire Fixation

To increase construct rigidity and stabilize the bone graft, wire fixation is added using either the Brooks or Gallie techniques (1,2). We prefer using titanium cables for their ease of passage, tensile strength, and image properties (28). A modified Brooks's technique is described next.

A 4-0 curette is used to subperiosteally dissect the superior and inferior edges of the posterior arch of C1 and lamina of C2. Using a suture passer, two sutures on each side are placed under the C1 and C2 lamina. Each suture is gently tied to the leader of a titanium cable and used to guide the cables around the posterior C1 arch. The caudal end of one of the cables is passed caudal to the C2 spinous process and secured with a temporary crimper device to maintain reduction of the C1–2 joint during screw placement. The other cable is clamped and directed out of the way for use later in the procedure. In general, placement of C1 and C2 sublaminar wires is safe as long as an anatomic reduction is obtained and stenosis is not present.

Screw Placement

The superior and medial borders of the C2 isthmus are identified with a Penfield #4 or an angled 4-0 curette. The starting point for the transarticular screw is 3 to 5 mm above the C2–3 facet joint and as medial as possible without breaking through the medial aspect of the C2 pedicle. Dissecting laterally increases the likelihood of vertebral artery injury due to the oblique course that the artery takes in the axis. Using a 3-mm burr, a starting hole is made at this critical location. We use a 2.5-mm AO Dynamic Hip Screw (AO, Paoli, Pennsylvania, U.S.A.) threaded guide pin to act as a drill for transarticular screws. A free guide pin is placed lateral to the neck and lateral C-arm images are used to estimate the appropriate skin entry point. A stab incision is made about 1 cm lateral to the T1 spinous process. The guide pin is inserted and advanced cranially through the paraspinous muscles until it reaches the prepared starting hole. This percutaneous method helps to minimize the length of the incision. Using anteroposterior and lateral C-arm imaging, the guide pin is advanced in a sagittal plane toward the center of the C1 lateral mass on the anteroposterior view and toward the middle of the anterior C1 arch on the lateral view. The drill and subsequent screws should not extend past the dorsal margin of the anterior arch of C1. Guide pins are placed on each side to help maintain the reduction during screw placement. A free guide pin is used to measure the screw length using a subtraction technique (Fig.4).

One guide pin is removed and a fully threaded self-tapping 3.5-mm cortical screw is placed confirming fluoroscopically that the C1–2 joint is not distracted as the screw traverses. A washer may be used if bone quality is questionable. The contralateral screw is placed in the same manner. We recommend passing a long screwdriver through the percutaneous incision first and then seating the screw on the screwdriver in the wound to avoid disengaging and losing the screw in the paraspinous muscles. Some screwdrivers lock the head of the screw to the screwdriver allowing easier percutaneous passage of the screw and screwdriver as a unit. The head of the screw should be tightened under direct vision and final anteroposterior and lateral films are obtained to confirm appropriate screws position and length.

Bone Graft

The posterior iliac crest is exposed and a 7- to 10-mm thick bicortical rectangular plate is harvested with an osteotome and mallet. Curettes are used to harvest separate pieces of cancellous graft. The structural graft is contoured with a Leksell rongeur. A notch is cut centrally on the caudal edge in which the C2 spinous process is seated. The posterior C1 arch and C2 are decorticated with a high-speed burr. After releasing the temporary crimper from the cable, the structural graft is seated on the posterior arch of C1 with the spinous process of C2 wedged in the notch of the graft. The additional cancellous bone is packed around the structural graft. The cables are looped around the caudal aspect of the C2 spinous process and passed around the cranial and caudal edges of the structural graft on each side. The caudal wires are passed through the cranial collars and the cables are tightened using a tensioning device. The cables are secured by crimping the collars and cable cutters cut the excess cable flush with the collar. The wounds are closed in layers with or without a drain based on the preference of the surgeon. It is important to reattach the short occipital rotator muscles to the C2 spinous process.

Postoperative immobilization is in a hard cervical collar for 8 to 10 weeks or until there is radiographic evidence of healing.

COMPLICATIONS AND THEIR MANAGEMENT

Placement of transarticular screws is a technically demanding procedure and even in the hands of experienced surgeons the incidence of malpositioned screws has been reported to be as high

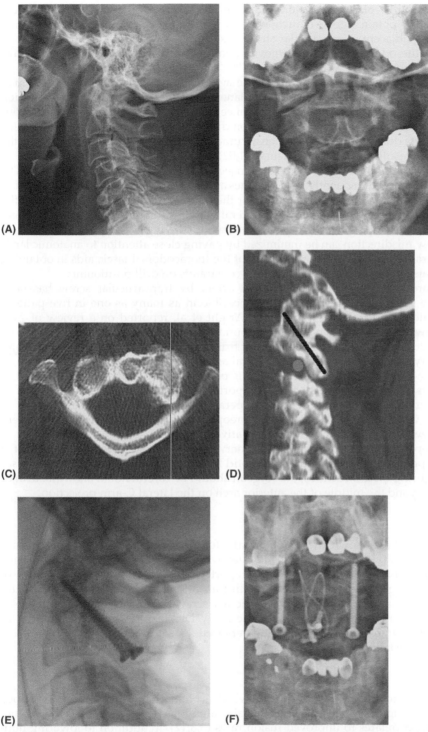

FIGURE 4 (**A**) Lateral cervical spine of a 75-year-old female with severe suboccipital pain, which is increased with left head rotation. (**B**) Open-mouth view showing severe degenerative arthritis of left C1–2 facet articulation. (**C**) Degenerative facet arthritis is seen on axial computed tomography (CT). (**D**) Sagittal CT reconstruction indicates excellent path for transarticular screw. (**E**) Intraoperative lateral after C1–2 transarticular screw insertion. Note screws are located at mid position of the anterior C1 arch and do not penetrate past its dorsal margin. (**F**) Six-month follow-up open-mouth radiograph. Good position of screws in the center of C1 lateral masses is seen. The sublaminar cables were used to secure bone graft blocks to the laminae.

as 15% (29). Proper screw placement requires anatomic reduction of the C1–2 during patient positioning. Failure to obtain a good reduction greatly increases the likelihood of misplacing screws and injuring adjacent neurovascular structures. Impediments to reduction such as an ossicle anterior to the odontoid or large synovial pannus can be identified on preoperative imaging.

High-quality biplanar intraoperative C-arm imaging is required to minimize screw malposition. Poor fluoroscopic visualization in either plane will increase the chance of misdirection during drilling and screw placement. Image guidance systems are an alternative (30). In our opinion, these lack reliability because of registration difficulties and position change between C1 and C2 that occurs during surgery. Although accuracy as high as 98% has been reported, the false-negative could result in catastrophic injury (31,32).

Careful attention should be given to the drill trajectory in both planes prior to drilling. The trajectory should be checked frequently in both planes as the drill is advanced across the joint. If the angle is too steep the tip of the screw may enter the occipitoatlantal joint, while a very flat trajectory may leave the screw inferior to the C1 lateral mass resulting in inadequate purchase. Medial deviation may leave a screw in the spinal canal, while straying laterally puts the vertebral artery at risk. Screw misdirection can be minimized by paying close attention to anatomic landmarks and radiographic images. A liberal incision of the thoracodorsal fascia aids in obtaining the appropriate trajectory by minimizing soft tissue constraints on drill positioning.

Although rare, penetration of the vertebral artery by transarticular screw has been reported (26). Safe screw placement may not be possible in as many as one in five patients because of anomalous vertebral artery anatomy. Wright et al. reported on a review of 2492 transarticular screws placed in 1318 patients and found the risk of vertebral artery injury to be 4.1% per patient (26). The risk of neurologic injury from vertebral artery injury was 0.2% and the risk of mortality was 0.1%. Fortunately, vertebral artery injuries rarely result in neurologic injury as long as the contralateral vertebral artery is patent and the posteroinferior cerebellar artery blood flow is preserved. Demetriades (33) reports that most vertebral artery injuries can be treated by observation rather than requiring operation or embolization. The best way to avoid injury to the vertebral artery is to recognize preoperatively when the course of the artery precludes safe screw placement and perform alternative fixation.

Grob has reported unilateral hypoglossal nerve paresis from excessive length of a screw (11). The hypoglossal nerve and internal carotid lie directly anterior to the lateral masses of C1. To avoid injuring these structures, the surgeon should be careful not to allow the drill or screw tip to pass beyond the middle of the anterior arch on the lateral C-arm projection.

OUTCOMES

Several clinical studies have shown low nonunion rates for transarticular screws despite the use of less external immobilization. Pseudarthrosis rates with posterior wiring techniques have been reported from 10% to 15% (3). Grob et al. reported only one nonunion in a series of 161 patients undergoing C1–2 posterior fusion with transarticular screws (11). Dickman and Sonntag reported a 2% nonunion rate for transarticular screw fixation compared with a 14% nonunion rate for posterior wiring (3). In a separate study, Dickman reviewed the repair of 16 C1–2 nonunions with transarticular screws and reported 13 solid bony fusions, two stable fibrous unions and one failure (34).

CONCLUSION

Transarticular screws provide three-point fixation which is biomechanically superior to various popular posterior wiring techniques. Several clinical evaluations have proved that this biomechanical advantage correlates to improved fusion rates (3,8,12). In addition to lowering nonunion rates, the increased stiffness of transarticular screws allows for less postoperative immobilization. Despite its many advantages, this technique is very technically demanding and should be performed by experienced surgeons. Comprehensive knowledge of the local anatomy and thorough understanding of potential pitfalls and how to avoid them will result in safe and successful placement of this screw.

REFERENCES

1. Brooks AL, Jenkins EB. Atlanto-axial arthrodesis by the wedge compression method. J Bone Joint Surg Am 1978; 60:279–284.
2. Gallie WE. Fractures and dislocations of the cervical spine. Am J Surg 1939; 46:494–499.
3. Dickman CA, Sonntag VK. Posterior C1-C2 transarticular screw fixation for atlantoaxial arthrodesis. Neurosurgery 1998; 43:275–280.
4. Moskovich R, Crockard HA. Atlantoaxial arthrodesis using interlaminar clamps. An improved technique. Spine 1992; 17(3):261–267.
5. Magerl F, Seeman PS. Stable posterior fusion of the atlas and axis by transarticular screw fixation. In: Weidner PA, ed. Cervical Spine. New York: Springer-Verlag, 1987:322–327.
6. Farey ID, Nadkarni S, Smith N. Modified Gallie technique versus transarticular screw fixation in C1-C2 fusion. Clin Orthop 1999; 359:126–135.
7. Grob D, Crisco JJ, III, Panjabi MM, Wang P, Dvorak J. Biomechanical evaluation of four different posterior atlantoaxial fixation techniques. Spine 1992; 17(5):480–490.
8. Hurlbert RJ, Crawford NR, Choi WG, Dickman CA. A biomechanical evaluation of occipitocervical instrumentation: screw compared with wire fixation. J Neurosurg Spine 1999; 90:84–90.
9. Naderi S, Crawford NR, Song GS, Sonntag VK, Dickman CA. Biomechanical comparison of C1-C2 posterior fixations. Cable, graft, and screw combinations. Spine 1955; 23:1946–1955.
10. Henriques T, Cunningham BW, Olerud C, et al. Biomechanical comparison of five different atlantoaxial posterior fixation techniques. Spine 2000; 25:2877–2883.
11. Grob D, Jeanneret B, Aebi M, Markwalder TM. Atlanto-axial fusion with transarticular screw fixation. J Bone Joint Surg Br 1991; 73:972–976.
12. Tokuhashi Y, Matsuzaki H, Shirasaki Y, Tateishi T. C1-C2 intra-articular screw fixation for atlantoaxial posterior stabilization. Spine 2000; 25:337–341.
13. Campanelli M, Kattner KA, Stroink A, Gupta K, West S. Posterior C1-C2 transarticular screw fixation in the treatment of displaced type II odontoid fractures in the geriatric population—review of seven cases. Surg Neurol 1999; 51:596–600.
14. McGuire RA Jr, Harkey HL. Primary treatment of unstable Jefferson's fractures. J Spinal Disord Tech 1995; 8(3):233–236.
15. Ohsawa T, Izawa T, Kuroki Y, Ohnari K. Follow-up study of atlanto-axial instability in Down's syndrome without separate odontoid process. Spine 1989; 14(11):1149–1153.
16. Boden SD, Dodge LD, Bohlman HH, Rechtine GR. Rheumatoid arthritis of the cervical spine. A long-term analysis with predictors of paralysis and recovery. J Bone Joint Surg Am 1993; 75(9):1282–1297.
17. Ghanayem AJ, Leventhal M, Bohlman HH. Osteoarthrosis of the atlanto-axial joints. Long-term follow-up after treatment with arthrodesis. J Bone Joint Surg Am 1996; 78(9):1300–1307.
18. Ebraheim NA, Misson JR, Xu R, Yeasting RA. The optimal transarticular c1-2 screw length and the location of the hypoglossal nerve. Surg Neurol 2000; 53:208–210.
19. Currier BL, Todd LT, Maus TP, Fisher DR, Yaszemski MJ. Anatomic relationship of the internal carotid artery to the C1 vertebra: a case report of cervical reconstruction for chordoma and pilot study to assess the risk of screw fixation of the atlas. Spine 2003; 28(22):E461–E467.
20. Ebraheim NA, Xu R, Ahmad M, Heck B. The quantitative anatomy of the vertebral artery groove of the atlas and its relation to the posterior atlantoaxial approach. Spine 1998; 23(3):320–323.
21. Young JP, Young PH, Ackermann MJ, Anderson PA, Riew DK. The arcuate foramen: implications for C1 lateral mass screw insertion. J Bone Joint Surg Am 2005; 87:2495–2498.
22. Mandel IM, Kambach BJ, Petersilge CA, Johnstone B, Yoo JU. Morphologic considerations of C2 isthmus dimensions for the placement of transarticular screws. Spine 2000; 25(12):1542–1547.
23. Paramore CG, Dickman CA, Sonntag VK. The anatomical suitability of the C1-2 complex for transarticular screw fixation. J Neurosurg 1996; 85(2):221–224.
24. Song GS, Theodore N, Dickman CA, Sonntag VK. Unilateral posterior atlantoaxial transarticular screw fixation. J Neurosurg 1997; 87:851–855.
25. Taitz C, Arensburg B. Vertebral artery tortuosity with concomitant erosion of the foramen of the transverse process of the axis. Possible clinical implications. Acta Anatomica 1991; 141(2):104–108.
26. Wright NM, Lauryssen C. Vertebral artery injury in C1-2 transarticular screw fixation: results of a survey of the AANS/CNS section on disorders of the spine and peripheral nerves. J Neurosurg 1998; 88:634–640.
27. Sasso R, Doherty BJ, Crawford MJ, Heggeness MH. Biomechanics of odontoid fracture fixation. Comparison of the one- and two-screw technique. Spine 1993; 18:1950–1953.
28. Dickman CA, Crawford NR, Paramore CG. Biomechanical characteristics of C1-2 cable fixations. J Neurosurg 1996; 85(2):316–322.
29. Gebhard JS, Schimmer RC, Jeanneret B. Safety and accuracy of transarticular screw fixation C1-C2 using an aiming device. An anatomic study. Spine 1998; 23(20):2185–2189.
30. Herz T, Franz A, Giacomuzzi SM, Bale R, Krismer M. Accuracy of spinal navigation for magerl screws. Clin Orthop 2003; 409:124–130.

31. Kamimura M, Ebara S, Itoh H, Tateiwa Y, Kinoshita T, Takaoka K. Cervical pedicle screw insertion: assessment of safety and accuracy with computer-assisted image guidance. J Spinal Disord Tech 2000; 13(3):218–224.
32. Richter M, Amiot LP, Neller S, Kluger P, Puhl W. Computer-assisted surgery in posterior instrumentation of the cervical spine: an in-vitro feasibility study. Eur Spine J 2000; 9(suppl 1):S65–S70.
33. Demetriades D, Theodorou D, Asensio J, et al. Management options in vertebral artery injuries. Br J Surg 1996; 83(1):83–86.
34. Dickman CA, Sonntag VK. Posterior C1-C2 transarticular screw fixation for atlantoaxial arthrodesis. Neurosurgery 1998; 43:275–280.

17 | Submuscular Instrumentation for Spinal Deformities

Douglas G. Armstrong and George H. Thompson
Division of Pediatric Orthopedics, Rainbow Babies and Children's Hospital, Case Medical Center, Case Western Reserve University, Cleveland, Ohio, U.S.A.

INTRODUCTION

The surgical treatment of scoliosis usually involves instrumentation for acute correction followed by arthrodesis to maintain long-term correction and spinal balance. These techniques are effected by both anterior, posterior, and combined surgical methods. Standard posterior methods involve extensive soft-tissue stripping and bony exposure. Recently, a less-invasive method of posterior instrumentation for gradual correction of scoliosis has been developed. It involves limited dissection in the upper and lower ends of a construct with insertion of spanning "growing" rod or rods placed through a submuscular or subcutaneous plane. The proposed advantages, in addition to its minimally invasive nature, are that it can allow considerable spinal growth during correction prior to definitive fusion. It is the authors' purpose to describe the application and outcomes of this technique for the treatment of idiopathic scoliosis.

INDICATIONS

Severe progressive scoliosis during infancy and early childhood (early onset scoliosis) that has failed orthotic or serial risser cast management or those who have a contraindication to this form of treatment. The etiology of such deformities include idiopathic (infantile and juvenile) scoliosis; congenital scoliosis; neuromuscular scoliosis; and spinal deformity secondary to various syndromes.

SINGLE GROWING ROD
Surgical Technique

With baseline spinal cord monitoring signals established when appropriate, the patient is placed in the prone position. Two short vertical incisions are made, one at the cranial and one at the caudal limits of the proposed instrumentation site, leaving a bridge of intact skin and fascia between them. Alternatively, a single long incision can be made, but the spine is exposed subperiosteally only at the proposed sites for the proximal and distal anchor sites. Using the single incision technique, the fascia is opened between the proximal and distal sites but the underlying paraspinal muscles are left intact. At either end of the construct, a one-level or two-level claw hook construct may be used. At the proximal end of the construct, a supralaminar hook is preferable when possible, as the lamina of the upper thoracic spine is considerably stronger than the transverse processes. At the distal end, a claw configuration is also used. If a pedicle screw is placed instead of a hook, it may be desirable to protect the screw with an infra laminar hook in some cases.

Next, the rod is inserted. It is tunneled beneath the paraspinal muscular layer to arrive at the proximal and distal sites. The initial length should be long enough so that it will project 4 to 5 cm beyond the proximal or distal claw construct. Once the rod is contoured and in position, the proximal or distal claw is compressed to achieve stabilization. Distraction is then carried out and the remaining foundation is tightened. Bone graft, usually allograft, can be placed about the anchor sites. An intraoperative radiograph is obtained prior to skin closure.

Patients are usually managed postoperatively with a thoracolumbosacral orthosis (TLSO). Additional rod lengthenings are performed at six-month intervals as an outpatient. This is accomplished by exposing the anchor site adjacent to the long end of the rod. The existing set of screws is loosened or exchanged and the rod is distracted. At the completion of each session of lengthening, about 1 cm of the rod will have been pushed proximally. The distraction force is gentle to avoid laminar fracture. When the patient reaches a suitable age or size a posterior spinal fusion is performed (Fig. 1A–D). It is recommended the implants be exchanged for standard dual rod segmental spinal instrumentation.

Pitfalls and Bailouts

In the event of rod breakage, which usually occurs after 1.5 to 2 years, a longitudinal tandem connector can be placed to connect the broken rod, if the surgeon prefers not to exchange it. This device also allows the surgeon to continue to lengthen through the connector itself. The set screws at one end of the connector are loosened and the construct lengthened. The set screws are then tightened.

DUAL GROWING RODS

In the same manner as described before, the patient is placed in the prone position with spinal cord monitoring in place. One long incision or two incisions with a vertical skin bridge between them may be used and the proximal and distal anchor sites are exposed subperiosteally out to the transverse processes. Small-diameter, pediatric-sized rods may be used for the smaller weight patients. The instrumentation may be placed subcutaneously or subfascially. The upper foundation is over two or three vertebrae.

If supralaminar hooks are chosen, two to three vertebrae should be exposed. The supralaminar hooks are staggered, with only one per level to avoid canal stenosis. The facet/infralaminar hooks may be both placed at one vertebra or staggered across two levels (Figs. 2–3). At the lower foundation, hooks or pedicle screws may be used. Two pairs of rods are used at each end of the construct; these are connected vertically by tandem connectors. The tandem connectors should not be proximal to the thoracolumbar junction as they cannot be contoured and must remain straight. The surgeon should plan for the appropriate lengths of rods at the cephalad anchors. Occasionally, side-to-side connectors can be necessary if the rods will overlap. Once the two proximal and two distal rods are through their respective hooks, the transverse connectors are placed. These must be left loose so that the tandem connectors can be applied. The rods cannot be contoured at the thoracolumbar junction as this would prevent them from passing into the tandem ("growth") connector. The first tandem connector is slid along the upper rod on the concavity of the curve. Once it has passed the upper end of the distal rod that rod may be brought into it. Once the two tandem connectors are in place tightening of the hooks and transverse connectors is carried out. Distraction is then applied, typically by using the smaller distraction tool that fits inside the tandem connector. Distraction should be alternated from one side to the other until completed. The set screws are then tightened.

Lengthening is performed by exposing only the tandem connectors. The previous set screws are loosened or exchanged. Distraction is carried out and the set screws re-tightened. When the patient reaches the appropriate size or age the growing rods are exchanged for a standard dual rod segmental spinal instrumentation and a posterior spinal fusion performed.

Pitfalls and Bailouts

If the construct seems to have become too short then the tandem connectors can be exchanged for longer ones. Rod exchange can be accomplished when necessary; again, one should make certain that the growth connectors are at the thoracolumbar junction to avoid prominence and deleterious effects on the sagittal profile.

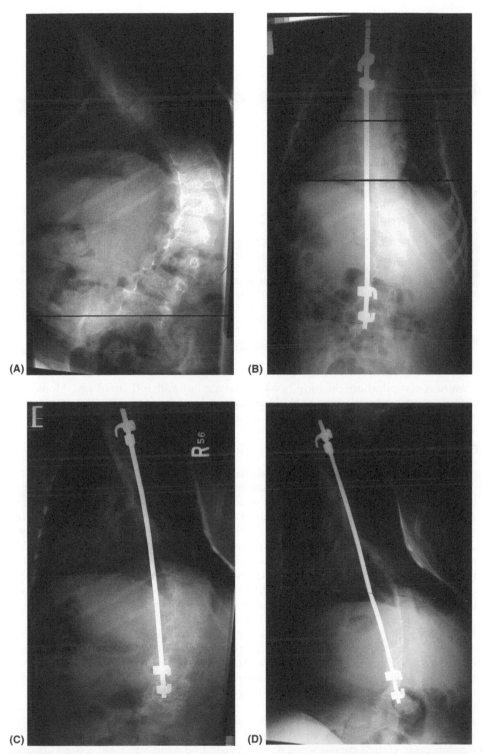

FIGURE 1   Single-rod instrumentation for neuromuscular scoliosis. (**A**) Preoperative radiograph showing a 78° thoracolumbar curve in a seven-year-old boy with spinal muscle atrophy. (**B**) Postoperative radiograph following initial procedure showing a single submuscular rod in place. The curve now measures 26°. Note the claw configuration of the cranial and caudal anchors. (**C**) Four years after the initial procedure, five lengthenings were made. The curve magnitude is 42°. (**D**) At final follow-up, the curve measured 62°. Because of the patients' underlying disease, a posterior fusion was performed without revision of instrumentation.

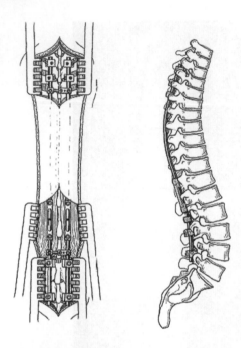

FIGURE 2   Dual-rod instrumentation. Note the use of hooks in a claw configuration at the cranial ends of the construct. Pedicle screws are frequently used at the caudal end, either two pairs or one pair of screws with a pair of sublaminar hooks. Transverse rod connectors are used next to the upper and lower anchors to connect each pair of rods. The tandem connectors are located at the thoracolumbar junction.

COMPLICATIONS

The most common complications include hook dislodgement and rod breakage. Hook dislodgement often necessitates replacement. Rod breakage can be managed with placement of an additional tandem connector to bridge the site of discontinuity.

OUTCOMES

Blakemore et al. reported the results or submuscular Isola segmental spinal instrumentation for 29 patients treated over a six-year period (1). The proximal anchors were placed in a claw configuration. Eleven children had a short apical fusion or convex hemi-epiphysiodesis in addition to placement of a single submuscular rod. The diagnoses were varied, and the mean age at the time of the initial procedure was 6.7 years (range: 1–11 years). Mean follow-up was 41 months (range: 11–65 months). Instrument lengthening was performed when the curve progressed 15° to 20°, usually every 6 to 12 months. All patients were managed with an orthosis postoperatively. Nine patients had undergone a definitive fusion by the time of the report. Seven patients had nine complications including hook dislodgement, rod breakage, and superficial infection. The best correction of the scoliosis was noted after the initial procedure. Postoperatively, curves averaged 38° (range: 16–70°) compared with 66° (range: 42–112°) preoperatively.

In a study comparing single rod with dual rods, Thompson et al. found that dual rods resulted in better initial correction and improved long-term maintenance of correction (2). Their study retrospectively analyzed 28 patients with various diagnoses, who had a minimum of two years follow-up following the definitive spinal fusions. Group I consisted of five patients who had a short apical fusion and a single Isola rod. Group II consisted of 16 children treated with a single submuscular rod alone. Group III consisted of seven patients who had undergone dual-rod instrumentation. The mean age at initial surgery was seven years (range: 2.9–9.3 years); 8.7 years (range: 5.9–11.6 years), and 6.9 years (range: 2.1–14 years), respectively, for groups I, II, and III. The mean preoperative curves were: 85° ± 23°, 61° ± 13°, and 92° ± 21°. Correction just prior to final fusion was 77° ± 20°, 55° ± 15°, and 33° ± 16°, respectively. Final curves after definitive fusion were 65° ± 22°, 39° ± 15°, and 26° ± 18°. The group with dual rods had been lengthened routinely every six months, which caused those patients to have a significantly greater number or lengthenings (six compared with three in the other two groups). The other two groups had undergone rod elongation only when there had been curve progression.

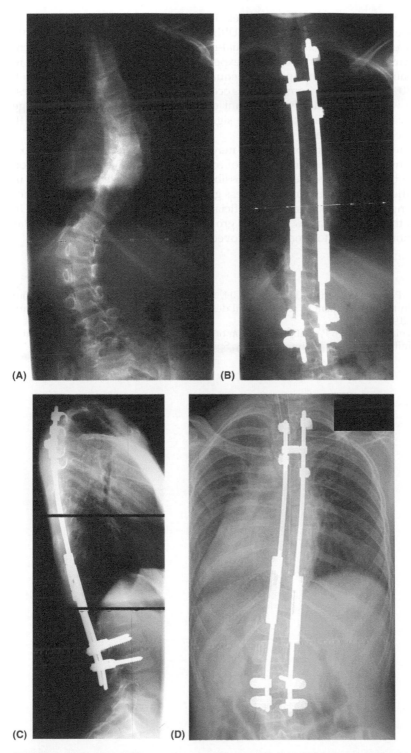

(A)

(B)

(C)

(D)

FIGURE 3 Case presentation: a nine-year-old girl with progressive juvenile idiopathic scoliosis. (**A**) Preoperative radiograph showing a 62° right thoracic and 60° left lumbar curves. (**B** and **C**) Curve appearance following placement of submuscular dual-rod instrumentation with pedicle screw caudal foundation. Curve measurements are 47° and 30°. (**D**) Following three lengthenings, 1.5 years after the index procedure, the curve measurements were 35° and 30°. There is normal saggital plane alignment. Note that the tandem connectors are in proper position at the thoracolumbar junction, and that the rods had been distracted through those devices.

Elongation was achieved over the instrumented levels in each group and corresponded to approximately 1 cm for each lengthening procedure. Ultimately, there was significantly more T1 to S1 height gained, averaging 11. 8 ± 4.0 cm, in the dual-rod group compared with 6.4 ± 1.4 cm in group I and 7.6 ± 4.7 cm in group II. As a percent of expected growth, calculated according to Dimeglio's growth remaining data for the spine, this equated to 25% of expected for group I, 80% for group II, and 130% for group III. Complications occurred in each group, with the lowest rate in group II. There were no statistically significant differences in rates of rod breakage between groups. However, hook displacements were significantly less frequent in group III. Group I had the highest complication rate.

The authors concluded that a short apical fusion may stiffen the spine thereby predisposing to crankshaft phenomenon and increasing the risk of complications. However, apical fusion was used in an effort to treat stiff curves so it was possible that surgeon selection resulted in group I having more patients with stiffer curves and less growth potential. The authors further concluded that either single or dual rods can be beneficial for control of spinal deformities in the very young and that they do in fact allow for spinal growth. Dual rods with frequent regular lengthening every six months appear to produce improved outcomes.

REFERENCES

1. Blakemore LC, Scoles PV, Poe-Kochert C, Thompson GH. Submuscular Isola rod with or without limited apical fusion in the management of severe spinal deformities in young children: preliminary report. Spine 2001; 26:2044–2048.
2. Thompson GH, Akbarnia BA, Kostial P, et al. Comparison of single and dual growing rod techniques followed through definitive surgery. A preliminary study. Spine 2005; 30(17 suppl):S94–99.

18 | Anterior Thoracoscopic Release/Fusion and Instrumentation for Spinal Deformities

Peter O. Newton
Department of Orthopedics, Children's Hospital San Diego, San Diego, California, U.S.A.

Vidyadhar V. Upasani
Department of Orthopedic Surgery, University of California, San Diego, California, U.S.A.

INTRODUCTION

Video-assisted thoracoscopy has recently evolved as an effective technique for multilevel anterior thoracic release and fusion in the treatment of spinal deformity. This minimally invasive approach was reintroduced in the early 1990s and has since become the standard approach to the anterior thoracic spine at many medical centers (1–5). The thoracoscopic approach uses a limited chest wall dissection to access the anterior spine. Several viable alternatives to specific aspects of the thoracoscopic technique have been developed to accommodate a variety of patient and surgeon preferences or needs. Once mastered, video-assisted thoracoscopy affords several advantages over the open approach, including (1): reduced postoperative pain, reduced pulmonary morbidity, access to more vertebral levels, and improved cosmesis.

INDICATIONS

The thoracoscopic approach in patients with spinal deformity (scoliosis or kyphosis) is appropriate for release and fusion between the T4 and T12 vertebral levels. As additional experience is gained, the procedure may be extended both proximally to T2 and distally to L1. As with any open spinal deformity correction procedure, the goal of video-assisted thoracoscopy is to obtain complete exposure and thorough disc excision so as to allow grafting and ultimately solid interbody arthrodesis.

In patients with scoliosis, anterior release and fusion is generally indicated for the treatment of large or rigid curves that require increased flexibility to obtain maximal correction during posterior instrumentation and fusion. Although the upper limits of curve magnitude and flexibility have not been concretely identified, it has been shown that anterior removal of the disc increases curve flexibility, and provides greater coronal and sagittal plane correction with posterior implant systems (6). The degree to which flexibility can be increased is dependent on the complete removal of both the annulus fibrosis and internal disc material. In the most severe cases of scoliosis, resection of the rib head and/or the costovertebral joint may also be required to optimize mobility.

A second indication for anterior disc excision and fusion is the prevention of crankshaft growth, which has been reported to occur following an isolated posterior instrumentation and fusion procedure in skeletally immature patients (7,8). The status of the triradiate cartilage may be a reasonable marker to identify patients who would benefit from an anterior procedure. Thus, patients with an open triradiate cartilage who are Risser 0 could be treated with an anterior release and fusion in an effort to limit future anterior growth.

A third indication may exist in patients at increased risk for pseudarthrosis formation; for example, patients diagnosed with neurofibromatosis or Marfan syndrome, or with a prior history of irradiation. An adequate anterior discectomy and fusion generally provides a large cancellous bony surface for increasing the likelihood of solid arthrodesis formation.

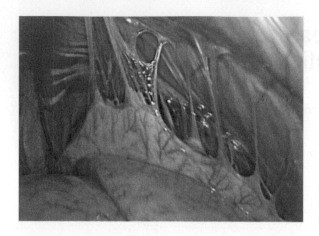

FIGURE 1 Pleural adhesions that limit the ability of the lung to adequately collapse can be a contraindication to the anterior thoracoscopic approach.

CONTRAINDICATIONS

Primarily, any medical history of compromised pulmonary status or intrathoracic pleural adhesion formation secondary to a prior thoracotomy or pulmonary infection should be considered a relative contraindication. The thoracoscopic approach requires adequate space within the chest cavity to manipulate both the endoscope and the working instruments. This generally requires selective ventilation of the lungs, and collapse of the lung on the side of the chest cavity being operated in. As such, the pulmonary status of the patient must allow single lung ventilation. Pleural adhesions between the lung and chest wall limit the ability of the lung to adequately collapse. Minor adhesions can be divided, however a nearly complete pleural symphysis between the chest and lung can make adequate lung collapse extremely challenging (Fig. 1).

Curves in which the spine has become closely approximated to the rib cage may be another relative contraindication due to the necessity of an adequate working space. A working distance of 2 to 3 cm should be considered the minimum when reviewing preoperative radiographs. This can be challenging to accomplish in young children with single-lung ventilation. Although children weighing less than 30 kg have been safely treated with the anterior thoracoscopic approach, the relative benefit of this minimally invasive technique seems to be reduced in very small patients (9). Visualization in larger patients is most often limited by excessive bleeding or inconsistent lung deflation. If visualization is inadequate at any point during the endoscopic procedure, conversion to an open approach must be considered.

SURGICAL TECHNIQUE
Patient and Surgeon Positioning

Lateral positioning of the patient allows anterior placement of ports on the chest wall, enabling greater circumferential visualization and access to the vertebral bodies and discs. The prone position, on the other hand, requires port placement to be more posterior than would be ideal for circumferential disc exposure. Similarly, as anterior exposure is the goal, positioning the surgeon and the assistant on the anterior side of the patient allows both of them to work and view the spine from the most natural perspective. It is also important to recognize that maintaining spatial orientation is easiest when the image on the video monitor is properly aligned and oriented, such that if the chest wall of the patient were made transparent, the image on the monitor would match what the surgeon would "see." In addition, an axillary roll should be placed under the patient, and the legs should be scissored to prevent excessive pressure on the down-side leg. Somatosensory-evoked potential monitoring in the upper and lower extremities can also be valuable.

Port Location and Spacing

Skin incisions (1.5 cm in length) are used to place rigid tubular ports between the ribs along the anterior axillary line. Port placement along the anterior axillary line, optimizes the exposure

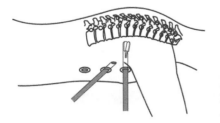

FIGURE 2 Port placement along the anterior axillary line optimizes visualization of the anterior spine and provides an adequate working distance. The working instrument is placed in a port parallel to the disc and the endoscope is placed one level proximal or distal.

and visualization of the anterior spine, and affords both a larger field of view with the scope, and an increased working distance for the instruments (Fig. 2). In cases of scoliosis, this port placement is ideal because disc angulation tends to converge anteriorly with kyphosis, and parallel access to several disc spaces is possible with a single port. This facilitates access into each disc space, minimizes the number of ports required to achieve inline access of the working instruments, and focuses the exposure on the anterior soft tissues (anterior longitudinal ligament) that require release. The opposite condition exists however, when the ports are placed posteriorly in patients with scoliosis, as the disc spaces are divergent.

The necessary number of ports is dictated mainly by the deformity being treated and the number of levels that require treatment. Four ports are typically sufficient to perform a six- to eight-level release and fusion. Care should be taken in placing the portals, particularly when placing them distally to avoid penetration below the diaphragm. Port spacing is dependent on the working distance from the chest wall to the spine, and angulation of the endoscopic viewing optics. This distance is also one of the most important determinants of the degree of endoscope angulation required to see within the depths of the disc. The higher the viewing angles of the endoscope, the greater the possible spacing of the ports while maintaining a view in line with the disc space. Typically, the instrument for discectomy is placed in the port that is parallel to the discs, and the endoscope is placed either one port proximal or distal to this level (Fig. 2).

Exposure of the Spine

Optimal port placement, camera orientation, and scope angulation are all required to ensure the best view of the spine. Maintaining ideal visualization throughout the video-assisted thoraco-scopic approach is critical to the success and safety of the procedure. The first step to ensure opti-mal visualization is to achieve complete lung deflation. This enables improved line of sight from the port to the spine, and reduces the risk of lung tissue perforation by an instrument. Selective lung ventilation is best managed with the placement of a double-lumen endotracheal tube.

A 10-mm endoscope, with both straightahead and angled optics, is inserted into the chest cavity and is used for visualization. The initial exposure of the spine can be increased with a fan retractor placed on the lung. The segmental vessels lying beneath the parietal pleura, as well as an oblique crossing sympathetic nerve, can be visualized overlying the spine (Fig. 3). After establishing the levels of release by counting from the proximal ribs, a harmonic scalpel is used

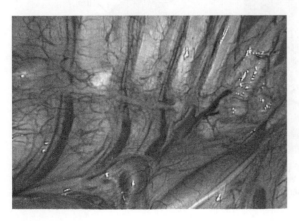

FIGURE 3 On initial exposure, the segmental ves-sels can be visualized beneath the parietal pleura.

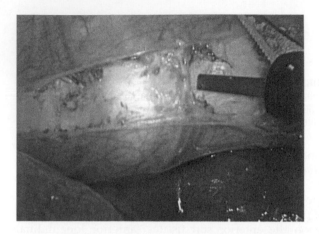

FIGURE 4 The segmental vessels are coagulated and divided with the harmonic scalpel to broaden the exposure and minimize bleeding, which can lead to occlusion of the field of view.

to create a longitudinal opening of the pleura. The initial pleural opening is performed superficial to the segmental vessels. Limited exposure of the discs is accomplished by retracting the pleura between the vessels. To broaden the exposure anteriorly, the segmental vessels are coagulated and divided with the harmonic scalpel (Fig. 4). This can be best accomplished if energy is applied slowly, over a 3- to 5-mm length of the vessel at a time. This allows excellent hemostasis and allows the pleura and vessels to be retracted together for circumferential exposure of the spine. It also facilitates pleural closure at the conclusion of the procedure.

Once the loose areolar tissue is divided, the pleura, the azygos vein, the esophagus, and the aorta are reflected anteriorly off the spine, and a space between the anterior longitudinal ligament and these structures is created, and maintained by packing sponges within the interval (Fig. 5). This creates a safe working area and provides retraction of the great vessels away from the spine, exposing the far side of the annulus for dissection and excision. Clear visualization of the discs circumferentially from the rib head on the convex side, to the rib head on the concave side is now accomplished. Distal exposure to the T12–L1 disc space requires division of the diaphragm insertion by extending the longitudinal incision of the pleura onto the inferiorly retraced diaphragm and by blunt stripping of the diaphragm from the anterior aspect of the spine.

Once an optimal dissection of the spine is accomplished, the surgical field must be maintained with as little blood as possible to maximize visualization. Ultrasonic dissectors are

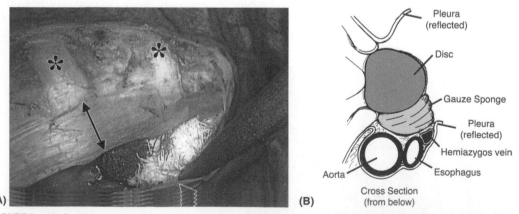

FIGURE 5 (A) Packing sponges are used to retract the great vessels and expose the entire disc. The *asterisk* identifies the intervertebral disc, an *arrow* is drawn across the width of the anterior longitudinal ligament, and the *open arrow* identifies the cut pleural edge. (B) A line drawing is used to show these relationships in cross-section, as a view from below.

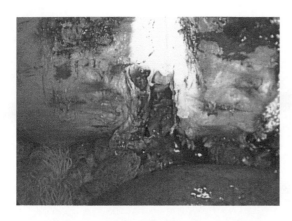

FIGURE 6 The most anterior and concave aspect of this annulus and disc is removed by an up-biting rongeur.

extremely useful in dissecting around the spine and controlling bleeding, as oozing from even the smallest vessels can obscure the anatomy.

Disc Excision and Bone Grafting

Disc excision is initiated anteriorly on the side farthest from the surgeon. Initial entrance into the disc space is facilitated by a circumferential annulotomy using the ultrasonic blade. An up-biting rongeur is used to remove the most anterior and concave aspect of the annulus of the disc first (Fig. 6). Complete disc removal requires optimal visualization deep into the disc space. During the discectomy, an attempt should be made to clear disc tissue as deeply as possible without disrupting the vertebral body endplate until the discectomy is essentially complete. The deep aspects of the disc should only be taken under direct visualization, maintaining the integrity of the posterior longitudinal ligament to protect the neural elements. With the disc space clearly identified, the removal of the disc progresses toward the convex side to the level of the rib head.

Clear identification of the direction and path of discectomy is required to avoid removing excessive bone, which will result in additional bleeding and difficulties in visualization. The endplate cartilage from the superior and inferior aspects of the vertebrae can be peeled off the bone with very little bleeding in most cases of idiopathic scoliosis (Fig. 7). However, in patients with osteopenia or when the disc excision inadvertently involves portions of the vertebral body, bleeding can make visualization more problematic. An angled curette or rongeur is useful in removing the endplate cartilage, and once it is excised, hemostasis can be aided by immediate cancellous bone grafting or with placement of hemostatic agents such as Surgicel®. The endoscopic retractor and working instruments are varied from port to port to maintain ideal visualization and access to the different levels of the spine. If exposure to the T12–L1 disc is required, an additional distal port may be required for greater retraction of the diaphragm.

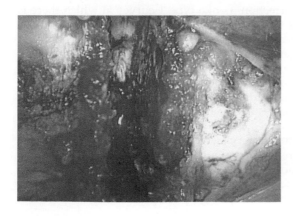

FIGURE 7 The endplate cartilage is then removed from the superior and inferior aspects of the vertebrae, after excision of the entire disc.

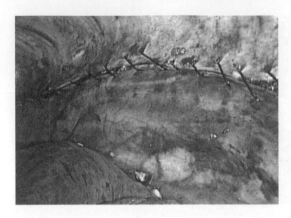

FIGURE 8 The EndoStitch® device is used to suture the pleura. Securing the suture proximally requires tying an internal knot with a series of half hitches.

Cancellous grafting of each evacuated disc space is recommended since arthrodesis is the ultimate goal of treating spinal deformities surgically. This may be autologous from the patient's ribs or ileum, allogenic (freeze dried or frozen), or artificial bone graft substitute. Enough morselized graft to fill the disc space is delivered through a tubular plunger device. A critical look at the postoperative radiographs will often demonstrate the extent of discectomy and grafting that was performed.

Pleural Closure

Following completion of the discectomy and bone grafting, or anterior spine instrumentation, endoscopic closure of the parietal pleura is undertaken. With practice this procedure can be relatively straightforward, and should not be any more time consuming that open pleural closures. The EndoStitch® device can be used to simplify this task by allowing the pleura to be reapproximated with a running closure. Beginning distally, the needle is passed through both sides of the cut pleura, or diaphragm if this was opened. A knot tied externally can be slid down the suture to secure the initial internal knot distally. The suturing device then passes a double-ended needle from one jaw to the other and a simple running closure of the pleura is performed (Fig. 8). Securing the suture proximally requires tying an internal knot with a series of half hitches. The advantages of the pleural closure are debated, but this may limit bleeding, maintain the bone graft in position, and decrease bleeding and pleural scarring.

THORACOSCOPIC ANTERIOR SCOLIOSIS INSTRUMENTATION

Endoscopic multilevel anterior thoracic instrumentation is becoming increasingly popular in the treatment of scoliosis for the selective fusion of a structural thoracic curve (10–12). The thoracoscopic minimally invasive approach has been developed in an effort to limit the morbidity associated with the open anterior thoracotomy and in some cases may provide a completely endoscopic option for scoliosis correction. Lenke type 1 curves in which there is reduced or normal kyphosis are ideal for this technique, as the anterior approach tends to be kyphogenic. Also curves less than 70° with greater than 50% flexibility are ideally amenable to the thoracoscopic approach. Even though larger curves have been instrumented, the challenges associated with thoracoscopy favor a posterior approach. The thoracoscopic approach is also contraindicated in obese patients (greater than 60 to 70 kg) who have an increased likelihood of overstressing a single rod anterior construct. In addition, the approach is contraindicated in very small patients in whom the vertebral bodies are unable to maintain the purchase of a vertebral body screw.

The patient is positioned and prepared for surgery just as for a thoracoscopic release and rigidly stabilized in the direct lateral position. An image intensifier is used to ensure perfect spatial orientation of each vertebra in the coronal plane, which is critical during vertebral body screw insertion. In this way, the trajectory of each screw can be anticipated before making a skin incision for screw placement. Generally, a series of three portals are required along the posterior

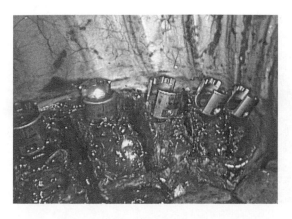

FIGURE 9   Appropriate screw alignment is important to facilitate rod insertion.

axillary line to place transvertebral body screws and connect them to a rod. This is supplemented by two anterior axillary line portals, which are used during disc excision and endoscope placement.

The procedure is initiated by thoracoscopic exposure of the spine and disc excision as described previously. All the segments of the measured Cobb angle are generally instrumented. The disc spaces are packed with an oxidized cellulose hemostat to reduce bleeding from the vertebral end plates. Next, screw insertion is initiated proximally. A 15-mm Thoracoport® (US Surgical, Norwalk, Conn.) is placed between the ribs through the proximal skin incision. The starting point for the screw is in the mid to superior aspect of the vertebral body just anterior to the rib head articulation with the vertebral body. An awl is used to initiate the hole, followed by a tap. The screw path is tapped through the far cortex, and using a ball-tipped calibrated probe the exact length of the screw is determined. Typically, 6.5-mm diameter screws are used. Moving the portal one rib space distally, the adjacent screw is placed in similar fashion, with care being taken to appropriately align each screw to make later rod insertion as straightforward as possible (Fig. 9). Each of the screws should be placed with bicortical purchase. However, given the location of the aorta on the left side of the vertebral bodies, excessive screw penetration should be avoided.

Following screw placement, each of the disc spaces should be grafted with autogenous bone, from either the iliac crest or rib. An interbody device or cortical allograft is used at the more distal levels where the interspace may require structural support. Deformity correction is accomplished by cantilevering a rod into position, beginning by engaging the proximal screws first. Segmental compression is performed at each of the levels with an endoscopic compressing device (Fig. 10). This combination of rod cantilevering facilitated with an approximating device and segmental vertebral body compression provide coronal plane correction of the scoliosis, sagittal restoration of kyphosis, and axial plane derotation of the spine (Fig. 11). Following rod insertion, the pleura may be closed as described previously using the EndoStitch® device.

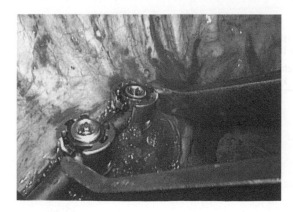

FIGURE 10   Segmental compression is performed with an endoscopic compressing device.

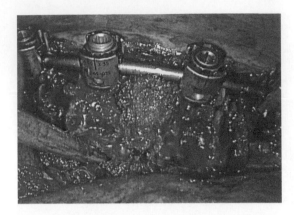

FIGURE 11 Rod cantilevering and segmental vertebral body compression provides coronal plane correction, sagittal restoration of kyphosis, and axial plane derotation of the spine. Autologous bone graft/morselized iliac is next used to fill each disc space.

OUTCOMES OF THORACOSCOPIC RELEASE AND FUSION

The thoracoscopic release and fusion technique continues to grow in popularity, particularly for pediatric spinal deformity indications, and has been shown to be comparable to the open thoracotomy approach (13). The learning curve for video-assisted thoracoscopy is substantial and requires a committed team to develop the skill required to perform these procedures safely and efficaciously (1). Attention to detail particularly in obtaining and maintaining visualization by limiting bleeding and optimizing scope position/orientation, is crucial as in most endoscopic procedures, and will limit complications. When compared to the open approach, several previously published studies demonstrate similar degrees of disc excision in both clinical series and animal models (6,14–16). In addition, evaluation of the safety of the thoracoscopic approach has demonstrated relatively few perioperative complications and rates equivalent to those for open procedures (1).

Potential complications after anterior thoracoscopy include excessive bleeding, lung parenchymal injury, spinal cord injury, chylothorax, and nonunion. In general, postoperative pulmonary complications and surgical times (2 to 2.5 hours) have been found to be similar compared to those experienced after open anterior thoracic surgery (9). This is especially true in patients with idiopathic scoliosis. However, in most series neuromuscular patients present the greatest challenge because of increased curve magnitude, small patient size, preoperative pulmonary compromise, and osteopenia (17).

Assessment of anterior fusion rates after thoracoscopic procedures demonstrate that in a majority of the disc spaces treated with either autograft or allograft, some degree of fusion exists. In our series of 112 consecutive cases of spinal deformity treatment, with more than two years follow-up, thoracoscopic anterior release and fusion of the thoracic spine was found to be a safe and effective procedure when combined with posterior instrumentation and fusion (17). The perioperative and postoperative data for these 112 patients, organized according to their diagnosis, is shown in Table 1. The primary goals of increasing the flexibility of a rigid spine,

TABLE 1 Perioperative and Postoperative Data by Diagnosis for 112 Patients with Spinal Deformity Treated with Thoracoscopic Release/Fusion and Posterior Instrumentation

	Adolescent idiopathic scoliosis	Scheuermann kyphosis	Neuromuscular	Other
Number of cases	23	19	50	20
Operative time (min)	166 ± 46	166 ± 30	162 ± 44	143 ± 34
Anesthesia time (min)	67 ± 14	67 ± 15	78 ± 27	83 ± 20
Estimated blood loss per kg (cc)	6 ± 7	4 ± 3	10 ± 13	8 ± 9
Number of discs excised	6 ± 1	7 ± 1	7 ± 2	6 ± 2
Intensive care unit stay (days)	1 ± 1	1 ± 1	5 ± 5	2 ± 2
Hospital stay (days)	7 ± 1	8 ± 2	12 ± 7	8 ± 3

Source: From Ref. 17.

TABLE 2 Perioperative and Postoperative Data from 50 Patients with Thoracic Scoliosis Treated with Thoracoscopic Instrumentation

Number of cases	50
Operative time (min)	350 ± 50
Estimated blood loss (mL)	430 ± 75
Number of levels fused	7.3 ± 0.8
Hospital stay (days)	6 ± 1.2
Blood transfused (mL)	500 ± 360

Source: From Ref. 29.

and achieving a solid arthrodesis occurred in the vast majority of cases, and clinical failures were exceedingly rare.

OUTCOMES OF THORACOSCOPIC ANTERIOR SCOLIOSIS CORRECTION

The worldwide experience with thoracoscopic anterior scoliosis systems has been increasing since Picetti first reported on its clinical use (18–22). Today, anterior thoracoscopic scoliosis correction remains a relatively new procedure with limited follow-up data. Comparative studies of anterior thoracoscopic and open posterior approaches to scoliosis correction have suggested similar degrees of deformity correction when curve patterns were matched (23–28). Complication rates, however, have been consistently greater for all inexperienced surgeons, as this approach remains technically demanding and requires thorough disc excision and grafting to obtain early solid union. Several functional advantages have been associated with the thoracoscopic approach, when compared with open procedures, suggesting that benefits may be realized once the surgeon becomes more experienced and is able to master the technique. For example, shoulder girdle strength and range of motion have been found to return to normal within three to six months following surgery, and a more rapid return to normal activity and less severe decrease in pulmonary function has been noted in patients compared with after open anterior instrumentation. Figure 12 demonstrates pre- and postoperative stand radiographs of a patient with the typical thoracic adolescent idiopathic scoliosis curve, corrected with a thoracoscopic instrumentation system.

In the primary author's initial experience with a series of 50 consecutive patients, curve correction averaged 60%, with an average operating time of 5.8 hours (29). The number of vertebra instrumented in such constructs ranged from six to nine levels, with the uppermost instrumented vertebra being T4 and the distal most level being L1. Table 2 shows the perioperative and postoperative data for these 50 patients who underwent anterior thoracoscopic scoliosis correction, and Table 3 shows their radiographic measurements and Scoliosis Research Society (SRS) Outcomes Questionnaire scores (range 0–5). The results of this initial series of patients

TABLE 3 Radiographic Measures and SRS Outcomes for 50 Patients with Thoracoscopic Instrumentation

	Preop	First erect	One year	Two years	Most recent follow-up
Thoracic cobb (°)	53 ± 9.1	20 ± 7.1	22 ± 6.5	24 ± 7.5	24 ± 7.6
Upper thoracic cobb (°)	28 ± 6.0	17 ± 6.6	18 ± 6.0	17 ± 5.6	17 ± 5.6
Lumbar cobb (°)	33 ± 11	20 ± 10	17 ± 8.5	17 ± 9.5	18 ± 9.1
Thoracic apical translation (mm)	4.2 ± 2.5	0.4 ± 1.5	0.9 ± 1.2	1.3 ± 1.1	1.4 ± 1.1
T5–T12 Cobb (°)	19 ± 9.6	24 ± 7.7	27 ± 9.3	29 ± 9.3	29 ± 9.1
Pain	3.9	3.8	4.4	4.4	4.1
General self-image	4.1	3.7	4.5	4.2	4.3
General function	4	3.2	4.3	4.4	4.3
Patient satisfaction after surgery	—	4.3	4.5	4.5	4.8
Function after surgery	—	1.4	2.7	3.4	4.3
Self-image after surgery	—	3	3.5	3.5	3.4

Source: From Ref. 29.

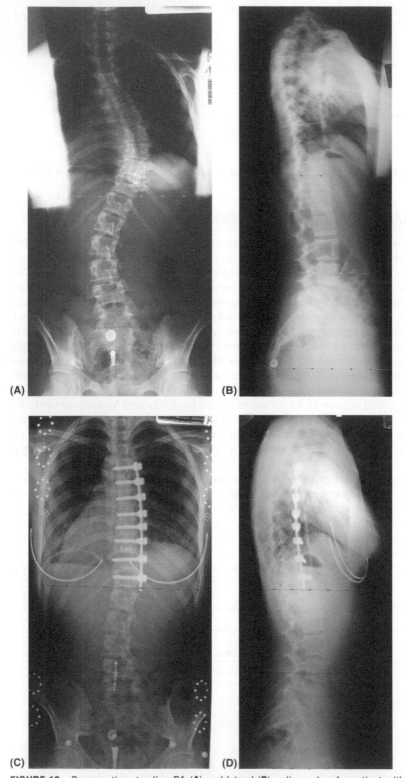

FIGURE 12 Preoperative standing PA (**A**) and lateral (**B**) radiographs of a patient with a typical thoracic adolescent idiopathic scoliosis curve. Postoperative standing PA (**C**) and lateral (**D**) demonstrate the correction achieved with a thoracoscopic instrumentation system.

suggest that the thoracoscopic approach is a viable option in the treatment of adolescent idiopathic scoliosis, however success remain dependent of patient selection and technical ability.

CONCLUSIONS

Video-assisted thoracoscopy is an evolving technology gaining acceptance in the treatment of pediatric spinal deformity. Early reports of this approach suggest its safety and efficacy; however, refinements in the technique and instrumentation continue to develop. Currently, the approach requires careful selection of patients and a surgeon with the appropriate temperament and judgment to negotiate the challenges of the early learning curve. Advancements in this technique in the near future will likely reduce the learning curve and increase the indications of its use. Long term follow-up and a comprehensive comparison of outcomes will ultimately define the role of thoracoscopic treatment of spinal deformities.

REFERENCES

1. Newton PO, Shea KG, Granlund KF. Defining the pediatric spinal thoracoscopy learning curve: sixty-five consecutive cases. Spine 2000; 25:1028–1035.
2. Mack MJ, Regan JJ, Bobechko WP, et al. Application of thoracoscopy for disease of the spine. Ann Thorac Surg 1993; 56:736–738.
3. Regan JJ, Mack MJ, Picetti GD III. A technical report on video-assisted thoracoscopy in thoracic spinal surgery. Preliminary description. Spine 1995; 20:831–837.
4. Lenke LG. Anterior endoscopic discectomy and fusion for adolescent idiopathic scoliosis. Spine 2003; 197:777–779.
5. Picetti GD III, Pang D, Bueff HU. Thoracoscopic techniques for the treatment of scoliosis: early results in procedure development. Neurosurgery 2002; 51:978–984.
6. Newton PO, Cardelia JM, Farnsworth CL, et al. A biomechanical comparison of open and thoracoscopic anterior spinal release in a goat model. Spine 1998; 23:530–535.
7. Dubousset J, Herring JA, Shufflebarger H. The crankshaft phenomenon. J Pediatr Orthop 1989; 9:541–550.
8. Sanders JO, Little DG, Richards BS. Prediction of the crankshaft phenomenon by peak height velocity. Spine 1997; 22:1352–1356.
9. Early SD, Newton PO, White KK, et al. The feasibility of anterior thoracoscopic spine surgery in children under 30 kilograms. Spine 2002; 27:2368–2373.
10. Newton PO, Faro FD, Lenke LG, et al. Factors involved in the decision to perform a selective versus nonselective fusion of Lenke 1B and 1C (King-Moe II) curves in adolescent idiopathic scoliosis. Spine 2003; 28:S217–S223.
11. Lenke LG, Betz RR, Clements D, et al. Curve prevalence of a new classification of operative adolescent idiopathic scoliosis: does classification correlate with treatment? Spine 2002; 27:604–611.
12. Lenke LG, Betz RR, Bridwell KH, et al. Spontaneous lumbar curve coronal correction after selective anterior or posterior thoracic fusion in adolescent idiopathic scoliosis. Spine 1999; 24:1663–1671.
13. Newton PO, Wenger DR, Mubarak SJ, et al. Anterior release and fusion in pediatric spinal deformity: a comparison of early outcome and cost of thoracoscopic and open thoracotomy approaches. Spine 1997; 22:1398–1406.
14. Wall EJ, Vylski-Austrow DI, Shelton FS, et al. Endoscopic discectomy increases thoracic spine flexibility as effectively as open discectomy: a mechanical study in a porcine model. Spine 1998; 23:9–15.
15. Huntington CF, Murrell WD, Betz RR, et al. Comparison of thoracoscopic and open thoracic discectomy in a live bovine model for anterior spinal fusion. Spine 1998; 23:1699–1702.
16. Connolly PJ, Ordway NR, Sacks T, et al. Video-assisted thoracic discectomy and anterior release: a biomechanical analysis of an endoscopic technique. Orthopedics 1999; 22:923–926.
17. Newton PO, White KK, Faro F, et al. The success of thoracoscopic anterior fusion in a consecutive series of 112 pediatric spinal deformity cases. Spine 2005; 30:392–398.
18. Sucato D, Flohr R. Accurate preoperative rod length measurement for thoracoscopic anterior instrumentation and fusion for idiopathic scoliosis. J Spinal Disord Tech 2005; 18:S96–S100.
19. Sucato DJ, Kassab F, Dempsey M. Analysis of screw placement relative to the aorta and spinal canal following anterior instrumentation for thoracic idiopathic scoliosis. Spine 2004; 29:554–559, discussion 559.
20. Picetti GD III, Ertly JP, Bueff HU. Endoscopic instrumentation, correction, and fusion of idiopathic scoliosis. Spine 2001; 1(3):190–197.
21. Newton PO, Marks M, Faro F, et al. Use of video-assisted thoracoscopic surgery to reduce perioperative morbidity in scoliosis surgery. Spine 2003; 28:S249–254.

22. Sucato DJ. Thoracoscopic anterior instrumentation and fusion for idiopathic scoliosis. J Am Acad Orthop Surg 2003; 11:221–227.
23. Lowe T, Betz R, Lenke L, et al. Anterior single-rod instrumentation of the thoracic and lumbar spine: saving levels. Spine 2003; 28(20):S208–S216.
24. Sweet FA, Lenke LG, Bridwell KH, et al. Prospective radiographic and clinical outcomes and complications of single solid rod instrumented anterior spinal fusion in adolescent idiopathic scoliosis. Spine 2001; 26:1956–1965.
25. Betz RR, Harms J, Clements DH, et al. Comparison of anterior and posterior instrumentation for correction of adolescent thoracic idiopathic scoliosis. Spine 1999; 24:225–239.
26. Remes V, Helenius I, Schlenzka D, et al. Cotrel-Dubousset (CD) or universal spine system (USS) instrumentation in adolescent idiopathic scoliosis (AIS): comparison of midterm clinical, functional, and radiographic outcomes. Spine 2004; 29:2024–2030.
27. Asher M, Lai SM, Burton D, et al. Safety and efficacy of Isola instrumentation and arthrodesis for adolescent idiopathic scoliosis: 2- to 12 year follow-up. Spine 2004; 29:2013–2023.
28. Edwards C, Lenke L, Peele M, et al. Selective thoracic fusion for adolescent idiopathic scoliosis with C modifier lumbar curves: 2 to 16 year radiographic and clinical results. Spine 2004; 29:536–546.
29. Newton PO, Parent S, Marks M, et al. Prospective evaluation of 50 consecutive scoliosis patients surgically treated with thoracoscopic anterior instrumentation. Spine 2005; 30(17 Suppl):S100–S109.

19 | Intervertebral Stapling for Spinal Deformity

Linda Park D'Andrea
Brandywine Institute of Orthopedics, Pottstown, Pennsylvania, U.S.A.

Randal R. Betz
Shriners Hospitals for Children, Philadelphia, Pennsylvania, U.S.A.

INTRODUCTION

Although there have been many recorded treatments for scoliosis over the centuries, the search for easier, alternative treatments continues. Nonoperative treatment is the preferred course to control curve progression in growing children. Several papers have stated that curve progression is more likely to occur in patients who are skeletally immature. The risk of progression for curves of 10° or more for skeletally immature patients is 15.4% (1). The risk of progression in untreated curves measures 20° to 29° if Risser 0 or 1 is 68% to 79% (2,3). Exercises, manual spinal manipulation, electrical stimulation, and prayer have been tried. Only full-time orthotic brace wear has been shown to possibly alter the natural history of scoliosis progression in growing children (2,4,5). For curves of 20° to 40°, many physicians believe that the standard treatment for juvenile and adolescent idiopathic scoliosis (AIS) is full-time brace wear. Sometimes, in spite of full-time brace wear, the scoliosis progresses (5).

Patients would, of course, prefer a less restrictive treatment regimen. A cervicothoracic lumbosacral orthosis (CTLSO) or a thoracolumbosacral orthosis (TLSO) is semi-custom or fully custom-made for the patient's specific scoliosis pattern and body dimensions. These braces successfully prevent curve progression of more than 5° in 74% to 89% of patients depending on brace wear schedule and compliance. Eighteen to 50% of these curves will progress in spite of bracing (4,6–13). In patients with flexible AIS, if full-time brace wear is initiated and complied with over several years, curve correction of 5° to 7° can occur (5,14).

According to most of our patients, wearing a CTLSO or a TLSO for 16 hours or more per day is not an enjoyable experience. Some patients complain of discomfort or nausea while wearing a brace. Unfortunately, the population most frequently affected by scoliosis consists of adolescent girls, who often have self-image issues (12,13,15–21). This may explain why there is such poor compliance with brace wear. For psychosocial reasons, patients often do not want to wear a brace, or they have claustrophobic feelings while wearing it. Some patients cannot wear an orthosis because of physical limitations, body habitus, or occasionally for environmental or climactic reasons. Full-time brace wear of 14 to 23 hours per day is often necessary for several years (6), prompting some parents to voice concern over the restrictions of physical activity. Boys may need to wear a brace for a longer period of time as they frequently grow until their mid- to late-teens. A few studies suggest that in some patients, bracing may be psychologically detrimental.

The search for an alternative to brace treatment reintroduced an old concept to the research forefront. Angular limb deformity in skeletally immature patients can be corrected with asymmetric physeal compression using metal staples on the convex side of the limb. This is a widely accepted, standard method of treatment. The amount of correction that is possible is calculated based on the patient's remaining growth (22–24).

Vertebral body stapling for scoliotic deformity was attempted many years ago. Nachlas and Borden (25) published results of vertebral stapling in a canine scoliosis model. The convex physeal endplates and discs were compressed as the dogs grew. Curve correction was obtained in many dogs, and in some the curve progression was arrested. In dogs in which two interspaces were spanned, the staples failed by breaking or loosening. The shape, metallurgy, and mechanical design of those staples also contributed to their failure.

Smith et al. (26) attempted to correct congenital scoliosis in humans using the vertebral stapling technique shortly after the animal results were published. The outcome was poor. Patient selection was, perhaps, not ideal, as the children had severe curves and were nearly mature. Failure was probably because of similar causes as in the dogs: loosening because of poor design and breakage because the stainless steel staples did not have the fatigue properties necessary for a highly mobile area such as spanning the vertebral disc space.

More recently, the concept of scoliosis treatment by modification of anterior vertebral body growth has been revisited. With newer technology in metallurgy and better engineering, the Nitinol® (Nickel Titanium Naval Ordinance Laboratory) bone staple was designed (Medtronic Sofamor Danek, Memphis, Tennessee, U.S.A.). Its curved prong design and shape changing abilities allow for easy insertion parallel to the cartilaginous vertebral apophyses to provide physeal compression. When the staples are cooled by immersion in a sterile ice-bath and the prongs are straightened manually, they remain straight. When the staple begins to return to normal body temperature, the prongs return to their curved shape as when manufactured. If the staple is completely seated within the vertebral bodies when the prongs deploy, then the staple position is secure.

To prove the safety and utility of the Nitinol® staple in vivo, an animal model was needed. Braun et al. (27) used the staples in a goat scoliosis model to halt progression of iatrogenic curves up to 70°. Our experience with the treatment of AIS using vertebral body stapling, including feasibility, safety, utility, and technique has already been reported (28,29).

The design of the vertebral body staples has undergone two major changes over the last several years, with tine length decreasing as the "intertine" distance becomes shorter. The technique changes made over the last four years has dictated the need for smaller, more compact staples. The staples are presently manufactured in two- and four-prong styles, with the prong tines being proportional to the length between the tines. Each style is available in lengths from 2 mm to 5 mm in 1-mm increments, and 6 mm to 12 mm at 2-mm increments. Most of the staples which have been inserted over the last few years have been small, from 4 mm to 8 mm.

INDICATIONS

The small nature of the instrumentation lends itself well to the use of a minimally invasive surgical technique. Surgeons choosing minimally invasive techniques should be familiar with them, or have an access surgeon able to assist. Thoracoscopic-assisted insertion of the vertebral body staples is a natural use of an existing technology. Lenke 1 right thoracic scoliosis curves occur 51% of the time (30). In most patients, if the compensatory upper thoracic or lumbar curve is less than 25°, the mid-thoracic curve is the only one to be addressed surgically. We will consider a patient to be a candidate for the stapling procedure if the curve(s) would be considered for bracing, or have failed bracing already.

PREOPERATIVE PLANNING

Once the surgeon has determined that the patient is going to have the stapling procedure, the levels to be instrumented are determined. The recommended guideline for choosing the levels is to include all vertebrae that lie within the Cobb angle of the curve. The levels that we have been able to safely staple include T3 to L4.

SURGICAL TECHNIQUE
Anesthesia and Positioning

Patients undergo the procedure while under general anesthesia. If video-assisted thoracoscopy is being utilized for insertion, then one-lung ventilation will be necessary. Sometimes this is not possible, perhaps because the patient's endotracheal diameter is too small or between sizes of the available endotracheal tubes, or one-lung ventilation is not tolerated. Exact placement of the dual-lumen endotracheal tubes and the univent tubes can be challenging, especially in very young children. A combination of endoscopic and fluoroscopic assistance often helps if there is

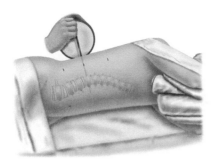

FIGURE 1 The patient is placed in a lateral decubitus position. Using fluoroscopic imaging, the levels of the spine to be stapled are confirmed.

difficulty with this part of the procedure. Without some collapse of the lung, placement of the staples is difficult without extra time and risk of injury to the lung or great vessels from the sharp staple tines. The patient is positioned on the operating table in the lateral decubitus position with the convex side of the scoliosis facing up.

Approach

Biplanar fluoroscopy is used to determine the exact location of the intercostal portals (Figs. 1 and 2). Most incisions will be within the area of the posterior axillary line (Fig. 3). The incisions used for staple insertion are slightly larger than the staples themselves. An alternative in making several portals is to make two mini-thoracotomies of less than 5 cm. This allows several levels to be stapled and accommodates the size of the instruments and implants.

INSERTION TECHNIQUE

The insertion device, which holds the single, two-prong staples, is 10 mm × 14 mm wide. As discussed previously, the staples now come in many sizes, with some being quite small; however, the 12-mm four-prong, double staple is the widest, longest object (at 14 mm × 12) that has to pass between the ribs (Figs. 4–7). As the staples themselves are designed to pass through bone, the prongs are quite sharp. The staples must pass quickly from the sterile ice-water bath to the vertebral body to allow insertion prior to the staples warming, allowing tine deployment. The complete tine transformation may take a few minutes to occur. If the staple touches anything that is close to body temperature, the tines may deploy before the staple is placed. Rigid, autoclavable plastic portals have been custom-made (Medtronic Sofamor Danek, Memphis, Tennessee, U.S.A.) for this specific use. They allow for the intercostal portal space to be maintained while protecting the muscle and pleura from repeated trauma. They allow rapid removal

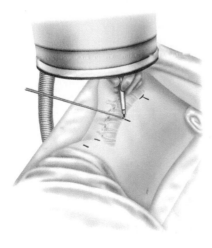

FIGURE 2 A lateral/medial fluoroscopy image is used to confirm the vertebral levels to be stapled and also to center the portals in the posterolateral line.

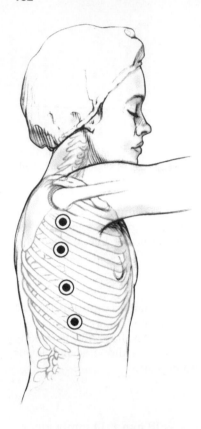

FIGURE 3 Generally, three to four portals in the intercostal spaces are placed over the levels to receive the staple instrumentation. They are in the posterolateral line.

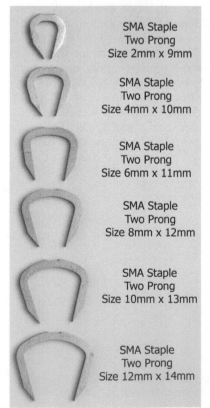

SMA Staple
Two Prong
Size 2mm x 9mm

SMA Staple
Two Prong
Size 4mm x 10mm

SMA Staple
Two Prong
Size 6mm x 11mm

SMA Staple
Two Prong
Size 8mm x 12mm

SMA Staple
Two Prong
Size 10mm x 13mm

SMA Staple
Two Prong
Size 12mm x 14mm

FIGURE 4 Photograph comparing two- and four-prong staples.

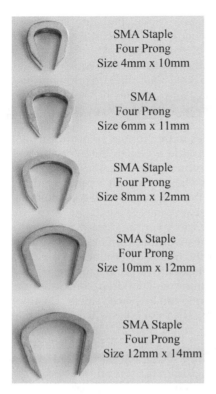

SMA Staple
Four Prong
Size 4mm x 10mm

SMA
Four Prong
Size 6mm x 11mm

SMA Staple
Four Prong
Size 8mm x 12mm

SMA Staple
Four Prong
Size 10mm x 12mm

SMA Staple
Four Prong
Size 12mm x 14mm

FIGURE 5   Photograph comparing two- and four-prong staples.

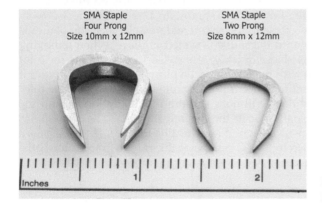

FIGURE 6   Photograph comparing two- and four-prong staples.

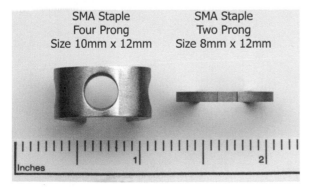

FIGURE 7   Photograph comparing two- and four-prong staples.

of the staple trial and placement of the appropriate-sized staple. Small pediatric Finochetto retractors or nasal speculum distractors can also be used to enlarge the intercostal skin portals and may be used in place of collapsible or rigid portals.

If the staples are being placed thoracoscopically, the addition of carbon dioxide (CO_2) gas allows for collapse of the lung without single-lung ventilation. Specialized equipment and portals are needed for this technique. The low-pressure gas also promotes hemostasis in the bleeding bone. The CO_2 pressure should be kept low to prevent a lateral shift of the mediastinum, which may cause a drop in blood pressure.

Minimal access surgery can also be used to place staples in the lumbar spine. Segmental vessels or other regional veins may need to be ligated to provide access to the intervertebral discs and endplates. We have used nerve stimulation (NeuroVision SE nerve locator; NeuroVision Medical, Ventura, California, U.S.A.) to identify the lumbar plexus through a psoas-splitting lateral approach. MaxCess®, a specialized retractor system (NuVasive, Inc., San Diego, California, U.S.A.), can aid with the minimal incision surgery of the lumbar spine.

Using fluoroscopy, the appropriate size trial is selected to span the distance across the disc, apophyses, and physes. The desired location of the tines is in the vertebral body but as close to the apophyses as possible. Once the correct size for the trial is determined, it is placed in the position where the staple will be located. Two single staples (two prongs) or one double staple (four prongs) will be placed at each level. In very young, small children, sometimes the most proximal vertebra is very small, and only one single staple can be placed safely. The tines of the trial are used to create the pilot holes for the staple tines. The pilot holes will act as a guide for the staple to ensure that the tines start in the correct position (Fig. 8). Once the desired position is achieved (Fig. 9), the staple inserter is removed, and if the staple is not flush against the bone, an impactor is used to push the staple further. The dull staple trial can be used to help push at the apex of the convexity to further reduce the curve during the procedure.

Staples are placed anterior to the rib heads and if the patient has severe hypokyphosis or thoracic lordosis, the staples can be placed more anterior on the vertebrae to help produce kyphosis. In the lumbar spine, the staples should be placed as far posteriorly on the vertebral body as possible, at least in the posterior half of the body, to maintain a normal lordosis.

If the tines of the staple will extend too close to the segmental vessels, then the pleura is incised and the vessels are retracted gently until the staple is seated in place. When removing the trial from the vertebral body, the staple is placed quickly; otherwise, bleeding from the pilot holes obscures them. Bone wax or gel foam with thrombin can be placed over the pilot holes if bleeding is excessive. Staple tine deployment may occur if the staple is not placed in the pilot holes quickly. The "compressed," deployed tines will not fit in the trial's pilot holes, and the track that the curved tines will create is usually not in the desired position. The staple tines must be distracted apart using the instrument designed specifically for this. If the tines are overdistracted, they may not be able to return to the "C" shape. If they are distracted too little, they may deploy before the staple is completely seated, often resulting in asymmetric tine posi-

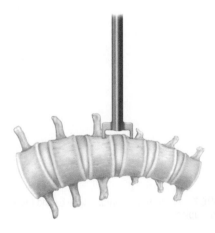

FIGURE 8   The appropriate sized staple trial is selected and used to create the pilot holes for the actual staple.

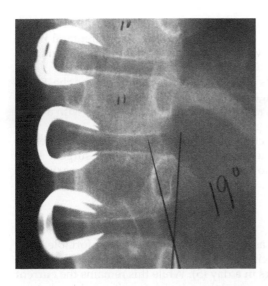

FIGURE 9 After the staple is inserted, the position is confirmed with fluoroscopic image.

tion. If the tines deploy early, the staple can be removed, rechilled, the tines distracted, and the staple reinserted. Once the staple is tamped into position, biplanar fluoroscopy is used to check the position. If the tine tips are not in a desired position, such as in the disc, the staple can be removed, rechilled, and repositioned. To reposition a staple, new pilot holes must usually be made or the tines will follow the previous channels in the bone.

While the patient is in the lateral decubitus position, often the flexible, mid-thoracic curve reduces. To further reduce the curve while placing the staples, lateral pressure to the apical ribs can be applied, similar to the corrective pressure used by a TLSO brace. This may be important, because preliminary evaluation of data from patients who have already undergone the procedure suggests that patients who had the greatest correction at the time of surgery maintained that correction best.

To minimize the total number of portals, the thoracoscope can be placed in the portals being used to insert the staples. A more or less angled scope may need to be used to improve visualization of the segmentals and other vessels during creation of the pilot holes and insertion of the staples. There are straight and offset staple holders for the single (two tine) staples. The double staples presently have only a straight holder for insertion. Even with a straight inserter, two or three levels can usually be instrumented through a single skin portal. The technique is similar to that used for inserting vertebral body screws during a thoracoscopic instrumented fusion, in which two or more intercostal portals can be made through each skin incision.

Intrathoracic stapling may require partial incision and retraction of the diaphragm. Repair is, of course, needed to prevent postoperative rupture or eventration. While it is possible, we do not incise the pleura longitudinally and then repair it afterward, to cover the instrumentation.

COMPLICATIONS

The procedure now has been performed in over 50 patients at our institution. As was previously reported, complications occurred after six of the surgical procedures (29), including one major complication (2.6%) and five minor complications (13%). The major complication occurred in a four-year-old patient with infantile idiopathic scoliosis who underwent an uncomplicated thoracoscopic stapling from T5 to T12. At six weeks postsurgery, she developed a rupture of a pre-existing, unrecognized diaphragmatic eventration that necessitated emergent repair. Five patients had minor complications. One early patient had a segmental spinal vein that was punctured by a staple prong, requiring conversion of the thoracoscopic portal to a mini-incision, and ligation of the vein. This resulted in an estimated blood loss (EBL) of 1500 cc, which is significantly more than the EBL of the collective surgeries (average: 247 cc ± 285 cc). A second patient developed a chylothorax from a staple prong puncture of the thoracic duct at T12 that was not noticed at surgery and was treated conservatively with chest tube and total parenteral nutrition. Another patient developed mild pancreatitis which resolved with a low-fat diet, and two patients had clinically significant atelectasis.

The use of a chest tube is left to the surgeon's discretion. At our institution, the chest tube is removed when there is less than 2 mL of drainage per kilogram of body weight for 24 hours. The early average hospital stay was 6.6 ± 2.6 days, and the average number of days with a chest tube was 3.8 ± 2.8 days; both have decreased with greater clinical experience.

Early in our series, patients wore a noncorrecting TLSO brace postoperatively. Currently, we ask patients to restrict their activities until the muscles incised during the surgery have healed for four to six weeks. After this there are no restrictions; patients are able to participate in dancing and most sports, including gymnastics.

SUMMARY

Patients with progressive scoliosis are frequently asked to use restrictive, uncomfortable body bracing until skeletal maturity. The results of bracing studies show that bracing is not always successful (2,4,6,8,9), even when worn for 23 hours in a day (5). While this remains the current standard of care for skeletally immature patients to control the spinal deformity, we have helped to develop this alternative treatment. The vertebral body stapling technique for the treatment of scoliosis described here continues to be studied retrospectively. It can be performed safely and has yielded good results in some patients.

REFERENCES

1. Rogala EJ, Drummond DS, Gurr J. Scoliosis: incidence and natural history. A prospective epidemiological study. J Bone Joint Surg Am 1978; 60(2):173–176.
2. Lonstein JE, Carlson JM. The prediction of curve progression in untreated idiopathic scoliosis during growth. J Bone Joint Surg 1984; 66A:1061–1071.
3. Bunnell WP. An objective criterion for scoliosis screening. J Bone Joint Surg, 1984; 66A:1381–1387.
4. Nachemson AL, Peterson LE. Effectiveness of treatment with a brace in girls who have adolescent idiopathic scoliosis. A prospective, controlled study based on data from the Brace Study of the Scoliosis Research Society. J Bone Joint Surg Am 1995; 77(6):815–822.
5. Rahman T, Bowen JR, Takemitsu M, et al. The association between brace compliance and outcome for patients with idiopathic scoliosis. J Pediatr Orthop 2005; 24(4):420–422.
6. Allington NJ, Bowen JR. Adolescent idiopathic scoliosis: treatment with the Wilmington brace. A comparison of full-time and part-time use. J Bone Joint Surg Am 1996; 78(7):1056–1062.
7. Lonstein JE. Idiopathic scoliosis. In: Lonstein JE, Bradford DS, Winter RB, et al., eds. Moe's Textbook of Scoliosis and Other Spinal Deformities. 3rd ed. Philadelphia, PA: W.B. Saunders, 1995.
8. Peterson LE, Nachemson AL. Prediction of progression of the curve in girls who have adolescent idiopathic scoliosis of moderate severity. Logistic regression analysis based on data from the Brace Study of the Scoliosis Research Society. J Bone Joint Surg Am 1995; 77(6):823–827.
9. Rowe DE, Bernstein SM, Riddick MF, et al. A meta-analysis of the efficacy of non-operative treatments for idiopathic scoliosis. J Bone Joint Surg Am 1997; 79(5):664–674.
10. Roach JW. Adolescent idiopathic scoliosis: nonsurgical treatment. In: Weinstein SL, ed. The Pediatric Spine: Principles and Practice. New York, NY: Raven Press, 1994:479.
11. Bridwell KH. Adolescent idiopathic scoliosis: surgical treatment. In: Weinstein SL, ed. The Pediatric Spine: Principles and Practice. New York, NY: Raven Press, 1994:511.
12. Karol LA. Effectiveness of bracing in male patients with idiopathic scoliosis. Spine 2001; 26: 2001–2005.
13. Noonan KJ, Dolan LA, Jacobson WC, et al. Long-term psychosocial characteristics of patients treated for idiopathic scoliosis. J Pediatr Orthop 1997; 17:712–717.
14. Landauer F, Wimmer C, Behensky H. Estimating the final outcome of brace treatment for idiopathic thoracic scoliosis at 6-month follow-up. Pediatr Rehabil 2003; 6(3–4):201–207.
15. Bengtsson G, Fallstrom K, Jansson B, et al. A psychological and psychiatric investigation of the adjustment of female scoliosis patients. Acta Psychiatr Scand 1974; 50(1):50–59.
16. Clayson D, Luz-Alterman S, Cataletto MM, et al. Long-term psychological sequelae of surgically versus nonsurgically treated scoliosis. Spine 1987; 12(10):983–986.
17. Fallstrom K, Cochran T, Nachemson A. Long-term effects on personality development in patients with adolescent idiopathic scoliosis. Influence of type of treatment. Spine 1986; 11(7):756–758.

18. Andersen MO, Andersen GR, Thomsen K, et al. Early weaning might reduce the psychologic strain of Boston bracing: a study of 136 patients with adolescent idiopathic scoliosis at 3.5 years after termination of brace treatment. J Pediatr Orthop B 2002; 11:96–99.
19. Climent JM, Sanchez J. Impact of the type of brace on the quality of life of adolescents with spine deformities. Spine 1999; 24:1903–1908.
20. Lindeman M, Behm K. Cognitive strategies and self-esteem as predictors of brace-wear noncompliance in patients with idiopathic scoliosis and kyphosis. J Pediatr Orthop 1999; 19(4):493–499.
21. MacLean WE, Green NE, Pierree CB, et al. Stress and coping with scoliosis: psychological effects on adolescents and their families. J Pediatr Orthop 1989; 9(2):257–261.
22. Moseley CF. A straight-line graph for leg-length discrepancies. J Bone Joint Surg 1977; 59A:174–179.
23. Beumer A, Lampe HI, Swierstra BA, et al. The straight line graph in limb length inequality. A new design based on 182 Dutch children. Acta Orthop Scand 1997; 68(4):355–360.
24. Eastwood DM, Cole WG. A graphic method for timing the correction of leg-length discrepancy. J Bone Joint Surg 1995; 77B:743–747.
25. Nachlas JW, Borden JN. The cure of experimental scoliosis by directed growth control. J Bone Joint Surg Am 1951; 33:24–32.
26. Smith AD, von Lackum HL, Wylie R. An operation for stapling vertebral bodies in congenital scoliosis. J Bone Joint Surg Am 1954; 36:342–348.
27. Braun JT, Ogilvie JW, Akyuz E, et al. Experimental scoliosis in an immature goat model: a method that creates idiopathic-type deformity with minimal violation of the spinal elements along the curve. Spine 2003; 28(19):2198–2203.
28. Betz RR, Kim J, D'Andrea LP, et al. An innovative technique of vertebral body stapling for the treatment of patients with adolescent idiopathic scoliosis: a feasibility, safety, and utility study. Spine 2003; 28(20S):S255–S265.
29. Betz RR, D'Andrea LP, Mulcahey MJ, et al. Vertebral body stapling procedure for the treatment of scoliosis in the growing child. Clin Orthop 2005; 434:55–60.
30. Lenke LG, Betz RR, Clements DH, et al. Curve prevalence of a new classification of operative adolescent idiopathic scoliosis: does classification correlate with treatment? Spine 2002; 27(6):604–611.

20 | Endoscopic Techniques for Stabilization of the Thoracic Spine

Max C. Lee
Department of Neurosurgery, Milwaukee Neurological Institute, Milwaukee, Wisconsin, U.S.A.

Bernard A. Coert
Department of Neurosurgery, Stanford University Medical Center, Stanford, California, U.S.A.

Se-Hoon Kim
Department of Neurosurgery, Korea University Medical Center, Seoul, Republic of Korea

Daniel H. Kim
Department of Neurosurgery, Baylor College of Medicine, Houston, Texas, U.S.A.

INTRODUCTION

The technological advancements made within spinal surgery have increased dramatically within the last two decades. Innovative techniques, from the use of the operating microscope to image guidance, have changed our approach to problems within the operating room. In addition, improved instrumentation (from odontoid screws and lateral mass screws to sacropelvic fixation) has improved the surgical management of countless patients. It is these changes that have collectively led to the advancement of spinal surgery and subsequent improved outcomes. One of the major advancements within the last decade has been the development of minimally invasive spinal surgery. Within this arena, development of thoracoscopic spinal surgery has skyrocketed.

The thoracoscopic approach was first described by Jacobaeus in 1922 for removal of tuberculosis adhesions (1,2). Further developments in endoscopic technology have greatly refined the technique and expanded its indications. In the early 1990s, Mack et al. first applied thoracoscopic techniques for the management of spinal diseases (3). This group was the first to describe the thoracoscopic transdiaphragmatic approach (TTA) for adrenal biopsy (3). This approach has since been used by various authors for adrenalectomy, nephrectomy, and microwave coagulation therapy for hepatic tumors (4–6). In parallel, and partly based on these reports, others carried out the first endoscopic operations to treat fractures of the thoracic and lumbar spine in 1996, after a preparation period of one year (1,2). Both the TTA to thoracolumbar junction (TLJ) approaches have been used for spinal injuries (1,7,8).

INDICATIONS
General Indications for Anterior Surgery of the Thoracic Spine

In general, anterior approaches are indicated in the restoration of anterior column support after significant injury to the anterior column and neurological deficits associated with retropulsed bony fragments (9). They can be performed by conventional open or endoscopic approaches. In recent years, less invasive open microscopic approaches have been developed that can often minimize the size of the operative access to 6 to 10 cm using special retractors. These minimally invasive open techniques ("mini-thoracotomy" and "mini-laparotomy") can be an effective alternative to endoscopic techniques (Fig. 1).

Indications and Contraindications for Endoscopic Techniques

Endoscopic techniques can be used for anterior decompression, reconstruction, and instrumentation of the entire thoracic spine and TLJ. However, they cannot be performed in patients with restricted cardiopulmonary function, acute post-traumatic lung failure, severe pleural adhesions,

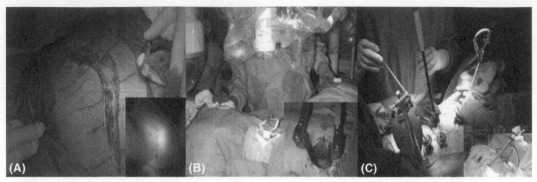

FIGURE 1   (**A**) Incisional length for a thoracotomy. (**B**) Mini-thoracotomy with a self-retaining retractor. (**C**) Thoracoscopic approach to a thoracic decompression and instrumentation.

and severe medical instability. When the lesion is located above the T12–L1 disc, thoracoscopic reconstruction and instrumentation can be performed without detachment of the diaphragm. Various techniques have been described for accessing lesions of the TLJ.

The advantages of endoscopic surgery include reduced operative pain, excellent cosmetic effect, lower perioperative morbidity, and an earlier return to work. Its disadvantages include the need for single-lung ventilation requiring increased anesthetic monitoring during the surgery. As the endoscopic image is two-dimensional with a longer working distance between the surgeon and the target area, a certain degree of difficulty is encountered in mastering the technique in the initial stages.

OVERVIEW OF VARIOUS ENDOSCOPIC APPROACHES TO THE THORACOLUMBAR JUNCTION

Endoscopic exposure of the TLJ is particularly challenging. A number of techniques have been reported, which include: (*i*) the thoracoscopic approach without diaphragmatic detachment, (*ii*) TTA, (*iii*) the combined thoracoscopic and laparoscopic retroperitoneal approach, (*iv*) the endoscopic retroperitoneal approach to TLJ, and (*v*) the retropleural-retroperitoneal endoscopic-assisted approach.

Thoracoscopic Approach Without Diaphragmatic Detachment

When the lesion is located above the T12–L1 disc, thoracoscopic reconstruction and instrumentation is quite feasible without detachment of the diaphragm (10). The diaphragm can be gently pushed with a traditional sponge forceps to improve the exposure at TLJ. Additional portals may be required for diaphragmatic retraction to facilitate the procedure (4). However, as most TLJ injuries require instrumentation of L1, diaphragmatic detachment is often required for satisfactory placement of instrumentation. Compromise in achieving adequate exposure may result in suboptimal placement of the implants.

Transthoracic Transdiaphragmatic Approach

TTA provides excellent access to the entire TLJ, thus permitting a safe and effective spinal decompression, reconstruction, and instrumentation. It facilitates the optimal placement of bone graft and instrumentation down to the L2 vertebra. The instrumentation of L3 vertebrae is also possible through the thoracoscopic approach. However, this usually requires extensive splitting of the diaphragm, and possibly an additional portal placement below the diaphragm. This is a borderline indication that should be reserved for long instrumentation constructs requiring thoracic access. Otherwise, preference should be given to a laparotomy or retroperitoneoscopic access. The major disadvantage of this approach lies in the steep angle required to work at the TLJ. This awkward angle can make instrumentation at the TLJ difficult and time-consuming.

Combined Thoracoscopic and Retroperitoneoscopic Approach

Regan et al. (11) reported a combined thoracoscopic and retroperitoneoscopic approach to perform L1–L2 discectomy or L1 corpectomy. Burgos et al. (12) also suggested this combined approach with diaphragmatic detachment for satisfactory and safe exposure of TLJ. This approach requires three laparoscopic portals in addition to the usual thoracoscopic portals. This procedure may be more useful for longer instrumentation constructs extending to L3 vertebrae. It has the disadvantages of entering both thoracic and abdominal cavities and greatly increasing surgical time. The major problem encountered during retroperitoneal endoscopic exposure of the spine is inadvertent peritoneal injury.

Endoscopic Retroperitoneal Approach to the Thoracolumbar Junction

Endoscopic retroperitoneoscopy was first developed for performing lumbar sympathectomy (13). This technique became more popular after the development of balloon-guided retroperitoneal dissections for urological procedures. Olinger et al. (13) described the first successful endoscopic retroperitoneal approach for management of spinal fractures involving TLJ and lumbar spine. They reported successful outcomes in a short series of 12 patients, six of them involving L1. No major complications were encountered except for one case of pneumothorax (8.3%) as result of inadvertent pleural injury.

The procedure is performed with the patient positioned in the right lateral decubitus position. Balloon-guided retroperitoneal dissection is performed using four abdominal endoscopic ports. In contrast to urological procedures, the renal (Gerota's) fascia is not incised. Following CO_2 insufflation, the left kidney together with the pararenal fat is gently pushed medially by the pressure of the gas and support of a sponge-bearing forceps. Care must be taken during mobilization of the peritoneal sac ventrally in the area of the diaphragm to prevent inadvertent opening of the peritoneal cavity. The diaphragm is split for cases requiring instrumentation of the T12 vertebral body.

The major advantage of this technique is that it avoids entering the thoracic cavity and the various associated pulmonary complications. It also obviates the need for a postoperative chest tube drain. The major disadvantages of this technique include: (*i*) the possibility of pleural injury while making the diaphragmatic opening; (*ii*) the possibility of peritoneal injury during retroperitoneal dissection or trocar placement; (*iii*) risk of injury to the kidney during trocar placement for CO_2 insufflation; (*iv*) requires the surgeon to work under the rib cage to reach the TLJ because the ribs are angled forward and downward the lower ribs extend over the TLJ; (*v*) the working space in the retroperitoneum is small and limits the number of ports one can insert as well as the dissection angle (6); (*vi*) procedures cannot be performed in patients who previously had abdominal surgery due to dense retroperitoneal adhesions (6). Although this technique appears promising, it needs to be evaluated further in larger numbers to prove its efficacy.

Retropleural Retroperitoneal Endoscopic-Assisted Surgery

Recently, Hovorka et al. (14) reported a retropleural retroperitoneal endoscopic-assisted approach in management of the 11 cases of TLJ injuries. This is a minimally invasive open procedure requiring costal resection. They were able to reach the upper part of the L1 vertebra via a supradiaphragmatic retropleural approach. Larger exposures required release of diaphragmatic insertions. The major advantage of this approach is to avoid pleural opening and its consequent morbidity. Because it is an open endoscopic-assisted approach, it is associated with all the complications of an open procedure except that the size of the incision is decreased.

PREOPERATIVE CONSIDERATIONS

As many of these patients have multiple orthopedic and visceral injuries, all major injuries should be addressed and appropriately stabilized prior to spine surgery. Thoracoscopic procedures are contraindicated in patients with previous cardiopulmonary disease with restricted cardiopulmonary function, acute post-traumatic lung failure, severe pleural adhesions, and severe medical instability (2,7,15). Routine bowel preparation is required to reduce intra-abdominal pressure and facilitate the retraction of the diaphragm. A detailed informed consent is obtained after explaining the various risks involved in the procedure, such as visceral injury, vascular injury, blood loss, instrumentation failure, failed fusion, and possible conversion to open procedure (2,7,15).

SURGICAL TECHNIQUE

Operative techniques for thoracoscopic spine surgery have been described in detail by various authors (2,7,15). Early in our experience, we often reserved the thoracoscopic approaches for thoracic fractures involving the T4 to T10 vertebrae. With increasing experience, we extended the indications to TLJ injuries. Here we describe the technique for stabilizing fractures with special attention toward the TTA to TLJ injuries.

Anesthetic Considerations

With the patient in a supine position, double-lumen endotracheal intubation is performed. The position of the double-lumen endotracheal tube is checked endoscopically. A foley catheter, central venous line, and arterial line for continuous blood pressure monitoring are inserted.

Patient Positioning

The patient is placed in a stable right lateral decubitus position and fixed with a four-point support at the pubic symphysis, sacrum, scapula, and upper arm. A left-sided approach is chosen to facilitate mobilization of the diaphragm. On the right side, the liver causes the right hemidiaphragm to be higher than the left. The top-lying arm is placed flat on an arm support and raised to 90° elevation to avoid a collision during placement and manipulation of the endoscope. Before starting the operation, the position and free tilt of the C-arm should be checked. Sterile draping extends from the middle of the sternum anteriorly to the spinous processes posteriorly as well as from axilla down to about 8 cm caudal to the iliac crest. Monitors are placed at both lower ends of the operating table on opposite sides to enable free vision for the surgeon and the assistant. The surgeon and the assistant holding the camera stand behind the patient. The C-arm monitor and the second assistant are placed on the opposite side (Fig. 2).

Unique Anatomical Considerations of the Thoracoscopic Transdiaphragmatic Approach

TTA presents several unique challenges to spine surgeons that necessitate a clear understanding of the diaphragmatic, thoracic, and retroperitoneal anatomy (16). Anatomically, the diaphragm originates from three locations: a sternal, a costal, and a lumbar part, which arises by means of crura and from arcuate ligaments.

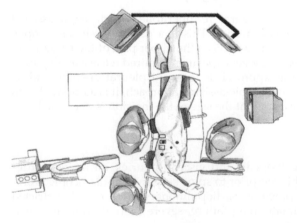

FIGURE 2 Operating room set up for thoracoscopic spine surgery. Note that the surgeon and the assistant holding the camera stand behind the patient, with the video and fluoroscopic monitor in front of them.

The sternal part arises by two fleshy slips from the dorsum of xiphoid process. The costal part arises from inner surfaces of cartilages and adjacent portions of the last six ribs on either side. The right crus arises from the sides of the bodies of L1–L3 bodies. The left crus arises from the sides of L1 and L2 bodies. The medial arcuate ligament covers the upper part of the psoas major muscle, attaching from the sides of first and second lumbar vertebrae to the tip of the L1 transverse process. The lateral arcuate ligament covers the quadratus lumborum and attaches from the tip of L1 transverse process to the lower border of the 12th rib. Thus, both the crura and arcuate ligaments of the diaphragm are inserted below the T12–L1 disc space (8,10,17), so lesions located above the T12–L1 disc can be approached thoracoscopically from above without dividing the diaphragm. Below the T12–L1 disc space the spine is surrounded by the diaphragmatic crura, psoas muscles, and arcuate ligaments, and so injuries here require diaphragmatic detachment for adequate exposure.

The entire TLJ can be exposed thoracoscopically with minimal diaphragmatic detachment. This is made possible by an anatomic peculiarity of the pleural cavity and the diaphragmatic insertion, the lowest point of which, the costodiaphragmatic recess, is projected onto the spine perpendicularly just above the base plate of the second lumbar vertebrae (8). Thus, with a diaphragmatic opening of about 6 to 10 cm the entire L2 vertebral body can be exposed, a much smaller opening than that is required for conventional open techniques.

Operative Technique
Localization and Placement of Portals
Under direct fluoroscopic guidance, the target fractured vertebra is projected onto the skin level. The borders of the fractured vertebra are marked on the skin (Fig. 3). The working channel (10 mm) is centered over the target vertebrae. The optical channel (10 mm) is placed two or three intercostal spaces cranial to the target vertebra. The position of the suction/irrigation (5 mm) and retractor (10 mm) channels is placed approximately 5 to 10 cm anterior to the working and optical channel.

To avoid inadvertent injury to lungs, the diaphragm, and the organs beneath it, the most cranial portal is inserted first by a mini-thoracotomy approach. Through a 1.5-cm skin incision placed above the intercostal space, the muscle layers of thoracic wall are cut through in a zigzag fashion following the direction of the fibers. The opening is gradually widened by the insertion of Langenbeck hooks. After collapsing the lung through single-lung ventilation, the pleura is perforated under direct visualization to introduce the first trocar. The 30° scope is introduced through the portal and the other trocars are inserted under direct thoracoscopic vision (Fig. 4). The endoscopic image is rotated to obtain an orientation of the spine parallel to the lower edge of the video monitor screen. The cephalocaudal axis of the camera is oriented to the view of the primary operative surgeon to allow for normal translation of his or her hand movements to the monitor.

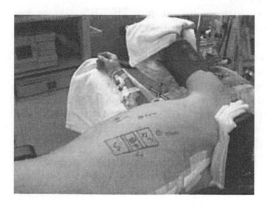

FIGURE 3 Localization. The target vertebra(e) is (are) projected and marked on the skin and marked under a fluoroscopic table.

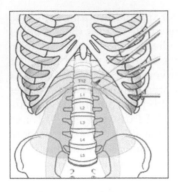

FIGURE 4   Diagram demonstrating the placement of the thoracoscopic portals for approaching the thoracolumbar junction.

Prevertebral Dissection and Diaphragm Detachment

The fractured area is now exposed with the help of a fan retractor inserted through the anterior port. The fan retractor performs the dual function of holding down the diaphragm and exposing the insertion of the diaphragm on the spine.

Exposure of the spine below L1 usually requires detachment of the diaphragm. To expose the entire TLJ for endoscopic surgery, we have been able to reduce to a minimum the previous total detachment of the diaphragmatic insertion performed in the open procedure. With a blunt probe, the anterior aspect of the spine along with its diaphragmatic insertion and course of the aorta are identified. The line of incision for the diaphragmatic detachment is identified and marked with monopolar cautery or ultrasonic knife. We prefer a semicircular incision along the spine and ribs parallel to the diaphragmatic insertion, leaving a 1- to 2-cm rim of the attachment to facilitate closure. The diaphragm is already thinner here than in the immediate area of insertion, which makes subsequent suturing easier. Radial incisions over the diaphragm are avoided, as they are associated with increased risk of diaphragmatic hernia. Under close thoracoscopic visualization, the different layers of the diaphragm are often easily observed, dissected, and incised with a pair of endoscissors (Fig. 5).

After the diaphragm has been split, the fan retractor is now placed into the diaphragmatic opening. Retroperitoneal fat and the peritoneal sac are exposed and mobilized in an anterior-to-posterior direction along the psoas bulk to avoid injury to the lumbosacral plexus. The psoas muscle with its tendinous insertions is dissected carefully from the vertebral bodies, avoiding any damage to the segmental vessels hidden underneath. A 4-cm incision is usually sufficient for the instrumentation of the first lumbar vertebrae. It has to be lengthened to 10 cm for the instrumentation of L2. The instrumentation of L3 is possible through thoracoscopic approach. This usually requires extensive splitting of the diaphragm and may require an additional portal below the diaphragm.

Corpectomy and Decompression of the Spinal Canal

The extent of the planned corpectomy is defined with an osteotome. The disc spaces are opened to define the borders. Trauma can obscure normal anatomic landmarks. Therefore, extreme caution must be exercised during removal of the disc or the vertebral body to avoid violation of segmental vessels. Bipolar cautery and back-up suction and sponges must be available for insertion if bleeding vessels need tamponade. After resection of the intervertebral discs, the fragmented parts of the vertebra are removed carefully with rongeurs. Radical removal of nonfractured parts of the vertebral body should be avoided. Resection close to the spinal canal is facilitated with the use of high-speed burrs. If decompression of the spinal canal is necessary, the lower border of the pedicle should first be identified with a blunt hook. The base of the pedicle is then resected in a cranial direction with a Kerrison rongeur and the thecal sac can be identified. Finally, the posterior fragments, which occupy the spinal canal, are removed (2,7).

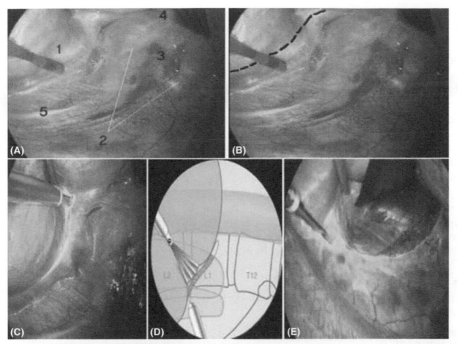

FIGURE 5 Operative steps in the thoracosopic detachment of the diaphragm. (**A**) Thoracoscopic view showing the anatomy of the thoracolumbar junction (1, diaphragm; 2, vertebral bodies; 3, segmental vessel; 4, aorta; 5, rib). (**B**) Thoracoscopic view showing the line of diaphragmatic insertion. (**C**) Diaphragmatic opening with hook diathermy electrode. (**D**) Diagram demonstrating the diaphragmatic opening with diathermy with gentle retraction of the diaphragm with a fan retractor. (**E**) The fan retractor is introduced into the diaphragmatic opening and retroperitoneal fat tissue is mobilized from the anterior surface of the psoas muscle. Later, the psoas muscle is gently dissected from the anterior aspect of the lumbar vertebrae.

Bone Grafting/Cage Placement
The preparation of the graft bed is completed by aggressive preparation of the adjacent endplates and complete removal of all soft tissue. The length and depth of the bone graft/spacer required are measured with a caliper. For vertebral fracture replacement, autologous iliac crest was used in most patients. Distractible titanium cages [Synthes, Paoli, Pennsylvania, U.S.A. or Vertebral Body Replacement (VBR), Osteotech, New Jersey, U.S.A.] were also used in some cases. The graft or cage are mounted on the graft holder and inserted through the working portal incision. Longer bone grafts (>2 cm) are inserted along their long axis through the opening and then mounted onto the graft holder inside the thoracic cavity. It is best to place the graft/cage under distraction. With the distractible titanium cages, additional reduction can be achieved by further increasing the height of the cage within the graft site.

Instrumentation
We have previously reported our technique of thoracoscopic instrumentation (1,2). We used the Z-Plate® (Medtronic Sofamor Danek, Memphis, Tennessee, U.S.A.) from May 1996 to October 1999. The MACS-TL system (AESCULAP, Germany) was exclusively used from November 1999 to June 2002 as it was specially designed for endoscopic placement and greatly facilitates the instrumentation.

Screw Insertion Preparation
Next, Insert a self-tapping screw under fluoroscopic control in the vertebra superior to the fractured one, as well as in the fractured vertebra. Next, insert the first screw of the MACS-TL system (AESCULAP, Germany) into the caudal vertebral body. Open the cortical surface with

a sharp trephine—1 to 1.5 cm from the posterior border of the vertebral body infra- and supr-adjacent to the fracture.

K-Wire Insertion
Next, insert the K-wire in the distal cannulated end of the instrument, and connect it with the K-wire impactor. Position the K-wire under fluoroscopic control.

The patient must be placed in a lateral position to expose the posterior edge of the corresponding vertebral body. It is important to confirm the perpendicular position of the patient to the beam.

If the instrument charged with the K-wire is well aligned, a dark inner point and a concentric ring will be observed, and the correct placement is ensured. If a line is observed on X-ray, the K-wire is not positioned parallel. Following alignment, the K-wire is impacted until it is stopped by the gray ring of the instrument (20 mm).

For safe screw implantation, the K-wire should be inserted ~10 mm away from the posterior edge of the vertebral body and 10 mm away from the endplate. Afterwards, release the K-wire by turning the knob of the impactor counterclockwise. The complete instrument can then be pulled back, with the K-wire remaining in place.

Decortication
A cannulated punch is used for a slight removal of cortical bone to prepare the entry hole for the polyaxial screw.

Centralizer Attachment
The twin screws and the polyaxial clamp have to be preassembled before insertion. The centralizer has to be attached either to the polyaxial plate or to the twin screws. It then has to be screwed into the inner thread. This is accomplished by using the hex key for the centralizer. For rotational locking, the centralizer has two flanges, which correspond to the slots of the clamp. When fully seated, the centralizer should be snug but not overtightened.

Assembly of Insertion Instrument
The handle must be connected to the proximal end, the external hex, of the insertion sleeve. The cannulated screwdriver has to be positioned through the insertion sleeve until it locks in position. The ratchet handle is connected to the cannulated screwdriver, and the ring of the Harris connector has to be pushed proximally. The assembled insertion instrument is then connected to the hexagonal end of the centralizer. The spring of the insertion sleeve snaps into the corresponding groove of the centralizer. The orientation of the polyaxial plate should correspond to the direction of the handle to ease the orientation, especially in endoscopic procedures. The polyaxial screw is put into a straight direction to attach the screwdriver.

Screw Insertion
Next, place the polyaxial, posterior screw over the K-wire. The direction of the polyaxial clamp can be controlled by the handle. The clamp has to be oriented so that the hole for the anterior stabilization screw comes to lie anteriorly. After the fast turns of the screw into the vertebral body, the K-wire has to be removed to avoid the risk of tissue perforation by pushing the K-wire forward during screw insertion (Fig. 6).

K-Wire Removal
After partial insertion of the polyaxial screws, the K-wire has to be removed. Insert the removal instrument through the insertion instrument, and attach it to the K-wire by turning the removal instrument clockwise and screwing it onto the wire. The K-wire can then be pulled out through the cannulated instrument.

Insertion Instrument Removal
Push the slide of the insertion instrument, then release the instrument from the centralizer by pulling backward. The segmental vessels of the fractured vertebra are then mobilized, closed with vascular clips, and dissected.

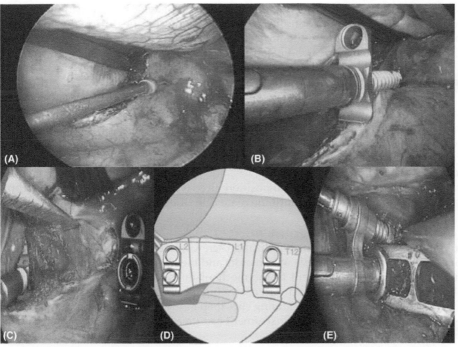

FIGURE 6 Placement of instrumentation. (**A**) Decortication to prepare the entry hole for the polyaxial screw (thoraco-scopic view). (**B**) Endoscopic view demonstrating the technique of screw insertion over the K-wire. (**C**) Thoracoscopic view showing a corpectomy and decompression of the spinal canal. (**D**) Graphical representation of polyaxial screws placed above and below the decompression site. (**E**) Thoracoscopic view demonstrating anterior screw placement.

Distraction Maneuvers

After discectomy or vertebrectomy and proper preparation of the graft bed, distraction can be applied to the vertebral bodies to insert a graft that is slightly larger than the prepared disc space and to achieve graft compression.

Place the distraction ratchet over the centralizers using holding forceps. According to the distance between the centralizers, choose the appropriate distraction bar. Before placing the ratchet onto the centralizers, unlock the bolt to allow the instrument to slide and be adjusted to the proper distance. After placing the distraction ratchets on the centralizers, engage the distraction forceps between the ratchet sleeves. Before applying the distraction forceps, lock the bolt.

Plate/Rod Placement

The distance between the polyaxial heads has to be measured. If plates are used, 30 mm must be added to select the proper plate length. The stabilization plate is then placed over the centralizer onto the polyaxial heads. The rounded side with the markings is on the upper side of the plate.

In cases of multisegmental assemblies, rod connection has to be chosen. Both rods have to be contoured in the same fashion. The anterior border of the polyaxial plate is slightly lower than the posterior. Thus, the posterior rod can be placed and temporarily closed by slightly tightening the nut to avoid rod loosening. A placement of the anterior rod is now still possible.

For both types of clamps, a degree of freedom should be preserved to allow angulation of the polyaxial heads. Final screw insertion is performed after the plates are placed and tightened with the fixation nuts.

Final Fixation

Next, the insertion sleeve is attached on the centralizer. After the plate or rod is placed and the polyaxial plate is well aligned, the assembly can be closed by using a fixation nut. The nut should be placed with the smooth part against the stabilization plate. Using the cannulated nut driver, the nut can be placed over the centralizer. To apply countertorque during the tightening process of the nut, attach the handle to the insertion sleeve. Prefixation can be achieved using the nut driver with the countertorque handle. For final fixation, the torque wrench is applied to the nut driver, and countertorque is again applied by using the handle on the insertion sleeve. Thus, no torque is applied to the spine. The tightening torque for final fixation is 15 nm.

Removal of the Centralizer
To remove the centralizer, attach the insertion sleeve with handle and hex key to the centralizer. Remove the centralizer from the polyaxial clamp by turning the screwdriver counterclockwise.

Tightening of the Polyaxial Screws
Next, the assembly must be brought into final position directly onto the surface of the vertebral bodies. To achieve this, insert the screws until the plate is in direct contact with the bone.

Insertion of the Anterior Screw
The screw-guiding sleeve for the anterior stabilization screw has to be attached to the polyaxial clamp. To do so, insert the insertion sleeve with handle and the hex key for the centralizer to the hexagonal end of the guiding instrument (same mechanism as for the centralizer). With the central punch, the cortex is then penetrated. After selecting the appropriate screw length, fix the anterior screw to the screwdriver with a retaining clip, then insert it through the guiding instrument into the vertebral body. The guiding instrument can then be removed (same mechanism as removal of the centralizer).

Insertion of Locking Screws
To lock the polyaxial mechanism, attach the yellow locking screw to the screwdriver with a retaining clip. The instrument has to be positioned perpendicular to the plate/rod. Tighten the locking screw with a torque of 10 nm. The torque wrench is applied to the screwdriver.

Closure and Postoperative Care

The gap in the diaphragm is closed with endoscopic suturing or hernia stapler. We prefer endoscopic suturing from the cost point of view. Smaller incisions less than 4 cm close by themselves without any approximating sutures. During diaphragmatic repair, care must be taken to avoid needle puncture of the lung, which may result in a bronchopleural fistula (4). The thoracic cavity is irrigated and blood clots are removed. A chest tube is inserted with the end placed in the costodiaphragmatic recess. The portals are closed with sutures or staples after removal of the trocars (Fig. 7).

Anteroposterior and lateral X-rays of the target area are obtained postoperatively. The majority of the patients are extubated immediately after the procedure. Elderly patients or those with pre-existing pulmonary or cardiovascular disease usually require ventilatory support for 24 hours. Low-dose, low-molecular weight heparin is given for thromboembolic prophylaxis. The chest tubes are usually removed on the first postoperative day. Mobilization and ventilation training are started on the first postoperative day. Physiotherapy is started on day two (1 hr/day) with gradual intensification after the first postoperative week. Follow-up X-rays are obtained two days, nine weeks, six months, and one year after surgery. Patients are allowed to return to work after 12 to 16 weeks.

COMPLICATIONS AND THEIR MANAGEMENT

Disadvantages of thoracoscopic procedures include slightly increased anesthetic monitoring and preparation because of the need for double-lumen ventilation, and the fact that the procedures require considerable training and practice to master. Because the endoscopic image is two-dimensional, a certain degree of difficulty may be encountered in obtaining adequate visual orientation during the initial experience. Further, as the thoracoscopic technique requires working through smaller portals at longer distances from the target area, it requires acquisition

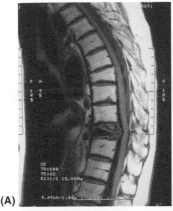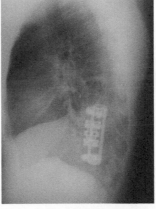

FIGURE 7   An illustrative case of pathologic fracture of T10 vertebra secondary to metastatic carcinoma. (**A**) Preoperative T1-weighted MRI. (**B**) Postoperative radiograph after thoracoscopic decompression and reconstruction of anterior column with MACS-TL system and an expandable vertebral body replacement cage.

of new cognitive, psychomotor, and technical skills to master the technique. Although difficult and challenging, the skills can be mastered with experience, and eventually operating times become shorter than the open thoracotomy procedures (2,8).

Our overall complication rate with thoracoscopic spinal surgery has been 11.4%. This compares favorably with the 29% rate reported in the multicenteric study of 1223 open anterior spinal procedures by Faciszewski et al. (of these, 707 were thoracotomies). Our incidence of vascular injury (0.5%) and neurological injury (0.5%) are reasonable compared with the 0.08% and 0.5% reported in Faciszewski's series (18). Our incidence of conversion to an open procedure (1.3%) is comparable with that reported by McAfee et al. (2.3%) on 100 cases of endoscopic surgery. Their incidence of pulmonary complications and intercostal neuralgia (11%) is much higher than in our series (5.4%) (19).

OUTCOMES

Morbidity associated with conventional open thoracotomy and laparotomy often limits the application of anterior approaches to thoracic and lumbar spine (18,20). As more than 50% of the fractures of the thoracic spine involve TLJ, they often require diaphragmatic detachment by combined thoracoabdominal approaches with possible complications such as post-thoracotomy syndromes, intercostals neuralgia, herniation of visceral contents into the chest cavity, and so on (20,21). These approaches require extensive exposures with incisions measuring about 20 cm, which can be cosmetically disfiguring. Most of the morbidity of these open procedures is not because of the exposure itself, but rather to injury inflicted to the chest or abdominal walls (2,8,21).

In recent years, minimally invasive open microscopic approaches using special retractors have been developed which can minimize the size of the operative access to 6 to 10 cm. These "mini approaches" are quite feasible in surgery on the upper and midthoracic spine. However, mini approaches to the TLJ require placement of retractors for the diaphragm, fan retractors for the lungs, and enough working space for suction and surgical instruments. The limited working space available through the small incisions at TLJ may block the microscopic view and result in collision of instruments. Thoracoscopy permits surgery at TLJ of the spine as effectively as the open approaches using four portals in the chest wall. Thoracoscopy provides a better view than the microscopic view, as its viewing distance is much closer to the target area. Unlike the open approaches, the surgeon's operative view is not obscured by his hands or operative instruments. Thus, thoracoscopic approach to TLJ is more practical than the mini approach, and has the biomechanical advantages of using an anterior approach without the disadvantages of high morbidity associated with open procedures (2,8,21).

Thoracoscopic approach has several other advantages over open procedures, including reduced pain, a better cosmetic effect, excellent direct visualization of the target area, lower perioperative morbidity, and an earlier return to normal activity.

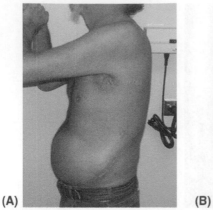
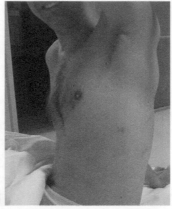

(A)   (B)

FIGURE 8   Postoperative scars following surgery after six months. (**A**) Open thoracotomy and retroperitoneal approach. (**B**) Thoracoscopic surgery.

Reduced Pain

As the thoracoscopic technique requires multiple smaller incisions without any need for major muscle dissection, rib resection, or retraction and can be performed in a shorter operating time, it reduces postoperative pain significantly. It reduces both the duration and dosage of analgesics required postoperatively. Reduction of postoperative pain was demonstrated in our previous study, in which we compared the 30 patients operated endoscopically in the first year with another group of 30 patients who had undergone open surgery. In the group treated endoscopically, the duration of analgesic medication was reduced by 31% and the overall dosage of analgesics by 42% relative to the group treated by open surgery (1,2).

It is well known that the intensity of acute postoperative pain correlates highly with the occurrence of chronic pain after thoracic surgery (1,2,20,21). Thus, the reported frequency of chronic postoperative pain ranges from 7% to 55% following thoracotomy compared with 4% to 35% reported with minimally invasive surgery.

Better Cosmetic Effect

Multiple smaller incisions without rib resection provide an excellent cosmetic outcome. Distressing operative scars because of open surgery are avoided (Fig. 8) (1,21).

Excellent Direct Visualization

Like thoracotomy, TTA provides direct full view of the entire anterior spine, anterior spinal cord, ipsilateral pedicle, and transverse process, permitting treatment of multisegmental lesions. The excellent magnified image provided by the thoracoscope is superior even to that afforded by open thoracotomy because the operative viewing distance is only a few centimeters from the injury. This view is far superior to the one achieved by posterolateral approaches (1,2,22).

Lower Perioperative Morbidity

Reduced wound pain, early extubation, reduced operating time, and diminished blood loss adds to the significant reductions in perioperative morbidity. Our present operating times are shorter than with open thoracotomy. The duration of pulmonary complications and ventilator support are three times higher with open thoracotomy (1,2,11).

Earlier Return to Normal Activity

Reduction of postoperative pain and perioperative morbidity reduce the hospital stay and hasten a return to normal activity. In our experience, 80% of our patients treated endoscopically were able to return to their previous employment, as compared with 66% of the open-thoracotomy patients (1,2,11,23).

SUMMARY

With increasing thoracoscopic/laparoscopic experience, improvements have been made in surgical techniques, implants, and instrumentation. While these improvements continue, so will the advancement of minimally invasive surgery (MIS) for anterior thoracoscopic surgery. Various technological advances will continue to improve the efficacy and safety of the thoracoscopic spine surgery. These will greatly facilitate TTA and improve its safety.

Improvements in Optical Imaging Technology

Future developments in optical imaging technology are likely to produce better resolution of the optical images, smaller diameter endoscopes, flexible endoscopes, three-dimensional (3D) endoscopic imaging, virtual reality endoscopy, and holographic imaging. An interactive, voice-controlled, 3D viewing headset that shows the endoscopic microsurgical operative anatomy is now available (Vista Technologies, Carlsbad, California, U.S.A.). Radiographic, computed tomography (CT), magnetic resonance imaging (MRI), and stereotactic guidance images are simultaneously projected onto a portion of the visual field. This permits the surgeon to examine the surgical pathology without turning away from the patient during the surgery (22).

Image-Guided Endoscopic Surgery

This technique requires CT scanning of the target area after percutaneous placement of a reference frame into vertebral pedicle from behind. The CT images are registered to the anatomy using the geometry of the frame as fiducials. This permits navigation of the endoscopic procedures and enhances the precision of dissection. It provides accurate information for guiding a surgical tool through the endoscope and thus facilitates the placement of spinal implants. It eliminates the need for multiple, tedious and time-consuming preoperative fluoroscopic images and thus reduces the radiation exposure. Compared with C-arm fluoroscopy, it provides 3D control of the surgical instrument in almost real time. In the future, it will be an effective tool for the endoscopic spine surgeon for improving safety and efficacy of the procedure.

Robotic Surgery

Voice-controlled robotic arms (automated endoscopic system for optimal positioning, AESOP) are currently available for use in thoracoscopic surgery. They are approved by the Food and Drug Administration (FDA) as endoscopic holder (Computer Motion, Golita, California, U.S.A.). Surgeons can verbally command the robotic arm to reposition the endoscope within the operative field. Intraoperatively, the robot can memorize several anatomical positions and immediately return to the designated positions. It provides the surgeon with direct control of the endoscope, resulting in a more stable and sustainable endoscopic image (22).

A surgical robotic arm is under clinical trial (Zeus, Computer Motion, Golita, California, U.S.A.). It performs the procedure with the surgeon guiding the robotic arm from a location in or adjacent to the operating room while viewing the surgery through a monitor showing magnified images. These robotic arms improve surgical dexterity by eliminating hand tremor. Potentially, with this technology, a surgeon can perform surgical dissection on a patient who is on the other side of the planet.

Another recent robotic development (HERMES, Computer Motion, Golita, California, U.S.A.) uses speech-recognition technology that gives the surgeon direct voice control over most equipments in the operating room, such as light sources, cameras, pumps, drills, energy sources, videocassette recording, suction, and the like. The status of the devices can also be displayed on the monitors to obtain feedback regarding the functioning of the device. This permits the surgeon to perform the procedure more effectively with a smaller surgical team (22).

REFERENCES

1. Beisse R, Potulski M, Buhren V. Endoscopic techniques for the management of spinal trauma. Eur J Trauma 2001; 27:275–291.
2. Khoo LT, Beisse R, Potulski M. Thoracoscopic-assisted treatment of thoracic and lumbar fractures: a series of 371 consecutive cases. Neurosurgery 2002; 51:S104–S117.

3. Mack MJ, Aronoff RJ, Acuff TE, et al. Thoracoscopic transdiaphragmatic approach for adrenal biopsy. Ann Thorac Surg 1993; 55:772–773.
4. Gill IS, Meraney AM, Thomas JC, et al. Thoracoscopic transdiaphragmatic adrenalectomy: the initial experience. J Urol 2001; 165:1875–1881.
5. Meraney AM, Gill IS, Hsu TH, et al. Thoracoscopic transdiaphragmatic nephrectomy: feasibility study. Urology 2000; 55:443–447.
6. Pompeo E, Coosemans W, De Leyn P, et al. Thoracoscopic transdiaphragmatic left adrenalectomy. An experimental study. Surg Endosc 1997; 11:390–392.
7. Beisse R. "Keyhole" surgery, even on the spine. Krankenpfl J 2000; 38:288–289.
8. Beisse R, Potulski M, Beger J, et al. Development and clinical application of a thoracoscopy implantable plate frame for treatment of thoracolumbar fractures and instabilities. Orthopade 2002; 31:413–422.
9. Kim D, Guiot B, Fessler R. Principles of spinal fixation, fusion and motion. In Crockard A, Hayward R, Hoff JT, eds. The Scientific Basis of Clinical Practice. Abingdon: Blackwell Science, 2000:1157–1169.
10. Huang TJ, Hsu RW, Liu HP, et al. Technique of video-assisted thoracoscopic surgery for the spine: new approach. World J Surg 1997; 21:358–362.
11. Regan J, Ben-Yishay A. Thoracolumbar discectomy. In: Regan J, McAfee P, Mack M, eds. Atlas of Endoscopic Spine Surgery. St. Louis: Quality Medical Publishing Inc, 1995:233–242.
12. Burgos J, Rapariz JM, Gonzalez-Herranz P. Anterior endoscopic approach to the thoracolumbar spine. Spine 1998; 23:2427–2431.
13. Olinger A, Hildebrandt U, Mutschler W, et al. First clinical experience with an endoscopic retroperitoneal approach for anterior fusion of lumbar spine fractures from levels T12 to L5. Surg Endosc 1999; 13:1215–1219.
14. Hovorka I, de Peretti F, Damon F, et al. Videoscopic retropleural and retroperitoneal approach to the thoracolumbar junction of the spine. Rev Chir Orthop Reparatrice Appar Mot 2001; 87:73–78.
15. Beisse R, Potulski M, Temme C, et al. Endoscopically controlled division of the diaphragm. A minimally invasive approach to ventral management of thoracolumbar fractures of the spine. Unfallchirurg 1998; 101:619–627.
16. Pait TG, Elias AJ, Tribell R. Thoracic, lumbar, and sacral spine anatomy for endoscopic surgery. Neurosurgery 2002; 51:S67–S78.
17. Huang TJ, Hsu RW, Liu HP, et al. Video-assisted thoracoscopic treatment of spinal lesions in the thoracolumbar junction. Surg Endosc 1997; 11:1189–1193.
18. Faciszewski T, Winter RB, Lonstein JE, et al. The surgical and medical perioperative complications of anterior spinal fusion surgery in the thoracic and lumbar spine in adults. A review of 1223 procedures. Spine 1995; 20:1592–1599.
19. McAfee PC, Regan JR, Zdeblick T, et al. The incidence of complications in endoscopic anterior thoracolumbar spinal reconstructive surgery. A prospective multicenter study comprising the first 100 consecutive cases. Spine 1995; 20:1624–1632.
20. Dajczman E, Gordon A, Kreisman H, et al. Long-term postthoracotomy pain. Chest 1991; 99:270–274.
21. Kalso E, Perttunen K, Kaasinen S. Pain after thoracic surgery. Acta Anaesthesiol Scand 1992; 36:96–100.
22. Dickman C, Rosenthal D, Perin N: Future directions for spinal thoracoscopy. In: Dickman C, Rosenthal D, Perin N, eds. Thoracoscopic Spine Surgery. New York: Thieme, 1999:355–360.
23. Landreneau RJ, Hazelrigg SR, Mack MJ, et al. Postoperative pain-related morbidity: video-assisted thoracic surgery versus thoracotomy. Ann Thorac Surg 1993; 56:1285–1289.

21 | Percutaneous Posterior Insertion of Thoracic Pedicle Screws

Daniel R. Fassett
Department of Neurosurgery, University of Utah, Salt Lake City, Utah, U.S.A.

Darrel S. Brodke
Department of Orthopedic Surgery, University of Utah, Salt Lake City, Utah, U.S.A.

INTRODUCTION

Pedicle screw fixation has been used in the thoracic spine for various clinical indications, including traumatic, deformity, and degenerative conditions. With its biomechanical superiority (1–5), pedicle screw fixation has supplanted wiring and hook-based techniques as the preferred method of posterior spinal fixation in the thoracic spine. In recent years, there has been a trend toward minimally invasive techniques in spinal surgery, including percutaneous pedicle screw fixation of the thoracic and lumbar spine. By reducing the extent of soft-tissue dissection, these percutaneous procedures have the potential benefits of lower blood loss, shorter hospital stays, earlier return to work, and reduced risk of infection in comparison with similar open procedures.

Percutaneous pedicle screw fixation is a challenging procedure that requires experience and an in-depth understanding of spinal anatomy to perform safely. The anatomical constraints of the thoracic vertebrae, which have generally smaller pedicles than the lumbar spine, can make this an especially challenging procedure. In addition, the presence of the spinal cord (vs. the cauda equina) in the thoracic spine makes the procedure a riskier one than that in the lower lumbar region, where misplacement into the spinal canal is better tolerated (6). The proximity of the great vessels to the thoracic spine also increases the risk for life-threatening complications from poor screw placement. These factors should be carefully considered before a percutaneous procedure in the thoracic spine is attempted.

INDICATIONS

Trauma is the most common indication for percutaneous pedicle screw fixation in the thoracic spine. Many fractures require treatment with anterior and posterior stabilization. If deformity is limited, these fractures can be treated via an anterior approach (open or thoracoscopically) with corpectomy or discectomy. With the placement of bone graft in the anterior column, there is no absolute need for bone grafting of the posterior elements, although percutaneous pedicle screws and rods may be placed to augment the anterior arthrodesis in situations where stability is a concern. The most common location for traumatic injury is the thoracolumbar junction, where the pedicles are most amendable to percutaneous placement of pedicle screws. Other potential indications may include degenerative conditions or spinal column tumors that are treated with an anterior approach first and need supplemental posterior instrumentation to provide additional stability.

Careful patient selection is a key factor for the successful use of this minimally invasive procedure. Placement of percutaneous pedicle screws relies primarily on fluoroscopic guidance to determine the location of the entry point and trajectory through the respective pedicle. Thus, patients with rotational deformities or other deformities that obscure the anatomy of the pedicles on fluoroscopy are not good candidates for this procedure. Other factors that can limit the quality of intraoperative fluoroscopy, such as obesity or osteopenia, should also be considered as relative contraindications to insertion of percutaneous pedicle screws.

Because of the anatomical constraints of the thoracic spine with small pedicles, percutaneous pedicle screw fixation is only recommended for the lower thoracic spine (T8–T12), depending on the individual anatomy. In open procedures, pedicle screws can be safely placed through small pedicles (7), but we do not recommend percutaneous placement for pedicles less than 5 mm in diameter. The transverse width of the pedicles is typically smallest in the T3 to T7 vertebrae (8), making this area challenging for safe placement of percutaneous screws. Although the pedicles are usually larger in the upper thoracic spine, issues with good fluoroscopic visualization of this region often limit the utility of the procedure in this region.

CONSIDERATIONS FOR PREOPERATIVE PLANNING
Preoperative Physical Examination

It is important to evaluate the spinal contour for abnormalities in spinal alignment and to observe the patient's body habitus closely when considering insertion of percutaneous thoracic pedicle screws. As in all spinal procedures, a thorough neurological examination is required preoperatively.

Imaging

We recommend preoperative computed tomography (CT) imaging with reconstructed images in the sagittal and coronal planes to assess the diameter and angles of the pedicles. Image guidance systems may help with placement of percutaneous screws and preoperative thin-cut CT images may be preloaded into these guidance systems. We also recommend plain anteroposterior (AP) and lateral radiographs to help assess whether intraoperative fluoroscopic visualization may be difficult. If there is any trouble appreciating the respective pedicles on the plain imaging, an open procedure should be seriously considered to provide direct visualization of the important anatomy.

SURGICAL TECHNIQUE
Operating Room Setup

A radiolucent table and modern fluoroscopy are recommended for percutaneous placement of thoracic pedicle screws. After the patient is positioned prone on a radiolucent table with padding of pressure points, the fluoroscopic equipment should be positioned. We recommend placing the fluoroscopic monitors above the head of the patient, contralateral to the primary surgeon. This allows the primary surgeon to maintain a comfortable body posture and directly view the fluoroscopic monitor throughout the procedure. It can also be beneficial to have another monitor on the other side of the room in view of the assisting surgeon and technicians. We recommend the use of neuromonitoring with somatosensory- and motor-evoked potentials as a surgeon is gaining experience with this procedure. Inadvertent screw trajectories into the spinal canal can have devastating consequences that may be minimized if neuromonitoring is able to detect early changes in spinal cord function.

Operative Approach/Relevant Anatomy

The thoracic pedicles are oval with a greater height than transverse diameter, making the transverse diameter the limiting feature in determining whether a pedicle screw can be placed safely and what size pedicle screw should be used. The average transverse diameter of the T8–T12 pedicles is 5.1 mm to 8.0 mm (Table 1) (9). The medial wall of the thoracic pedicle is typically thicker than the lateral wall, which helps minimize the risk for medial wall breakout and the possibility for spinal cord injury. The preoperative CT scan should be reviewed, and we recommend selecting a pedicle screw 0.5-mm diameter smaller than the transverse diameter of the pedicle.

The starting point for open (and percutaneous) pedicle screws in T11 and T12 is on a line bisecting the transverse process at a point 1 mm medial to the lateral aspect of the pars interarticularis. In T8, T9, and T10, the entry site is slightly more medial and more cephalad than the

TABLE 1 Pedicle Transverse Diameter and Angulation for T8–T12 Pedicles

Pedicle	Mean transverse diameter (mm)	Mean medial angulation (°)
T8	5.1 ± 1.2	6.9 ± 5.0
T9	5.8 ± 1.5	7.1 ± 4.6
T10	6.7 ± 1.6	4.1 ± 6.1
T11	8.0 ± 1.9	0.7 ± 3.3
T12	7.8 ± 2.0	0.3 ± 2.7

Source: From Ref. 9.

entry sites for T11 and T12 (Fig. 1) (7). Although these anatomic landmarks will not be directly visualized when placing percutaneous screws, they may be appreciated with fluoroscopy and palpation with the pedicle-probing needle. The angle of the pedicle can also be appreciated by reviewing the preoperative CT images and is usually less than 10° in the lower thoracic spine (Table 1) (9). Obviously, experience in open placement of thoracic pedicle screws helps significantly with the percutaneous placement of these screws.

Description of Procedure

Fluoroscopy in the lateral view is used to confirm the level of surgery, and the cephalad–caudal levels of the respective pedicles are marked on the patient's back with a marking pen. A perfect AP fluoroscopic image is used next to confirm both the superior and the lateral margins of the pedicles. With the minimal medial angulation of the pedicles in the lower thoracic spine, the intersection of these two lines (cephalad and lateral margin of pedicle) represents the entry point at the skin (usually 2 to 3 cm off midline) to access the pedicle. In the lumbar spine where there is greater medial angulation of the pedicles, a more lateral skin opening is optimal to gain the correct medial angulation through the pedicle.

A 1-cm vertical incision is made through the skin and dorsal fascia centered on the location of the pedicle based on fluoroscopy. A spinal-access needle (such as a Jamshidi needle, which is a cannulated device similar to a biopsy needle used in transpedicular biopsies) is placed through this stab incision and slowly directed toward the entry point for the pedicle (Fig. 2). It is recommended that this needle be advanced under direct lateral fluoroscopic visualization as the

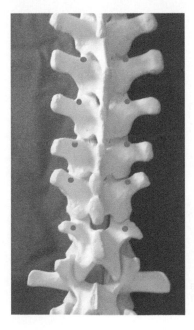

FIGURE 1 Starting points for thoracic pedicle screws for T8–T12 as visualized in an open procedure. *Source*: From Ref. 7.

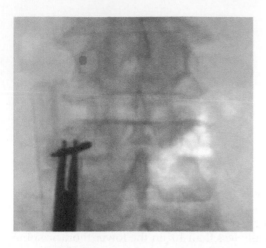

FIGURE 2 Anteroposterior fluoroscopic image showing a needle at the entry point on the pedicle. The *grey dot* at the level above shows the optimum entry point for the spinal-access needle into the pedicle.

surgeon is gaining experience with this technique to avoid interlaminar placement with possible dural violation and cord injury. On the lateral fluoroscopic view, the cephalad–caudal angulation of the spinal access needle can be adjusted for appropriate trajectory through the pedicle. Tactile feedback should allow the surgeon to determine when the spinal-access needle is on bone. Once the needle is docked on bone, fluoroscopy is adjusted to an AP image to determine the medial–lateral relationship of the spinal-access needle to the pedicle. We recommend adjusting the spinal-access needle to a point on the lateral margin of the pedicle to reduce the risk for medial pedicle breakout (Fig. 2).

Using a gentle twisting motion, the spinal-access needle (Fig. 3) is slowly advanced through the dense cortical bone. As the needle advances and enters cancellous bone, the resistance decreases significantly. At this point, AP and lateral fluoroscopy images are obtained to confirm appropriate trajectory through the pedicle. Adjustments in starting point and trajectory are made if needed. Once the trajectories are optimized, the spinal-access needle is slowly advanced through the pedicle with a gentle twisting motion similar to that of the pedicle probe used with open placement of thoracic pedicle screws. Lateral fluoroscopy is used to monitor the passage of the spinal-access needle through the pedicle and into the vertebral body. Sudden changes in resistance (plunging) likely signals breakout and the location of the instrument

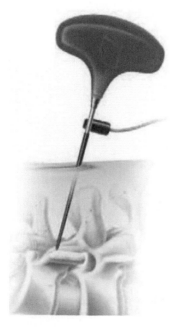

FIGURE 3 Lateral view of the spine with spinal-access needle ready to be slowly advanced through the pedicle (SpheRx™ DBR spinal access needle, Nuvasive). *Source*: Courtesy of Nuvasive, San Diego, California.

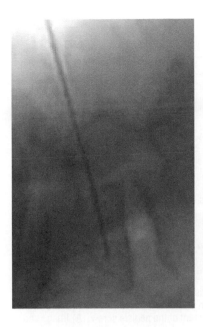

FIGURE 4 Lateral fluoroscopy showing a K-wire placed through the pedicle into the vertebral body. We recommend stopping the K-wire just as it passes through the pedicle and slightly into the vertebral body to decrease the risk of advancing the K-wire through the ventral aspect of the vertebral body during tapping and placement of pedicle screw. The K-wire in this picture is slightly deeper than we recommend, so extreme care would be necessary to ensure that the K-wire does not advance further as the procedure continues.

should be investigated fluoroscopically. Repetitive problems with pedicle breakout warrant close investigation and conversion to an open procedure.

Once the spinal access needle is at an appropriate depth in the vertebral body just past the posterior wall of the vertebra, a K-wire is placed through the spinal-access needle into the vertebral body. A lateral fluoroscopic image is obtained to confirm that the K-wire exits the tip of the spinal-access needle (Fig. 4). The K-wire should be placed with great care not to penetrate too deeply as the anterior cortex could be perforated and great vessel injury could occur with deep placement of K-wire.

After the K-wire is placed, the spinal-access needle is removed, without moving the K-wire. A series of dilators are then placed over the K-wire to dilate the posterior musculature and soft tissues to provide a space for insertion of tap and screw over the K-wire (Fig. 5A). The final dilators are typically left in place and a tap is placed over the K-wire and through the final dilator (Fig. 5B). We recommend tapping the pedicle with a tap 0.5 mm smaller than the anticipated screw diameter (e.g., 4.5-mm tap for 5.0-mm screw) to improve screw purchase in the pedicle. After tapping, the tap is removed without moving the K-wire, and a cannulated-pedicle screw is placed over the K-wire and screwed into position (Fig. 6). Care should be exercised not to advance the K-wire when placing instruments and the screw. Once all of the screws are in place, the rods between the screws are placed. The technique of rod insertion can vary with the respective instrumentation manufacturer.

Closure and Postoperative Management

The incisions for these procedures are small and can typically be closed with resorbably sutures in the fascia and subcutaneous layers, followed by sterile bandages (e.g., Steri-Strips) or skin adhesive. Activity restrictions relate to adequacy of fixation, general stability, and comorbidities. In general, we encourage early mobilization. In the authors' experience, pain control with minimally invasive approaches is typically easier. Some patients may experience painful muscle spasms in the posterior musculature and benefit from muscle relaxants in the postoperative course.

MANAGEMENT OF COMPLICATIONS
Pitfalls

Experience and good fluoroscopic technique are both extremely important to performing this procedure safely. We advocate performing this procedure multiple times on cadavers to gain

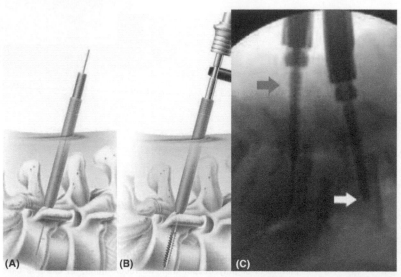

FIGURE 5 A series of dilators are placed over the K-wire to expand the soft tissues and provide a corridor for placement of the pedicle screw. The inner dilators are removed with the outer dilator left in place. Cannulated instruments and screws are placed over the K-wire and through the outer dilator to complete the placement of the pedicle screw. (**A**) Image showing dilators placed over K-wire dilating the soft tissues. (**B**) Image showing cannulated tap placed over the K-wire and through the outer dilator to tap the pedicle in preparation for placement of the pedicle screw. (**C**) Lateral fluoroscopic image showing a tap (*grey arrow*) going through the pedicle with a completed screw at the level above (*white arrow*) (SpheRx™ DBR percutaneous pedicle screw system, Nuvasive). *Source*: Courtesy of Nuvasive, San Diego, California.

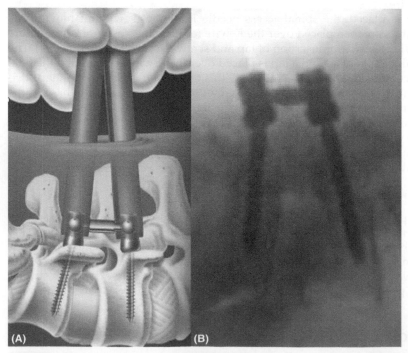

FIGURE 6 Cannulated pedicle screws are placed over the K-wire using lateral fluoroscopy to confirm positioning. Rods are then placed via various methods depending on the instrumentation manufacturer. (**A**) Rods can be inserted via various methods as shown here through slotted tubes. (**B**) Lateral fluoroscopy showing the final construct (SpheRx™ DBR percutaneous pedicle screw system, Nuvasive). *Source*: Courtesy of Nuvasive, San Diego, California.

experience and mastering placement of lumbar percutaneous screws before attempting insertion of thoracic screws. The lumbar pedicles are more forgiving, and poor trajectories are typically not as devastating in the lumbar spine. It is of utmost importance that the best fluoroscopic images be obtained. Perfect lateral and AP images are needed to place thoracic pedicle screws safely, and spending extra time to eliminate obliquity on the fluoroscopic images is justified.

Bailouts

If the surgeon is concerned about anatomical landmarks or possible screw breakout, the threshold for conversion to an open procedure should be low. In this scenario, we recommend closing the small paraspinous incisions and opening a midline exposure to gain the access needed to visualize the pertinent anatomy. Laminotomies may enable the surgeon to palpate and appreciate the location of the pedicle as well as determine if medial pedicle violation occurred. If breakout has occurred with a straight-forward trajectory (parallel to the endplate), a so-called anatomic trajectory (in the caudally angulated plane of the pedicle) can be used as a salvage procedure after conversion to an open technique (10). Hooks or additional levels of fixation may also be considered.

OUTCOMES

Outcome studies for insertion of percutaneous thoracic pedicle screws are lacking. Cadaveric studies have shown that percutaneous thoracic pedicle screws can be placed with greater than 90% accuracy (no breakout) with fluoroscopic image guidance (11), but in vivo studies have not been performed. Similarly, prospective studies of the potential clinical benefits of the percutaneous insertion of thoracic pedicle screws have not been reported.

SUMMARY

Percutaneous insertion of thoracic pedicle screws is a challenging procedure that can be performed safely by the experienced surgeon. Patient selection and surgeon experience are key factors in determining the success of this procedure. The indications for the procedure are limited and several contraindications should be considered before initiating percutaneous placement. Adequate clinical studies are lacking to determine whether the potential benefits of decreased blood loss, shorter hospital stay, and earlier return to work truly exist.

REFERENCES

1. Zindrick MR, Wiltse LL, Widell EH, et al. A biomechanical study of intrapeduncular screw fixation in the lumbosacral spine. Clin Orthop Relat Res 1986; 203:99–112.
2. Heller JG, Shuster JK, Hutton WC. Pedicle and transverse process screws of the upper thoracic spine. Biomechanical comparison of loads to failure. Spine 1999; 24(7):654–658.
3. Liljenqvist U, Hackenberg L, Link T, Halm H. Pullout strength of pedicle screws versus pedicle and laminar hooks in the thoracic spine. Acta Orthop Belg 2001; 67(2):157–163.
4. Hitchon PW, Brenton MD, Black AG, et al. In vitro biomechanical comparison of pedicle screws, sublaminar hooks, and sublaminar cables. J Neurosurg 2003; 99 (suppl 1):104–109.
5. Hackenberg L, Link T, Liljenqvist U. Axial and tangential fixation strength of pedicle screws versus hooks in the thoracic spine in relation to bone mineral density. Spine 2002; 27(9):937–942.
6. Wiesner L, Kothe R, Schultz KP, Ruther W. Clinical evaluation and computed tomography scan analysis of screw tracts after percutaneous insertion of pedicle screws in the lumbar spine. Spine 2000; 25(5):615–621.
7. Kim YJ, Lenke LG, Bridwell KH, et al. Free hand pedicle screw placement in the thoracic spine: is it safe? Spine 2004; 29(3):333–342, discussion 342.
8. Zindrick MR, Wiltse LL, Doornik A, et al. Analysis of the morphometric characteristics of the thoracic and lumbar pedicles. Spine 1987; 12(2):160–166.
9. Vaccaro AR, Rizzolo SJ, Allardyce TJ, et al. Placement of pedicle screws in the thoracic spine. Part I: morphometric analysis of the thoracic vertebrae. J Bone Joint Surg Am 1995; 77(8):1193–1199.
10. Lehman RA Jr, Kuklo TR. Use of the anatomic trajectory for thoracic pedicle screw salvage after failure/violation using the straight-forward technique: a biomechanical analysis. Spine 2003; 28(18):2072–2077.
11. Holly LT, Foley KT. Three-dimensional fluoroscopy-guided percutaneous thoracolumbar pedicle screw placement. Technical note. J Neurosurg 2003; 99(suppl 3):324–329.

22 | Laparoscopic Anterior Lumbar Interbody Fusion

Grigory Goldberg
Thomas Jefferson University, Philadelphia, Pennsylvania, U.S.A.

Alexander R. Vaccaro
Department of Orthopedic Surgery and Neurosurgery, Thomas Jefferson University and the Rothman Institute, Philadelphia, Pennsylvania, U.S.A.

INTRODUCTION

Prior to the 1980s, laparoscopic procedures were mainly used in the fields of gynecology and urology. In 1980s, the first laparoscopic appendectomy was performed in Germany. In 1991, only six years after the first laparoscopic cholecystectomy was performed by Muhe (1), Obenchain (2) reported the first laparoscopic lumbar discectomy for a herniated disc. In 1995, Cloyd (3) reported his results with 21 laparoscopic lumbar discectomies. Zucharman et al. (4) was the first one to describe the technique in detail, and subsequently published preliminary outcome data for laparoscopic anterior lumbar fusion. In 1999, Regan et al. (5) published a prospective study comparing open and laparoscopic methods of anterior lumbar fusion. They concluded that patients who had laparoscopic anterior lumbar interbody fusion (ALIF) had significantly lower blood loss and shorter postoperative recovery time. To date, the transperitoneal laparoscopic approach has never received widespread use outside the L5-S1 level due to the proximity of the great vessels at proximal levels.

Technically, the use of gas insufflation (carbon dioxide) in laparoscopic ALIF surgery prevented large tissue removal or the use of large instruments due to pressure decompression of the abdominal cavity. The presence of gas also interferes with the ability to suction blood in the vicinity of the surgical dissection and can lead to significant hemodynamic changes.

To address these issues, Thalgott et al. (6) described a gasless technique, referred to as the balloon-assisted endoscopic retroperitoneal gasless (BERG) method, which used an inflatable balloon to dissect and spread the retroperitoneal tissues. This method helped to eliminate some of the problems associated with gas-mediated approaches to the lumbar spine. Other authors described a mini-open technique (4-cm incision) which avoided the use of an endoscope altogether and allowed direct visual exposure of the spinal elements (7).

INDICATIONS

The indications and patient selection criteria are similar for open and laparoscopic ALIF. Patients with chronic mechanical lower back pain due to degenerative disc disease, internal disc disruption, spondylolisthesis (grades I and II), symptomatic posterolateral pseudarthrosis, and segmental instability are all candidates for laparoscopic ALIF if anterior interbody fusion is deemed necessary for symptom relief (8). The ideal patient for a laparoscopic fusion procedure is one who has radiographic degenerative disc changes that are isolated to one level on both plain films and magnetic resonance imaging (MRI).

Vascular anatomic blockade and pregnancy are considered absolute contraindications to a laparoscopic ALIF regardless of the spinal pathology. Laparoscopic approaches to the lumbar spine are contraindicated in patients with severe intra-abdominal adhesions from inflammatory conditions involving the peritoneum or from previous laparotomy or history of severe abdominal trauma. Morbid obesity should be considered a relative contraindication because the abdominal girth decreases the functional length of the instruments. These patients often require an open procedure to obtain adequate visualization of the disc space. Finally, patients who have severe osteoporosis should be considered relative contraindications to this procedure. Good end-plate bone is required to perform adequate interspace distraction. With severe osteoporosis, the distraction plugs collapse the end plate rather than distract.

Obviously, patient selection is a key. Patients with psychological problems, patients who exhibit chronic pain behavior or have imaging evidence of multilevel disease are not good candidates for the procedure.

PREOPERATIVE PLANNING

Preoperative planning should include standard plain films [anteroposterior (AP) and lateral] and advanced imaging studies detailing the level or levels of pathology [magnetic resonance imaging (MRI) with or without computed tomography (CT)/discography]. T2-weighted MRI images clearly demonstrate the level of the degenerative process. Discography is beneficial in symptomatic degenerative disc disease in order to understand the anatomic location of the presumed pain generator better.

MRI is also valuable in mapping the location of the vascular structures in the vicinity of the surgical field. The location of the vena cava, aorta, level of the aortic bifurcation and iliac vein confluence in relation to the pathologic disc space can be easily visualized.

It is imperative that preoperative planning is performed jointly with the access of general/laparoscopic surgeon in order to facilitate the procedure. A well-documented abdominal examination should be performed by the general surgeon to determine if any contraindications exist in performing the procedure. As referred to previously, patients who have had multiple previous transabdominal surgeries, previous abdominal mesh implant insertion, or retroperitoneal surgery may not be the appropriate candidates for laparoscopic ALIF. Patients should also undergo a preoperative mechanical large bowel preparation to empty the sigmoid colon.

SURGICAL TECHNIQUE FOR THE LAPAROSCOPIC
APPROACH TO L5–S1 DISC LEVEL

The technique most commonly described (9) involves the placement of the patient on a radiolucent operating table in the supine position with arms secured perpendicular to the patient's body to enable the spine surgeon and laparoscopic surgeon to stand on the opposite sides of the table (Fig. 1). The table should be positioned at 30° of Trendelenberg, so that the small intestine and the omentum are retracted cephalad by gravity, and the sigmoid colon is retracted laterally. To prevent the patient from sliding when in the Trendelenberg position, stirrups are used or the patient's knees may be flexed with pillows.

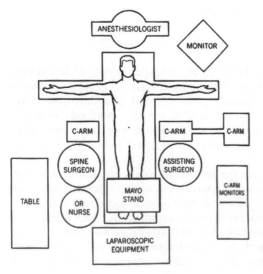

FIGURE 1   The patient is placed supine on a radiolucent operating table with the arms secured perpendicular to the body in order for the spine surgeon and laparascopic surgeon to stand on opposite sides of the table.

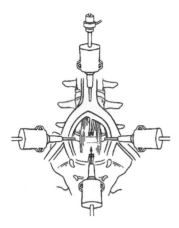

FIGURE 2 A 0° endoscope is placed at or slightly below the umbilicus. Under direct visualization, two working portals are then placed, one in the right lower quadrant for insertion of a retractor or suction tube, and one in the left lower quadrant for dissection tools. Other portals may be placed as necessary at the discretion of the surgeon. The lower quadrant portals should be in line with the L5–S1 disk space (intended level of surgery) as visualized on a pre-incision lateral fluoroscopy view.

Once the patient is under anesthesia, a Foley catheter and nasogastric (NG) tube should be placed. If the patient has had no previous abdominal surgeries then CO_2 insufflation can be performed using a Veress needle. For patients with previous abdominal surgery an open laparoscopy is performed with a Hasson cannula so that the initial trochars can be placed under direct vision. This minimizes the chance of injury to the small bowel. Other subsequent trochars are placed under direct vision as viewed from the insufflated abdominal cavity.

A small incision is made at the level of the umbilicus and an insufflation needle is introduced. The peritoneum is filled with CO_2 to approximately 15 mmHg. A blunt trochar is placed at or slightly below the umbilicus, thus allowing a 0° endoscope to be introduced into the abdominal cavity. Under direct visualization, two working portals are then placed: a 5-mm right lower quadrant port for the insertion of a retractor or suction tube, and a 10-mm left lower quadrant port for dissection tools. These ports should be in line with the L5–S1 disc space as visualized on a preincision lateral fluoroscopy view. This is extremely important as it allows for collinear placement of the interbody fusion cage without the need for significant soft-tissue retraction.

The location of the bifurcation of the great vessels is identified and the sigmoid colon mesentery is approached from the right side (Fig. 2). Before incising the sigmoid mesentery and posterior peritoneum in the midline, the location of the right and left ureter is confirmed. The right ureter courses over the right iliac artery and vein, and can be identified by peristalsis associated with the probing of this structure, whereas the left ureter lies deep in the sigmoid colon in the retroperitoneal space (10). After incising the posterior peritoneum longitudinally, blunt dissection is required to visualize the disc space of L5–S1 and the median sacral vessels. The median sacral vein and artery are ligated with vascular clips (Figs. 3 and 4) In male patients, the parietal peritoneum overlying the L5–S1 space is swept from the midline using a blunt dissection

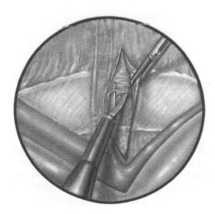

FIGURE 3 After incising the posterior peritoneum longitudinally, blunt and occasionally sharp dissection is used to visualize the disk space of L5–S1 and the median sacral vessels.

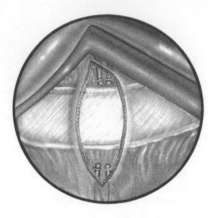

FIGURE 4   The median sacral vein and artery are ligated with vascular clips to access the L5–S1 disk space.

technique. Sharp dissection and monopolar cautery are avoided to prevent injury to the presacral sympathetic plexus, which might result in retrograde ejaculation.

SURGICAL TECHNIQUE FOR LAPAROSCOPIC APPROACH TO THE L2–L5 LEVELS

Trochar placement and positioning of the patient are identical to the technique used for the L5–S1 disc exposure, except that the trochars are placed 2 to 3 cm higher (11). In addition, the upper margin of the umbilicus is incised instead of the lower margin. The sigmoid colon is again retracted laterally. The midline posterior peritoneum is incised longitudinally approximately 3 cm more cephalad than for the L5–S1 disc exposure. The aortic bifurcation is identified with gentle blunt dissection. The L4–L5 disc space lies below the level of vessel bifurcation. The left iliac artery and vein are retracted to the right (Fig. 5). When retracting these vessels, it is imperative to initially dissect lateral to the iliac artery and vein and to ligate the ascending segmental vessels and lumbar or iliolumbar venous branches to allow vessel mobilization. The iliac vessels are retracted with Kitner forceps. If the aortic bifurcation lies cephalad to the L4–L5 disc space, the exposure is similar to that for the L5–S1 disc space.

For the L2–L4 levels, the surgical approach is similar to the exposure described for L4–L5 interspace. The posterior peritoneum is incised lateral to the aorta and medial to the left ureter and mesenteric vessels. A crossing lumbar vein and artery are usually located in the area of the

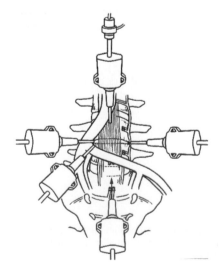

FIGURE 5   The L4–L5 disk space lies below the level of vessel bifurcation. The left iliac artery and vein are retracted to the right. When retracting these vessels it is imperative to initially dissect lateral to the iliac artery and vein and to ligate the ascending segmental vessels and lumbar or iliolumbar venous branches to allow vessel mobilization.

L3–L4 disc space. These vessels can be ligated and divided between hemoclips, but are best avoided if they do not interfere with access to the disc space.

An iliac crest autograft, if wanted, can be obtained at any point during the procedure. It is obtained through a standard anterolateral incision.

DISCECTOMY AND INTERBODY FUSION

After the appropriate disc space is exposed, a spinal needle or K-wire is passed percutaneously in the midline suprapubic region under direct visualization into the desired disc level. A cross-table lateral radiograph or preferably C-arm flouroscopy is performed to confirm that the diseased disc space has been identified properly. The needle also determines the angle of trajectory for the placement of the surpapubic operating trochar. The operating trochar should be parallel to the endplates of the disc space in the saggital plane. When the proper angle of trajectory has been determined, the final incision is made for the operating trochar (9).

The annulus over the disc space is then divided with an extended and protected scapel, and the disc is evacuated with curettes and pituitary instruments until bleeding subchondral bone is exposed (Fig. 6). A dilator and distraction plug are then driven into the interspace to restore native disc space height in preparation for bone graft or cage placement. The interspace graft should be sized greater than the distraction space to allow optimum restoration of disc height with good compression loading. The interbody prosthesis is then delivered by device-specific instrumentation into the disc space through the cannula. This is done under constant laparoscopic and fluoroscopic guidance.

Throughout the procedure, C-arm fluoroscopy is used intermittently to evaluate proper instrument and prosthesis placement. Cage failures may be minimized by avoiding placing the cage too far lateral, too deep, or not deep enough. It is easy to loose sight of the midline if one does not pay appropriate attention to the video or by not paying close attention to the positioning of the C-arm, which might deliver oblique images of the surgical site. To prevent this, one should consistently identify the relation of the midline spinal structures (pedicles and spinous processes) with the C-arm in the AP midline trajectory and make sure the endplates are parallel on the lateral fluoroscopic view (11).

Once the interbody cage is in place, the Trendelenburg position is reduced and the surgical field is copiously irrigated with bacitracin antibiotic solution. The pneumoperitoneum is slightly reduced to observe bleeding. Each port is observed for bleeding concurrent with surgical retreat. The posterior peritoneum is closed under visualization with sutures and clips. The fascia is closed with absorbable sutures and skin ports are closed with steri-strips.

BALLOON-ASSISTED ENDOSCOPIC RETROPERITONEAL GASLESS METHOD

As was mentioned previously, the laparoscopic approach has its limitations owing to the need for gas insufflation. The use of CO_2 gas can cause significant physiologic and hemodynamic

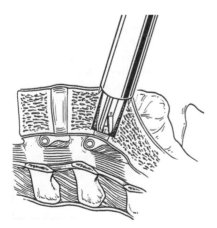

FIGURE 6 The anulus over the disc space is divided with an extended and protected scapel, and the disc is evacuated with curettes and pituitary instruments until punctate bleeding subchondral bone is exposed.

changes during the surgery (12). In addition, the suctioning of blood and irrigation fluid often outperforms the insufflation device's ability to pump an adequate amount of CO_2 gas. As a result, there is constant loss of the pneumoperitoneum with subsequent problem visualizing the surgical field. To address these and other problems, an alternative procedure was developed.

Thalgott et al. (6) suggested an endoscopic retroperitoneal approach using a balloon dissector to visualize the anterior spine. The patient is placed on a radiolucent table in the supine position. A radiolucent support may be placed under the patients left flank. The skin is marked to identify the level and angle of the pathologic disc space using fluoroscopic assistance. A transverse 20-mm flank incision is made over the left flank. This incision should be placed midway between the iliac crest and the coastal margin, along the midaxillary line. The external and internal oblique muscles are dissected bluntly with the clear-ended endoscopic dissection portal, as are the fibers of the transverses abdominus muscle. The dissection is taken down all the way to the pre-peritoneal fat layer. The retroperitoneal space is then gently insufflated with a bulb syringe and digitally dissected into the iliac fossa to allow balloon insertion. A dissecting balloon and cannula are advanced into the retroperitoneal space through the incision. Through the cannula, a 0° endoscope is inserted and the balloon is inflated to approximately 1 L. The endoscope is directed toward the anterior abdominal wall. This position allows the identification of the peritoneal reflection on the anterior abdominal wall, at the level of the rectus sheath. The reflection is a good landmark for anterior portal insertion. The anterior working portal is lateral to the peritoneal reflection on the rectus sheath.

A 2-cm paramedian incision is made about 2 cm off the anterior abdominal midline at the same level as the left flank incision, already described. The incision is made lateral to the peritoneal reflection, taking great care to avoid the peritoneal sac. Dissection is then taken down sharply though the fascia. This step creates the anterior working port that can also be used for retraction instruments. The balloon is removed after a malleable retractor is placed between the two ports under direct endoscopic visualization. A retroperitoneal endoscopic gasless working cavity has now been created. The next step is the physical retraction of the abdominal wall contents.

Thalgott et al. (6) described three steps used for adequate abdominal wall retraction in order to achieve good visualization of anterior lumbar spine. The first step is physical distraction of the anterior abdominal wall. This is done by the insertion of a fan retractor into the initial flank port. The fan retractor is expanded under endoscopic visualization and then attached to a mechanical lifting arm. By elevating the abdominal wall, the retroperitoneal space is developed, thus obviating the need for gas. A flexible nonvalved port is then placed directly below the fan retractor to provide a clear path for the endoscope.

The second step of the retroperitoneal exposure is to displace the peritoneal contents past the midline. A long retractor with an inflatable end is inserted through the newly created lateral working port in the initial left flank incision to push the peritoneal sac and intra-abdominal contents aside, creating the working space. This provides access to the anterior lumbar spine and vascular anatomy.

Finally, as with other laparoscopic approaches to the lumbar spine, the vascular structures must be identified and mobilized in order to safely approach the anterior aspect of the lumbar spine. The psoas muscle and vascular anatomy are used as landmarks. The psoas muscle should be bluntly dissected and retracted posteriorly to expose the pathologic disc space. During the dissection, the segmental vessels should be identified and ligated if required. Vascular retraction at the level of the L5-S1 disc space begins with the identification of the right iliac vein. A standard vein retractor is passed through the visualization/retraction port. It is used to retract the iliac vein laterally. Care must be taken in dissecting the anterior soft tissues to prevent damage to presacral plexus. Cauterization is not suggested to prevent injury to sympathetic presacral plexus.

The L4–L5 exposure is more complex. It begins by utilizing an anterior vessel retractor to retract the vena cava or left iliac vein to the right under tension. Next, the iliolumbar vein is ligated using a right-angled clip applier. After vessel ligation, the left iliac vein should be gently retracted past the midline to expose the L4–L5 interspace. Vascular retraction for the L3–L4 interspace is performed in a similar way, but it does not require ligation of the iliolumbar vein.

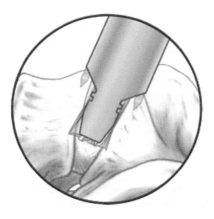

FIGURE 7 The vertebral end-plates are further denuded of cartilage with a protected circular rasp.

Following psoas dissection and vascular structure retraction, a needle should be placed in the diseased disc space to confirm the operative level under fluoroscopy. Once the exposure part of BERG method is done, the ALIF is performed in a standard way. The discectomy is performed with a long-handled protected scalpel. The vertebral end plates are then denuded of cartilage (Fig. 7). Following interspace distraction and implant placement (Fig. 8), the retroperitonium is inspected for any bleeding and the retractors are removed. The incision is closed in a standard fashion.

COMPLICATIONS AND MANAGEMENT
Vascular

Laceration of the great vessels is the most common reason for conversion to an open ALIF procedure. The most common reason for injury to the great vessels during an open ALIF procedure is excessive retraction. This is also the same for a laparoscopic procedure. What is unique to the laparoscopic approach, however, is the presence of a pneumoperitonium. As a result, the gas may compress or even collapse the iliac vein, making it difficult to identify the vascular injury during the dissection. If an injury to one of the vessels does occur, the surgeon should tomponade the bleeding with a gauze sponge placed through one of the large trochars. If this measure fails, the surgeon should proceed with an urgent laparotomy so that better access to the bleeding vessel can be achieved.

Retrograde Ejaculation

Retrograde ejaculation happens when the superior hypogastric plexus of the autonomic nervous system is injured. As a result, the seminal vesicles fail to contract, and the bladder neck does not close during ejaculation. The prevalence of retrograde ejaculation in laparoscopic ALIF

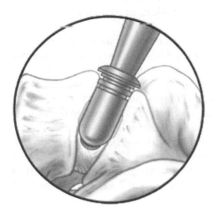

FIGURE 8 The interspace is distracted to get an objective understanding of implant size.

has been reported to be somewhere between 2.7% and 5.1% (11,13). The surgeon should avoid dissecting below the pelvic brim or using electrocautery, especially monoploar electrocautery, during the dissection. Injuries to the pelvic splanchic nerves or the pudendal nerves can result in impotence.

Deep-Venous Thrombosis and Pulmonary Embolism

The exact rate of deep-venous thrombosis (DVT) after laparoscopic ALIF is not well documented. Nonetheless, cases have been reported by several authors (14). A preventive measure should include the standard use of sequential pneumatic compression devices in all patients. Anticoagulation agents, such as aspirin or low-molecular-weight heparin may be used at the discretion of the surgeon.

Other complications that have been reported in the literature involve bone graft donor site infections; hernia, due to an enlarged trochar site; the need for open conversion owing to poor exposure; or abdominal or prediscal adhesions (5,14).

OUTCOMES

The first published series on the laparoscopic ALIF procedure reported encouraging results. Regan evaluated 34 patients who underwent laparoscopic fusion of L4–5 or L5–S1 at two medical centers in 1994. Laparoscopic lumbar fusion was successful in 30 of 34 patients. Four patients, early in the series, were successfully converted to an open procedure because of poor visualization (two cases) or iliac venous injury (two cases). Transfusion was required in one patient, and the average blood loss was 128 ml. The operative time averaged at 218 minutes, and the average hospitalization time was 3.67 days. In the authors' opinion, laparoscopic spinal surgery was a feasible means of accessing the anterior lumbar spine with minimal complications when a skilled laparoscopic surgeon is present for exposure. Preliminary results indicated an earlier discharge and return to work (three weeks) than that expected for standard open techniques.

In 1999, Regan reported the results of a large prospective multicenter study comparing laparoscopic transperitoneal ($n = 240$) and open retroperitoneal ($n = 305$) ALIF (5). They reported a shorter hospital stay (mean 3.3 days vs. 4.0 days), less blood loss (mean 141.7 ml vs. 207.2 ml) and longer operative times (mean 201.2 minutes vs. 144.9 minutes) in the laparoscopic group. There was also a 10% conversion rate to an open procedure. The reasons for the conversion included iliac vein injury ($n = 6$), obstructed access to the spine by the presence of bowel or one of the major vessels ($n = 5$), adhesions ($n = 8$), and technical reasons ($n = 6$). No significant difference was found in the postoperative complication rate (19.1% vs. 14.1%).

In another study, 14 patients were retrospectively reviewed who underwent a laparoscopic ALIF at either the L5–S1 or L4–L5 level (15). The average operative time was 300 minutes. The average blood loss was 60 ml. No intraoperative vascular or neurologic injuries were observed. Three patients were converted to open procedure (21%). One patient was noted to have an ovarian mass during the surgery, and the other two had a less-than-ideal graft position. The average hospital stay was 3.4 days. The patients were able to eat by postoperative day 1. Eighty percent ($n = 11$) of the patients achieved a solid interbody fusion, as assessed by plain X ray at three to six months.

The BERG procedure was developed because of the limitations of the laparoscopic anterior interbody fusion procedure, previously described. Thalgott reported his results with 202 patients (6). The rate of conversion was 24% for the first 101 patients and went down to 10% for the second 101 total cases. Six vessel lacerations required repair and there was one case of a ruptured diverticulum. Mean hospital stay was 1.95 days, with 47% of patients discharged in less than 47 hours following surgery. Clinical results at two-year follow up for the first 50 patients demonstrated a 92% fusion rate with 78% of patients reporting satisfactory pain relief.

Vazuez reported his series of 46 ALIF procedures performed with the BERG method (16). The conversion rate was reported to be 4%. The average blood loss was 223 ml and the mean hospital stay was four days (average two to four days). Operative complications included two venous vascular injuries which were managed with physical tamponade. One male patient reported retrograde ejaculation.

Finally, a number of studies have tried to compare the laparoscopic ALIF procedure with mini-open ALIF procedure. Zdeblick reported prospective data on 50 consecutive patients who underwent a L4–L5 anterior interbody fusion with a threaded device by either a laparoscopic or an open mini-ALIF approach (17). Twenty-five patients underwent a laparoscopic procedure and 25 an open mini-ALIF approach. For single-level L4–L5 fusions, there was no statistical difference in the operating time, blood loss, or the length of hospital stay between each group. For two-level procedures, only the operative time differed, with laparoscopic procedures taking 25 minutes longer. The rate of complications was significantly higher in the laparoscopic group (20% vs. 4%). This included DVT, disc herniation, ureter injury, retrograde ejaculation, and iliac vein laceration.

Kaiser performed a retrospective review of 98 patients who underwent an ALIF procedure either with laparoscopy or a mini-open laparotomy (18). Operative preparation and the procedure time were longer with the laparoscopic approach. There was no statistically significant difference in blood loss between the two methods. The average length of hospitalization was longer for the mini-open method by approximately one day. There were four intraoperative complications in the laparoscopic group and three in the mini-open group. These included vessel lacerations and bladder perforations.

The immediate postoperative complication rate was greater after the mini-open ALIF procedure (17.6 vs. 4.3%); however, the rate of retrograde ejaculation was higher in the laparoscopic group (45% vs. 6%).

Rodriques reported on a total of 65 anterior spinal access procedures. Thirty-one procedures were performed using a transperitoneal laparoscopic technique and 14 using an open mini-laparotomy (19). Mean follow-up was 12 months (range 1–50). No significant differences between the groups were found when comparing analgesia requirements, time to resumption of oral intake, length of hospitalization, and complication rates. Statistical analysis showed that the laparoscopic procedures were associated with shorter operating room times and less intraoperative blood loss. The laparoscopic approach was estimated to cost US$1374 more than the open technique.

It appears from the review of the literature that transperitoneal laparoscopic techniques for anterior spinal procedures are comparable in terms of the majority of the surgical indices assessed. Therefore, the use of a laparoscope or the BERG technique offers at this time no obvious advantage over a mini-open procedure in anterior lumbar spine surgery. What is evident is that the overall cost of laparoscopic spinal surgery is higher compared with conventional open procedures.

SUMMARY

The laparoscopic transperitoneal approach to the lumbar spine and the BERG method has been successfully applied in multiple centers. Each method has several clear benefits. There appears to be a faster recovery over open techniques, and some studies have demonstrated less blood loss. Nonetheless, it remains a very technically challenging procedure. There is a steep learning curve that must be maintained with surgical frequency. There also seems to be a higher incidence of operative complications. Recent studies comparing laparoscopic ALIF with a mini-open ALIF have concluded that the results of the two procedures are comparable. As compared with the laparoscopic ALIF method, the mini-open procedure has fewer complications and requires less time to master. It appears at this time that the mini-open laparotomy for the exposure of the anterior lumbar spine is the procedure of choice for an ALIF.

REFERENCES

1. Muhe E. Die erste cholecystektomie durch das laparoskop. Langenbeck's Arch Surg 1986; 369:804.
2. Obenchain TG. Laparoscopic lumbar discectomy: case report. J Laparoendosc Surg 1991; 1:145.
3. Cloyd DW, Obenchain TG, Savin M. Transperitoneal laparoscopic approach to lumbar discectomy. Surg Laparosc Endosc 1995; 5:85.
4. Zucherman JF, Zdeblick TA, Bailey SA, et al. Instrumented laparoscopic spinal fusion. Preliminary results. Spine 1995; 20:2029–2035.
5. Regan JJ, Yuan H, McAfee PC. Laparoscopic fusion of the lumbar spine: minimally invasive spine surgery. A prospective multicenter study evaluating open and laparoscopic lumbar fusion. Spine 1999; 24:402–411.

6.   Thalgott JS, Chin AK, Amerika JA, et al. Gasless endoscopic anterior lumbar interbody fusion utilizing the B.E.R.G. approach. Surg Endosc 2000; 14:546–552.
7.   McAfee PC, Reagan JJ, Geis WP, Fedder IL. Minimally invasive anterior retroperitoneal approach to the lumbar spine: emphasis on the lateral BAK. Spine 1998; 23:1476–1484.
8.   Zdeblick TA. Laparoscopic spinal fusion. Orthop Clin 1998; 29(4):635–645.
9.   Mathews HH, Long BH. The laparoscopic approach to the lumbosacral junction. In: Mayer HM, ed. Minimale Invasive Techniques in Spinal Surgery. Springer–Verlag: Springer, 2000:207–216.
10. Regan JJ, Guyer RD. Endoscopic techniques in spinal surgery. CORR 1997; 335:122–139.
11. Heniford BT, Matthews BD, Lieberman IH. Laparascopic lumbar interbody fusion. Surg Clin North Am 2000; 80(5):1487–1499.
12. Kent RB. Subcutaneous emphysema and hybercarbia following laparascopic cholecystectomy. Obstet Gynecol Surg 1975; 126:1154–1156.
13. Regan JJ, McAfee PC, Guyer RD, Aronoff RJ. Laparoscopic fusion of the lumbar spine in a multicenter series of the first 34 consecutive patients. Surg Laparosc Endosc 1996; 6(6):459–468.
14. Mahvi DM, Zdeblick TA. A prospective study of laparoscopic spinal fusion: technique and operative complications. Ann Surg 1996; 224:85.
15. Liu JC, Ondra SL, Angelos P, Ganju A, Landers ML. Is laparoscopic anterior lumbar interbody fusion a useful minimally invasive procedure? Neurosurgery 2002; 51(suppl 2):155–158.
16. Vazquez RM, Gireesan GT. Balloon-assisted endoscopic retroperitoneal gasless (BERG) technique for anterior lumbar interbody fusion (ALIF). Surg Endosc 2003; 17:268–272.
17. Zdeblick TA, David SM. A prospective comparison of surgical approach for anterior L4-L5 fusion: laparoscopic versus mini anterior lumbar interbody fusion. Spine 2000; 25(20):2682–2687.
18. Kaiser MG, Haid RW Jr., Subach BR, Miller JS, Smith CD, Rodts GE Jr. Comparison of the mini-open versus laparoscopic approach for anterior lumbar interbody fusion: a retrospective review. Neurosurgery 2002; 51(1):97–103.
19. Rodriguez HE, Connolly MM, Dracopoulos H, Geisler FH, Podbielski FJ. Anterior access to the lumbar spine: laparoscopic versus open. Am Surg 2002; 68(11):978–982.

23 | Minimally Invasive Anterior Lumbar Interbody Fusion Using the "Mini-Open" Technique

John M. Beiner
Department of Orthopedics, Yale University School of Medicine, New Haven, Connecticut, U.S.A.

Todd J. Albert
Department of Orthopedics, Thomas Jefferson University, Philadelphia, Pennsylvania, U.S.A.

INTRODUCTION

Lumbar fusion has become a commonly accepted method of treating a variety of disorders that require spinal stabilization to decrease pain from degenerative, traumatic, neoplastic, and infectious origins. The posterior approach to these disorders, however, has inherent drawbacks—extensive muscle stripping and limited access and visualization of the disc space, including possible suboptimal debridement or discectomy. In addition, the ability to restore the proper sagittal alignment is sometimes limited via the posterior approach, despite recent improvement in surgical techniques.

Anterior lumbar fusion was developed initially in the 1930s to treat tuberculosis and spondylolisthesis (1,2). The approach was either transperitoneal for lower lumbar levels or the flank retroperitoneal approach for upper lumbar levels. With time, the morbidity of incising the oblique musculature became apparent, and thus muscle-sparing retroperitoneal approaches were later developed (3,4). After the introduction of laparascopic techniques for gall bladder surgery in the late 1980s, endoscopic technology was adapted to approach the lumbar spine (5). As surgeons mastered the technique, laparoscopic anterior lumbar interbody fusion (ALIF) became much more common. In recent years, however, laparoscopic ALIF has been called into question. There appears to be no significant advantage compared with the more traditional open ALIF or the mini-open incision techniques as described in this chapter. In fact, some significant disadvantages with the laparoscopic procedure have been reported (6–9).

One of the first mini-open anterior approaches to the lumbar spine was described by Mayer in 1997 (10). It used a 4-cm incision with muscle-splitting techniques. It used the trans-peritoneal interval to approach the L5–S1 disc space and the retroperitoneal approach for the other lumbar segments. In the analysis of his results, Mayer found "negligible" postoperative wound pain. He concluded that the procedure was safe and effective, and reduced morbidity from the more traditional open approaches, without a long learning curve. A subsequent modification was described by DeWald et al. (11), using a 6- to 10-cm left lower quadrant transverse skin incision, with a Z-plasty of the fascia allowing extensile exposure of the lumbar spine. More modern techniques employ a variety of incisions, two of which will be described in this chapter.

INDICATIONS

The mini-open approach for ALIF should be considered for most nonobese patients in whom access to the anterior column is necessary. The most common diagnosis which brings surgeons to consider a mini-open ALIF is degenerative disc disease. Any anterior column instability, however, can produce symptoms of low back pain, referred pain into the pelvic girdle, and sometimes even "pseudoradicular" symptoms of pain into the posterior thighs. Depending on the diagnosis, most patients should be given a trial of extensive conservative management prior to the consideration for surgery. Spondylolisthesis (isthmic, degenerative, iatrogenic, or other) can be stabilized with either anterior or posterior fusion. Anterior fusion gives the advantage of a more thorough discectomy, better restoration of the lordotic sagittal alignment, and can obviate the need for posterior decompression via indirect neuroforaminal decompression (12). For anterior pathology, such as resistant discitis, fractures, and in some cases, herniated discs, the mini-open approach can offer the most direct means for debridement or discectomy.

In obese patients, the panus makes access to the front of the lumbar spine technically challenging, as the mini-open approach should be used with caution. Similarly, in patients with previous surgical procedures in the retroperitoneum, scarring can limit the surgeon's ability to mobilize the vascular structures. Although this was traditionally a contraindication to the anterior approach, the recent increase in the number of anterior lumbar procedures (in part due to the availability of interbody cage devices and total disc prostheses) has made it likely that this will be more of a relative than an absolute contraindication. In most cases, however, the mini-open approach should best be reserved for index cases, using a more extensile approach for the revision setting.

In patients in which multiple disc spaces are to be accessed (e.g., deformity), the mini-open approach may not be advisable. In particular, the Pfannensteil incision (see later) is not optimum for reaching discs above the L5–S1 level. The mini-open pararectus approach, however, can be extended to access discs from the L2–S1 levels if necessary.

CONSIDERATIONS FOR PREOPERATIVE PLANNING

Once the decision for ALIF has been made, patients should be screened by history and physical examination for body habitus, abdominal scars indicating prior surgery, and any nutritional depletion. Patients, regardless of their weight, should be encouraged to eat a healthy, balanced diet and to avoid dieting prior to any spinal surgery. Postoperative wound infections almost universally occur in malnourished patients (13), though the incidence is lower in anterior procedures.

Sagittal alignment should be specifically considered when planning a mini-open ALIF. In the setting of high-grade spondylolisthesis, for example, the angle of the disc space may preclude access via a mini-open incision or in some cases, via any anterior approach. In each case, the incision should be planned with the trajectory of the target disc space in mind (Fig. 1). This will avoid conversion to a more extensive incision. The position of the pubic symphysis relative to the L5–S1 interspace is particularly relevant.

Plain X rays, including flexion extension laterals, are beneficial in preoperative planning to uncover cases of dynamic spondylolisthesis, and for guiding the surgeon in terms of the overall approach to disc pathology. Entering a severely degenerative disc from the posterior approach can be quite challenging, and can be accomplished in some cases more easily via an anterior approach. Cross-sectional imaging via magnetic resonance imaging (MRI) or computed tomography (CT) gives information regarding neural compression. By restoring the normal disc space height, indirect decompression of the foramen, and in some cases, the central canal, can be accomplished. As the learning curve progresses, herniated disc material in the canal can be removed via the anterior approach. In general, however, the presence of significant radicular complaints in conjunction with the evidence of neural compression on MRI or CT warrants

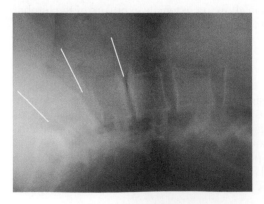

FIGURE 1   The trajectory of each disc space is different, and should be considered when placing the skin incision.

posterior decompression and might, in some cases, make the anterior approach superfluous (e.g., degenerative spondylolisthesis with stenosis).

The role of discography in evaluating low back pain is controversial, and beyond the scope of this chapter. Older literature has questioned the validity of the procedure, finding a high false-positive rate (14). More recently, however, Walsh indicated that false positives are distinctly rare (15). Carragee stresses that the psychologic makeup of the patient plays an important role in test interpretation (16,17). It remains, however, the only physiologic test for low back pain. At least one study has shown that the results of interbody fusion are improved in the subset of people with positive, concordant discograms at the surgical level, with negative injections at the other levels (18).

SURGICAL TECHNIQUE

The mini-open ALIF has been described using a variety of skin and fascial incisions, depending on the level of pathology, body habitus, gender, and surgeon preference. The two most common approaches—the pararectus approach and the Pfannensteil approach—will be described in the following sections. Other options include the midline vertical incision, transverse flank incision, and oblique flank incision used at the thoracolumbar area, which are less suited to the mini-open approach.

Pfannensteil Approach: L5–S1

For disc space pathology and access at the L5–S1 segment, the authors prefer to use a Pfannensteil incision. This can be hidden below the bikini line, just above the pubic symphysis, and allows the positioning of the surgical instruments at the best angle to enter a lordotic disc space at L5–S1.

Patients should be positioned supine on the operating table, with the lumbosacral junction at the break in the table, just over the kidney rest. Alternatively, or in conjunction, a half-moon gel roll can be placed under the lumbosacral junction. Each technique is used to hyperextend the disc space at the L5–S1 level, opening up anterior access (Fig. 2). The surgeon can stand on either side of the patient, or can stand between the abducted legs, allowing mid-line access, according to surgeon preference. Consideration should be given for preoperative or intraoperative administration of subcutaneous heparin to avoid deep vein thrombosis from vein retraction.

The skin should be shaved low into the pubic area to expose the pubic symphysis. The skin incision is placed transversely, approximately one-third of the distance between the symphysis and the umbilicus (Fig. 3). The inferior epigastric vessels are superolateral to the borders of this incision. The surgeon then encounters the anterior rectus sheath, and a transverse fascial incision is made of 4–5 cm in length, drawing the rectus muscle laterally away from the midline. The transversalis fascia is thicker here than above the arcuate line, and should also be incised transversely. The preperitoneal space is entered by bluntly dissecting the peritoneum superiorly. Alternatively, a transperitoneal approach may be used, though this carries a higher incidence of

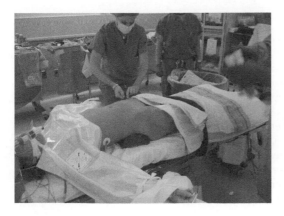

FIGURE 2   Supine positioning for a mini-open approach to the L5–S1 disc space.

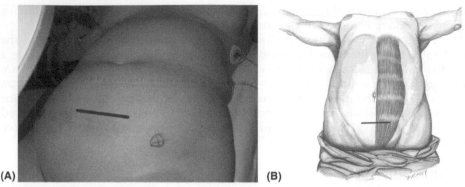

FIGURE 3 (A,B) Pfannensteil incision for access to the L5–S1disc space. *Source*: From Ref. 21.

complications, such as retrograde ejaculation and abdominal adhesions. The authors prefer to avoid the transperitoneal approach whenever possible.

The presacral fascia is then encountered enveloping the great vessels. The bifurcation is above the L5–S1 disc space, allowing a direct anterior approach to this disc. The middle sacral artery and vein should be ligated and transected to avoid traction on the iliac veins. Electrocautery should be minimized to avoid injury to the presacral plexus, which can result in retrograde ejaculation in males, or the so-called warm leg syndrome (loss of unilateral sympathetic tone resulting in hyperemia). Blunt dissection exposes the disc space to a wide extent. The authors prefer to use hand-held vessel retractors to ensure periodic release of the vessels, minimizing the risk of thrombi developing. Alternatively, some type of table-based retraction system is used.

The discectomy is then performed using scalpel, rongeurs, and curettes. The anterior, or the leading edge of the endplates, should be positively identified, particularly at S1, to avoid leaving the anterior aspect of the bone graft or cage proud or uncovered. Particular attention should be given to avoiding any anterior-directed force on the instruments to avoid "popping-out" of the disc space, with possible catastrophic injury to the great vessels. Side-to-side curettage, retaining the lateral-most extent of the annulus bilaterally, serves to protect against vessel injury. If a herniated disc is to be removed from the canal via this approach, the surgeon can consider a range of distraction instruments to facilitate visualization of the posterior disc space and ventral epidural space. Caution should prevail in this area, as repair of a dural tear in this area is difficult if not impossible. An analogous approach may be used in the case of disc replacement procedures, but a more meticulous bilateral lateral discectomy and exposure are necessary.

The surgeon can harvest autograft bone via a separate incision, or use one of the various bone graft substitutes to fill the center of the prosthesis. After insertion of the structural bone graft or cage, the wound is irrigated, and unless there is unexpected bleeding, a drain is usually not required. The closure of the incision begins with the anterior rectus sheath; the transversalis fascia can be closed, but is not necessary. Subcutaneous sutures and skin closure follow this.

Pararectus Approach: L4–L5 and Higher

Patients with pathology at the L4–L5 disc space or higher in the lumbar spine are positioned in the supine or semisupine position, depending on surgeon preference. Depending on body habitus, we prefer to use the half-moon gel roll under the lumbar spine. Following positioning, fluoroscopy can be used to localize the skin incision over the target disc, considering the angle of the disc and its closest overlying skin. A 4- to 6-cm vertical skin incision is made (Fig. 4), exposing the lateral border of the rectus sheath. The thick superficial fascia is incised and may be tagged for later closure. The posterior rectus fascia is then incised, entering the preperitoneal space, and blunt dissection used to peel away the peritoneum, allowing a retroperitoneal approach to the left side of the spine. The dissection is carried medial to the psoas muscle, lifting the ureter anterior and medial with the peritoneum. The left common iliac vein and artery are encountered. The iliolumbar vein (Fig. 5) should be recognized and ligated to allow mobilization of the iliac vessels toward the right side, exposing the disc space (Fig. 6). Table-based retractors may be inserted

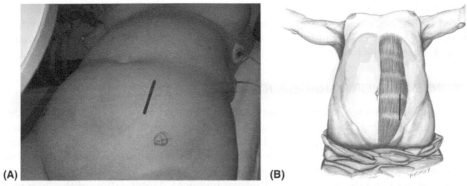

(A)   (B)

FIGURE 4 (**A,B**) Skin incision for the pararectus approach to the L4–L5 disc space. *Source*: From Ref. 21.

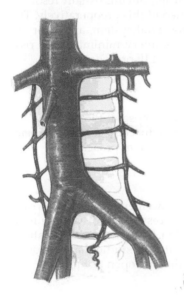

FIGURE 5 The iliolumbar vein constitutes a venous anastamosis between the iliac vessels, the lumbar radicular vessels, and the renal veins. It should be ligated and mobilized to gain access to the disc spaces above L5–S1. *Source*: From Ref. 21.

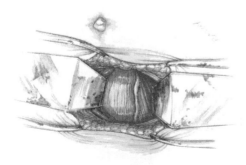

FIGURE 6 Dissection is carried medial to the psoas muscle, with the iliac vessels retracted medially, to allow access to the disc space. *Source*: From Ref. 21.

at this phase, or sharp Holman retractors may be anchored into the vertebral bodies above and below to provide exposure. The discectomy is now performed as described earlier. Most instrumentation companies supply structural allograft bone rings or cages which are machined to be inserted either from the straight anterior position or from an "anterolateral" position if exposure is difficult. Again, for disc replacement, meticulous bilateral exposure and discectomy is necessary to allow precise midline positioning of the prosthesis.

Closure is limited to the anterior rectus sheath, using a running, looped nonabsorbable suture, followed by subcutaneous sutures and a skin layer. A drain is usually not required, as blood loss is typically minimal. The authors use a lumbosacral orthosis for a period of six weeks to three months following the fusion.

COMPLICATIONS AND THEIR MANAGEMENT

Venous injury can be a catastrophic complication. Arterial injures may cause brisk bleeding but can be repaired after clamping the affected vessel. Venous injuries, by contrast, are much more difficult to repair and can necessitate grafting, bypass grafting, or ligation to control. Perhaps the most common pre-existing risk factor for venous injury is the presence of inflammation, such as in acute or chronic discitis. This may cause scarification with fusion of the posterior wall of the common iliac vein and the anterior longitudinal ligament. Mobilization of the ligament with the vein should be the approach in these cases.

Injury to the sympathetic trunk results in a warmer ipsilateral leg, but this usually resolves. Among other potential complications, patients should be informed of this preoperatively. The sympathetic hypogastric plexus provides innervation to the urogenital system, and injury to this can cause retrograde ejaculation. Avoiding the use of electrocautery minimizes the risk, with a reported complication rate of 0.42% in a series of 4500 open ALIF procedures (19).

OUTCOMES

Outcomes from the mini-open approach have been compared with those of the laparoscopic approach, with fewer complications (6–9,20). Decreased blood loss, reduced postoperative pain, and shorter hospital stay have been reported unlike the traditional open approach (6).

SUMMARY

The mini-open approach to the lumbar spine for ALIF and disc replacement procedures is safe, allowing full exposure of the neurovascular structures and full access to the disc space for a complete discectomy and interbody device placement and/or fusion. It has fewer complications than the laparoscopic equivalent, with a shorter learning curve. Outcome studies have reported shorter hospital stays and shorter overall recovery than with traditional open techniques.

Indications

- Discogenic low back pain
- Instability
- Inflammatory or infectious disease

Outcomes

- Fewer complications than laparoscopic approach
- Shorter hospital stays and reduced pain from open approach
- Faster relief of pain and return to work
- Avoids posterior muscle damage for intervertebral fusion

Complications

- Vascular injury
- Retrograde ejaculation
- Sympathetic chain injury—"warm leg syndrome"
- Ureter injury

REFERENCES

1. Capener N. Spondylolisthesis. Br J Surg 1932; 19:374–386.
2. Ito H, Tsuchiya J, Asami G. A new radical operation for Pott's disease. J Bone Jt Surg 1934; 16:499–515.

3. Allen BT, Bridwell KH. Paramedian approach to the anterior lumbar spine. In: Bridwell KH, DeWald RL, eds. The Textbook of Spinal Surgery. 2nd ed. Philadelphia: Lippincott-Raven, 1997:267–275.
4. Selby DK, Henderson RJ, Blumenthal S, Dossett D. Anterior lumbar fusion. In: White AH, Rothman RH, Ray CD, eds. Lumbar Spine Surgery: Techniques and Complications. St. Louis:C.V. Mosby Co., 1987.
5. Obenchain TG. Laparoscopic lumbar diskectomy: case report. J Laparoendosc Surg 1991; 1:145–149.
6. Liu JC, Ondra SL, Angelos P, et al. Is laparoscopic anterior lumbar interbody fusion a useful minimally invasive procedure? Neurosurgery 2002; 51(suppl. 2):155–158.
7. Kaiser MG, Haid RW, Subach BR, et al. Comparison of the mini-open versus laparoscopic approach for anterior lumbar interbody fusion: a retrospective review. Neurosurgery 2002; 51:97–105.
8. Zdeblick TA, David SM. A prospective comparison of surgical approach for anterior L4–L5 fusion; laparoscopic versus mini anterior lumbar interbody fusion. Spine 2000; 25:2682–2687.
9. Rodriquez HE, Connolly MM, Dracopoulos H, et al. Anterior access to the lumbar spine: laparoscopic versus open. Am Surg 2002; 11:978–983.
10. Mayer MH. A new microsurgical technique for minimally invasive anterior lumbar interbody fusion. Spine 1997; 15:691–699.
11. DeWald CJ, Millikan KW, Hammerberg KW, et al. An open, minimally invasive approach to the lumbar spine. Am Surg 1999; 1:61–68.
12. Lee SH, Choi WG, Lim SR, et al. Minimally invasive anterior lumbar interbody fusion followed by percutaneous pedicle screw fixation for isthmic spondylolisthesis. Spine J 2004; 4:644–649.
13. Beiner JM, Grauer JN, Kwon BK, Vaccaro AR. Postoperative wound infections of the spine. Neurosurg Focus 2003; 15:E14.
14. Holt E. The question of discography. J Bone Joint Surg [Am] 1967; 50:720–726.
15. Walsh T, Weinstein J, Spratt K, et al. Lumbar discography in normal subjects: a controlled prospective study. J Bone Joint Surg [Am] 1990; 72:1081–1088.
16. Carragee EJ, Tanner CM, Yang B, Brito JL, Truong T. False-positive findings on lumbar discography. Reliability of subjective concordance assessment during provocative disc injection. Spine 1999; 24:2542–2547.
17. Carragee EJ. Psychological and functional profiles in select subjects with low back pain. Spine J 2001; 1:198–204.
18. Derby R, Howard MW, Grant JM, et al. The ability of pressure-controlled discography to predict surgical and nonsurgical outcomes. Spine 1999; 24:364–371.
19. Flynn JC, Price CT. Sexual complications of anterior fusion of the lumbar spine. Spine 1984; 9:489–491.
20. Foley KT, Holly LT, Schwender JD. Minimally invasive lumbar fusion. Spine 2003; 28:S26–S35.
21. Albert TJ, Balderston MA, Northrup BE. Surgical Approaches to the Spine. W.B. Saunders Co., 1997.

24 | Percutaneous Lumbar Pedicle Screws

Daniel R. Fassett
Department of Neurosurgery, University of Utah, Salt Lake City, Utah, U.S.A.

Darrel S. Brodke
Department of Orthopedic Surgery, University of Utah, Salt Lake City, U.S.A.

INTRODUCTION

Lumbar pedicle screw fixation is a common procedure performed in spinal surgery. In traditional open approaches, extensive midline exposure extends above and below the instrumented levels allowing lateral retraction of the soft tissues to visualize the pedicle screw entry points at the intersection of the transverse process and facet complexes (Fig. 1). In addition, the open approach extends laterally to expose the transverse processes of the levels to be fused and requires wide retraction of the paraspinous muscles for extended periods of time. Extensile midline exposures can have significant morbidity, such as blood loss, wound infection, and denervation and atrophy of the paraspinal muscles. Possible advantages of percutaneous placement of pedicle screw include the reduction of these complications.

Magerl introduced percutaneous pedicle screw placement for external fixation of the spine in the treatment of fractures and osteomyelitis in 1977 (1). Indications for this procedure were expanded to include the so-called external fixation test, which was used to prognostically evaluate patients for possible arthrodesis for degenerative back pain (2–4). In 1995, Matthews and Long first used percutaneous pedicle screws connected by plates placed external to the dorsal muscular fascia (5). This construct acted as an internal fixation system; however, the long moment arms placed the instrumentation at a biomechanical disadvantage in comparison with traditional surgical pedicle screw systems. Since those early systems, percutaneous screw/rod systems have been developed that allow subfascial/submuscular placement of rods (6). Percutaneous pedicle screws, in combination with other minimally invasive spine procedures, have the potential benefits of less soft-tissue trauma, reduced blood loss, shorter hospital stays, and earlier return to work when compared with open procedures.

INDICATIONS

Percutaneous lumbar pedicle screws may be used to treat degenerative disc disease, spondylolisthesis, and spinal trauma. A number of different techniques have been developed, including transforaminal lumbar interbody fusion (TLIF), posterior lumbar interbody fusions (PLIF), and posterolateral fusion (PLf), utilizing small incisions and specialized retraction systems through a muscle-splitting approach (Fig. 1B,C) (7,8). Percutaneous pedicle screws are often used to augment such minimally invasive posterior fusions.

Percutaneous pedicle screws may also be used to supply additional stability to an anterior lumbar interbody fusion (ALIF) (Fig. 2). In the authors' experience, the most common indication for ALIF, combined with posterior percutaneous pedicle screw supplementation, has been low-grade (I and II) spondylolisthesis, though many other degenerative conditions may be treated in this manner (6,9). In addition to degenerative conditions, other potential indications for percutaneous lumbar pedicle screws include traumatic injuries or spinal tumors that have been treated via anterior reconstruction procedures.

As with all spinal procedures, careful patient selection is a key factor predicting success. Patients with rotational deformities or other deformities that obscure the anatomy of the pedicles on fluoroscopy are not the best candidates for this procedure. Other factors that can limit the quality of intraoperative fluoroscopy, such as obesity or osteopenia, should also be considered as relative contraindications to the insertion of percutaneous pedicle screws. Percutaneous

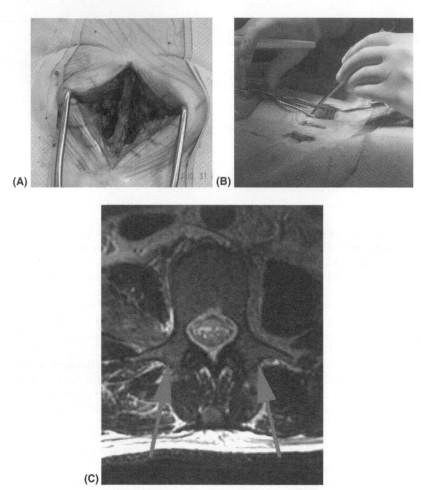

FIGURE 1 Comparison of open and minimally invasive (paramedian) incisions for single-level L4/L5 pedicle screw instrumentation. (**A**) Open approach for exposure for L4–L5 instrumentation requires a longer incision (8 cm) and significant retraction on paraspinous muscles to gain exposure laterally at the pedicle screw entry sites. (**B**) Small (2.5 cm) paramedian incisions allowing for percutaneous placement of pedicle screws and subfascial rod placement. (**C**) Axial magnetic resonance imaging image demonstrating the direct approach to pedicle with a paramedian approach as used in percutaneous pedicle screws.

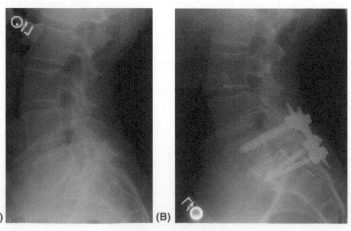

FIGURE 2 Preoperative (**A**) and postoperative (**B**) radiographs of a 42-year-old male with back pain and radiculopathy owing to L5–S1 spondylolisthesis, who was treated with mini-open anterior lumbar interbody fusion and posterior percutaneous pedicle screws.

pedicle screws are best limited to one- or two-level fusions. More extensive procedures are probably better performed through open techniques.

CONSIDERATIONS FOR PREOPERATIVE PLANNING
Preoperative Physical Examination

It is important to evaluate the spinal contour for abnormalities in alignment and to observe the patient's body habitus when considering percutaneous lumbar pedicle screws. As in all spinal procedures, a thorough neurologic examination is required preoperatively.

Imaging

We recommend preoperative computed tomography (CT) imaging with reconstructed images in the sagittal and coronal planes to assess the diameter and angles of the pedicles. Image guidance systems might help with the placement of percutaneous screws, and preoperative thin-cut CT images may be preloaded into these guidance systems. We also recommend plain anteroposterior (AP) and lateral radiographs to help assess whether intraoperative fluoroscopic visualization may be difficult. If there is any difficulty appreciating the respective pedicles on plain radiographs, an open procedure should be considered.

SURGICAL TECHNIQUE
Operating Room Setup

A radiolucent table and fluoroscopy are recommended for percutaneous placement of pedicle screws. After the patient is positioned prone on a radiolucent table with padding of pressure points, the fluoroscopes should be positioned. We recommend placing the fluoroscopic monitors in a position that is easily viewed by the primary surgeon, usually at the head or foot of the bed contralateral to the primary surgeon. This allows the primary surgeon to maintain a comfortable body posture and directly view the fluoroscopic monitor throughout the procedure. It can also be beneficial to have another monitor on the other side of the room in view of the assisting surgeon and technicians.

Operative Approach/Relevant Anatomy

In the upper lumbar spine, the pedicles are oval, with a greater height than transverse diameter, making the transverse diameter the limiting feature in determining the appropriate pedicle screw diameter. In the lower lumbar spine, the pedicles are larger and more round, with relatively equal transverse and vertical diameters. The transverse (medial) angulation of the pedicles increases from approximately 10° at L1 to 30° at L5. Sagittal angulation of the pedicles changes subtly from approximately 2° caudally cephalad angulation at L1 to 5° caudally at L5 (Table 1) (10–12).

The starting point for open (and percutaneous) pedicle screws in the lumbar spine is close to the junction of the transverse process and the facet complex. A line bisecting the transverse processes and a line at the lateral margin of the superior articular process is a good starting point throughout the lumbar spine. Small adjustments are usually made with a slightly more cephalad entry point in the upper lumbar spine and a slightly lower entry point in the lower

TABLE 1 Anatomic Characteristics of the Lumbar Pedicle

Level	Mean transverse diameter (millimeters)	Mean medial angulation (degrees)	Mean sagittal (caudal) angulation (degrees)
L1	8.0	14.5	2.6
L2	7.8	14.2	2.7
L3	10.2	18.5	2.7
L4	13.4	16.6	3.9
L5	18.0	24.6	5.5

Source: From Ref. 12.

lumbar spine (11). Although these anatomic landmarks will not be directly visualized when placing percutaneous screws, they may be appreciated with fluoroscopy and palpation with the pedicle-probing needle. Obviously, experience in the open placement of lumbar pedicle screws helps significantly with the percutaneous placement of these screws.

Description of Procedure

Fluoroscopy in the lateral view is used to confirm the level of surgery, and the cephalad–caudal levels of the respective pedicles are marked on the patient's back with a marking pen. A perfect AP fluoroscopic image is used next to confirm both the superior and the lateral margins of the pedicles. With the minimal angulation of the pedicles in the upper lumbar spine, the intersection of these two lines (cephalad and lateral margin of pedicle) represents the entry point at the skin (usually 2–3 cm off midline) to access the pedicle. In the lower lumbar spine, where the medial angulation of the pedicles is greater, a more lateral skin opening is optimal to gain the correct medial angulation through the pedicle (Fig. 3).

A 1-cm vertical incision is made through the skin and dorsal fascia centered on the location of the pedicle based on fluoroscopy. A spinal-access (e.g., Jamshidi) needle, a cannulated needle similar to a biopsy needle used in transpedicular biopsies, is placed through this stab incision and slowly directed toward the entry point for the pedicle. It is recommended that this needle be advanced under direct lateral fluoroscopic visualization as the surgeon is gaining experience with this technique to avoid interlaminar placement with possible dural violation and cord injury. On the lateral view, the cephalad–caudal angulation of the spinal-access needle can be adjusted for appropriate trajectory through the pedicle. Tactile feedback should allow the surgeon to determine when the spinal-access needle is on bone. Once the needle is docked on bone, fluoroscopy is adjusted to an AP image to determine the medial–lateral relationship of the spinal-access needle with the pedicle. We recommend adjusting the spinal-access needle to a point on the lateral margin of the pedicle to reduce the risk for medial pedicle breakout and allow for maximal medial angulation of the pedicle screws into the vertebral body to reduce the risk of lateral screw breakout from the vertebral body (Fig. 4).

Using a gentle twisting motion, the spinal access needle is slowly advanced through the dense cortical bone. As the needle advances and enters the cancellous bone, the resistance decreases significantly. At this point, AP and lateral fluoroscopy images are obtained to confirm appropriate trajectory through the pedicle. Adjustments in starting point and trajectory are made if needed. Once the trajectory is optimized, the spinal-access needle is slowly advanced through the pedicle with a gentle twisting motion similar to that of the pedicle finder in open placement of pedicle screws. Lateral fluoroscopy is used to monitor the passage of the

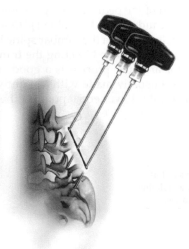

FIGURE 3 The skin entry points for percutaneous pedicle screws in the lumbar spine are typically 2.0 to 3.5 cm off midline. In the lower lumbar spine, the skin entry is more lateral to accommodate for increased medial angulation of the lower lumbar pedicles.

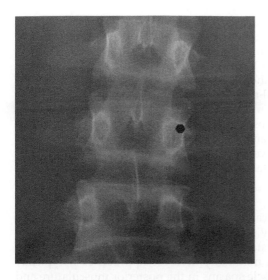

FIGURE 4 Target point for pedicle entry (*black circle*) is at the superior lateral border of the pedicle on a perfect antero-posterior image.

spinal-access needle through the pedicle and into the vertebral body. Sudden changes in resistance (plunging) likely signals a breakout, and the location of the instrument should be investigated fluoroscopically. Repetitive problems with pedicle breakout warrant close investigation and possible conversion to an open procedure.

Once the spinal-access needle is at an appropriate depth in the vertebral body (just past the posterior wall of the vertebra), a K-wire is placed through the spinal-access needle into the vertebral body. A lateral fluoroscopic image is obtained to confirm that the K-wire exits the tip of the spinal-access needle. The K-wire should be placed with care not to penetrate too deeply as the anterior cortex could be perforated and great vessel injury can occur (Fig. 5A).

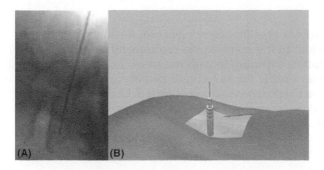

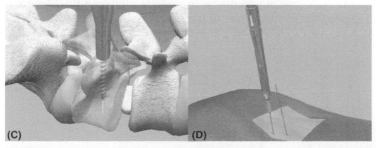

FIGURE 5 Percutaneous pedicle screws are placed with a series of short steps with the aid of anteroposterior and lateral fluoroscopy. A spinal-access needle is slowly advanced through the pedicle under direct fluoroscopic visualization and (**A**) a K-wire is left in place. (**B**) Soft tissues around the K-wire are dilated to prepare the soft tissues for cannulated instruments and cannulated pedicle screws. (**C**) A cannulated tap is placed over the K-wire and advanced through the pedicle to prepare the pedicle for screw. (**D**) Cannulated pedicle screws are placed over the K-wire and advanced through the pedicle into the vertebral body. *Source*: VIPER™ percutaneous pedicle screw system, Depuy Spine, Inc., Raynham, Massachusetts.

After the K-wire is placed, the spinal-access needle is removed, without moving the K-wire. A series of dilators are then placed over the K-wire to dilate the posterior musculature and soft tissues to provide a space for the insertion of tap and screw over the K-wire (Fig. 5B). The final dilators are typically left in place and a tap is placed over the K-wire and through the final dilator (Fig. 5C). We recommend tapping the pedicle with a tap 0.5-mm smaller than the anticipated screw diameter (e.g., 4.5-mm tap for 5.0-mm screw) to improve screw purchase in the pedicle. After tapping, the tap is removed without moving the K-wire, and a cannulated-pedicle screw is placed over the K-wire and screwed into position (Fig. 5D). Care should be exercised not to advance the K-wire when placing instruments and the screw. Once all the screws are placed for a respective hardware construct, the rods between the screws are placed. The technique of rod insertion varies with the respective instrumentation manufacturer (Fig. 6).

Closure and Postoperative Management

The incisions for these procedures are small and can typically be closed with Vicryl sutures in the fascia and subcutaneous layers, followed by strip bandages or skin adhesive. Activity restrictions relate to adequacy of fixation, general stability, and comorbidities, but generally, we encourage early mobilization. Pain control with minimally invasive approaches is typically easier. Some patients may experience painful muscle spasms in the posterior musculature and benefit from muscle relaxants in the postoperative course.

MANAGEMENT OF COMPLICATIONS
Pitfalls

Experience and good fluoroscopic technique are both extremely important to perform this procedure safely. We advocate performing this procedure multiple times on cadavers to gain experience. It is of utmost importance that the best fluoroscopic images be obtained. Perfect lateral and AP images are needed to place lumbar pedicle screws safely. Spending extra time to eliminate obliquity on the fluoroscopic images is justified.

Bailouts

If the surgeon is concerned over landmarks or possible screw breakout, the threshold for conversion to an open procedure should be low. In this scenario, we recommend closing the small paraspinous incisions and opening a midline exposure to gain the access needed to visualize the pertinent anatomy. Laminotomies may enable the surgeon to palpate and appreciate the location of the pedicle and determine if medial pedicle violation occurred. Lamina or transverse process hooks can be used if adequate pedicle screw fixation cannot be obtained, and additional levels of fixation may also be considered.

OUTCOMES

Limited data are available regarding the use of percutaneous pedicle screws in the literature. In 2002, Foley and Gupta (6) reported the results of one of the first percutaneous pedicle screw

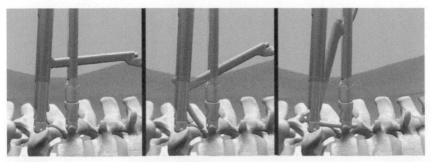

FIGURE 6 Subfascial pedicle screw rod insertion techniques can vary with the instrumentation manufacturer. *Source*: VIPER™, Depuy Spine, Inc., Raynham, Massachusetts.

systems to use a subfascial rod placement for stabilization. Most of their patients (10 of 12 patients) had the screws placed to supplement a mini-open ALIF procedure, with spondylolisthesis being the most common indication (10 of 12 patients). Good or excellent results were reported in 91% of patients, and 50% of patients were discharged on postoperative day 1 or 2.

In 2004, Lee et al. (9) reported similar results using a combination of a mini-ALIF with percutaneous pedicle screw instrumentation to treat low-grade spondylolisthesis. They reported good or excellent results in 95% (69/73) of patients and a 97% fusion rate. Although, only standard fluoroscopic imaging was used to assist with placement, only 6 of 146 (4%) pedicle screws were found to be misplaced. One patient experienced transient thigh numbness. No patients required a return to the operating room for hardware modifications.

The results of percutaneous pedicle screw instrumentation in combination with minimally invasive PLIF and TLIF procedures are limited. Khoo et al. (8) reported successful use of percutaneous pedicle screws with mini-PLIF to treat radiculopathy occurring in combination with mechanical low-back pain from single-level lumbar spondylosis in three patients. Schwender et al. (7) reported the results of a larger series of 47 patients who underwent percutaneous pedicle screw fixation as a part of a mini-TLIF procedure. The mean estimated blood loss was 140 mL and the mean hospital stay for this procedure was 1.9 days. Radiographic fusion was reported in all patients at the last follow-up. The mean score on the visual analogue pain scale was reduced from 7.2 preoperatively to 2.1 at final follow up; Oswestry disability index scores decreased from 46 preoperatively to 14 at final follow-up. Two cases required hardware revision for malposition of percutaneous pedicle screws.

SUMMARY

The popularity of minimally invasive spinal arthrodesis procedures is growing, and percutaneous pedicle screws are often used to minimize soft-tissue trauma. Given the relatively common frequency of lumbar spine degenerative conditions, the potential for the use of these procedures is sizable, especially in combination with ALIF, TLIF, or PLIF procedures, performed with minimally invasive techniques. Clinical studies have been limited to a few small retrospective series, but the results are encouraging for the ability to achieve a solid fusion, reduce hospital stays, and producing good clinical results.

REFERENCES

1. Magerl FP. Stabilization of the lower thoracic and lumbar spine with external skeletal fixation. Clin Orthop Relat Res 1984; 189:125–141.
2. Wiltse LL. A review of "stabilization of the lower thoracic and lumbar spine with external skeletal fixation" by Friedrich P. Magerl, M.D. Clini Orthop Relat Res 1984; 203:63–66.
3. Olerud S, Sjostrom L, Karlstrom G, Hamberg M. Spontaneous effect of increased stability of the lower lumbar spine in cases of severe chronic back pain. The answer of an external transpeduncular fixation test. Clin Orthop Relat Res 1986; 203:67–74.
4. Esses SI, Botsford DJ, Kostuik JP. The role of external spinal skeletal fixation in the assessment of low-back disorders. Spine 1989; 14(6):594–601.
5. Mathews H, Long B. Endoscopy assisted percutaneous anterior interbody fusion with subcutaneous suprafascial internal fixation: evolution, techniques, and surgical considerations. Orthop Int Ed 1995; 3:496–500.
6. Foley KT, Gupta SK. Percutaneous pedicle screw fixation of the lumbar spine: preliminary clinical results. J Neurosurg 2002; 97(1 suppl):7–12.
7. Schwender JD, Holly LT, Rouben DP, Foley KT. Minimally invasive transforaminal lumbar interbody fusion (TLIF): technical feasibility and initial results. J Spinal Disord Tech 2005; 18(suppl):S1–6.
8. Khoo LT. Minimally invasive percutaneous posterior lumbar interbody fusion. Neurosurgery 2002; 51(5 suppl):S166–1.
9. Lee SH, Choi WG, Lim SR. Minimally invasive anterior lumbar interbody fusion followed by percutaneous pedicle screw fixation for isthmic spondylolisthesis. Spine J 2004; 4(6):644–649.
10. Ebraheim NA, Rouins JR, Xu R, Yeasting RA. Projection of the lumbar pedicle and its morphometric analysis. Spine 1996; 21(11):1296–1300.
11. Weinstein JN, Rydevik BL, Rauschning W. Anatomic and technical considerations of pedicle screw fixation. Clin Orthop Relat Res 1992; 284:34–46.
12. Panjabi MM, Goel V, Oxland T, et al. Human lumbar vertebrae. Quantitative three-dimensional anatomy. Spine 1992; 17(3):299–306.

25 | Minimally Invasive Transforaminal Lumbar Interbody Fusion

Frank M. Phillips
Department of Orthopedic Surgery, Rush Medical Center, Chicago, Illinois, U.S.A.

Sameer Mather
Department of Orthopedic Surgery, University of North Carolina–Chapel Hill, Chapel Hill, North Carolina, U.S.A.

INTRODUCTION

Lumbar arthrodesis is a commonly performed surgical procedure for the treatment of spondylosis, trauma, infection, neoplasm, and spinal instability. A posterolateral fusion with autologous on-lay bone graft has traditionally resulted in acceptable clinical results; however, reported fusion rates have been inconsistent. With the addition of internal fixation using pedicle screw instrumentation, fusion rates have improved significantly, especially in cases of instability (1,2). Performing an interbody arthrodesis may further improve the clinical results by eliminating the disc as a potential pain generator, improving fusion rates, and restoring intervertebral height and lumbar lordosis (3–8). Techniques to achieve anterior column interbody fusion include anterior lumbar interbody fusion (ALIF), posterior lumbar interbody fusion (PLIF), or transforaminal lumbar interbody fusion (TLIF).

Over the last decade, TLIF has become a popular technique for achieving interbody fusion. The TLIF approach may reduce the risk of iatrogenic neurologic injury when compared with PLIF; provide a circumferential arthrodesis; and avoid anterior spinal exposure and its associated complications (9–14). Lowe et al. reported on 40 patients who underwent a TLIF and demonstrated that 85% of the patients had excellent or good results in terms of pain relief, return to work, and improvement in the daily activities (15,16). Similarly, Potter and Salehi concluded that TLIF is a safe and effective method of achieving lumbar fusion with a nearly 80% rate of patient satisfaction (17,18). Hackenberg et al. prospectively reviewed 52 patients who underwent an open TLIF with a three-year follow up. Patients had a significant decrease in the Visual Analog Scale (VAS) and the Oswestry Disability Index with an 89% fusion rate (6).

With advances in minimal access technology, TLIF can now be performed through a minimally invasive, unilateral approach, providing an adequate decompression and circumferential fusion, and avoid many of the disadvantages of the traditional posterior open approach (19,20).

ADVANTAGES OF MINIMAL-ACCESS TRANSFORAMINAL LUMBAR INTERBODY FUSION

Traditional open posterior approaches to the lumbar spine provide access to the posterior spinal structures, including the lamina, facet joints, transverse processes, and also to the intervertebral disc space. The posterior midline spinal exposure typically requires the paraspinal muscles to be separated from the bony spinal structures using a subperiosteal dissection technique. The dissection is carried over the facet joints and laterally to the tips of the transverse processes when concomitant posterolateral arthrodesis is required. Although providing wide access to the spine, the posterior approach is shown to result in significant paraspinal muscle injury that may be responsible for immediate postoperative morbidity and compromising the long-term surgical outcome. Kawaguchi demonstrated that the duration of muscle retraction during spinal surgery, pressure of the retractors, and the number of levels exposed, directly correlate with the postoperative elevation of serum creatinine phosphokinase isoenzymes, a marker of muscle injury (21). In a follow-up study, the authors demonstrated that muscle retractors increase the intrinsic paraspinal muscle pressure impeding local blood flow. As a direct result, the muscles showed extensive necrosis histologically (22,23).

Gejo obtained postoperative lumbar magnetic resonance images (MRIs) and measured the trunk muscle strength in 80 patients who previously had lumbar surgery. They concluded that the damage to the lumbar musculature was directly related to the duration of retraction. Furthermore, the incidence of low back pain was significantly increased in patients who had long surgical retraction times (24). Mayer studied the trunk muscle strength in patients who had lumbar spine surgery, concluding that muscles were weaker after open fusion procedures compared with discectomies (25). A postoperative electromyograph (EMG) study performed in patients following laminectomy revealed EMG abnormalities in the paraspinal muscles at multiple vertebral levels and at distances 1 and 3 cm from the midline (26).

EVOLUTION OF MINIMAL-ACCESS TRANSFORAMINAL LUMBAR INTERBODY FUSION

Minimal-access surgery has indeed become the standard of care for many surgical procedures. Today, open knee arthrotomy or cholecystectomy are rarely performed and have been surpassed by their minimally invasive counterparts. In the spine, the principal rationale for the development of minimally invasive approaches is to reduce the paraspinal muscle injury associated with traditional techniques. Recently, minimally invasive spinal systems have been developed based on the principle of using a series of dilators of different lengths to create a path between muscle fascicles to access the posterior spinal elements (27–30). This approach avoids stripping the paraspinal muscles and retains the midline ligamentous structures. A working channel is created through which spinal decompression and fusion can be accomplished. Most of the commercially available minimal access systems use this blueprint for access to the spine. Initial surgeries using these access portals involved simple decompressive procedures; however, over the last decade, these systems have been expanded to facilitate interbody and posterolateral arthrodesis in addition to the placement of pedicle screws in a less invasive fashion (31–33).

INDICATIONS AND CONTRAINDICATIONS

The indications for a minimally invasive TLIF do not differ from those for conventional open TLIF (Table 1) (25,34,35). In a number of situations, the minimally invasive TLIF provides an advantage over its open counterpart, especially in obese patients where the minimally invasive TLIF can be achieved via a small incision using a long tubular retractor. Minimal-access TLIF can also be performed in revision cases. When performing minimal-access TLIF after prior lumbar surgery, special care must be taken to clearly visualize bony and neural anatomy, and carefully dissect the scar tissue. The more lateral TLIF approach to the disc space avoids much of the midline scarring and may allow easier access to the disc space. The technical challenges associated with performing TLIF via a minimally invasive approach should mandate that the surgeon's technical expertise allow for accomplishing the surgery without compromising with the patient's safety or the ultimate result (12,13,36,37).

TABLE 1   Indications for Minimally Invasive Transforaminal Lumbar Interbody Fusion

Spondylolisthesis (grades I or II)
Degenerative disc disease causing discogenic low back pain
Recurrent lumbar disc herniation with significant mechanical back pain
Postdiscectomy collapse with neural foraminal stenosis and radiculopathy
Treatment of pseudoarthrosis
Treatment of postlaminectomy kyphosis
Treatment of lumbar deformity with coronal and/or sagittal imbalance

PREOPERATIVE PLANNING

Preoperative work up is geared toward ensuring that the patient is an appropriate mini-TLIF candidate. It is important to determine whether the patient has predominant axial back pain, radiculopathy, or a combination of symptoms. If neurogenic symptoms are present, the surgeon may perform a decompression of the involved neural structures at the time of TLIF surgery. A history of prior lumbar surgery is important as this may add to the difficulties of performing mini-TLIF. If there is concern for secondary gain, disproportionate pain behaviors, or symptom magnification, these issues should also be explored.

Imaging

Anteroposterior (AP) and lateral radiographs of the lumbar spine allow the evaluation of disc space geometry and height, osteophytes, and spinal alignment. In addition, flexion and extension views of the spine may be obtained to detect spinal instability (38,39).

The advent of MRI has greatly increased the sensitivity of imaging degenerative disc levels. Degenerative disc disease, characterized by a loss of signal intensity on T2 weighted sequences, is considered to be a possible source of back pain. In addition to demonstrating dark discs on T2-weighted images, MRI can demonstrate annular tears as evidenced by high-intensity zone (HIZ) and also modic end-plate changes (40). Magnetic resonance imaging would also allow for the visualization of the detailed neural anatomy. In patients who have had prior lumbar surgery, gadolinium-enhanced MRI is used to differentiate the scar tissue from the disc material or other anatomic structures causing neural compression. Lumbar discography remains controversial but is considered a useful test to assist in the diagnosis of discogenic pain (41).

SURGICAL TECHNIQUE
Anesthesia

General anesthesia is typically used for TLIF. However, when nerve monitoring is being performed, paralytic agents, muscle relaxants, or nitrous oxide, should be avoided, as these agents impede the direct monitoring of nerve-root stimulation. The authors routinely use EMG testing to confirm proper pedicle screw placement and believe this to be essential when the pedicle screws are placed percutaneously.

Positioning

The patient is placed prone on a Jackson table, which allows for easy multiplanar fluoroscopy. The elbows are placed at 90° to decrease traction on the brachial plexus. Pads are placed under the ulnar and peroneal nerves. In addition, pillows are placed under the lower extremities. Thromboembolic hose stockings and sequential compression devices (SCD) are placed on the lower extremities to reduce the incidence of deep vein thrombosis. Prior to starting the case, ensure that the Foley catheter is mobile; endotracheal tube is secure; and the fluoroscopic machine is draped into the operative field.

Surgical Procedure

After appropriate positioning, the skin is prepped with antiseptic paint. Under fluoroscopic imaging, a guide pin is advanced onto the ipsilateral facet joint at a trajectory parallel to the disc space. A paramedian incision is made around the guide pin and lateral to the facet joint to allow for medial direction of instruments in the disc space. The incision is then carried through the skin, soft tissue, and dorsal lumbar fascia. Under fluoroscopic guidance, serial dilators are placed docking on the facet joint and spreading the muscle fascicles. Once the largest dilator has been placed, a tubular retractor is placed over the dilator and locked in the correct position. The dilators are then removed. With certain systems, the final retractor is a fixed tube, whereas other systems have a split blade tubular retractor that can be expanded. The appropriate position of the retractor is on the facet joint and angled with a trajectory parallel to the intervertebral disc. Subsequently, loupe or microscope magnification can be used.

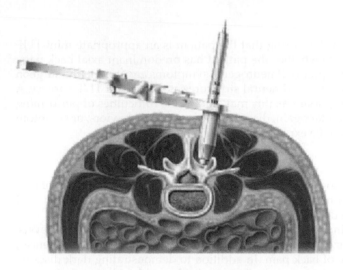

FIGURE 1 Serial dilators are advanced using a muscle-splitting approach and are docked on the facet joint. The working cannula is then positioned. *Source*: Courtesy of Nuvasive Inc.

The next step in the procedure is performing the facetectomy. The soft tissue over the facet is removed with a bovie cautery and rongeurs. The facet–lamina junction is delineated using curettes. Using an angled curette, the space between the lamina and the ligamentum flavum is defined. Using the Kerrison rongeur, the lamino–facet junction is removed. If there is no stenosis, then a small laminotomy can be done to allow the visualization of the neural elements in close proximity to the facet joint. If the patient has stenosis on the ipsilateral side, a complete laminectomy should be performed. In cases of bilateral stenosis, the spinous process can be undercut and a contralateral laminectomy and facetectomy accomplished. If stenosis is severe or there is a significant foraminal component on the contralateral side, we suggest direct decompression. Using a combination of Kerrison rongeurs and osteotomes, the facet joint is removed. The fragments of bone should be saved for autologous bone grafting. A burr may be used to remove the facet joint but this decreases the quantity of bone graft.

The next step involves identifying the disc space. If the laminectomy was already performed, dura and the nerve root are identified. If a laminectomy has not been done, remove the ligamentum flavum to expose the lateral edge of the dura and nerve root. In general, the traversing root is medial to the foramen and minimal if any retraction is required. The exiting nerve roots hug the pedicle as it exits the neural foramen and is generally cephalad to the level of the disc in the foramen. Although we do not necessarily dissect out the exiting root, it may be protected by placing a patty directed toward the cephalad pedicle in the foramen.

The annulus is incised with a long-handle blade directing the knife blade away from the nerve root and dura. A pituitary rongeur is used to initiate the discectomy. Subsequently, a series of curettes and disc shavers are used to loosen and remove the remainder of the disc from

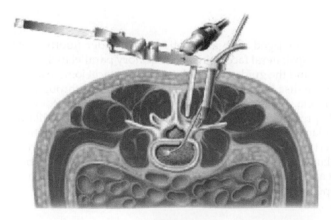

FIGURE 2 After performing facetectomy, a subtotal discectomy is performed. *Source*: Courtesy of Nuvasive Inc.

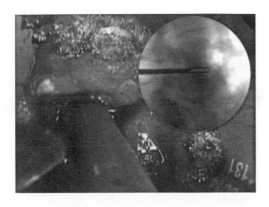

FIGURE 3 Disc cutters are placed into the disc space lateral to the thecal sac under lateral fluoroscopic guidance, and are used to facilitate thorough discectomy. *Source*: Courtesy of Nuvasive Inc.

the endplates. Under lateral fluoroscopy, a distractor and sizer are placed into the disc space. An end-plate scraper is utilized to complete the disc-space preparation. A chisel can be used to remove osteophytes from the posterior vertebral body cortex that can impede the placement of the interbody device. Care must be taken to place the chisel parallel to the superior and inferior endplates preventing damage to the vertebral body.

The appropriate size trial interbody cage is then placed into the disc space. After confirming proper placement on fluoroscopy, the trial is removed. The disc space is irrigated copiously and any fragment of bone and cartilage is removed. Bone graft is then packed into the anterior disc space. When bone morphogenic protein is used, we recommend placing this anterior to the interbody device to prevent posterior bony overgrowth toward the neural foramen. The interbody structural device is then advanced into the disc space under fluoroscopy. An AP and lateral fluoroscopic X-ray is used to verify appropriate implant positioning. If a concomitant intertransverse process arthrodesis is being performed, the transverse processes are decorticated using a burr until there is a bleeding bed and bone graft placed between the transverse processes (42).

Focus is now turned to placing percutaneous pedicle screws (discussed elsewhere in this book in more detail). In most cases, pedicle screws on the ipsilateral side are placed via the same retractor used for performing the TLIF. This usually requires a combination of direct visualization of bony landmarks and fluoroscopy. On the contralateral side to the TLIF, pedicle screws and rod may be placed percutaneously or via a second expandable retractor. During pedicle cannulation, tapping and placement of pedicle screws and dynamic EMG monitoring is performed. A static EMG is done after the placement of the pedicle screw at each level.

After the placement of the pedicle screw construct, the lumbosacral fascia is closed with an interrupted number one absorbable suture. The subcutaneous layer is closed with interrupted 2.0 absorbable suture, and the subcuticular skin is approximated with a running 3.0 monofilament stitch. Marcaine (0.5%) is injected into the subcutaneous layer for local analgesia. Steri-strips are placed and a sterile dressing is applied. No drains are placed (12).

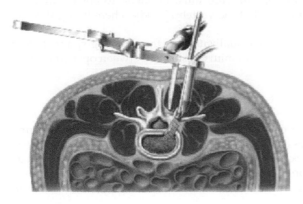

FIGURE 4 Placement of the interbody device. *Source*: Courtesy of Nuvasive Inc.

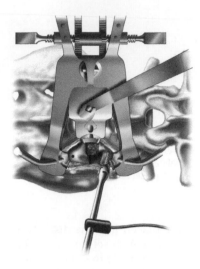

FIGURE 5 Placement of ipsilateral pedicle screws down the split-blade retractor with live dynamic electromyograph monitoring. *Source:* Courtesy of Nuvasive Inc.

POSTOPERATIVE CARE

The patient is mobilized into a chair on the night of surgery. On postoperative day 1, the Foley catheter is removed and the patient is converted to oral pain medication. The patient is typically discharged by postoperative day 2.

COMPLICATIONS AND MANAGEMENT

Although offering certain advantages, minimally invasive lumbar spine surgery has several limitations and potential complications. There is a learning curve associated with the development of technical skills necessary to perform this procedure. In contrast to open procedures, minimally invasive exposures are limited to the area of surgical interest with a narrow field of view so that an appreciation of the underlying three-dimensional spinal anatomy is mandatory. Surgeons must become adept using longer instruments that are bayoneted. In addition, intraoperative fluoroscopic imaging is frequently utilized (3,8,43). The ability to translate a two-dimensional radiographic image to three-dimensional anatomy can be challenging.

With the limited access intrinsic to minimally invasive surgery (MIS) approaches, the management of complications is more challenging. Inadvertent durotomy may occur and direct suture repair can be quite challenging down a tubular retractor. Dural sealants, such as Duragen and Tisseal, may be used when direct repair is impossible (30,32,33).

Percutaneous pedicle screw placement has been shown to be safe, with similar risks of misplacement to those reported for open-screw placement (5,44,45). The authors feel that EMG monitoring of the screws should further reduce the risks of neural injury.

During percutaneous pedicle screw placement, care must be taken to ensure that the K-wire does not advance through the anterior wall of the vertebral body where it might cause vascular or visceral injury.

Nerve-root injury can be avoided by direct visualization of the working space during interbody fusion. The reported incidence of nerve-root injury is similar between open and minimally invasive TLIF procedures (18,27).

OUTCOMES

There are no studies that directly compare minimally invasive TLIF with an open procedure. However, there are two retrospective studies analyzing the clinical outcomes and complications associated with minimally invasive TLIF. Schwender et al. reviewed 49 patients who underwent a minimally invasive TLIF with 18-month follow up (46). Patients had significant improvements in the VAS and Oswestry disability index. All patients had radiographic evidence of fusion, and there were two complications. The first was a malpositioned screw that was revised, and the second complication was new onset of radiculopathy postoperatively. Salerni et al. reviewed 13 patients who underwent a minimal-access TLIF and reported 11 excellent or good outcomes at one year using the McNab criteria. There were two complications related to the insertion of the interbody device (37).

CONCLUSION

The future of minimal-access surgery appears quite bright with the constant evolution of technology. A number of commonly performed open lumbar procedures, including TLIF, can now be effectively performed via a minimal-access approach. The early results demonstrate safety and efficacy. The preservation of the spinal musculature and midline ligaments may translate into shorter hospital stay, decrease in postoperative pain and narcotic use, and earlier mobilization.

Despite the early encouraging clinical results, it must be remembered that minimally invasive lumbar fusion techniques are in their infancy and the results are preliminary at best. There is a learning curve, and the development of technical skills requires time. Prospectively conducted outcome studies with long-term follow up will be the ultimate determinants of the safety and effectiveness of minimal-access lumbar fusion (27,47).

REFERENCES

1. Thomsen K, Christensen R. 1997 Volvo Award winner in clinical studies. The effect of pedicle screw instrumentation on functional outcome and fusion rates in posterolateral lumbar spinal fusion: a prospective, randomized clinical study. Spine 1997; 22(24):2813–2822.
2. Dickman C, Fessler RG, MacMillan M. Transpedicular screw-rod fixation of the lumbar spine: operative technique and outcome in 104 cases. J Neurosurg 1992; 77:860–870.
3. Brislin B, Vaccaro AR. Advances in posterior lumbar interbody fusion. Orthop Clin North Am 2002; 33(2):367–374.
4. Dewald CJ, Millikan, KW. An open, minimally invasive approach to the lumbar spine. Am Surg 1999; 65(1):61–68.
5. Figueiredo N, Martins JW. TLIF—transforaminal lumbar interbody fusion. Arq Neuropsiquiatr 2004; 62(3B):815–820.
6. Hackenberg L, Halm H. Transforaminal lumbar interbody fusion: a safe technique with satisfactory three to five year results. Eur Spine J 2005.
7. Harris BM, Hilibrand AS. Transforaminal lumbar interbody fusion: the effect of various instrumentation techniques on the flexibility of the lumbar spine. Spine 2004; 29(4):E65–70.
8. Javernick MA, Kuklo TR, Polly DW, Jr. Transforaminal lumbar interbody fusion: unilateral versus bilateral disk removal—an in vivo study. Am J Orthop 2003; 32(7):344–348; discussion 348.
9. Mayer HM. The ALIF concept. Eur Spine J 2000; 9 (suppl 1):S35–43.
10. Moskowitz A. Transforaminal lumbar interbody fusion. Orthop Clin North Am 2002; 33(2):359–366.
11. Mummaneni PV, Haid RW, Rodts GE. Lumbar interbody fusion: state-of-the-art technical advances. Invited submission from the Joint Section Meeting on Disorders of the Spine and Peripheral Nerves, March 2004. J Neurosurg Spine 2004; 1(1):24–30.
12. Phillips FM, Cunningham B. Intertransverse lumbar interbody fusion. Spine 2002; 27(2):E37–41.
13. Rosenberg WS, Mummaneni PV. Transforaminal lumbar interbody fusion: technique, complications, and early results. Neurosurgery 2001; 48(3):569–574; discussion 574–575.
14. Humphreys SC, Hodges SD, Comparison of posterior and transforaminal approaches to lumbar interbody fusion. Spine 2001; 26(5):567–571.
15. Lowe TG, Coe JD. Bioresorbable polymer implants in the unilateral transforaminal lumbar interbody fusion procedure. Orthopedics 2002; 25(10 suppl):s1179–1183; discussion s1183.
16. Lowe TG, Tahernia AD. Unilateral transforaminal posterior lumbar interbody fusion. Clin Orthop Relat Res 2002; 394:64–72.
17. Salehi SA, Tawk R. Transforaminal lumbar interbody fusion: surgical technique and results in 24 patients. Neurosurgery 2004; 54(2):368–374; discussion 374.
18. Potter B, Freedman BA. Transforaminal lumbar interbody fusion: clinical and radiographic results and complications in 100 consecutive patients. J Spinal Disord 2005; 18(4):337–346.
19. An HS, Andersson G. Minimally invasive surgery for lumbar degenerative disorders: Part II. Degenerative disc disease and lumbar stenosis. Am J Orthop 2000; 29(12):937–942.
20. Deen HG, Fenton DS, Lamer TJ. Minimally invasive procedures for disorders of the lumbar spine. Mayo Clin Proc 2003; 78(10):1249–1256.

21. Kawaguchi Y, Matsui H, Tsuji H. Changes in serum creatine phosphokinase MM isoenzyme after lumbar spine surgery. Spine 1997; 22(9):1018–1023.
22. Kaiser MG, Haid RW, Jr. Comparison of the mini-open versus laparoscopic approach for anterior lumbar interbody fusion: a retrospective review. Neurosurgery 2002; 51(1):97–103; discussion 103–105.
23. Kawaguchi Y, Matsui H, Tsuji H. Back muscle injury after posterior lumbar spine surgery. A histologic and enzymatic analysis. Spine 1996; 21(8):941–944.
24. Gejo R, Kawaguchi Y. MRI and histologic evidence of postoperative back muscle injury in rats. Spine 2000; 25(8):941–946.
25. Mayer HM. A new microsurgical technique for minimally invasive anterior lumbar interbody fusion. Spine 1997; 22(6):691–699; discussion 700.
26. Kraft G. Electromyography in paraspinal muscles following surgery for root compression. Arch Phys Med Rehabil 1975; 56:80–83.
27. Foley KT, Holly LT, Schwender JD. Minimally invasive lumbar fusion. Spine 2003; 28(15 suppl): S26–35.
28. Jahng TA, et al. Endoscopic instrumented posterolateral lumbar fusion with Healos and recombinant human growth/differentiation factor-5. Neurosurgery 2004; 54(1):171–180; discussion 180–181.
29. Kambin P, Foley KT, Holly LT, Schwender JD. Minimally invasive lumbar fusion. Spine 2003; 28:S26–35. Spine 2004; 29(5):598–599.
30. Khoo LT, et al. Minimally invasive percutaneous posterior lumbar interbody fusion. Neurosurgery 2002; 51 (5 suppl):S166–S178.
31. Kim DH, Albert TJ. Update on use of instrumentation in lumbar spine disorders. Best Pract Res Clin Rheumatol 2002; 16(1):123–140.
32. Kim DH, Jaikumar S, Kam AC. Minimally invasive spine instrumentation. Neurosurgery 2002; 51(5 suppl):S15–25.
33. Mathews HH. Percutaneous interbody fusions. Orthop Clin North Am 1998; 29(4):647–653.
34. Moskovitz PA. Minimally invasive posterolateral lumbar arthrodesis. Orthop Clin North Am 1998; 29(4):665–667.
35. Regan JJ, Yuan H. Laparoscopic fusion of the lumbar spine in a multicenter series of the first 34 consecutive patients. Surg Laparosc Endosc 1996; 6(6):459–468.
36. Radek M, Zapalowicz K, A. Radek. Minimally invasive percutaneous transpedicular lumbar spine fixation. Operative technique and a case report. Neurol Neurochir Pol 2005; 39(2):150–156.
37. Salerni AA. A minimally invasive approach for posterior lumbar interbody fusion. Neurosurg Focus 2002; 13(6):e6.
38. Boden SD. The use of radiographic imaging studies in the evaluation of patients who have degenerative disorders of the lumbar spine. J Bone Joint Surg Am 1996; 78(1):114–124.
39. Frobin W, Brinckmann P. Height of lumbar discs measured from radiographs compared with degeneration and height classified from MR images. Eur Radiol 2001; 11(2):263–269.
40. Vital JM, Gille O. Course of Modic 1 six months after lumbar posterior osteosynthesis. Spine 2003; 28(7):715–720; discussion 721.
41. Willems PC, Jacob SW. Lumbar discography: should we use prophylactic antibiotics? A study of 435 consecutive discograms and a systematic review of the literature. J Spinal Disord Tech 2004; 17(3):243–247.
42. Benz RJ, Garfin SR. Current techniques of decompression of the lumbar spine. Clin Orthop Relat Res 2001; 384:75–81.
43. Haaker RG, Senkal M. Percutaneous lumbar discectomy in the treatment of lumbar discitis. Eur Spine J 1997; 6(2):98–101.
44. Beaubien BP, Mehbod AA. Posterior augmentation of an anterior lumbar interbody fusion: minimally invasive fixation versus pedicle screws in vitro. Spine 2004; 29(19):E406–412.
45. Folman Y, Lee SH. Posterior lumbar interbody fusion for degenerative disc disease using a minimally invasive B-twin expandable spinal spacer: a multicenter study. J Spinal Disord Tech 2003; 16(5):455–460.
46. Schwender JD, Holly LT. Minimally invasive transforaminal lumbar interbody fusion (TLIF): technical feasibility and initial results. J Spinal Disord Tech 2005; 18 (suppl):S1–6.
47. Fessler RG. Minimally invasive percutaneous posterior lumbar interbody fusion. Neurosurgery 2003; 52(6):1512.

26 | Minimally Invasive Translaminar Facet Screw Fixation

K. B. Wood and A. A. Mehbod
Department of Orthopedic Surgery, Massachusetts General Hospital, Boston, Massachusetts, U.S.A.

INTRODUCTION

The concept of spinal arthrodesis is based on experience with other regions of the body in which arthrodesis has been used to treat painful joints by elimination of motion. Initially, spinal fusion was used to treat instability due to infectious conditions, tumors, and trauma. Later, the indications were expanded to include deformities such as scoliosis, kyphosis, and spondylolisthesis, and subsequently for the more controversial indication of discogenic back pain. The outer annulus is thought to be the painful tissue in most cases of low back pain (1), and thus by limiting motion or removing the intervertebral disc, lumbar arthrodesis could potentially eliminate or reduce the pain.

Posterior spinal fusion is a popular treatment for discogenic low back pain; however, pain and dysfunction have been reported to persist despite solid posterior fusion (2,3). Anterior lumbar interbody fusion (ALIF) using structural allograft spacers has become a widely used alternative method for the treatment of discogenic low back pain and instability (4). However, the incidence of pseudarthrosis remains as high as 10% to 25% in some cases (5). Even with the use of bone morphogenic proteins, standalone ALIF has been shown to have an unacceptably high rate of pseudarthrosis (6,7). As supplementing the ALIF with posterior fixation yields increased fusion success, circumferential procedures have been advocated.

Transpedicular fixation is currently the most widely used method of supplementation of an ALIF construct. Standard pedicle screw insertion techniques can increase the operative time, blood loss, reoperation rates, and the rate of complications (8–12). Furthermore, "posterior fusion disease" is a term commonly used to describe the pain and disability that can often accompany long incisions, muscle stripping and denervation, infection, bursitis, or other complications that can be associated with pedicle screws (12,13). The increased morbidity associated with pedicle screw fixation has led surgeons to search for less-invasive techniques for posterior fixation. One such technique is translaminar facet screws.

Transfacet screws were first described by King (14), who inserted a cortical screw across the facet joint. Subsequently, Boucher (15) used longer screws directed toward the pedicle to cross joint. Magerl (16) altered the technique to a translaminar approach. In this technique, the screw is inserted from the base of the spinous process transversely across the contralateral lamina to transfix the facet joint and extend into the base of the transverse process. Clinical findings have suggested that translaminar facet screw fixation is less invasive with decreased perioperative morbidity compared with pedicle screw fixation (17). Additionally, in comparison with the pedicle screw systems, the potential risk for infection may possibly be reduced by the relatively smaller size of the screw. Furthermore, the relatively smaller size of the screw allows ample space for the placement of the graft material for the posterior fusion.

INDICATIONS

The indication for translaminar screws is to augment the stability provided by a one- or two-level ALIF construct. It is the author's opinion that more than two levels of fixation may well require more rigid transpedicular fixation. Adding translaminar screws increases the stability of the construct as compared with standalone ALIF, and does so to a similar extent as pedicular fixation (18). The use of translaminar screws to augment an ALIF should be avoided in cases of deformities, such as scoliosis, spondylolisthesis, and kyphosis, where the spatial relationship between the facets may be altered. Additionally, this technique may not be possible in cases that have previously undergone or presently require extensive decompression in which the lamina and/or facets are totally or partially removed. In these cases, alternative methods of posterior fixation such as pedicle screws should be sought.

SURGICAL TECHNIQUE
Patient Positioning

After administration of general anesthesia and intubation, the patient is placed either supine or lateral decubitus position for performance of the ALIF. The technique for the mini-open approach for ALIF is described in a previous chapter. After the performance of a one- or two-level ALIF, the patient is positioned prone on the Jackson table or four-poster frame which is beneficial in maintaining lumbar lordosis as opposed to other tables or positions (19,20). At this point, one can perform minimally invasive translaminar screw insertion or a totally percutaneous translaminar screw insertion (21,22).

Insertion Technique

The minimally invasive technique with open midline exposure of the posterior spine allows the surgeon to visualize the translaminar passage of the screws under direct vision and enable a posterior spinal fusion, if desired, for a true circumferential arthrodesis. The totally percutaneous technique is more demanding, requiring fluoroscopy and does not allow for additional posterior fusion.

An appropriate midline incision is made over the spinous process of the level to fix. The supraspinous ligament is maintained at the same time as careful paraspinal muscle dissection is carried out subperiosteally down the spinous process of cephalad vertebra, exposing the lamina and the facet-joint capsule. The facet joint should be the lateral extent of the dissection. The entry point of the screws are at the superior junction of the cephalad lamina and spinous process (Fig. 1A). A 3.2-mm drill bit is used and placed at the starting hole. Commonly, it is necessary to insert the drill and screw percutaneously via a separate and more lateral incision (lateral to the midline incision) to be able to get the proper insertion trajectory. The hole is drilled toward and through the opposite lamina, between its tables, and across the facet joint to the base of the caudal vertebra's transverse process (Fig. 1B). Subsequently, the hole is palpated and its length measured. A 4.5-mm fully threaded screw is then placed though the hole without tapping to prevent splitting of the lamina.

The second screw should be inserted in a similar fashion. The entry hole of the second screw should be more inferior and deep or more proximal and superficial in order to avoid penetration into the first screw (Fig. 1). In an anatomical study (23), measurements for screw path length, caudal and lateral angles, and superior and inferior lamina border thicknesses from L1 to L5 were measured with regard to translaminar facet screw fixation in 30 dried lumbar spines. The mean values of the length of the screw (41–54 mm) and lateral angle (39–60°) gradually

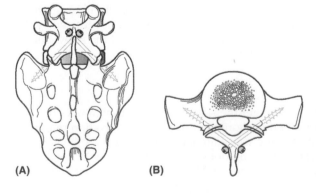

(A)   **(B)**

FIGURE 1   (**A**) Anteroposterior (AP) view of the spine demonstrating translaminar screw fixation across the L5-S1 facet joint. (**B**) Axial images demonstrating the passage of the screws across the facet joints toward the caudal vertebra's transverse process or ala (S1).

increased from L1–2 to L5–S1 levels. Additionally, this study showed that a translaminar facet screw of 4.5-mm diameter, should be inserted through the lumbar facet joint at an angle of 40° to 50° laterally and 35° to 40° caudally at L1–L5 levels; at L5–S1, these angles should be 50° to 55° laterally and 35° to 40° caudally.

Once both the screws are inserted, intraoperative radiographs should be used to verify the position of the screws (21). Then, if fusion is desired, the posterior elements of L4 and L5 should be decorticated and the appropriate bone graft should be placed. Additionally, one may elect to remove the facet capsule at L4–L5 level, followed by decortication and fusion, prior to the insertion of the screw across the facet joint. This provides the benefits of facet fusion. Extensive decompressive laminotomies should be avoided to evade compromising with the stability of the screws.

COMPLICATIONS

Complications may arise intraoperatively or postoperatively. One is malplacement of the screw within the spinal canal and neural impingement. The minimally invasive (mini-open) technique of translaminar screw insertion under direct vision can aid the surgeon in detecting any posterior lamina wall violations. Mild violation of the posterior laminar wall is not necessarily a cause for concern as long as the screw has crossed the facet joint, and if the surgeon determines the screw purchase of bone to be adequate. Unfortunately, one cannot visualize any inner (anterior) lamina wall violations. However, under direct vision, a narrow probe can be inserted into the pilot hole prepared by the drill. The patency of the inner lamina wall can be palpated similar to the palpation of a pilot hole for pedicle screw insertion. If there is a violation of the inner lamina wall, the surgeon must determine the extent of the violation and can accept the hole if it re-enters the lamina, redirect the pilot hole, or look for salvage options. In a recent study (22), 65 translaminar screws were placed and evaluated with CT scans postoperatively. Seven screws (11%) were found to have violated some portions of the walls of the laminae: five at the outer lamina and two at the inner lamina. No direct neural injury or neural compression by the screws occurred. Facet purchase was successful in all screws. Another rare complication is the fracture of the facet as the screw is being inserted. This can be noticed intraoperatively and salvaged with pedicle screw fixation. Certainly, placing a smaller trans-facet screw avoids the risk of intracanal penetration.

Postoperative complications can occur similar to any other procedure. Postoperative radiculopathies may be attributed to misplaced screws or facet fractures as well. This can be evaluated with CT scans and appropriately managed with the removal of the screw, decompressions, and salvage with pedicle screws. In cases of pseudarthrosis, the translaminar screws may fatigue and break, usually at the level of the facet joint (24). These cases can be salvaged with revision surgeries for the pseudarthrosis and placement of pedicle screw instrumentation. The proximal broken translaminar facet screws can be removed. The distal broken tips can be removed if they prevent pedicle screw instrumentation. Otherwise, they can be left in place with little risk of migration (24).

CLINICAL RESULTS

The advantages of using translaminar facet screws are that a relatively small incision is used with minimal muscle dissection. The technique is safe, feasible, and effective (22,24–27). Clinical findings have indicated that translaminar facet screw fixation was a less invasive spinal fixation method with decreased perioperative morbidity compared with pedicle screw fixation (17). The arthrodesis rates and clinical outcomes have been favorable with the use of this technique. Kornblatt (25), in 1986, retrospectively reviewed 30 patients who underwent posterior fusion with the use of translaminar screws. Their radiographic fusion rate was 70% with a clinical success rate of 63%. The underlying diagnosis was not clear in this study. In 1998, Humke (24) retrospectively studied his case series of 173 patients who had undergone posterior spinal fusion with translaminar screws. The preoperative diagnosis included a variety of disorders, the most common of which were degenerative disc disease and spinal stenosis. A solid bony fusion was observed radiographically in 94% of patients. The pain rating improved from a preoperative average of 7.6 to 2.9 at final follow up. When comparing one- and two-level fusions, there was no significant difference in the outcomes. Reoperations for symptomatic pseudarthrosis was necessary in eight (5%) patients, and they were revised to pedicle screw systems.

In a more recent study (22), the authors studied 20 patients with symptomatic degenerative disc disease who had a percutaneously placed translaminar facet screw augment their ALIF with Peek anterior cages, allograft, and bone-marrow aspirate. Radiographic fusion occurred in all cases (100%). The average operation time for the ALIF was 94 minutes and 79 minutes for the posterior-screw placement. The Oswestry disability index improved from a preoperative value of 52 to 26 postoperatively. There was one complication, which was a fractured tip of a superior articular process of the S1 segment that was compressing the exiting L5 nerve root.

SUMMARY

The aforementioned studies show that over time, the techniques for fusion have improved, especially with the addition of anterior structural grafting. The clinical results are acceptable in terms of fusion rate and complications. Level I evidence consisting of prospective randomized trials using this technique of translaminar screws augmenting anterior lumbar interbody graft, compared with other posterior augmentation methods, are needed to demonstrate its benefits. Until then, we believe that the advantages of the use of translaminar screws include relatively smaller incision with less dissection, less risk to neural structures, and smaller screws that allow more space for bone grafting.

REFERENCES

1. Kuslich SD, Ulstrom CL, Michael CJ. The tissue origin of low back pain and sciatica: a report of pain response to tissue stimulation during operations on the lumbar spine using local anesthesia. Orthop Clin North Am 1991; 22:181–187.
2. Barrick WT, Schofferman JA, Reynolds JB, et al. Anterior lumbar fusion improves discogenic pain at levels of prior posterolateral fusion. Spine 2000; 25:853–857.
3. Weatherley CR, Prickett CF, O'Brien JP. Discogenic pain persisting despite solid posterior fusion. J Bone Joint Surg Br 1986; 68:142–143.
4. Buttermann GR, Glazer PA, Hu SS, et al. Revision of failed lumbar fusions. A comparison of anterior autograft and allograft. Spine 1997; 22:2748–2755.
5. Hanley EN Jr, David SM. Lumbar arthrodesis for the treatment of back pain. J Bone Joint Surg Am 1999; 81:716–730.
6. Burkus JK, Gornet MF, Dickman CA, et al. Anterior lumbar interbody fusion using rhBMP-2 with tapered interbody cages. J Spinal Disord Tech 2002; 15:337–349.
7. Burkus JK, Transfeldt EE, Kitchel SH, et al. Clinical and radiographic outcomes of anterior lumbar interbody fusion using recombinant human bone morphogenetic protein-2. Spine 2002; 27:2396–2408.
8. Bjarke Christensen F, Stender Hansen E, Laursen M, et al. Long-term functional outcome of pedicle screw instrumentation as a support for posterolateral spinal fusion: randomized clinical study with a 5-year follow-up. Spine 2002; 27:1269–1277.
9. Esses SI, Sachs BL, Dreyzin V. Complications associated with the technique of pedicle screw fixation. A selected survey of ABS members. Spine 1993; 18:2231–2238; discussion 8–9.
10. Fritzell P, Hagg O, Wessberg P, et al. Chronic low back pain and fusion: a comparison of three surgical techniques: a prospective multicenter randomized study from the Swedish lumbar spine study group. Spine 2002; 27:1131–1141.
11. Jutte PC, Castelein RM. Complications of pedicle screws in lumbar and lumbosacral fusions in 105 consecutive primary operations. Eur Spine J 2002; 11:594–598.
12. Lonstein JE, Denis F, Perra JH, et al. Complications associated with pedicle screws. J Bone Joint Surg Am 1999; 81:1519–1528.
13. Benini A, Magerl F. Selective decompression and translaminar articular facet screw fixation for lumbar canal stenosis and disc protrusion. Br J Neurosurg 1993; 7:413–418.
14. king D. Internal fixation of lumbosacra fusion. J Bone Joint Surg Am 1948; 30:559–565.
15. Boucher H. A method of spine fusion. J Bone Joint Surg Am 1959; 41:248–259.
16. Magerl FP. Stabilization of the lower thoracic and lumbar spine with external skeletal fixation. Clin Orthop Relat Res 1984; 189:125–141.
17. Tuli SK, Eichler ME, Woodard EJ. Comparison of perioperative morbidity in translaminar facet versus pedicle screw fixation. Orthopedics 2005; 28:773–778.

18. Beaubien BP, Mehbod AA, Kallemeier PM, et al. Posterior augmentation of an anterior lumbar inter-body fusion: minimally invasive fixation versus pedicle screws in vitro. Spine 2004; 29:E406–412.

19. Stephens GC, Yoo JU, Wilbur G. Comparison of lumbar sagittal alignment produced by different operative positions. Spine 1996; 21:1802–1806; discussion 7.

20. Tribus CB, Belanger TA, Zdeblick TA. The effect of operative position and short-segment fusion on maintenance of sagittal alignment of the lumbar spine. Spine 1999; 24:58–61.

21. Phillips FM, Cunningham B, Carandang G, et al. Effect of supplemental translaminar facet screw fixation on the stability of stand-alone anterior lumbar interbody fusion cages under physiologic compressive preloads. Spine 2004; 29:1731–1736.

22. Shim CS, Lee SH, Jung B, et al. Fluoroscopically assisted percutaneous translaminar facet screw fixation following anterior lumbar interbody fusion: technical report. Spine 2005; 30:838–843.

23. Lu J, Ebraheim NA, Yeasting RA. Translaminar facet screw placement: an anatomic study. Am J Orthop 1998; 27:550–555.

24. Humke T, Grob D, Dvorak J, et al. Translaminar screw fixation of the lumbar and lumbosacral spine. A 5-year follow-up. Spine 1998; 23:1180–1184.

25. Kornblatt MD, Casey MP, Jacobs RR. Internal fixation in lumbosacral spine fusion. A biomechanical and clinical study. Clin Orthop Relat Res 1986; 203:141–150.

26. Rathonyi GC, Oxland TR, Gerich U, et al. The role of supplemental translaminar screws in anterior lumbar interbody fixation: a biomechanical study. Eur Spine J 1998; 7:400–407.

27. Sasso RC, Best NM, Potts EA. Percutaneous computer-assisted translaminar facet screw: an initial human cadaveric study. Spine J 2005; 5:515–519.

27 | Spinal Cord Stimulation for Chronic Pain

T. Desmond Brown
*Department of Orthopedic Surgery, Boston University School of Medicine,
Boston, Massachusetts, U.S.A.*

INTRODUCTION

The use of electricity for medical purposes has a long and colorful history, beginning with the application of electrified fish to treat gout and headache in ancient Rome, and flourishing in various forms in 19th-century Europe and America as a treatment for neuralgia and back pain. During this "golden age" of medical electricity, electrical stimulation was eagerly adopted by both conventional and alternative practitioners. By the early 20th century, however, these methods had fallen into disrepute, and the use of electricity for medical purposes was largely abandoned (1).

The gate theory of pain, as described by Melzak and Wall in 1965 (2), renewed interest in electro-analgesia. The theory predicted that stimulating low-threshold afferent nerve fibers could block the central transmission of pain. Shealy implanted the first spinal cord stimulation (SCS) device in 1967, placing a subdural electrode over the dorsal columns and connecting it to an external power source (3). Complications and treatment failures were common with the early stimulators, but research by individuals and the medical device industry led to refinements in the technique, with improved results.

Current practice uses epidural electrodes placed percutaneously or with a limited open exposure, and is referred to as spinal cord stimulation rather than dorsal column stimulation. The electrodes are activated by an implanted, programmable pulse generator, which may have an internal or external power supply. Despite uncertainty about its mechanism of action (4), SCS has been used increasingly for a variety of painful conditions, and there is a growing evidence base for its effectiveness.

A consulting report stated that more than 24,000 spinal cord stimulators were implanted in the United States in 2002, and that the projected annual revenue growth was 13.1% for the industry (5). Devices are implanted by neurosurgeons, orthopedic surgeons, anesthesiologists, or other pain management specialists. Patient selection and technical issues remain important concerns, and recent literature reviews stress the need for further evaluation in clinical trials (6,7).

INDICATIONS

Spinal cord stimulation is used primarily for chronic pain of neuropathic origin. It is less effective for mechanical or nociceptive pain, and ineffective for acute pain. The most common indication in North America is axial and lower extremity pain that persists after back surgery, sometimes called the failed back surgery syndrome (FBSS). Because SCS is more effective for leg pain than back pain, patients with primarily low back pain may be less suitable for SCS. Other indications include chronic regional pain syndrome, type 1 (reflex sympathetic dystrophy) or type 2 (causalgia). It has been used with limited effectiveness for postherpetic neuralgia (8) and painful diabetic neuropathy (9). Outside North America, it has been used in the treatment of refractory angina pectoris (10) and ischemic leg pain from peripheral vascular disease (11).

Patients who are considered for SCS should have chronic pain that has failed to respond to medical and rehabilitative management, and which interferes substantially with normal daily activities or employment. In previously operated patients with an identifiable surgically correctable problem, SCS may be considered as an alternative to repeat surgery (12). Patients who are candidates for SCS should undergo a period of trial stimulation and should demonstrate at least 50% relief of pain, to be considered for permanent implantation. However, this commonly used criterion may not correspond well with the desires and expectations of patients, and is only moderately successful at predicting a good outcome (13).

Coexisting infection or coagulopathy are medical contraindications to SCS. Patients with coexisting psychiatric illness or diminished mental capacity may be unable to cooperate sufficiently during the trial stimulation period and afterward, and should not be considered for implantation. Patients with active drug-seeking behavior or who are heavily influenced by a desire for secondary gain are poor candidates. An anatomic block that restricts the passage of an epidural electrode may necessitate an open rather than percutaneous approach. Patient who do not benefit from trial stimulation are considered unlikely to benefit from a permanent implant.

PREOPERATIVE PLANNING

Most patients who are being considered for SCS would have undergone a lengthy evaluation process, often through a multidisciplinary pain management clinic. Nevertheless, it is imperative for the implanting physician to identify the factors that precipitate or worsen pain, and the character and location of the pain, as these may affect electrode placement and programming. Plain radiographs should be reviewed to look for deformity or severe degenerative changes, and a computed tomography (CT) scan or magnetic resonance imaging (MRI) should be reviewed to look for evidence of severe spinal stenosis, which can make electrode placement more difficult. A formal psychologic assessment should be done to identify factors that may portend a poor result from SCS (14).

The most important aspect of preoperative planning is the period of trial stimulation, which should be considered an integral part of the surgical procedure. During the trial, one or more electrodes are placed percutaneously or through a small incision, with an externalized wire connected to a pulse generator. The location of the lead and the stimulation parameters are adjusted in an attempt to "cover" the area of pain with paresthesias that are tolerable to the patient. The trial may last from a few days to more than a week, and is considered successful if there is at least 50% reduction in pain using the Visual Analog Scale; ideally, there should be improvements in physical function as well (15).

SURGICAL TECHNIQUE
Trial Implant Insertion

The trial is done in a standard operating room equipped with C-arm image intensifier. The patient lies prone on a radiolucent operating room table, and the entire back from T1 to sacrum, including both flanks, is prepared and draped. Prophylactic antibiotics are given. Local anesthesia and intravenous sedation are used, but the patient must remain sufficiently alert to cooperate in identifying areas of paresthesia.

A Tuohy needle is inserted percutaneously, with the bevel directed cranially and dorsally, via a paramedian approach (Fig. 1). The needle is angled at 30° to 45° from the skin and directed cranially toward the L1–L2 or T12–L1 interspace. The image intensifier is used to guide needle placement, and epidural location is verified with the "loss of resistance" technique. The wire electrode is introduced through the Tuohy needle and advanced with C-arm guidance to the T9–T10 level (Fig. 2). The electrode can be steered by adjusting the position of the needle or by placing a small bend in the wire stiffener within the electrode. For a patient with low back pain or bilateral leg pain, a midline position is preferred; however, the anatomic midline may not correspond to the physiologic midline in terms of stimulating paresthesias. For patients with unilateral symptoms, a single electrode may suffice; for those with axial or bilateral leg pain, a second electrode should be placed using the same technique in order to maximize the potential for paresthesia coverage and pain relief (Fig. 3). The optimum position of the electrode for patients with lower extremity pain is usually at the T9–T10 interspace.

The electrode is connected to a screening wire that is passed off the surgical field and connected to the trial stimulator. The position of the electrodes and the parameters of stimulation are adjusted until the patient confirms that paresthesias cover the areas of pain. A 3- to 4-cm incision is made around the needle, and dissection is carried down to the lumbodorsal fascia. The needle and stiffener are withdrawn and the electrode is secured to the fascia using a silastic anchor and nonabsorbable suture (Fig. 4). The electrode is connected to an extension wire which

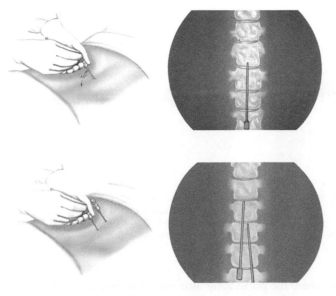

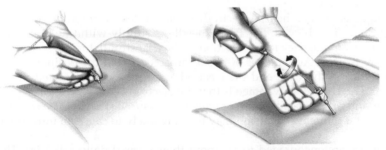

FIGURE 1 The Tuohy needle is inserted by a paramedian approach using the image intensifier and directed toward the L1–L2 or T12–L1 interspace. A second needle may be inserted in the same manner.

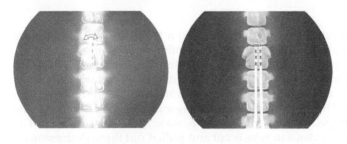

FIGURE 2 The wire electrode is introduced through the Tuohy needle and advanced with C-arm guidance to the T9–T10 level. The electrode can be steered by adjusting the position of the needle or by placing a small bend in the wire stiffener within the electrode.

FIGURE 3 Two electrodes may be placed near the midline to assist in providing bilateral paresthesias and pain relief.

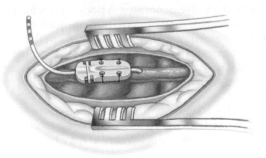

FIGURE 4 The electrode is secured to the fascia using a silastic anchor and nonabsorbable suture.

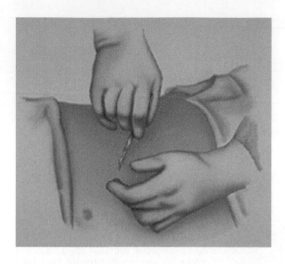

FIGURE 5 A 10 cm incision is made over the abdomen (shown here) or buttock. A pouch is created in the subcutaneous fat 5 mm below the skin surface, and the pulse generator is placed into the pouch.

is tunneled laterally toward the side where the pulse generator would be implanted if the trial is successful. The wire is brought out through a stab wound in the skin. The posterior wound is closed and both wounds are dressed.

An alternative technique is to treat the trial electrode or electrodes as temporary devices. When proper electrode position is achieved, the Tuohy needle is simply withdrawn and the lead wires are left protruding from the back for connection to the trial stimulator. No incision is made and no extension wire is used. Advantages of this approach are that the position of the electrodes can be adjusted during the trial, and the electrodes can be easily removed in the office at the end of the trial. The chief disadvantage is that the electrodes must be replaced if a permanent implant is done, and proper positioning for pain relief assured. There is also concern that a temporary lead without a tunneled extension may be more likely to cause an intraspinal infection.

During the trial, patients are encouraged to go about their normal daily activities. The patient or physician adjusts the stimulation parameters to maximize pain relief. The physician should meet the patient during the trial in order to assess pain relief, use of analgesics, and functional improvement, and to decide if permanent implantation is indicated.

Permanent Implant

If the trial is successful, the patient returns to the operating room for placement of the pulse generator. Common sites for implantation include the lower abdominal wall or superior buttock. For placement in the buttock, the patient may be positioned prone as during the trial; for abdominal wall placement, the lateral decubitus position is used. Generous local anesthesia and intravenous sedation are given, although general anesthesia may be used if there is to be no adjustment in electrode position. The previous midline posterior incision and the site for the pulse generator are prepared and draped. The externalized wire is excluded from the field. The posterior incision is reopened and the extension wire is cut and pulled out through the skin by an unscrubbed assistant.

A 10-cm incision is made at the site selected for the pulse generator. A pocket is created in the subcutaneous fat 5 mm below the skin; deeper placement may impede communication with the external programmer (Figs. 5 and 6). A malleable tunneling device is directed from the posterior wound to the pocket, and a wire from the generator brought back into the posterior wound and connected to the electrode. The wounds are irrigated and complete hemostasis is obtained. The pulse generator is placed in the pocket, with any redundant wire coiled deep to it. The wounds are closed and dressings applied.

Although percutaneously placed wire electrodes have been used successfully in trials and as permanent implants, there are circumstances in which a different electrode design may be preferred. If there is scarring of the epidural space from previous surgery, it may be difficult

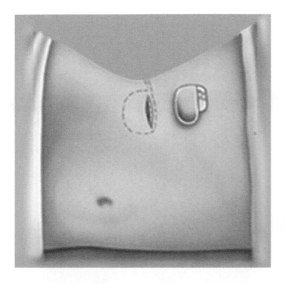

FIGURE 6 A 10 cm incision is made over the abdomen (shown here) or buttock. A pouch is created in the subcutaneous fat 5 mm below the skin surface, and the pulse generator is placed into the pouch.

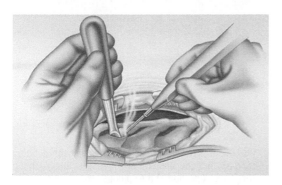

FIGURE 7 A 6–8 cm midline incision is made over the interspace one level distal to the desired level of stimulation. The supraspinous ligament is resected and the paraspinous muscles elevated from the lamina as necessary to expose the ligamentum flavum.

to place an electrode percutaneously. Percutaneous electrodes may migrate, leading to loss of paresthesia coverage and pain relief. Modern wire electrodes have multiple contacts (sites where electric current is applied) and reprogramming the contacts may restore effectiveness. However, if lead migration recurs, it may be necessary to replace the wire electrode with a paddle-style electrode placed via a small laminotomy. Besides having greater resistance to migration, paddle electrodes are insulated such that current is channeled more directly toward the spinal cord. As less current is used, there is less risk of undesired nerve root stimulation, and battery life is prolonged. Some surgeons prefer to use laminotomy leads as a permanent implant for all patients.

To place the paddle-style electrode, either general anesthesia or local anesthesia with sedation may be used. The patient is positioned prone, and the vertebral level at which effective trial stimulation was achieved is identified using the image intensifier. The electrode is inserted at the next interspace, and hence the incision is made just distal to this level. A 6- to 8-cm midline incision is made, and dissection is carried down to the spinous process and supraspinous ligament. The ligament is released, and the paraspinous muscles are elevated from the spinous process and lamina to expose the ligamentum flavum (Fig. 7). The ligamentum is opened with a biting rongeur and the opening enlarged with the Kerrison rongeurs. A portion of the spinous process and lamina may be resected with the Kerrison rongeur if necessary (Figs. 8 and 9). The paddle electrode is inserted over the dura with contacts facing the spinal cord and passed up to the desired level (Figs. 10 and 11). The location of the electrode is verified with the image intensifier and the electrode is secured to the lumbodorsal fascia with a silastic anchor. Tunneling of the wire extension and placement of the pulse generator are done as described for the percutaneous leads.

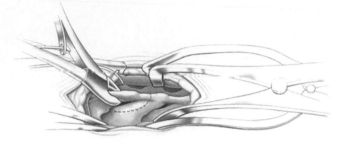

FIGURE 8 The ligamentum is opened with a biting rongeur and the opening enlarged with the Kerrison rongeurs. A portion of the spinous process and lamina may be resected with the Kerrison rongeur if necessary.

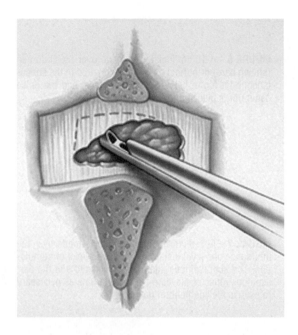

FIGURE 9 The ligamentum is opened with a biting rongeur and the opening enlarged with the Kerrison rongeurs. A portion of the spinous process and lamina may be resected with the Kerrison rongeur if necessary.

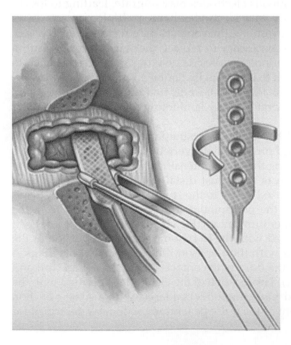

FIGURE 10 The paddle electrode is inserted over the dura with contacts facing the spinal cord and passed up to the desired level.

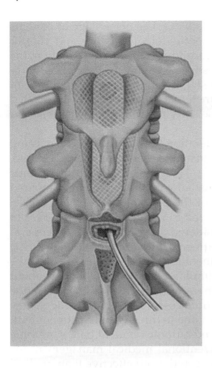

FIGURE 11 The paddle electrode is inserted over the dura with contacts facing the spinal cord and passed up to the desired level.

COMPLICATIONS

A systematic review of published studies of SCS for FBSS and chronic regional pain syndrome found an overall complication rate of 34% (16). Superficial infection occurred in 4.5% of the patients, and deep infection in 0.1%. Pain associated with the stimulator components, usually the pulse generator site, occurred in 5.8%. The most common reason for reoperation was for stimulator revision (23.1%), usually to reposition electrodes that had migrated or lost effectiveness. Other complications included cerebrospinal fluid leakage and failure of the pulse generator. Reviews of SCS for other indications, such as intractable angina and critical limb ischemia have found similar complications, although occurring at somewhat lower rates (17).

Superficial infections most commonly involve the pulse-generator site and may resolve with intravenous or oral antibiotics and local wound care. Deep infection requires the removal of the pulse generator and electrodes. Methods to reduce the likelihood of infection include giving peri-operative antibiotics to cover gram-positive skin flora, minimizing dead space and hematoma around the pulse generator, and reducing operative time and handling of the implants (18).

The most common equipment-related problem is the loss of pain relief due to the movement of the epidural electrode. Some movement undoubtedly occurs when patients go from the prone position assumed at implantation to the erect position, and additional side-to-side and cranial–caudal movement may occur over time. Contemporary multi-polar electrodes can be reprogrammed to change the location and pattern of stimulation, which may restore effective pain relief (19). If a lead has broken or cannot be rendered effective by reprogramming, it should be removed and replaced with a percutaneous or laminotomy-type electrode. The broad plate-shaped laminotomy electrode is thought to be more resistant to migration. As the laminotomy electrode is more effective at focusing current on the spinal cord, there are fewer problems with unwanted nerve-root stimulation and lower energy consumption (20).

OUTCOMES

A systematic review of SCS for chronic back and leg pain and FBSS identified 72 case series, one controlled study, and one randomized clinical trial (6). In over 3400 patients receiving

SCS implants, there was at least 50% pain relief in 62% of patients. The percentage of patients reporting pain relief was higher in studies with poorer methodologic quality and shorter follow-up. Although 53% of patients took no analgesic medication after SCS implantation, the ten studies that compared analgesic use before and after surgery found no difference. Forty percent of patients returned to work after receiving SCS, a significant increase compared with the preoperative value. The few studies that reported on functional capacity and health-related quality of life found significant improvements with SCS. Seventy percent of patients reported satisfaction with the procedure.

A randomized clinical trial comparing SCS with reoperation for patients with persisting leg and back pain after surgery, and in whom a surgically treatable lesion could be identified, found that SCS was more successful than reoperation (12). Forty-seven percent of patients randomized to SCS had at least 50% pain relief and were satisfied with the treatment, compared with 12% of those randomized to reoperation. Only 21% of the patients randomized to SCS crossed over to require reoperation; 54% of those randomized to reoperation crossed over to receive SCS. The authors suggested that SCS could be considered as an alternative to reoperation in patients with FBSS who have exhausted other treatment options. An ongoing clinical trial is comparing SCS with conventional medical management for FBSS (21).

The high initial cost of implanting a spinal cord stimulator has led to concerns about cost-effectiveness. A study comparing SCS plus physical therapy with physical therapy alone found clinical benefits from adding SCS, with reduced lifetime costs (22). A systematic review of published economic evaluations of SCS found that within one to three years, treatment with SCS is less costly than other forms of treatment for FBSS and chronic regional pain syndrome (23). A decision-analytic model comparing SCS with conventional medical management for FBSS found that over a lifetime, SCS was both less expensive and more effective than medical management (24). The incremental benefit of SCS, as measured in quality-adjusted life years, was high but within the range generally accepted as reasonable.

SUMMARY

Spinal cord stimulation is a minimally invasive treatment for FBSS, chronic regional pain syndrome, and other painful conditions. Treatment is more effective for leg pain than for back pain. The mechanism of action is unknown. Hardware-related complications, such as migration of the stimulating electrodes, are common and may necessitate reoperation; major complications are infrequent. The high initial cost may be offset by reduced expenditure on health care afterward. Careful preoperative assessment, including a screening trial, is necessary to identify patients most likely to benefit from this procedure.

REFERENCES

1. Rossi U. The history of electrical stimulation of the nervous system for the control of pain. Pain Res Clin Manag 2003; 15:5–16.
2. Melzack R, Wall PD. Pain mechanisms: a new theory. Science 1965; 150(699):971–979.
3. Shealy CN, Mortimer JT, Reswick JB. Electrical inhibition of pain by stimulation of the dorsal columns: preliminary clinical report. Anesth Analg 1967; 46(4):489–491.
4. Oakley JC, Prager JP. Spinal cord stimulation: mechanisms of action. [Review] [43 refs]. Spine 2002; 27(22):2574–2583.
5. Krames E. The right place at the right time. Neuromodulation 2005; 8(3):149–152.
6. Taylor RS, van Buyten JP, Buchser E. Spinal cord stimulation for chronic back and leg pain and failed back surgery syndrome: a systematic review and analysis of prognostic factors. Spine 2005; 30(1):152–160.
7. Harney D, Magner JJ, O'Keeffe D. Complex regional pain syndrome: the case for spinal cord stimulation (a brief review). [Review] [47 refs]. Injury 2005; 36(3):357–362.
8. Harke H, Gretenkort P, Ladleif HU, Koester P, Rahman S. Spinal cord stimulation in postherpetic neuralgia and in acute herpes zoster pain. Anesth Analg 2002; 94(3):694–700.
9. Tesfaye S, Watt J, Benbow SJ, Pang KA, Miles J, MacFarlane IA. Electrical spinal-cord stimulation for painful diabetic peripheral neuropathy. [see comment]. Lancet 1996; 348(9043):1698–1701.
10. Mannheimer C, Eliasson T, Augustinsson LE, et al. Electrical stimulation versus coronary artery bypass surgery in severe angina pectoris: the ESBY study. [see comment]. Circulation 1998; 97(12):1157–1163.

11. Erdek MA, Staats PS. Spinal cord stimulation for angina pectoris and peripheral vascular disease. Anesthesiol Clin N Am 2003; 21(4):797–804.
12. North RB, Kidd DH, Farrokhi F, Piantadosi SA. Spinal cord stimulation versus repeated lumbosacral spine surgery for chronic pain: a randomized, controlled trial. Neurosurgery 2005; 56(1):98–106.
13. Simpson BA. Electrical stimulation and the relief of pain: selection of patients and assessment of outcome. Pain Res Clin Manag 2003; 15:237–249.
14. Doleys DM, Dinoff BL. Psychological aspects of interventional therapy. Anesthesiol Clin N Am 2003; 21(4):767–783.
15. Oakley JC. Spinal cord stimulation: patient selection, technique, and outcomes. [Review] [48 refs]. Neurosurg Clin N Am 2003; 14(3):365–380.
16. Turner JA, Loeser JD, Deyo RA, Sanders SB. Spinal cord stimulation for patients with failed back surgery syndrome or complex regional pain syndrome: a systematic review of effectiveness and complications. [Review] [36 refs]. Pain 2004; 108(1–2):137–147.
17. Ubbink DT, Vermeulen H, Spincemaille GH, Gersbach PA, Berg P, Amann W. Systematic review and meta-analysis of controlled trials assessing spinal cord stimulation for inoperable critical leg ischaemia. [see comment]. [Review] [39 refs]. Br J Surg 2004; 91(8):948–955.
18. Follett KA, Boortz-Marx RL, Drake JM, et al. Prevention and management of intrathecal drug delivery and spinal cord stimulation system infections. [Review] [65 refs]. Anesthesiology 2004; 100(6):1582–1594.
19. North RB, Ewend MG, Lawton MT, Piantadosi S. Spinal cord stimulation for chronic, intractable pain: superiority of "multi-channel" devices. [see comment]. Pain 1991; 44(2):119–130.
20. North RB, Kidd DH, Olin JC, Sieracki JM. Spinal cord stimulation electrode design: prospective, randomized, controlled trial comparing percutaneous and laminectomy electrodes-part I: technical outcomes. Neurosurgery 2002; 51(2):381–389.
21. Kumar K. Spinal cord stimulation vs. conventional medical management: a prospective, randomized, controlled, multicenter study of patients with failed back surgery syndrome (PROCESS Study). Neuromodulation 2005; 8(4):213–218.
22. Kemler MA, Furnee CA. Economic evaluation of spinal cord stimulation for chronic reflex sympathetic dystrophy. Neurology 2002; 59(8):1203–1209.
23. Taylor RS, Taylor RJ, Van Buyten JP, Buchser E, North R, Bayliss S. The cost effectiveness of spinal cord stimulation in the treatment of pain: a systematic review of the literature. [Review] [28 refs]. J Pain Symptom Manag 2004; 27(4):370–378.
24. Taylor RJ, Taylor RS. Spinal cord stimulation for failed back surgery syndrome: a decision-analytic model and cost-effectiveness analysis. Int J Technol Assess Health Care 2005; 21(3):351–358.

28 | Radiofrequency Neurotomy of the Cervical Facet Joints

Jay Govind
Department of Anesthesia and Pain Medicine, The Canberra Hospital and The Australian National University, Canberra, Australian Capital Territory, Australia

INTRODUCTION

As a therapeutic technique for the relief of pain, thermal radiofrequency (RF) creates a mechanical barrier that prevents the transmission of nociceptive information from a source that is responsible for the patient's pain. By passing a low-energy, high-frequency alternating current (100,000 to 500,000 Hertz) between the exposed tip of a Teflon covered electrode ("active" electrode) and a large dispersive ground plate ("passive" electrode), heat is generated in the tissues immediately surrounding the active tip. At a certain temperature, the surrounding tissue coagulates and the resulting thermal lesion incorporates the targeted nerve. In the treatment of chronic cervical spinal pain, thermal radiofrequency neurotomy (RFN) has a special application in the treatment of proven zygapophysial joint pain and where the target nerve is the medial branch of the dorsal ramus.

Following its introduction by Kirschner in 1932 for the treatment of trigeminal neuralgia (1), controlled thermal coagulation achieved prominence due to the pioneering work of Sweet and White (2,3). By 1996, radiofrequency neurotomy was the procedure of choice for most patients undergoing first surgical treatment for trigeminal neuralgia (4). With respect to spinal pain, radiofrequency neurotomy was first used for the treatment of low back pain ostensibly arising from the lumbar zygapophysial joints (5) and the first successful application of radiofrequency neurotomy for the treatment of cervical zygapophysial joint pain was reported by Schaerer in 1978 (6). Two years later Schaerer described its favorable application for the treatment of headaches emanating from the upper cervical joints (7,8). In contrast, the aggregate outcomes from subsequent descriptive studies over the next 10 years were inconsistent, mixed and generally not compelling (9–12). While in some patients, RFN had conferred significant relief, in others the spectrum of outcomes ranged between modest and failure. An independent review attributed inconsistent results and poor success rates to inadequate patient selection, inaccurate surgical and radiographic anatomy, and technical errors in the application of radiofrequency neurotomy (13). In Schaerer's series (6–8), the presurgical confirmation of zygapophysial joint pain by selective diagnostic blocks would have accounted for the higher success rate reported. Other investigators presumed the diagnosis of zygapophysial joint pain based on history and physical examination (11,12). Given that there were and still are no valid clinical or radiological features unique for cervical zygapophysial joint pain, the poor outcomes reported were commensurate with the tenuous selection criteria; as exemplified in a recent study (14). Historically, not all studies had selected patients on the basis of diagnostic blocks and when used, single blocks were relied upon (14–17) and the techniques described may have been inaccurate. These factors might have explained why the reported results were only fair in terms of the proportion of patients relieved and the degree of relief that they obtained.

Prompted by these inconsistencies, a pilot study was undertaken in 1995 to assess the efficacy of RFN in the management of proven cervical zygapophysial joint pain (13). It showed that where patients were properly selected and a more precise technique applied, complete relief of pain was achievable in a large proportion of patients in whom the source of chronic neck pain resided in the lower zygapophysial joints. However, similar outcomes were elusive when the third occipital nerve (TON) was targeted for the treatment of upper neck pain and headaches.

This was followed by the first-ever randomized double blind placebo controlled trial in which Lord et al. (18) established RFN to be an efficacious and effective mode of treatment for chronic neck pain emanating from the lower zygapophysial joints. Long-term follow-up studies have since attested to the efficacy of these procedures (19,20) irrespective of litigation (21). A recently completed study showed that with certain modifications and with meticulous application, the procedure could be successfully performed for the treatment of third occipital (cervicogenic) headache emanating from the C2/3 zygapophysial joint (22).

Compared with electrocautery and neurolytic agents such as phenol, radiofrequency generates lesions that are smooth, regular, well-circumscribed, and confined to restricted areas. By monitoring the rate of heating, temperature can be maintained under 85°C thereby preventing gas formation, boiling, vaporization, explosive reactions, and cavitation (23,24). The lesion size can be reproducibly quantified. Successful execution of the procedure ensures long lasting effects with no major sensory or motor complications, unlike surgical neurectomy. No permanent damage has been reported and, when indicated, the procedure can be repeated. The electrodes are robust and easily made to different configurations to suit specific anatomical usage (12,25). The procedure can performed under local anesthetic and postoperative recovery time is minimized.

INDICATIONS

The only indication for cervical radiofrequency medial branch neurotomy is the total abolition of pain following controlled diagnostic blocks of the target nerve. Given that there are no valid clinical or radiological manifestations pathognomonic for zygapophysial joint pain, this caveat is absolute if RFN is being offered. RFN should not proceed in the absence of positive diagnostic blocks (26). Partial relief to diagnostic blocks may suggest a placebo or false positive response or that the targeted joint may not be the source of pain and that residual pain may reside in some other cervical structure. Neurotomy in such cases will fail (14,27). Cervical medial branch blocks have a false-positive rate of about 30% (28) and hence diagnostic blocks must be either placebo controlled or comparative (29–31). Studies have confirmed that the cervical zygapophysial joints are a common source of chronic neck pain (32). Given the neurology of chronic neck pain (33), discogenic pain and zygapophysial joint pain are clinically indistinguishable (8,20,34). Hence, any deviation from the diagnostic algorithm will incur poor outcomes (26,29).

Absolute contraindications might include an inability to secure informed consent, untreated infection either systemic or local, bleeding diathesis, patient medically or psychologically unstable, inconclusive diagnostic blocks, patient using anticoagulants, and pregnancy. Relative contraindications include an uncooperative patient, patients on anticoagulants but whose treatment could be temporarily suspended, patients using pacemakers, variations in normal anatomy (congenital or postsurgical) which may compromise the safety of the procedure, accompanying comorbidities which may affect the safe and comfortable conduct of the procedure, immunosuppression, unrealistic expectations by patient or family members, and inadequate relief pain of less than three months duration following previous neurotomy.

PREOPERATIVE PLANNING
Assessment

As with any major surgical procedure, a preoperative risk analysis checklist is advisable. Accurate history taking is essential to evaluate the impact of attending comorbidities such as cardiac or respiratory disorders, or any other medical condition that would impede the safety of the procedure. Adverse reactions to previous operations including general and local anesthetics should be established. Any clinical and anatomical variation of the cervical spine must be carefully evaluated and from the operator's perspective, the proposed trajectory for the insertion of the electrode should be accurately conceptualized. In patients with short muscular necks or high shoulders, denervating the lower facet joints may pose certain physical difficulties including distortion on imaging and electrode placement.

Imaging

Generally, plain X rays should suffice unless there any specific indications for advanced imaging studies. Anatomical variations should be factored in when planning the insertion of the electrode and block needle. Bony outlines may be difficult to visualize in the presence of severe osteopenia or osteoarthrosis. Resolution on fluoroscopic screens may not be optimal, and hence familiarization with the idiosyncrasies associated with RFN is essential both for the surgeon and the radiographer.

Other Considerations

Previous surgery is not an absolute contraindication. RFN can be performed provided controlled diagnostic blocks are positive and the target sites accessible. Distortion on imaging due to postsurgical anatomical changes must be evaluated preoperatively and the procedure planned accordingly. In those patients where radiofrequency neurotomy has been successful, the procedure could be repeated should pain recur (22). How often the procedure can be repeated is not known. With successful coagulation of the target nerve a proportion of the cervical musculature will be denervated. Although it is not known how many nerves could be coagulated, it is inadvisable in the first instance to coagulate more than two nerves either ipsilaterally or bilaterally. It would be prudent not to coagulate any more than three nerves and if additional radiofrequency is indicated, confirmatory diagnostic blocks should be completed to ascertain not only whether the patient's remaining pain is relieved but also to exclude any severe side effects they may suffer when these nerves are blocked.

Bilateral neurotomies of the third occipital nerves deserve special consideration. Unilateral third occipital neurotomy patients do demonstrate a higher level of ataxia; this would be compounded if performed bilaterally. While some patients may tolerate bilateral third occipital neurotomies, in others profound ataxia would be distressing (22). A recommendation would be to treat one side first, and in the absence of severe adverse effects, a subsequent prognostic block of the untreated side should be performed. If the patient suffers no severe side effects, neurotomy may be considered.

Equipment and Personnel

Surgery must be performed in an aseptic environment comparable to an operating theatre. Surgery cannot proceed in the absence of an image intensifier (C-arm or bi-planar) and a complementary radiolucent operating table.

While the newer operating tables can be adjusted for height, it is essential that the width of the operating table permits a free rotation of the C-arm so that the cervical spine could be visualized from any angle within a 270-degree arc. Having the X ray tube encased in a transparent sterile plastic bag would preserve sterility of the operative field. The final placement of each block needle and the electrode must be recorded onto an appropriate device (thermal paper, radiographic plates, or digitally).

It is imperative that the operator is skilled in the use of a fluoroscopic C-arm, and is familiar with the surgical and radiographic anatomy of cervical RFN. Appropriate credentials attesting to the operator's expertise is always advantageous. An assistant should be available to attend to the patient and record the events during the procedure. A certified X ray technician (radiographer) should be well-versed in the idiosyncrasies of imaging for RFN. By anticipating the surgeon's intentions, and by providing the desired projections accurately in a timely manner exposure to radiation, operative times, and patient discomfort can be minimized.

A calibrated radiofrequency generator not only must adequately and unobtrusively illuminate temperature, amperage, voltage, and impedance readings, but it must also be compatible with the attachments including the electrodes (solid-state or a cannula thermocouple combination) and the dispersive/ground plate. The electrical circuit is completed by attaching a ground plate to a large body surface area and by means of a reference lead attached to the generator. Spinal needles must not be used to complete the circuit as the heat generated along the shaft of the needle will cause burns.

The operator and assistant should be surgically gowned complete with mask, headgear, and sterile gloves as they would for any major aseptic procedure. Protective lead-lined cervical collars and aprons should be provided for all personnel within the theatre complex and each individual should be provided with a personalized X ray dosimeter.

For the surgical procedure, generally a basic pack will suffice but the equipment can be assembled to suit the individual operator. By cleansing the skin with approved agents such as an iodine base, or an alcohol preparation for patients allergic to iodine, an optimal aseptic operating field can be secured and shielded by surgical drapes.

Local anesthetic is usually administered using a 2 mL syringe (e.g., containing 2% lidocaine) and a 5 mL syringe (containing 0.5% bupivacaine). To access the target sites including the intended tract of the electrode either a 23 or 25 gauge spinal needle (90 mm/3.5 inches) is generally recommended. A minimal volume extension tubing (6 inches long) connected to the spinal needle, among other things allows the operator to work with the X tube optimally elevated. Maintaining the X ray tube close to the operative field, minimizes the effects of magnification on the monitor screen, reduces scatter radiation and improves radiographic resolution. A number eleven-scalpel blade is used to puncture the skin and the subcutaneous tissue to facilitate an easier introduction of the electrode, particularly if the electrode is equipped with a blunt tip.

BASIC TECHNIQUE
Preoperative Sedation

As a general rule, preoperative medication either systemic analgesics or hypnotics is not required. In the majority of cases, the procedure can be quite safely and comfortably conducted under local anesthetic on the proviso that the patient has been adequately informed during the pre-surgical consultation. Throughout the operation, the patient must be informed as to what is occurring and what might be expected. The patient is encouraged to report any adverse or unpleasant effects. This is not only reassuring for the patient but generates ongoing vigilance on the part of the operator.

Should the patient be unduly apprehensive or agitated, mild sedation may be considered. Under such circumstances a minimal effective dose, which allows the patient to be lucid and conversant throughout the procedure, may be administered. For this reason, general anesthetic is not recommended. Whilst intravenous solutions are not required, maintaining an open venous channel and having the patient connected to a monitoring device including pulse oxymeter would be advantageous and is strongly recommended.

Patient Position

Depending on operator preference, the patient may be positioned either prone or in the lateral position with the target site upper most. Patients find the lateral position more comfortable and less claustrophobic (Fig. 1). In the lateral position the posterior cervical muscles are more relaxed and allows for an easier insertion of the electrode. Visual contact with theatre personnel is often reassuring to the patient. The opportunity to converse allows the operator to extract

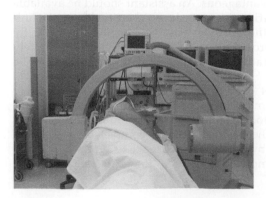

FIGURE 1   Fluoroscope positioned for anteroposterior view.

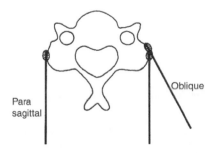

FIGURE 2 Axial view showing electrode placement for the oblique and sagittal insertions. The objective is to create a matrix of lesions along the length of the nerve. *Source*: From Ref. 18.

appropriate feedback whilst the patient's facial features may assist in determining the level of relaxation or distress.

Electrode Placement

The primary objective is to maximally coagulate the target nerve lengthwise by creating a matrix of lesions. This is achieved by placing the exposed tip of the electrode contiguous with (or at least within 1 mm) and parallel to the target nerve so that the entire width of the nerve can be incorporated in the lesion generated. In this regard knowledge of the surgical anatomy (35) and an appreciation of the radiographic anatomy cannot be overstated (26).

Anatomical Considerations

At typical levels (C3-4 to C5-6 inclusive), the zygapophysial joints are innervated by the medial branches of the dorsal rami (35). Emerging from the intervertebral foramen, the dorsal ramus soon divides into a lateral and a medial branch: the latter assumes a curvilinear geometry conforming to the lateral convexity presented by the superior articular process (SAP) in its anterolateral one-third. At about the middle-third of the SAP, the medial branch assumes a more linear trajectory and descends obliquely and posterocaudally. To accommodate these geometrical perturbations, cervical medial branch neurotomy is by necessity a two-stage procedure comprising an oblique and a sagittal insertion ("pass") of the electrode (Fig. 2). The purpose of the oblique pass is to accommodate the curvilinear course of the nerve as it emerges from the intervertebral foramen. This ensures that the exposed tip is no more than 1 mm away from and is parallel to the target nerve along the anterior one-third of the SAP. Likewise the sagittal pass endeavors to coagulate the nerve in the middle-third of the SAP. By maximizing the length of nerve coagulated, rapid regeneration is impeded and duration of relief lengthened. Conversely, single lesions are associated with more rapid recovery and consequent shorter duration of relief (26). RFN is technically demanding and accurate placement of the electrode onto the target nerve is essential.

LEVEL-SPECIFIC DENERVATION TECHNIQUES
Denervation of the C3/4, C4/5, and C5/6 Synovial Joints

The course of the medial branch of the dorsal ramus is determined by the shape of the SAP. The archetypical relationship between nerve and bone is illustrated at the C5 level (19). In the lateral view (Fig. 3A) (19) the C5 medial branch runs obliquely across the centroid of the C5 articular pillar. Topographic variations of the nerve are generally distributed across the middle-fifth of the height of the pillar. In the anteroposterior (AP) view (Fig. 3B), the C5 medial branch occupies the lateral concavity of the articular pillar (Fig. 3).

The C4 medial branch runs slightly higher across the articular pillar. In the lateral projection the nerve may lie anywhere in the upper half of the middle two-quarters of the height of the pillar: in the AP view, it is located in the concavity of the C4 articular pillar (26,35).

In the lateral projection, the C6 medial branch may be located anywhere across the middle two-quarters of the C6 articular pillar; or it may cross the lower end of the C5/6 zygapophysial joint. In the AP view, it often occupies the concavity of the articular pillar: and at times it may lie lateral to the lower half of the convexity of the C5/6 zygapophysial joint (Fig. 3).

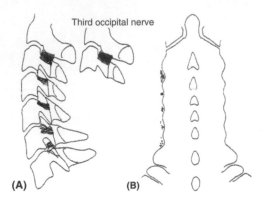

FIGURE 3 Variations in topographical distributions of cervical medial braches. (**A**) Lateral view C5 medial branch is fairly constant but at C3,C4 may occupy higher levels. Insert shows location of the third occipital nerve. (**B**) Anteroposterior view shows the nerves as dots. *Source*: From Ref. 19.

At the C3 level two medial branches are present: the deep C3 medial branch, which innervates the C3/4 joint, and the superficial branch, known as the third occipital nerve (TON), which innervates the C2/3 zygapophysial joint. In the lateral view (Fig. 3), the deeper branch usually runs across the upper half of the C3 articular pillar. Occasionally it may cross the lower half of the C2/3 zygapophysial joint (19,35).

To optimize the outcomes of RFN, these topographical variations in the location of the cervical medial branches have to be considered and accommodated. Single lesions created with small gauge electrodes may not adequately denature the nerve and it is very likely that the nerve will escape coagulation With the exception of the third occipital nerve, all other medial branches are less than 1.0 mm in diameter. Additionally a zone of areolar tissue may displace the nerve from the bone surface by 1 or 2 mm. Hence, with smaller electrodes, multiple lesions are essential to achieve maximal coagulation.

The Oblique Pass

The oblique pass is designed to create a matrix of lesions over the anterior one-third of the SAP as seen in lateral profile, commencing at a level opposite the bottom of the intervertebral foramen and extending cranially to cover at least two-thirds of the height of the SAP.

The size of the nerve, its topographical variations, the size of the electrode and the height of the SAP determines the number of lesions generated. As a rule consecutive placements of the electrode should be no further than one electrode width apart. With a large electrode the SAP could be adequately covered with three lesions. In some cases, two lesions may suffice provided the electrodes are placed no more than one electrode width apart. With smaller diameter electrodes, a greater number of lesions may be required.

The oblique pass is considered to be more difficult. Radiographically, the oblique creates a number of composite shadows. So that the safety of the procedure is not compromised, operators should be well-versed with the radiographic images.

Surgical anesthesia for the oblique pass encompasses two maneuvers:

- Anesthetization of the target sites
- Anesthetization of the tract for the electrode.

Anesthetization of the Target Sites

Preoperatively the C-arm is preferably inverted and elevated such that the concavity of the "C" lies above the patient and all subsequent excursions of the C-arm in the vertical plane are executed above the patient (Fig. 1). From this position a more accurate angulation of the fluoroscope is achievable. Having the C-arm above the patient also overcomes the constraints of the operating table.

Once an aseptic field has been secured, a routine medial branch block is completed (29). Given that the primary objective of an oblique pass is to coagulate the nerves along the anterior one-third of the articular pillar, supplementary local anesthetic is injected onto the target sites to anesthetize the proximal end of the target nerve. The muscles immediately overlying the target sites are similarly anesthetized by withdrawing the needle 2 to 3 mm and reinjecting. Usually, a total volume of 0.5 to 1.0 mL at each site secures adequate anesthesia. Bupivacaine (0.5%) is preferred because of its longer duration of action.

This lateral block needle is repositioned to rest on the bony surface constituting the anterolateral aspect of the target articular pillar. This will serve as a radiographic marker or the "target point" for the insertion of the electrode along the oblique pass.

Anesthetization of the Posterior Cervical Musculature (Electrode Tract)

In a fully conscious patient, who has received no premedication, it is advantageous to adequately anesthetize the projected trajectory within the posterior cervical musculature through which the electrode must pass. Securing muscle relaxation in this manner, facilitates an easier insertion of the electrode, obviates unnecessary distress, ensures greater patient comfort, and prevents movements of the cervical spine during insertions: thus by controlling for image distortion, fewer C-arm maneuvers will minimize exposure to radiation.

With the patient in the lateral position a true anteroposterior projection is initially obtained (Fig. 1). In this view, the odontoid peg should be centralized, asymmetry between the lateral atlantoaxial joints from the midpoint rectified, and the cervical spinous processes should bisect the tracheal shadow.

The patient maintains this position, as the fluoroscope is rotated 30° above the horizontal (Fig. 4) giving an oblique view of the marker needle left in situ, on the anterolateral aspect of the articular pillar and resting on bone. There should be no transparency between the lateral bony outline of the articular pillar and the point of the block/marker needle. This is because if the bony outlines were obscured, then a clearly visible needle tip would serve as the target point.

To anesthetize the entire length of projected tract through the posterior cervical musculature, a 23-gauge 90 mm (3.5 inches) long spinal needle is recommended. The point of entry on the skin overlies, but is slightly lateral to the tip of the marker needle. If the point of entry is medial, the electrode inserted towards the marker needle will be deflected laterally by the edge of the articular pillar and hence some distance away from the target nerve. If the insertion is too medial, interlaminar penetration is likely.

The spinal needle is inserted through the designated point in line with the X-ray beam ("down the beam") thereby maintaining the 30-degree obliquity (Fig. 5). Progression towards the target point should occur in small increments and checked frequently by repeat screening so that the needle does not stray away from its intended path. Any correction in the trajectory is best performed whilst the needle tip is still in the deeper layers of the subcutaneous tissue. In order to prevent too deep an insertion, at the first instance the needle tip should be directed to strike the articular pillar slightly medial to where the block needle rests on the pillar: but at all times the depth of insertion should not exceed the depth of the lateral block/marker needle. On contacting bone, the fluoroscope is rotated to secure a true lateral projection: in this view the track needle is advanced anteriorly along the lateral surface of the SAP, to meet the marker needle or lie in close proximity. Approximately 2 to 3 mL of 2% lidocaine is infiltrated as the

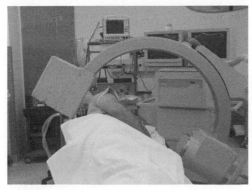

FIGURE 4   Thirty degree oblique projection.

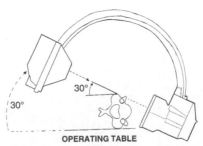

FIGURE 5   Fluoroscope elevated 30° above horizontal for the oblique projection.

tract needle is gently withdrawn through the posterolateral cervical muscles, ensuring that the skin is adequately anesthetized prior to withdrawing the track needle.

Insertion of the Electrode for the Oblique Pass

Before inserting the electrode, radiographic alignment must to be rechecked and reinstated as the patient may have moved. With the patient in the lateral position, a true AP projection is once more secured (Fig. 1). The position of the block/marker needle is reaffirmed ensuring that the marker needle remains in contact with bone. The fluoroscopic tube is elevated 30 degrees above the horizontal, as for the tract needle (Figs. 4 and 5). If the skin is sufficiently anesthetized, a stab incision is made through the skin and subcutaneous tissue to facilitate an easier introduction of the electrode. Maintaining the fluoroscope in a 30-degree oblique projection, the electrode is inserted through the puncture wound in line with the X ray beam. The electrode is advanced in small increments through the posterior neck muscles, towards the tip of the marker needle, its progress monitored by repeated screening. The electrode tip should be directed to strike the articular pillar immediately medial to the tip of the marker needle, thereby avoiding too deep an insertion. Once contact has been established, the electrode is redirected so as to "gently slip" past the lateral margin of the pillar, by gliding anteriorly a few millimeters only; throughout maintaining contact medially with the articular pillar. A lateral projection is now reinstated. The anterior border of the SAP must be sharply defined, errors of parallax rectified and the tip of the electrode resting on the SAP. Advancement of the electrode tip anterior to the posterior edge of the articular pillar or its placement should always be performed under lateral fluoroscopy. To prevent overinsertion, the electrode is gently advanced by simultaneously oscillating the shaft within minor excursions, and applying gentle forward movements, rather than "a thrusting motion." Throughout, the tip should remain in contact with the articular pillar medially whilst covering the anterolateral aspect of the pillar. At no stage should the tip of the electrode advance beyond the anterior margin of the articular pillar.

Conventionally the first placement should be opposite the trough of the intervertebral foramen and once achieved, the electrode is held in place whilst the position is checked, confirmed and recorded on both lateral and AP films prior to generating the lesion. The lateral projection should ensure that the electrode has not been inserted too far forwards or inadvertently expelled. The tip of the electrode should coincide with the anterior margin of the articular pillar (Fig. 6). Contact with the articular pillar is confirmed in the AP view and because of its the oblique introduction, the tip of the electrode lies in front of the anterolateral aspect of the SAP, and hence on the AP projection the electrode tip may appear just medial to the lateral silhouette of the articular pillar (Fig. 7). There should be no gray or white shadows between the electrode and the lateral margin of the articular pillar.

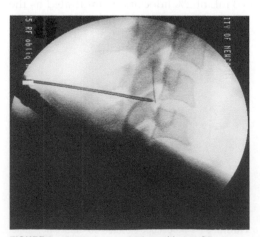

FIGURE 6   Oblique pass, high position at C5.

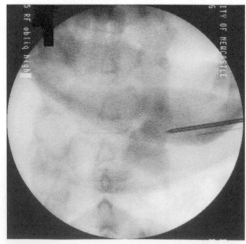

FIGURE 7   Anteroposterior view C5. Note close contact with lateral surface of superior articular process.

The marker needle is withdrawn about 5 mm to avoid contact with the electrode, lest coagulation occurs also along the marker needle causing superficial burns.

Prior to generating a lesion, ensure the circuit is complete, the patient is attached to the generator by a large dispersive plate, and the marker needle adequately withdrawn and the generator records body temperature.

Once correct placement has been achieved, confirmed and recorded, a lesion is created by raising the temperate one degree per second to no less than 80°C and no more than 85°C. For the oblique pass, temperature should not exceed 80°C. Once this level has been reached, the temperature is maintained for 90 seconds. From the moment heating commences, the operator maintains a firm hold on the electrode (by hand) lest the electrode is expelled by muscle tension. If larger electrodes are used, the weight of the hub if left unsupported may cause the electrode tip to rotate or displace laterally. Hence, the position of the electrode should be checked periodically by lateral fluoroscopy to ensure that it has not moved.

If during the procedure the patient reports symptoms of any kind, the operation should be terminated, nature of symptoms ascertained, interpreted, and rectified. The sensation of local pain or heat at the site of electrode tip may warrant supplementary local anesthetic through the marker needle. If other symptoms occur, the position of the electrode should be checked and rectified accordingly. Once remedial action has been effected and there are no contraindications, coagulation can proceed. If symptoms recur, and which cannot be adequately addressed or rectified by the above measures, the procedure should be abandoned.

With the completion of the first lesion, the electrode is carefully and only slightly withdrawn, at all times avoiding a sudden expulsion of the electrode. Preferably the electrode should not be withdrawn beyond the posterior margin of the articular pillar, as contact with the pillar will be lost. The entire process must be monitored under lateral fluoroscopy. Usually the electrode is withdrawn, no further than the middle of the articular pillar from where it is redirected to a new position. Under lateral projection, the electrode is readjusted to each of the subsequent positions. It is essential that placements be confirmed by repeated imaging. Should the electrode loose contact with the articular pillar readjustment should be completed under AP screening so as to ensure its lateral relationship to the articular pillar. With each subsequent placement the same precautions apply. Once the final lesion has been completed, the electrode is completely withdrawn and slight pressure is maintained over the surgical site to minimize bleeding and hematoma formation.

The Sagittal Pass

The objective of the sagittal pass is to coagulate the nerve as it passes along the middle two-thirds of the articular pillar as seen in the lateral projection. Segmentally, the relationship of the nerve to the height of the pillar shows slight variation. The C5 medial branch normally occupies the middle two-fourths whilst the C3, C4, and C6 are somewhat higher (Fig. 3).

Not dissimilar to the oblique pass, the number of lesions required depends on the size of the electrode and the height of the pillar. With large gauge electrodes, two or three lesions may suffice where as with smaller electrodes a larger number of lesions may be required. As for the oblique pass, lesions should be placed no greater than one electrode width apart.

Surgical anesthesia for the sagittal pass includes:

- Anesthetization of the target sites and
- Anesthetization of the proposed tract.

Anesthetization of the Target Sites

In the lateral projection the block/marker needle used during the oblique pass is readjusted and supplementary aliquots of 0.5% bupivacaine (0.5 mL) are deposited onto each of the designated target site. The marker needle then rests firmly upon the centroid of the articular pillar and the AP projection reinstated.

Anesthetization of the Posterior Cervical Musculature (Electrode Tract)

For the sagittal pass, a new tract is established through the posterior neck muscles. To avoid the flanges of the zygapophysial joints, the electrodes are inserted in a cephaloanterior direction,

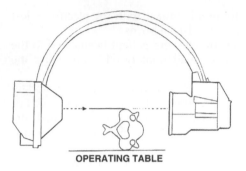

OPERATING TABLE

FIGURE 8   Position of fluoroscope to obtain anteroposterior view. Axial view of C spine showing trajectory for parasagittal pass.

and as parallel as possible to the plane of the zygapophysial joint. Consequently the point of entry for the electrode is caudal to the target point for the nerve.

To locate this caudal point of entry on the lateral projection, the tip of a metallic marker (e.g., spinal needle) is placed on the skin and over the target articular pillar with its shaft parallel to the slope of the targeted zygapophysial joint. The point at which the shaft of the metallic marker intersects with the skin of the back at the neck, establishes the posteroanterior trajectory and the level of the puncture point on the skin.

In the AP projection, the mediolateral entry point lies on the transverse line established for the caudocephaloid trajectory and on a horizontal line that passes just lateral to the lateral margin of the target pillar. Positioning is always confirmed by repeat fluoroscopy. Having localized the puncture point, the track needle is advanced in an anterocephalad direction towards the marker needle, the latter firmly resting on the target site (Fig. 8). To prevent over-insertion, it is essential to periodically monitor the progress of the block needle with a view of striking bone immediately medial to the tip of the marker needle. A minor readjustment thereafter would allow the block needle to enter the lateral concavity of the articular pillar. At this juncture lateral fluoroscopy is advisable. This would ensure that the block needle has not advanced beyond the anterior margin of the articular process and remains in close proximity to the marker needle. The tract needle is gently withdrawn while simultaneously injecting 2 to 3 mL of 2% lidocaine and ensuring adequate anesthetization of the skin at the designated point of entry.

Electrode Insertion for the Sagittal Pass
As for the oblique pass, a stab incision creates an entry portal for the electrode. With the patient in the lateral position, a true anterior posterior projection is secured. To prevent distortion of the image on the convex screen, the target area is centralized on the active monitor. The electrode is inserted through the puncture point and is advanced in small increments through the posterior neck muscle. At inception the electrode should be directed to land on the articular pillar immediately medial to the tip of the marker needle thereby preventing too deep an insertion (Figs. 2 and 8). Upon contact, the electrode is redirected so as to "just slip past" the lateral margin of the pillar by a few millimeters only. Using fine pincer movements, the shaft of the electrode is supported between the tips of the thumb and index finger, just one centimeter away from the skin so that as the electrode is advanced anteriorly over the edge of the articular pillar. Overinsertion is prevented by contact of the operator's fingers with the patient's skin. To prevent dislodgment, the electrode is held firmly in the operator's hand, and the C-arm rotated to secure a lateral projection.

Under lateral fluoroscopy, the electrode is gently advanced so that the tip remains in contact with the articular pillar medially. Often, a distinctive tactile quality is perceptible as the electrode slides across bone. At all times, and particularly where pointed electrodes are used, forceful thrusting motions are best avoided, lest the sudden propulsive motion causes an avulsive fracture of the target nerve. The retracted nerve ends may not be amenable to lesioning and a functional neuroma is likely. At the first instance, the electrode should cover the center of the lateral aspect of the articular pillar and the first placement could be opposite the geometric center of the articular pillar. In the lateral view, the uninsulated tip of the electrode should

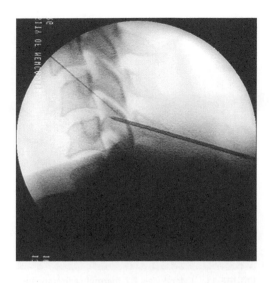

FIGURE 9 C5 sagittal pass. Electrode inserted parallel to nerve. Active tip lies on the centroid of the SAP.

cover at least the middle-third of the articular pillar as measured from front to back (Fig. 9). Once adequate placement has been achieved, the operator holds the electrode in place, and on the AP projection contact with the articular pillar is confirmed. The electrode is seen end-on with no gray or white shadows (transparencies) between it and the lateral margin of the articular pillar. Prior to generating a lesion, lateral projection is reinstated and the position of the electrode confirmed, ensuring that the tip has neither advanced beyond the anterior margin of the pillar, nor has it been expelled posteriorly. The block needle is withdrawn 5 to 10 mm, the electrode placement is recorded appropriately on both the lateral and AP projections and the lesion is generated by raising the temperature one degree per second to no less than 80°C and no more than 85°C. The temperature is maintained at 85 degrees for 90 seconds. Throughout the period of lesion generation, the electrode should be held firmly in place, and position confirmed by periodic screening in the lateral projection. The same precautions, caveats, and conditions apply as for the oblique pass.

Once the first lesion has been created, the electrode is carefully withdrawn by oscillating the shaft within small excursions: but not beyond the posterior margin of the articular pillar. The electrode is then readjusted to any of the subsequent positions (Fig. 9). Provided the electrode tip maintains contact with the articular pillar, all adjustments are usually completed under the lateral projection. Should the electrode loose contact with the articular pillar (slip off the posterior margin), it should be reinserted under AP projection and once secured further adjustments must be completed under lateral fluoroscopy. The same precautions apply for every lesion created. A permanent record of each placement must be secured.

Denervation of the C6/7 Zygapophysial Joint

The C6/7 zygapophysial joint is also dually innervated, receiving fibers from the C6 and C7 dorsal rami (35). To effectively coagulate the medial branch of the C6 dorsal ramus, both the oblique and sagittal placements, as described are essential.

At the C7 level, the same technical principles and precautions apply. Because the C7 SAP is small, only a sagittal pass is required. Unlike a typical medial branch (e.g., C6), the C7 medial branch most often crosses the triangular SAP of C7 and not the waist. It may also occupy a more lateral and inferior location, crossing the superior surface of the proximal end of the C7 transverse process (Fig. 10). On the AP projection; the nerve is most often located in the groove formed by the junction of the C7 SAP and the root of the C7 transverse process. Occasionally it may be displaced more cephalad towards the tip of the SAP or further lateral over the root of the transverse process. Hence, to accommodate these topographical variations, multiple placements of the electrode are essential (Fig. 11).

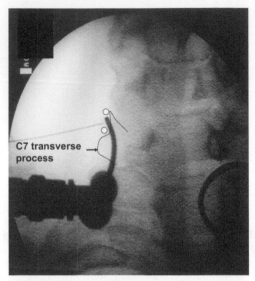

FIGURE 10   Anteroposterior view for C7 thermal radiofrequency neurotomy. Note variable position of the nerve and the relationship to the transverse process and the superior articular process.

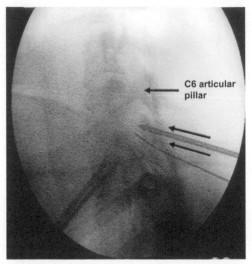

FIGURE 11   Lateral view C7 thermal radiofrequency neurotomy. Electrode occupies mid position of the superior articular process. *Arrows* indicate additional two positions.

Securing an optimal operating field can be difficult, particularly in patients with a short muscular neck or tall shoulders. The ideal radiographic depiction of the C7 articular pillar may not always be easily acquired. Prior to attempting RFN at the C7 level, practitioners should familiarize themselves with the radiographic idiosyncrasies encountered at this level. Operators should be aware that the SAP of C7 is small, triangular in shape and unlike the diamond shape encountered at typical levels. Counting from C1 should always identify the seventh cervical vertebrae.

Surgical Anesthesia for C7 Medial Branch Neurotomy
As with other levels, both the target sites and the posterior cervical musculature are anesthetized separately.

Anesthetization of the Target Sites
The lateral block/marker needle is landed onto the superior articular pillar just below its apex: prior to injecting the local anesthetic, check position of the needle on the AP view, lest the needle tip is far too lateral, having landed on lateral border of the transverse process. Should this eventuate, needle repositioning must always be performed in the lateral projection: for, in the AP projection there is always the danger of entering the intervertebral foramen. Once adequate placement has been achieved, a small aliquot (1 mL) of 0.5% bupivacaine is injected. To accommodate the possibility that the medial branch may cross the root of the transverse process, the marker needle is repositioned to land at the base of the triangular SAP: needle tip position rechecked in the AP projection to ensure needle placement is not too far lateral: ideally the needle tip should firmly rest on bone, in a groove formed by the root of the transverse process and the base of the SAP (29).

Anesthetization of the Posterior Cervical Musculature (Electrode Tract)
For the sagittal pass, the posterior cervical muscles are anesthetized as described previously. In the AP projection, a point of entry is selected on the skin to overlie the junction between the SAP and the transverse process of C7. The spinal needle is introduced until it strikes the rear of either the SAP or the transverse process Two milliliters of 2% lignocaine is injected as the needle is slowly withdrawn and a puncture wound is created as described previously.

Electrode Insertion for the Sagittal Pass

Only a sagittal pass is required. With the patient in the lateral position a true AP projection is secured. The electrode is inserted through the point of entry, initially directed to strike the back of the SAP, while the tip of the marker needle rests at a point just below the apex of the triangular SAP. As for the other levels, once contact is made with the bony surface, the electrode is redirected laterally so as to just slip onto the lateral surface of the SAP. Once the posterior border of the SAP has been engaged, further anterior advancement is completed under lateral projection.

As a matter of convenience, the tip is directed to cover the apex of the SAP, ensuring at all times that the tip of the electrode does not venture anterior to the posterior margin of the C6/7 intervertebral foramen (Fig. 11). Once adequate placement is achieved, the electrode is held firmly in place, and the position checked in the AP view. The electrode must lie snugly against the lateral surface of the SAP. Soft tissue interposing between the electrode and bony surface may promote a too smooth or a too rapid an insertion and hence thrusting motions are best avoided. The lesion is generated following the same precautions and protocols and permanent record is obtained.

Subsequent placement should ensure that the entire height of the lateral surface of the SAP has been adequately covered by lesions, (Fig. 11) and the electrode is thereafter repositioned across the superior aspect of the transverse process until about 5 mm of the proximal transverse process has been covered with lesions. It is essential that a number of lesions be generated so as to accommodate all possible variations in the location of the nerve (Fig. 10).

Denervation of the C2/3 Zygapophysial Joint (Third Occipital Nerve Neurotomy)

The C2/3 zygapophysial joint is innervated by a single nerve, the superficial medial branch of the C3 dorsal ramus, known as the third occipital nerve (TON). A large nerve, with a diameter of 1.5 to 2.0 mm, it furnishes an articular branch to the C2/3 facet joint as it initially winds around the lateral and subsequently the posterior aspect of the joint (Fig. 12). The joint may also receive articular branches from a communicating loop formed between the third occipital nerve and the C2 dorsal ramus (35). Unlike the medial branches at typical levels, the third occipital nerve has a transverse trajectory and it is the only dorsal ramus that crosses a zygapophysial joint.

The nerve may lie anywhere from opposite the apex of the C3 SAP to opposite the bottom of the trough formed by the C2/3 intervertebral foramen (Fig. 13). In the AP view, either the deep medial branch or the third occipital nerve may occupy the concavity of the C3 articular pillar (Fig. 3). More often, the third occipital nerve courses along the lower half of the convexity of the C2/3 zygapophysial joint, but an overlap in locations is not uncommon (35). Given its transverse trajectory, the plane of insertion of the electrodes is a critical factor and the target points are different. Irrespective, both the oblique and the sagittal insertions are essential.

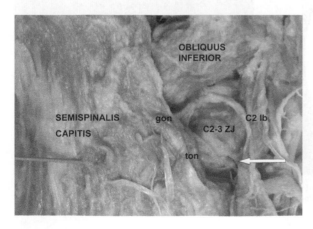

FIGURE 12 Dissection specimen at the C2/3 level. *Arrow* points to the large third occipital nerve. *Source*: Courtesy of Department of Clinical Research, University of Newcastle.

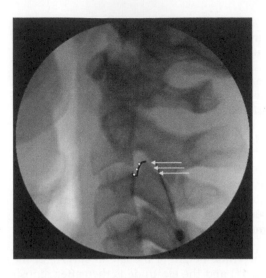

FIGURE 13 Lateral cervical spine. The *white* dots represent three possible positions of the third occipital nerve. *Arrows* indicate the transverse trajectory of the electrode for the oblique and sagittal pass. The anterior margin of the superior articular process has been highlighted to show the "j" curve.

For the oblique pass, the primary objective is to create as many lesions as possible that would cover the entire anterolateral surface of the SAP of C3, from the apex, to a point, which lies opposite to the bottom of the trough of the C2/3 intervertebral foramen, the bony contours of which form a "j" curve (Fig. 13). On the lateral projection, the uninsulated portion of electrode should cover the anterior third of the SAP of C3 so that the pointed tip coincides with the anterior margin of the SAP but not projecting beyond (Fig. 14). Because of its oblique introduction, the tip of the electrode on the AP projection lies just medial to the lateral silhouette of the C2/3 zygapophysial joint, given that the electrode lies anterolateral to the lateral edge of the SAP (Fig. 15).

With respect to the sagittal pass, the primary objective is to cover the entire lateral surface of the joint and as many lesions as necessary are generated to cover entirely the middle third of the SAP from the apex to the base as for the oblique pass. In the lateral projection, the uninsulated portion of the electrode lies over the middle third of the C2/3 zygapophysial joint (Fig. 13). In the AP view, the electrode abuts against the lateral convexity of the joint.

By slightly rotating or extending the neck, superimposed mandibular and dental silhouettes can be overcomed. Occasionally an open-mouth view will offer greater clarity of the target area (Fig. 15).

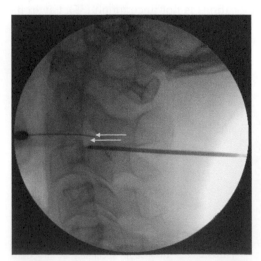

FIGURE 14 The three electrode placements for thermal radiofrequency neurotomy of the third occipital nerve oblique pass.

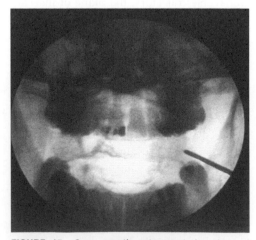

FIGURE 15 Open mouth anteroposterior view, of Figure 14, depicting electrode in close contact with lateral margin of C3 superior articular process.

Anesthetization of the Target Sites (Oblique Pass)

So that the proximal end of the third occipital nerve is adequately anesthetized, the lateral block/marker needle is aimed over the anterolateral aspect of the C3 SAP and an appropriate volume of long acting local anesthetic is injected onto the target sites where lesioning would occur. Upon completion, the lateral block needle is left in place, preferably midway between the apex of the C3 SAP and at a point opposite the trough of the "j" shaped intervertebral foramen: the marker needle at all times maintaining firm contact with bone.

Anesthetization of the Posterior Neck Musculature (Electrode Tract)

With the patient in the lateral position, a true AP projection is once more secured: from this position the X-ray tube is elevated 30 degrees above the horizontal, which allows for the completion of the oblique pass. The posterior neck muscles are anesthetized as previously described and the block needle is inserted "down the beam." Once the needle tip makes contact with the lateral margin of the articular pillar, further advancements across the pillar are executed in the lateral projection, so that the tip of the tract needle meets the tip of the marker needle. About 2 to 3 mL of 2% lidocaine is injected to anaesthetize the intended tract as the needle is slowly withdrawn.

Insertion of the Electrode

In the oblique projection, a stab incision facilitates the easier introduction of the electrode. Its progress through the posterior cervical muscles should occur in small increments and in the first instance the electrode is projected slightly medial to the block needle so as to abut against the rear of the C3 SAP. This safety measure prevents the electrode from being inserted too far. Upon contact, the electrode is readjusted to gently "slip past" by a few millimeters and whilst the operator secures the electrode with his hand, the C-arm is rotated and further adjustments of the electrode are executed on the lateral projection.

    The third occipital nerve is a relatively large nerve and the number of lesions generated would depend on the height of the articular pillar, electrode size, and topographic variations of the nerve. With a large electrode, sufficient coagulation can be achieved with three or four lesions.

    Conventionally, the high placement should be opposite the apex of the C3 SAP, that is, the apex of the "j" curve: whilst the low placement would be opposite the bottom of C2/3 intervertebral foramen or the trough of the "j" curve (Fig. 13). The mid placement is between these two positions. As always, prior to lesion creation, the electrode position should be checked in the AP projection (Fig. 15). Because of its oblique insertion, the tip of the electrode projects just medial to the lateral margin of the silhouette of the C3 SAP. A lesion is created in the usual manner and as a precautionary measure lesion temperature must not extend beyond 80°C lest excess heat extends ventrally.

    For the sagittal pass, the same protocol is adopted and lesions are generated over the lateral aspect of the C2/3 joint. As for the oblique pass, the electrode is inserted transversely, in order to maintain parallelility with the target nerve (Figs. 13 and 14). At the first instance, contact is established with the posterior aspect of the joint and thereafter the electrode is gently advanced anteriorly by a few millimeters. All further placements of the electrode are executed on a lateral projection. With each placement, the active tip of the electrode should cover the middle third of the lateral aspect of the C2/3 zygapophysial joint.

    The target sites along the height of the pillar are as for the oblique pass. In the high position, the tip of the electrode lies opposite the apex of the C3 SAP (or the apex of the "j curve"): in the low position, the electrode lies opposite the bottom of the C2/3 intervertebral foramen (the trough of the "j" curve): and in the mid position the electrode lies in-between (Fig. 13). Frequent scanning in both the AP and lateral projections should ensure that the electrode has not strayed away and lies in close apposition with the bony margin. When viewed in the AP projection, in the "high position" the electrode normally lies opposite the mid point of the rounded eminence of the C2/3 zygapophysial joint. In the mid position, it lies opposite of the middle of the lower half of the joint whilst in the low position, it is normally just above the waist of the C3 SAP. For the sagittal pass, lesions can be generated at 85°C and this temperature is maintained for 90 seconds. Permanent records are maintained for each electrode placement.

Postoperative Care

Upon completion, needles and electrodes are removed, the skin is cleansed with antiseptic alcohol preparation, and a small adhesive pressure dressing is applied.

Before arising, the patient should be warned and reminded that they might experience ataxia or unsteadiness, more so when third occipital neurectomy is performed. They should be encouraged to engage visual cues and preferably should not be allowed to ambulate for at least the next 30 minutes.

Patients are always discharged into the care of a responsible adult who would be able to escort and drive the patient home. At no stage must the patient be allowed to drive a motor vehicle, as there is the danger that sudden turning may cause an episode of light headiness or ataxia. Cold packs are applied for at least a day or two and simple analgesics prescribed on a time contingent basis. Very occasionally, patients may require opioid medications for postoperative pain. Postsurgical progress is monitored closely on an outpatient basis, at least for the first three weeks and thereafter on a need basis. The operating practitioner should always be available to address any unusual symptoms or side effects. Patients should be provided with contact telephone numbers.

CLINICAL OUTCOMES

Proper patient selection and the operator's proficiency in executing the procedure are the cardial prerequisites in determining the efficacy of cervical medial branch RFN. In the earlier observational studies (6–12), "success' was a variable commodity and the relief of pain was described either numerically (percentage reduction) or descriptively (excellent, good, and fair). The aggregate data suggested that between 50% and 90% of patients secured 40% relief of their index pain (13,19): only a few studies reporting total relief of pain for greater than two months (12).

Later investigators adopted a more stringent definition, and "success" was deemed to include the complete relief of pain, the restoration of the impaired activities of daily living and requiring no other form of health services (18,20–22). If diagnostic blocks conferred total relief of pain, then RFN properly executed must also generate the same outcome and for a lasting period. A response other than complete relief of pain infers incorrect patient selection and/or imperfect execution of the procedure.

If patients are properly selected and the procedure meticulously applied, then complete relief of pain for a durable period can be achieved. Lord et al. (13) showed that the complete relief of the patient's index pain following controlled diagnostic blocks was the cardinal indication. In a double blind controlled trial, 24 patients were equally randomized to receive either the active treatment or a placebo. In the control group, the median time for recurrence of pain was eight days: whereas in the active group, the mean duration for total relief of pain was 263 days (18). Long-term studies by the same group, confirmed that at least 64% of the patients continued to report complete relief of pain for a median duration of 421 days (20), and litigation did not affect the outcome (20–22).

Comparable outcomes were recently reported for the treatment of third occipital headaches (22). Based on the anatomical and radiographic variations of the third occipital nerve, a larger electrode was placed such that consecutive lesions were generated no further than one electrode width apart and the electrode was held in position throughout the period of coagulation. Of the 49 patients operated upon, 86% reported complete relief of pain. At the time of publication, the median duration for the complete relief of pain was 297 days with eight patients still reporting complete relief. Fourteen patients underwent repeat neurotomy when their index pain returned. Complete relief was reinstated in 12 (86%), following confirmatory diagnostic blocks.

Three independent reviews have not only unambiguously confirmed the efficacy of RFN as a valid treatment for proven cervical zygapophysial joint pain (36–38), but also reinforced the cardinal precepts that proper patient selection and accurate application of the procedure is paramount.

COMPLICATIONS

In addition to the more common side effects associated with this procedure (Table 1), RFN to the third occipital nerve generates a different set of side effects (Table 2). This nerve has a

TABLE 1 Incidences of Side Effects Following Neurotomy at Typical Cervical Levels (C3–C7)

Side effect	Incidence[a]
Vasovagal syncope	2%
Dermoid cyst	1%
Kobner's phenomenon	1%
Neuritis	2%
Numbness in the cutaneous territory of one of the coagulated nerves	29%
Dysesthesia in the cutaneous territory of one of the nerves coagulated	19%

[a]The neurological side effects were neither lasting nor required treatment.
Source: From Refs. 18–20, 39.

TABLE 2 Incidence of Side Effects Following
Third Occipital Nerve Neurotomy

Side effect	Incidence
Numbness	97%
Ataxia	95%
Dysesthesia	55%
Hypersensitivity	15%
Itch	10%

Source: From Ref. 22.

significant role in maintaining cervical proprioception and also has a small but constant cutaneous distribution. Table 2 lists the incidence of the known side-effects. The ataxia is not disabling provided the patient is encouraged to rely on visual cues to locate horizontal objects. Dysesthesia and hypersensitivity to touch resolve within one to two weeks; in one case, it lasted for six weeks. In the referenced study, none required any treatment (Table 2) (22).

The following are potential complications:

- Anaphylaxis or allergic reactions to latex, skin cleansing agents, and local anesthetics.
- Infection and hematoma.
- Injury to the spinal cord, dorsal root ganglion, ventral ramus, vertebral, and radicular arteries. By introducing the electrode in a posterior to anterior direction, the trauma of insertion is limited to the skin and the posterior cervical musculature. Ensuring that the tip of the electrode remains behind the posterior margin of the intervertebral foramen and lateral to the lateral surface of the SAP, injuries to the vital structures are avoided. Hence from inception to the moment of final electrode placement, frequent fluoroscopic monitoring remains paramount.
- Burns. Provided that a compatible dispersive/ground plate of a large surface area is correctly applied, skin burns should not occur. Spinal needles or similar are best avoided: this would act like an antenna and current density would concentrate along the uninsulated portion causing burns along its length.

Charcot's joints. The concept of Charcot's joints is often raised as a theoretical consideration in discussion forums (40); yet Charcot's joints are an unlikely event. Commonly encountered in tertiary syphilis and diabetes, neuropathic joints are primarily neurovascular in origin and not due to neurotrauma (41,42). Charcot's joints principally occur in weight bearing joints in which the muscles and other tissues are anesthetic. Manifestations indicate an injury to the afferent pathways of pain and proprioception, which can occur in fibers ranging from peripheral nerves to the spinal cord (43). RF does not render the functional cervical unit insensate. Within the three joint complex, the contralateral zygapophysial joint, the ipsisegmental intervertebral disc and the surrounding muscle retain their innervation, while the orientation of the articular facet maintains the mechanical stability (44). For each nerve coagulated only about 16% to 20% of the multifidus and the semispinalis cervicis are denervated (29). Coagulation is not permanent and in some experimental animals, the nerve begins to regenerate within two weeks of injury (45–47). Arthropathy may also develop in advance of neurological changes (48). No such complications have been reported.

REFERENCES

1. Rovit RL. Percutaneous radiofrequency thermal coagulation of the gasserian ganglion. In: Rovit RL, Murali R, Jannetta PL, eds. Trigeminal Neuralgia. Baltimore: Williams and Wilkins, 1990:109–136.
2. White JC, Sweet WH. Pain and the Neurosurgeon. Illinois: Thomas Springfield, 1969:184:603.
3. Sweet WH, Wespic JG. Controlled thermocoagulation of the trigeminal ganglion and rootlets for differential destruction of pain fibers. J Neurosurg 1975; 43:143–156.
4. Taha JM, Tew JM. Comparison of surgical treatments for trigeminal neuralgia: re evaluation of radiofrequency rhizotomy. Neurosurgery 1996; 38:865–871.
5. Shealy CN. Percutaneous radiofrequency denervation of the lumbar facets. J Neurosurg 1975; 43:143–156.
6. Schaerer JP. Radiofrequency facet rhizotomy in the treatment of chronic neck and low back pain. Int Surg 1978; 63:53–59.
7. Schaerer JP. Radiofrequency facet denervation in the treatment of persistent headache associated with chronic neck pain. J Neurol Orthop Surg 1980; 1:127–130.
8. Schaerer JP. Treatment of prolonged neck pain by radiofrequency facet rhizotomy. J Neurol Orthop Med Surg 1988; 9:74–76.
9. Hildebrandt J, Argyrakis A. Percutaneous nerve block of the cervical facets—a relatively new method in the treatment of chronic headache and neck pain. Manual Medicine 1986; 2:48–52.
10. Sluijter ME, Koetsveld-Baart CC. Interruption of pain pathways in the treatment of the cervical syndrome. Anaesthesia 1980; 35:302–307.
11. Sluijter ME, Mehta M. Treatment of chronic neck and back pain by percutaneous thermal lesions. In: Lipton S, Miles J, eds. Persistent Pain: Modern Methods of Treatment. London: Academic Press and New York: Grune & Stratton, 1981:3:141–179.
12. Vervest ACM, Stolker RJ, Groen GJ. Radiofrequency lesioning for pain treatment: a review. Pain Clinic 1995; 8:175–189.
13. Lord SM, Barnsley L, Bogduk N. Percutaneous radiofrequency neurotomy in the treatment of cervical zygapophysial joint pain: a caution. Neurosurgery 1995; 36:732–739.
14. Stovner LJ, Kolstad F, Helde G. Radiofrequency denervation of facet joints C2–6 in cervicogenic headaches: a randomised double blind sham controlled study. Cephalalgia 2004; 24:821–830.
15. McCulloch JA. Percutaneous radiofrequency lumbar rhizolysis (rhizotomy). Appl Neurophysiol 1976/77; 39:87–96.
16. Mehta M, Sluijter ME. The treatment of chronic back pain. Anaesthesia 1979; 34:768–775.
17. Ogsbury JS, Simon RH, Lehman RAW. Facet denervation in the treatment of low back syndrome. Pain 1977; 3:257–263.
18. Lord SM, Barnsley L, Wallis B, McDonald GJ, Bogduk N. Percutaneous radiofrequency neurotomy for chronic cervical zygapophysial joint pain. N Eng J Med 1996; 335:1721–1726.
19. Lord SM, McDonald GJ, Bogduk N. Percutaneous radiofrequency neurotomy of the cervical medial branches: a validated treatment for cervical zygapophysial joint pain. Neurosurgery Quarterly 1998; 8:288–308.
20. McDonald GJ, Lord SM, Bogduk N. Long -term follow-up of patients treated with cervical radiofrequency neurotomy for chronic neck pain. Neurosurgery 1999; 45:61–68.
21. Sapir DA, Gorup JM. Radiofrequency medial branch neurotomy in litigant and nonlitigant patients with cervical whiplash. Spine 2001; 26:E268–E273.
22. Govind J, King W, Bailey B, Bogduk N. Radiofrequency neurotomy for the treatment of third occipital headache. J Neurol Neurosurg Psychiat 2003; 74:88–93.
23. Organ LW. Electro physiologic principles of radiofrequency lesion making. Appl Neurophysiol 1976; 39:69–76.
24. Zervas NT, Kuwayama A. Pathological characteristics of experimental thermal lesions. Comparison of induction heating and radiofrequency electrocoagulation. J Neurosurg 1972; 37:418–422.
25. Cosman ER, Blaine S, Nashbold MD, Ovelman-Levitt J. Theoretical aspects of radiofrequency lesions in the dorsal root entry zone. Neurosurgery 1984; 15:945–950.
26. International Spine Intervention Society. Percutaneous radiofrequency: cervical medial branch neurotomy. In: Bogduk N, ed. Practice Guidelines for Spinal Diagnostic and Treatment Procedures. San Francisco: International Spine Intervention Society, 2004:249–284.
27. Bogduk, N. Cervicogenic headache (editorial). Cephalalgia 2004; 24:819–820.
28. Barnsley L, Lord SM, Wallis B, Bogduk N. False positive rates of cervical zygapophysial joint blocks. Clin J Pain 1993; 9:124–130.
29. International Spine Interventional Society. Cervical medial branch blocks. In: Bogduk N, ed. Practice Guidelines for Spinal Diagnostic and Therapeutic Procedures. San Francisco: International Spine Intervention Society, 2004:112–137.
30. Barnsley L, Lord S, Bogduk N. Comparative anaesthetic blocks in the diagnosis of zygapophysial joint pain. Pain 1993; 55:99–106.
31. Bogduk N. Diagnostic blocks. In: Clark CR, ed. The Cervical Spine. The Cervical Spine Research Society. 4th ed. New York: Lippincott Williams & Wilkins, 2005:255–260.

32. Bogduk N. The anatomy and pathophysiology of neck pain. Phys Med Rehabil Clin N Am 2003; 14:455–472.
33. Barnsley L, Lord S, Bogduk N. The pathophysiology of whiplash. Spine: State of the Art Reviews 1993; 7:329–353.
34. Aprill C, Bogduk N. On the nature of neck pain, discography and cervical zygapophysial joint blocks. Pain 1993; 54:213–217.
35. Bogduk N. The clinical anatomy of the cervical dorsal rami. Spine 1982; 7:319–330.
36. British Columbia Office of Health Technology Assessment. Percutaneous radio-frequency neurotomy treatment of chronic cervical pain following whiplash injury. Vancouver: The University of British Columbia, 2001.
37. Cousins MJ, Walker S. Chronic pain: management strategies that work. Anaesthesia and Analgesia 2001; 92(suppl 3):15–25.
38. Boswell MV, Shah RV, Everett CR, et al. Interventional techniques in the management of chronic spinal pain; evidence—based practice guidelines. Pain Physician 2005; 8:1–47.
39. Lord SM, McDonald GJ, Bogduk N. Side effects and complications of cervical percutaneous radiofrequency neurotomy—an audit of 83 procedures.(abstract). Anaesth Intensive Care 1998; 26:322–328.
40. Drinka PJ, Jaschob K. Treatment of chronic cervical zygapophysial joint pain (letter). N Eng J Med 1997; 336:1530.
41. CW Hutton. Osteoarthritis. In Weatherall DJ, Ledingham JGG, Warrell DA, eds. Oxford Textbook of Medicine. 3rd ed. Oxford: Oxford University Press, 1996:2979.
42. Allman RM, Brower AC, Kotlyarov EB. Neuropathic bone and joint disease. Radiol Clin North Am 1988; 26:1373–1381.
43. Mohit AA, Mirza S, James J, Goodkin R. Charcot arthropathy in relation to autonomic dysreflexia in spinal cord injury. J Neurosurg Spine 2005; 2:476–480.
44. Lord SM, Bogduk N. treatment of chronic zygapophysial joint pain (letter) N Eng J Med 1997; 336:1531.
45. Hamann W, Hall S. Acute effect and recovery of primary afferent nerve fibers after graded radiofrequency lesions in anaesthetized rats (abstract). Proceedings of the Anaesthetic Research Society. Br J Anaesth 1992; 68:1238.
46. Podhajsky RJ, Sekiguchi Y, Kikuchi S, Myers RR. The histologic effects of pulsed and continuous radiofrequency lesions at 42°C to rat dorsal root ganglion and sciatic nerve. Spine 2005; 30:1008–1013.
47. Louw AJA de, Vles HSH, Freling G, Herpers MJHM, Arends JW, Kleef M van. The morphological effects of a radiofrequency lesion adjacent to the dorsal root ganglion (RF-DRG)—an experimental study in the goat. Eur J Pain 2001; 5:169–174.
48. Norman A, Robins H, Milgram JE. The acute neuropathic arthropathy—a rapid severely disorganising form of arthritis. Radiology 1968; 90:1159–1164.

29 | Percutaneous Radiofrequency Neurotomy of the Lumbar Facet Joints

Jay Govind
Department of Anesthesia and Pain Medicine, The Canberra Hospital and The Australian National University, Canberra, Australian Capital Territory, Australia

INTRODUCTION

Devised as a therapeutic technique for the relief of chronic low back pain emanating from the lumbar zygapophysial joint, thermal radiofrequency neurotomy (RFN) coagulates the targeted nerve responsible for the transmission of nociceptive information, thereby creating a mechanical barrier. This is achieved by the passage of a low-energy, high-frequency alternating current between the exposed tip of a Teflon-covered electrode and a large dispersive ground plate. In this instance the target nerve is the medial branch of a lumbar dorsal ramus.

For the treatment of chronic lumbar zygapophysial joint pain, RFN or facet denervation was first promoted by Shealy in 1973 (1–4). The anticipated results did not eventuate, and by 1976, Shealy had abandoned the procedure in favor of 0.4% phenol injected in the same location (4). Undeterred, a number of subsequent investigators, who had based their observational studies on Shealy's description of RFN, reported good outcomes (5,6). These included those studies in which diagnostic blocks were not performed (7–10). In the late 1970s, the most impressive outcomes were reported by Oudenhoven (11). In his series of 268 non-compensable patients, 222 had experienced good to excellent relief of pain and returned to work. Of 69 non-compensable patients, 51 returned to work. These outcomes were not replicated by contemporary investigators (6,12–15). Inconsistency in outcomes was attributed most likely to the indiscriminate application of RFN for all cases of back pain, poor patient selection, and inaccurate placement of the active electrode. The target zones advocated in Shealy's original surgical technique (3–5,11) were shown to be anatomically incorrect (16), and thus a reliable denervation could not be expected. The electrode had been placed some distance away from the target nerve, and adequate coagulation was not achievable. The correct target points were anatomically redefined and a modified technique was described (17). By applying these modifications in properly selected patients, better outcomes were reported by later investigators (18,19). Conversely, poor and inconsistent outcomes were a quantifiable and reproducible feature where the Shealy technique was performed in patients inappropriately selected (15,20,21).

Failure to appreciate the electrophysiologic principles and the inherent technical limitations of RFN provided the third rider in the generation of inconsistent outcomes. Laboratory studies had disproved the prevailing misconception that thermal RFN was synonymous with or behaved in a manner analogous to electrocautery. Lesions generated by an RF electrode did not extend distal to the tip of the electrode, but instead spread radially above the long axis of the electrode (22) and assumed the shape of a "prolate spheroid" (23). Consequently, electrodes placed perpendicular to the target nerve would fail to coagulate the nerve adequately, even though they might be correctly placed directly onto the nerve. For the target nerve to be sufficiently and effectively coagulated, it is paramount that the electrode is placed contiguous with and parallel to the target nerve (22,24–27).

Contrary to published evidence, subsequent studies continued to replicate both the technical and surgical errors. Gallagher (28) used the erroneous technique of Shealy (3–5,11), whereas LeClaire (21) modified Shealy's technique in a manner not explicitly described. Although van Kleef et al. (29) identified the correct target points, they failed to place the electrodes parallel to the target nerve. One study dispensed with diagnostic blocks and relied on history, physical examination, and imaging studies to determine the level of neurotomy (20). In contrast, Dreyfuss et al. (19) reaffirmed the efficacy of RFN by placing the electrodes parallel to the target nerves, in their correct anatomical locations and in patients properly selected.

The sole indication for the procedure is complete relief of pain following controlled diagnostic blocks of the target medial branches (24,26,27,30,31). Shealy (3–5,11) neither described the method for patient selection nor advocated the use of diagnostic blocks. Assertions that zygapophysial joint pain can be clinically and unambiguously diagnosed in the absence of diagnostic blocks have no validation (9,10,20). There are no features either in the history, physical examination, or imaging studies that are unique or pathognomic for lumbar zygapophysial joint pain (24,30–38). Single blocks are unreliable (37,38), given that some two-thirds are false-positive (39), whereas venous uptake accounts for about 8% to 11% false-negative rate (35,40). Unlike comparative medial branch blocks (41), the sensitivity and specificity for intra-articular blocks, as in the LeClaire study (21), have not been determined—that intra-articular injections may not effectively block subchondral nociceptors has been raised elsewhere (42).

INDICATIONS

The only known indication for lumbar medial branch RFN is the complete relief of pain following controlled diagnostic blocks of the target medial branches (19,24,26,27,31,37). These blocks may be either placebo-controlled (43) or comparative local anesthetic blocks (38,44). No other treatment has been shown to be as effective. Given that the prevalence of lumbar zygapophysial joint pain ranges between 15% and 40% (32,33,45), the procedure has considerable application if properly executed. If pain returns and is of sufficient intensity, the procedure can be repeated (46).

PREOPERATIVE PLANNING
Patient Selection

Lumbar zygapophysial joint pain cannot be validly diagnosed by clinical impression, physical examination, computerized tomography or magnetic resonance imaging. Clinical features, putatively "classical" for lumbar zygapophysial joint pain (10,13), have not been validated (24,32,33). It is an absolute requirement that diagnostic blocks be undertaken according to proven guidelines (24,26,27,44). Although complete relief of pain (100% relief) may not be achievable due to extraneous factors, such as procedural pain, it is nevertheless noteworthy that the benchmark study on lumbar medial branch neurotomy (19) used at least 80% relief following medial branch blocks as the criterion for a positive response.

Anatomical Considerations

The L1–L4 dorsal rami are short nerves that arise almost at right angles from the lumbar spinal nerves, each nerve measuring about 5 mm in length (47). These are directed backwards and caudally toward the upper border of the transverse process below (Fig. 1). The L5 dorsal ramus differs in that it is a longer nerve and travels over the top of the ala of the sacrum.

Near the transverse processes, the L1–L4 dorsal rami divide primarily into the medial and lateral branches, with a variable intermediate branch arising from the lateral branch. A medial and lateral branch is always represented at every level. The L5 dorsal ramus forms only a medial branch and a branch that is equivalent to the intermediate branches of the other lumbar dorsal rami.

Anatomical studies have confirmed that the medial branches of the dorsal rami at segmental levels L1–L4 ("typical levels") assume a constant and similar course (48–51). As it emerges from the intervertebral foramen, each medial branch courses around the lateral surface of the neck of the superior articular process (SAP) below the foramen from which it issues (Fig. 1). Closely applied to the SAP, the medial branch passes caudally and dorsally to disappear under a fibro-osseous canal, the roof of which is formed by the mamilloaccessory ligament (50). This ligament fixes the medial branch and permits very little variation in the location or orientation of the nerve (Fig. 1). Emerging from this fibro-osseous canal, the medial branch divides into a proximal segment, which innervates the ipsi-segmental joint from its caudal aspect, and a distal segment, which supplies the joint at the next lower level. Thus, any given zygapophysial joint receives a dual innervation (16), for example the L4/L5 zygapophysial

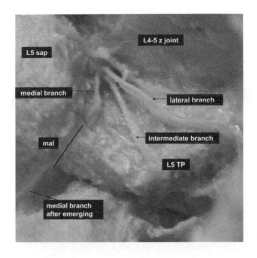

FIGURE 1 Posterior view of the branches of the right L4 dorsal ramus. *Abbreviations*: MAL, mammillo-accessory ligament; SAP, superior articular process; TP, transverse process.

joint would be supplied by the L3 and L4 dorsal rami, and the L5/S1 joint by the L4 and L5 dorsal rami.

Because the articular branches are either too small or inaccessible for RF coagulation, the parent medial branch is targeted. As it hugs the lateral surface of the SAP, only a limited length of the nerve is accessible, the optimal location being opposite the middle two-fourths of the neck of the SAP, in its postero-anterior width. Distal to this zone, the mamillo-accessory ligament protects the nerve from coagulation: proximally, the electrode is close to the origin of the lateral branch (Fig. 1). The lateral branches are spared by placing the electrode posterior to the ventral fourth of the neck of the SAP.

When accurately positioned, a 10-mm active tip would coagulate the nerve along its maximum accessible length. With a 5-mm active tip, two placements of the electrode are recommended: initially, in an area opposite the junction of the first and second ventral quarters (deeper insertion) and a second posterior placement corresponding to the middle of the neck of the SAP. Anteriorly, the electrode tip should not venture beyond the ventral fourth of the neck of the SAP, lest the lateral branches are denatured.

From the L5/S1 intervertebral foramen, a rather long L5 dorsal ramus courses along the groove formed between the ala of the sacrum and the root of the first sacral (S1) SAP. The medial branch of the L5 dorsal ramus hooks medially around the lower end of the SAP, deep to some fibrous tissue. A communicating branch to the S1 dorsal ramus constitutes the longitudinal course of the dorsal ramus (51).

Correlation of Anatomy to Radiographs

Studies in cadavers illustrate that when the electrodes are correctly placed, certain distinctive features are evident on imaging. Recognition of these features may assist in the proper execution of the procedure. The appearances are characteristic for each projection (51).

The "declined view" or caudal–cephalad projection attempts to simulate the axial view of computerized tomography (Fig. 2). In this view, the electrode placed parallel and close to the nerve, crosses the neck of the SAP, and it lies against the lower level of the lateral surface of the SAP rather than on the root of the transverse process.

In the lateral view, the electrode crosses the neck of the SAP (Fig. 3). In the deeper position the electrode tip extends anteriorly to the extent but not beyond the anterior quarter of the neck; withdrawn 3 to 5 mm, the tip lies opposite the middle of the neck.

In the anteroposterior (AP) projection, the following features are evident (Fig. 4):

- The electrode lies obliquely at about 20° from the sagittal plane and appears to hug the SAP. If the electrode is introduced parasagittally, the accessory process, the mamillo-accessory ligament, and/or the lateral flange of the SAP may either obstruct the course of the electrode or displace the electrode laterally, and the nerve would escape coagulation.

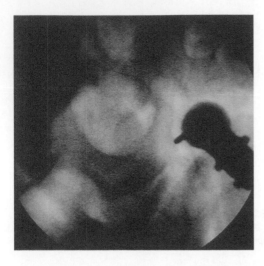

FIGURE 2 Declined view, L4 neurotomy. Note how the electrode rides up the wall of the superior articular process.

- The electrode is seen lying medial to the silhouette of the lateral margin of the SAP and medial to the lateral margin of the superior vertebral end plates, at the ipsi-segmental level.
- As the root of the transverse process expands along the neck of the SAP, the tip of the electrode may appear to project into the intervertebral canal, but when seen on the lateral view, it lies behind the root of the transverse process (Fig. 5).

The L5 dorsal ramus is a long nerve and accessible for a substantial length of its course where it crosses the ala of the sacrum. Electrodes can be placed deeply onto this nerve or in a more withdrawn position. Here, too, by placing the electrode parallel and onto the nerve, certain distinctive features are evident on imaging.

In the declined view, the electrode lies across the groove between the medial wall of the ala and lateral surface of the root of the SAP of S1, where the nerve lies deep to the electrode (Fig. 6).

In the lateral view, the electrode crosses the neck of the SAP of S1. When fully inserted, the electrode tip lies at the junction of the anterior and middle thirds of the neck of the SAP. Slightly withdrawn, the tip lies at the junction of the middle and posterior thirds of the neck.

In the AP view, the electrode is contiguous with the lateral aspect of the S1 SAP, and the tip projects over the superior margin of the ala when fully inserted, slightly withdrawn, the tip lies opposite the caudal half of the L5/S1 zygapophysial joint.

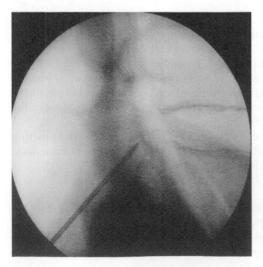

FIGURE 3 Lateral view, L4 neurotomy. Electrode crosses the neck of the superior articular process and lies behind the intervertebral foramen.

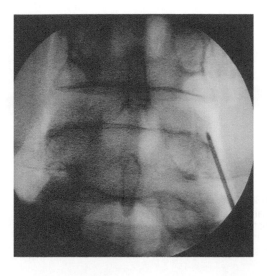

FIGURE 4   Anteroposterior view, L4 neurotomy (see text).

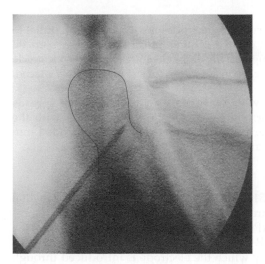

FIGURE 5   Lateral view, L4 neurotomy. Outline of the superior articular process (SAP). Note how the SAP mushrooms above the neck of the SAP.

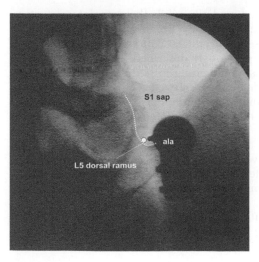

FIGURE 6   Declined view for L5 neurotomy. *Abbreviation*: SAP, superior articular process.

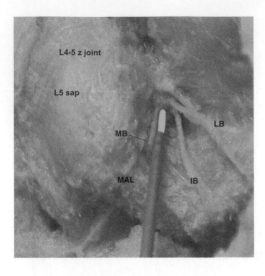

FIGURE 7 Electrode inserted as deep as possible along medial branch, superior to the mal. *Abbreviations*: IB, intermediate branch; LB, lateral branch; MAL, mammillo-accessory ligament; MB, medial branch; SAP, superior articular process.

Electrode Size and Placement

For an RF lesion to fully incorporate the target nerve, the electrodes must be placed parallel to and in contact with the nerve (Fig. 7). The lesion created is an elliptical sphere or a "prolate spheroid" (23), the maximum coagulation occurring radially along the long axis of the electrode rather than distal to the tip. This is not a hypothetical consideration (52). If inaccurately placed, a less-than-optimal lesion will be generated.

When a larger electrode is in close contact with the nerve, a wider lesion that spreads beyond the nerve is generated, thereby ensuring optimal coagulation. In contrast, with the smaller Sluijter-Mehta Kit (SMK), there is very little room for error—placing the electrode 1 mm away from the target nerve would fail to incorporate the nerve.

Anatomical Variations

More recent anatomical dissections by Lau et al. (51) redefined the course of the lumbar medial branch and its relationship with the bony structures. Rather than crossing the transverse process or lying in the groove constituted by the SAP and the root of the transverse process, the medial branches cross the lateral aspect of the SAP. Even though the surgical anatomy remains unchanged, what does change is the angulation by which the electrode is introduced through the skin, its course through the posterior back muscles, and its final placement on the lateral surface of the SAP.

The ventrolateral aspect of the SAP is inclined medially, while the dorsolateral surface, enhanced by the mamillary process, is inclined more laterally. Because of its relationship to the SAP, the emerging medial branch assumes a semi-curvilinear course. This redefinition of the surgical anatomy invalidates the techniques previously described. Parasagittally introduced electrodes placed on the transverse process would either miss the nerve or encounter the nerve "end-on." Even if the tip of the electrode lies near or even on the nerve, because of the tapering shape of the lesion ("prolate spheroid"), the nerve may escape coagulation or may be partially coagulated. The less the target nerve is coagulated, the more rapidly it is likely to regenerate.

By carefully placing the electrode parallel to and contiguous with the nerve, as it crosses the lateral surface of the SAP, the lesion generated would incorporate a substantial length of the nerve (Fig. 7) (51). Each medial branch innervates two joints, and two consecutive medial branches innervate each zygapophysial joint. Consequently, both medial braches have to be denatured in order to denervate a joint.

Given these redefined anatomical configurations, better visualization of the landmarks can be achieved by maneuvering the fluoroscopic tube along certain planes (51). Securing an unambiguous view of the target zones ensures precise placement of the electrode. The "declined

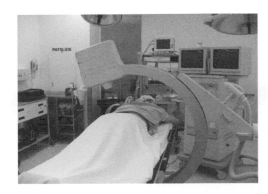

FIGURE 8 Fluoroscope aligned 20° off sagittal, to project the left-sided facet joint.

view" is obtained initially by tilting the X ray beam laterally by 20° from an AP view (Fig. 8), and from this position, the X-ray tube is declined caudally, along the length of the patient's body (Fig. 9), until the transverse process appears "edge-on" and the SAP is seen to arise cephalad from the transverse process (Fig. 9). In this projection, the medial branch crosses the lateral surface of the SAP and the electrode is seen "end-on" as it lies parallel to the nerve (Fig. 6).

A lateral view should confirm the relation of the electrode with the neck of the SAP, the depth of insertion, and the distance between the tip of the electrode and the intervertebral foramen (Figs. 3 and 10). The target zone lies between the posterior quarter and the anterior quarter of the neck of the SAP. Closely approaching the anterior quarter are the lateral and intermediate branches (Fig. 7), whereas over the posterior quarter, the mamillo-accessory ligament shields the medial branches (Figs. 1 and 12). Hence, by placing the electrode in the middle two quarters of the neck of the SAP, not only is the accessible medial branch adequately denatured but also, the lateral and intermediate branches are spared the effects of thermal coagulation (Fig. 7).

When placed parallel to the target nerve, in the AP view, the electrode is seen closely applied to the SAP at an angle to the sagittal plane. This angulation prevents the electrode tip from being laterally displaced by the mamillary protuberance, the accessory process, and the mamillo-accessory ligament (Figs. 4 and 12).

For the L5 dorsal ramus, the target zone lies opposite the middle and posterior thirds of the neck of the S1 SAP. The declined view, which sharply outlines the groove between the ala and the SAP, facilitates electrode placement along this groove and parallel to the nerve (Fig. 6).

For RFN to be of clinical benefit, it is crucial that the target zones are properly identified, and that the electrode is placed accurately and parallel to the target nerve (51). These prerequisites are not "hypothetical" (52). Placements recommended in the Lau study (51) have been vindicated in a benchmark observational study (19). Stringent selection criteria and precise surgical technique ensured good and lasting outcomes with postoperative electromyographic (EMG) studies confirming the coagulation of the target nerves.

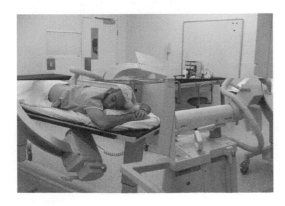

FIGURE 9 Fluoroscope aligned for the declined view.

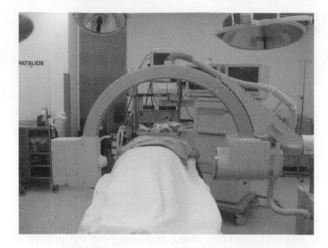

FIGURE 10 Alignment of the fluoroscope for the lateral view.

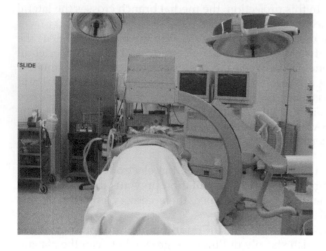

FIGURE 11 Alignment of the fluoroscope for the anteroposterior projection.

SURGICAL TECHNIQUES
Patient Positioning

With the patient prone, pillows are provided under the abdomen to reverse the lumbar lordosis—the knees and feet are similarly insulated against the tabletop. Generous infiltration of local anesthetic secures good anesthesia and the operation can be safely conducted, without sedation or premedication. A regular commentary as to what happens as the procedure evolves is reassuring to the patient.

Preoperative Sedation

Sedatives may be indicated only if the patient is particularly apprehensive or agitated, and in such instances, a minimal effective dose is administered so that the patient remains fully conversant and lucid throughout the procedure and is able to report concisely unexpected symptoms or discomfort.

Procedural Technique

At "typical levels" (L1–L4), the surgical technique is the same. However, to denervate the L5/S1 zygapophysial joint, in addition to the L4 medial branch, it is the L5 dorsal ramus that is coagulated, rather than the latter's medial branch. The lesion is created where it crosses the ala of the sacrum and not on the transverse process.

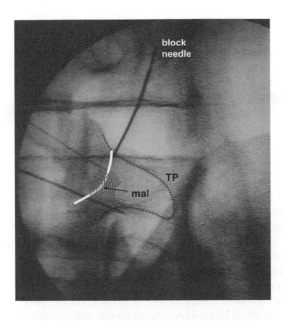

FIGURE 12 Oblique view of the right L4 facet joint showing topography of the L4 medial branch in relation to the superior articular process, transverse process (TP), the mamillo-accessory ligament (mal) and optimal placement of the block needle.

Radiographic Orientation at the L1–L4 Levels

The active tip of the electrode is placed on the lateral surface of the neck of the SAP where the target nerve runs, just above its junction with the root of the transverse process. In the lateral projection, this narrow portion of the SAP appears as a short stalk from which the remainder of the SAP expands like the head of a mushroom (Fig. 5) (51).

One or more lesions are created at a point opposite the central two-thirds or the central two-fourths of the neck so that the maximum length of the target nerve is denatured. Proximal to this zone lie the lateral and intermediate branches of the dorsal rami; hence, lesions should not be made over the ventral quarter of the neck of the SAP. Distally, the mamillo-accessory ligament insulates the medial branch from coagulation (Figs. 7 and 12).

Radiographic Orientation at the L5 Level

Because the mamillo-accessory ligament is vestigial, a greater length of the L5 dorsal ramus is accessible as the target area across the neck of the S1 SAP is longer. The number of lesions required depends on the electrode size and the relative size of the SAP.

Surgical Anesthesia

Using the same standard technique as for a medial branch block, the generous deposition of local anesthetic renders the target area sufficiently anesthetic to allow lesioning to proceed without sedation or systemic analgesia. Because large diameter electrodes will heat tissues several millimeters away from the active tip, it is imperative that the surrounding tissues and the overlying back muscles are also adequately anesthetized by injecting local anesthetic as the block needle is slightly withdrawn. Upon completion of the block, the needle is left in situ, over the designated target zone. This will serve as a convenient marker during the passage of the electrode and also a conduit for supplementary local anesthetic. From a true AP (sagittal) position, obtain a 20° oblique projection and from here, decline the fluoroscope caudally. This maneuver creates a number of composite and ambiguous shadows, and familiar bony landmarks are either obstructed or become indistinct. Placement of the block needle accurately and firmly onto the target area will ensure that the tip of the needle will always be pointing toward the target nerve.

Prior to inserting the block needle, maneuver the C-arm such that the point of entry through the skin overlies the target zone. To achieve this, the fluoroscope is adjusted so as to obtain an oblique declined view of the target area (Figs. 2,8,9). The transverse process is seen "edge-on" and the SAP is seen arising cranially from the base of the transverse process. The junction between the two becomes more apparent, and the block needle now points to the target zone. It is along this projection/trajectory that the intended track of the electrode should be anesthetized.

The spinal needle is inserted in line with the X ray beam until it reaches the target point. Once 2 to 3 ml of long-acting local anesthetic is injected at the intended surgical site, the track for the electrode can be anesthetized by injecting a total of about 2 to 4 ml of local anesthetic, at the same time as slowly withdrawing the needle. Ensure that the skin is sufficiently anesthetized to permit a painless stab incision and the introduction of a large/blunt electrode.

Insertion of the Electrode

To avoid any bony obstacles during the passage of the electrode, not only must the entry point be carefully selected, but also the plane of insertion through the posterior back muscles must be a direct linear extension of the X ray beam. At the L1–L4 levels, a large accessory process or the mamillo-accessory ligament would impede the accurate placement of an electrode inserted parasagittally. Generally, in the lower lumbar vertebrae, the mamillary process and the SAP project laterally so as to overhang the root of the SAP. This overhanging bone, often difficult to visualize when seen end-on in the oblique-declined view, deflects the sagittally introduced electrode laterally and away from the nerve. The accessory process lies just caudal and lateral to the caudal edge of the SAP. The size of the accessory process varies from a tiny tubercle to a large prominent mass and may be associated with substantial bony overgrowth on the dorsal surface of the root of the transverse process. Large accessory processes are frequent in the L4 and L5 vertebrae (16).

To circumvent these obstacles and to secure an accurate placement, it is essential that:

- At the L1–L4 levels, the electrode is inserted along a plane that is 15° to 20° oblique to the sagittal plane (Fig. 8). This plane of insertion allows the tip of the electrode access to the anterolateral aspect of the curved neck of the SAP where the nerve is most accessible (Figs. 3 and 12). With respect to the L5 dorsal ramus, a vestigial mamillo-accessory ligament offers no obstruction at the S1 level, and given that a substantial length of the nerve is available for coagulation, a more parasagittal pass should achieve the desired effect.
- At all levels, the electrode must be close to and parallel to the nerve (Fig. 7).
- The electrode must be able to reach the target point. In patients with a flat lordosis and small sacral angle, the target zones may be almost axial in their orientation and the entry point on the skin invariably would be below the targeted level. This oblique approach in the sagittal plane increases the length of the proposed trajectory, and hence the length of the electrode in order to achieve maximal coagulation. Conversely, in patients with steep sacral angles, and a normal pronounced lordosis, the target groove will point somewhat backward and would facilitate the placement of the electrode parallel to the target nerve from an insertion point that is only moderately caudal to the target level.

Preoperatively, by plotting the coordinates for each target level onto a lateral radiograph of the patient's lumbar spine, the required line of insertion is projected onto the patient's skin, and this, in turn, will determine the point of entry and the length of electrode required to reach the target nerve and still be parallel to it. In certain instances, a longer electrode may be necessary. Conversely, where the trajectory is too steep, a modified approach may be considered. Where such modifications compromise the degree of parallelism and proximity to the target nerve, generating a matrix of lesions would ensure adequate and optimal coagulation.

Outcomes can be optimized not only by precise placement but lesion size and hence electrode size. Preferably, electrodes should not be less than 18G. With an 18G or higher caliber electrode, the length of the nerve coagulated can be maximized using a 10-mm active tip. With a 5-mm tip, extra lesions would be required along the length of the target nerve.

Insertion of a Solid Electrode: The Declined View

The anesthetized skin over the designated entry point is stabbed with a number 11-scalpel blade, which allows an easier insertion of the electrode through the skin and fascia. The electrode is maintained parallel to the X ray beam and is directed to the target zone through the muscles of the back. In this view, the electrode is seen "end on" (Fig. 2). The electrode is advanced in small increments, and throughout, periodic screening should monitor its progress in order to ensure that it does not stray from the required course. To prevent an insertion anterior to the target zone, at the onset, the electrode is directed to contact bone, either the base of the SAP, or the root of the transverse process close to the target point. Upon contact, the depth of the insertion is noted and the electrode is withdrawn slightly. It is readjusted such that the tip, lying close to the neck of the SAP, is advanced anteriorly beyond the point of initial contact by no more than a few millimeters further than the depth at which the bone was contacted.

Subsequent Radiographic Projections: The Anteroposterior View

At this stage, an AP projection is secured. In this view, the electrode is seen lying snugly against the lateral surface of the SAP, and that the lateral margin of the head of the SAP overhangs the tip of the electrode, laterally (Fig. 4). With respect to the L5 dorsal ramus, the electrode assumes an analogous position in relation to the ala of the sacrum.

The Lateral Projection

Two important features are confirmed on the lateral projection, namely, the orientation of electrode, that is, it lies parallel to the nerve, and the depth of insertion (Figs. 3 and 5). Preferably, the electrode tip should lie opposite the middle two-thirds of the neck of the SAP so that a segment of the bone intervenes between the point of the electrode and the edge of the foramen (or about one-quarter of the AP width of the neck of the SAP). Final placement is always executed in the lateral projection, lest the electrode advances too far anteriorly, thus exposing the lateral and intermediate branches to the effects of RF.

The Oblique View and the Concept of Squaring

An oblique view also ensures that the electrode tip does not encroach upon the lateral and intermediate branches (Fig. 7). Prior to securing an oblique view, it is essential that the X-ray beam passes parallel to the disc space and the vertebral end plates at the target level. This is achieved by declining the fluoroscope either caudally (for the lower two lumbar vertebrae) or cranially (for those above) from a true AP projection so that the inferior end plates of the target vertebrae overlap; otherwise, the apparent location of the nerve may not be its actual location. This is especially evident when evaluating the placement of an electrode for L5 dorsal ramus neurotomy. If the L5/S1 disc space is not squared off, the tip of the electrode in an oblique view may appear to be in a high position.

As a final check prior to lesioning, the placement of the electrode in all projections should be reviewed simultaneously and confirmed to be correlating. In the AP (Fig. 4) and oblique views, the tip of the electrode should lie snugly against the neck of the SAP; however, because of the rostral expansion of the base of the transverse process, the tip of the electrode may project slightly beyond the superior margin of the transverse process. Thus, to prevent an extreme anterior insertion of the electrode, the SAP, and not the transverse process, should be used as a reference mark. A permanent record is created for all final placements.

Lesion Creation

Because of their weight, large-gauge electrodes have a propensity to displace spontaneously; hence, it is essential that the electrode be firmly held in position by the operator. During the process of lesion generation, the position of the electrode should be checked periodically on the lateral view to ensure that it has not migrated either away from the target zone or toward the ventral ramus.

The temperature of the electrode is raised slowly at about 1°C per second, and rapid escalation is avoided at all times. If the patient complains of any untoward side effects, lesion generation can be aborted and remedial action instituted. Where the target zone has been insufficiently or inadequately anesthetized, patients may report pain as the temperature reaches 65°C or more. In such instances, supplementary anesthesia can be provided through the block needle.

If the patient reports sensation in the territory of the ventral ramus or any other region, lesion generation can be interrupted, the position of the electrode checked, and the procedure could recommence if there are no contraindications. Any other problem should be appropriately addressed. If, despite these measures, heating is still painful and the cause of discomfort cannot be ascertained, the procedure should be aborted and adjourned appropriately.

If no untoward sensations are encountered, the temperature is raised until it reaches 80–85°C. This temperature is maintained for 90 seconds. Retaining the block needle has a useful purpose. Occasionally, the prominence of the contralateral SAP may act as a surrogate operative field that may inadvertently cause the tip of the electrode to be advanced too anteriorly. The composite shadows created in a lateral projection makes it difficult to distinguish the dorsal superior aspect of the SAP in question. By securing an oblique position, the block needle should move with and in the same direction as the operative site.

Creating Multiple Lesions

Whether additional lesions are required depends on the size of the active tip of the electrode and the size of the target zone. With an 18G electrode, a 10-mm active tip would generally denature an appreciable length of the target nerve and, consequently, only one lesion may suffice. With a 5-mm active tip or where the target zone is longer than the active tip, a second lesion along the same trajectory can be created by withdrawing the electrode to about 50–75% of the length of the active tip. In this manner, a second lesion, which slightly overlaps the first, is generated, thus increasing the length of the nerve coagulated.

If a tall SAP is encountered, the electrode should then be reinserted further up the SAP and parallel to the first trajectory. This ensures that the nerves that run somewhat higher on the SAP are adequately coagulated.

Postoperative Care

As with any invasive procedure, the surgical field is thoroughly cleaned with a suitable antiseptic and a pressure dressing is applied. Side effects are investigated and rectified appropriately. Vasovagal episodes may occur and the treatment is largely conservative, monitoring vital signs.

Controlling the volume and the pressure at which the injectate is deposited at the surgical site should ensure its minimal dissemination. Nevertheless, seepage closer to the intervertebral foramen is likely to occur with anesthetization of the other branches of the spinal nerve. Lateral spread within muscle planes may incorporate the ventral ramus. Hence, before arising from the operation table, patients should be reminded that they might experience some numbness and/or unsteadiness, and unassisted ambulation is best avoided until full motor function is restored. Patients must be discharged into the care of an accompanying adult, who would safely transport the patient home. At no stage must the patient be allowed to drive a motor vehicle until the neurologic deficits, affecting the lower extremity, are completely reversed and the patient regains preoperative status. Cold packs are recommended for a day or two. Appropriate analgesics for postoperative pain may include a short course of opioids. In the absence of contraindications, early mobilization is encouraged and the patient counseled to report any unusual symptoms. Unless otherwise clinically indicated, the patient's progress is closely monitored for the first two or three weeks and thereafter as required.

OUTCOMES

For the treatment of lumbar zygapophysial joint pain, unambiguously diagnosed by controlled diagnostic blocks, medial branch RFN is the single most effective mode of treatment. When meticulously executed in patients who are properly selected, RFN confers more than 80% relief of the index pain for a considerable period (19), and in a substantial proportion, total relief is achievable. No other form of treatment has been shown to be equally or more effective. Given that the prevalence of lumbar zygapophysial joint pain can be as high as 40% (33,39), the role of RFN in the management of proven zygapophysial joint pain cannot be discounted. It has the potential to reduce the burden of chronic low back pain safely and effectively. When compared with the side effects and complications of nonsteroidal anti-inflammatory medications, the efficacy and cost-effectiveness of RFN is not inconsequential.

COMPLICATIONS

The theoretical risks have been considered under cervical RFN. Specific to the lumbar spine, no major complications have been reported. Complications may arise due to misplacement of the electrode. General anesthetic is not recommended as accurate patient feedback is essential for the safe conduct of the procedure.

Commonly reported side effects include reaction to local anesthetic, superficial infections, and skin burns from inadequate dispersive plates and broken or poorly insulated electrodes (8,24). Some patients may develop dysesthetic symptoms, presumably due to "post-denervation neuritis" (53). It may manifest as a sunburn-like feeling, and usually requires no treatment, symptoms resolving spontaneously within six to eight weeks. The exact pathomechanism remains unclear. Severe symptoms may warrant medial branch blocks and/or membrane stabilizers, such as pregabalin.

In an unrelated study of 92 patients in whom 616 RF lesions were generated, 0.25% complained of localized pain lasting more than two weeks, and three patients were thought to have "neuritic pain" lasting less than two weeks (54). Neither infection nor any new neurologic deficits were reported.

Efficacy Studies

Prior to 1994, there were no randomized controlled trials (RCT) to attest to the efficacy of lumbar RFN for the treatment of chronic back pain ostensibly emanating from the zygapophysial joint. Despite a lack of uniformity in patient selection and surgical techniques, a number of observational studies reported favorable outcomes (1–15,55,56). By 2001, three RCT and one observational study appeared in the medical literature, each reflecting its own idiosyncratic nuances. Contrary to published evidence, inadequate selection criteria and an inaccurate execution of the procedure prevailed in the three RCTs. Notwithstanding this inherent therapeutic heterogeneity and methodologic flaws in each study, some commentators denounced the procedure based on questionable outcomes (57). Consequently, clinicians should maintain vigilance when treatment is denounced on the basis of pooled estimates associated with unexplained heterogeneity.

Based on the Shealy technique, the first reported placebo-controlled trial showed that active treatment was more effective than placebo, and at six months, 24% of the treated patients reported on going relief (28). Relief of pain from an average of 58 (pre-treatment) to 44 (post-treatment) on a 100-point visual analogue scale (VAS) was considered to be clinically effective.

In the second RCT, van Kleef et al. (29) showed that where the target zones were correctly identified, active treatment was more effective than placebo, but the outcomes were compromised by not having the electrodes parallel to the nerve. These investigators reported only a three-point improvement in a 10-point VAS.

The construct and internal validity of the third RCT was not declared (21). In this study, the cardinal indication for RFN was the patient's response to intra-articular deposition of corticosteroids and lignocaine. A positive response was defined as "significant relief" of their back pain for not less than 24 hours. Neither medial branch nor controlled blocks were performed. Unlike other studies, "significant relief" was not assigned a numerical value. The rationale in utilizing a therapeutic agent, steroid (58), as a surrogate diagnostic utility, was not explained, nor were the paradoxical effects of lignocaine considered (59–61). Randomized in blocks of four, patients received either a modified Shealy's or sham treatment. At 12 weeks, none in the active group benefited. Paradoxically, outcomes in the active group were slightly worse than those in the placebo group. A lack of response to active treatment must suggest that the patients were either misdiagnosed, poorly selected, or incorrectly treated. When critically appraised, it becomes evident that the LeClaire study (21), in essence, compared one sham treatment against another, which ironically invalidated the Cochrane review (62).

Conversely, a well-designed observational study showed that substantial and lasting relief of pain is achievable if the procedure is properly executed (19). Stringent selection criteria minimized selection bias, and only those patients who reported at least 80% relief of their index pain to comparative diagnostic blocks were eligible for treatment. Placing the electrodes close to and parallel to the targeted nerves secured optimal coagulation. At 12 months follow-up, 30% continued to enjoy 100% relief of their index pain; 50% reported 90% pain relief, whereas in 80%, pain was reduced by 60%. The subjective relief of pain was corroborated by significant and sustained improvements in physical function, even as EMG studies confirmed denervation of the appropriate segments of the multifidus muscle, normally innervated by the medial branches.

The Dreyfuss study (19) reaffirms that sustainable relief is feasible by placing the electrodes parallel and close to accurately identified target zones in patients who are positive to comparative diagnostic blocks. Independent commentators have reasserted that the RCTs, upon which some of the Cochrane reviews are based, are contradictory and inconsistent (25–27,53). Contrary to the Cochrane review, there is strong evidence for the efficacy of RFN in the management of lumbar zygapophysial joint pain (24,63–65).

A number of unrelated studies have countered the misconception that observational studies may overestimate the magnitude of treatment effects (66–68). Many RCTs lack external validity (69, 70), and when critically appraised (71), both RCTs and systematic reviews generate conflicting results (72,73). Flaws in the basic methodology of systematic reviews can lead to incorrect and biased conclusions with serious implications for the quality of patient care (74). Denouncing a treatment based on questionable methodology (57,62), is simply providing a misguided conclusion and a significant disservice to patient care (69).

CONCLUSIONS

The prevalence of cervical and lumbar zygapophysial joint pain is not insignificant. Unlike certain visceral disorders, there are no specific biologic markers that are either unique or pathognomonic for zygapophysial joint pain. Equally, neither the history, physical examination, nor imaging can distinguish zygapophysial joint pain from other sources/causes of chronic neck or low back pain. In the management of chronic spinal pain, the only indication for RFN is the complete relief of the patient's index pain following controlled diagnostic medial branch blocks. The primary objective of RFN is the relief of pain emanating from the zygapophysial joint.

The prerequisites for a successful outcome include an appreciation of the surgical and radiographic anatomy, accurate identification of the target zones, placement of the electrodes close to and parallel to the target nerve, proper patient selection, and operator proficiency.

SUMMARY

- Radiographic target points for neurotomy are based on anatomical studies.
- Because of a high false-positive rate of single blocks, controlled diagnostic blocks that result in complete relief of pain are paramount.
- RFN should only proceed if controlled blocks confer total relief of the patient's index pain.
- Unlike medial branch blocks, the sensitivity and specificity of intra-articular blocks have not been determined.
- The anatomical course of the target nerve determines the trajectory of the electrode. In the cervical spine, topographic variations of the nerve necessitate the creation of multiple lesions
- RFN is relatively free of side effects and no serious complications have been reported.
- Where appropriate, the procedure can be repeated.
- RFN is the only known treatment for proven zygapophysial joint pain that provides complete relief of pain for a lasting period.
- Standardization of surgical techniques may improve therapeutic homogeneity and hence better outcomes.

ACKNOWLEDGMENT

For access to electronic data and the anatomical dissections, I am greatly indebted to P. Powis and Prof N. Bogduk of the Newcastle Bone and Joint Institute, Newcastle, Australia.

REFERENCES

1. Shealy CN. Facets in back and sciatic pain. Minn Med 1974; 57:199–203.
2. Shealy CN. The role of the spinal facets in back and sciatic pain. Headache 1974; 14:101–104.
3. Shealy CN. Percutaneous radiofrequency denervation of spinal facets. J Neurosurg 1975; 43:448–451.
4. Shealy CN. Facet denervation in the management of back sciatic pain. Clin Orthop 1976; 115:157–164.
5. Oudenhoven RC. Articular rhizotomy. Surg Neurol 1974; 2:275–278.
6. Anderson KH, Mosdal C, Vaernet K. Percutaneous radiofrequency facet denervation in low back and extremity pain. Acta Neurochir 1987; 87:48–51.
7. McCulloch JA, Organ LW. Percutaneous radiofrequency lumbar rhizolysis (rhizotomy). Can Med Ass J 1977; 116:30–32.
8. Burton CV. Percutaneous radiofrequency facet denervation. Appl Neurophysiol 1976/1977; 39:80–86.
9. Cho J, Park YG, Chung SS. Percutaneous radiofrequency lumbar facet rhizotomy in mechanical low back pain syndrome. Stereotact Funct Neurosurg 1997; 68:212–217.
10. Koning HM, Mackie DP. Percutaneously radiofrequency facet denervation in mechanical low back pain syndrome. Pain Clinic 1994; 7:199–204.
11. Oudenhoven RC. The role of laminectomy, facet rhizotomy and epidural steroids. Spine 1979; 4:145–147.
12. Scherer JP. Radiofrequency facet rhizotomy in the treatment of chronic neck and low back pain. Int Surg 1978; 63:53–59.
13. Mehta M, Sluijter ME. The treatment of chronic back pain. Anaesthesia 1979; 34:768, 775.
14. Sluijter ME, Mehta M. treatment of chronic back and neck pain by percutaneous thermal lesions. In: Lipton S, Miles J, eds. Persistent Pain: Modern Methods of Treatment, vol. 3. London: Academic Press, 1981:141–179.
15. Ogsbury JS, Simon RH, Lehman RAW. Facet denervation in the treatment of low back syndrome. Pain 1977; 3:257–263.
16. Bogduk N, Long DM. The anatomy of the so-called "articular nerves" and their relationship to facet denervation in the treatment of low back pain. J Neurosurg 1979; 51:172–177.
17. Bogduk N, Long DM. Percutaneous lumbar medial branch neurotomy. A modification of facet denervation. Spine 1980; 5:193–200.
18. Rashbaum RF. Radiofrequency facet denervation. A treatment alternative in refractory low back pain with or without leg pain. Orthop Clin North Am 1984; 14:569–575.
19. Dreyfuss P, Halbrook B, Pauza K, Joshi A, McLarty J, Bogduk N. Efficacy and validity of radiofrequency neurotomy for chronic lumbar zygapophysial joint pain. Spine 2000; 25:1270–1277.
20. Pevsner Y, Shabat S, Catz A, Folman Y, Gepstein R. The role of radiofrequency in the treatment of mechanical pain of spinal origin. Eur Spine J 2003; 12:602–605.
21. Leclaire R, Fortin L, Lambert R, Bergeron YM, Rossignol M. Radiofrequency facet joint denervation in the treatment of low back pain. A placebo controlled clinical trial to assess efficacy. Spine 2001; 26:1411–1416.
22. Bogduk N, Macintosh J, Marsland A. Technical limitations to the efficacy of radiofrequency neurotomy for spinal pain. Neurosurgery 1987; 20:529–535.
23. Organ LW. Electrophysiologic principles of radiofrequency lesion making. Appl Neurophysiol 1976; 39:69–76.
24. Hall DJ. Facet joint denervation: a minimally invasive treatment for low back pain in selected patients. In: Herkowitz HN, Dvorak J, Bell GR, Nordin M, Grob D, eds. The Lumbar Spine, 3rd Ed. The International Society for the Study of the Lumbar Spine. Philadelphia: Lippincott Williams and Wilkins, 2004:307–311.
25. Van Zundert J, Raj P, Erdine S, van Kleef M. Application of radiofrequency treatment in practical pain management: state of the art. Pain Practice 2002; 2:269–278.
26. Slipman CW, Bhat AL, Gilchrist RV, Isaac Z, Chou L, Lenrow DA. A critical review of the evidence for the use of zygapophysial injections and radiofrequency denervation in the treatment of low back pain. Spine J 2003; 3:310–316.
27. Hooten WM, Martin DP, Huntoon MA. Radiofrequency neurotomy for low back pain: evidence based procedural guidelines. Pain Med 2005; 6:129–138.
28. Gallagher J, Petriccione di Valdo PL, Wedley JR, et al. Radiofrequency facet joint denervation in the treatment of low back pain: a prospective controlled double blind study to assess its efficacy. Pain Clin 1994; 7:193–198.
29. Van Kleef M, Barendse GAM, Kessels A, Voets HM, Weber WEJ, de Lange S. Randomized trial of radiofrequency lumbar facet denervation for chronic low back pain. Spine 1999; 24:1937–1942.

30. Whitmore LA, Feler CA. Application of spinal ablative techniques for the treatment of benign chronic painful conditions. Spine 2002; 27:2607–2612.

31. International Spine Intervention Society. Percutaneous radiofrequency lumbar medial branch neurotomy. In: Bogduk N, ed. Practice Guidelines for Spinal Diagnostic and Treatment Procedures. San Francisco: International Spine Intervention Society, 2004:188–210.

32. Schwarzer AC, Aprill CN, Derby R, Fortin J, Kine G, Bogduk N. Clinical features of patients with pain stemming from the lumbar zygapophysial joints. Is the lumbar facet syndrome a clinical entity? Spine 1994; 19:1132–1137.

33. Schwarzer AC, Wang S, Bogduk N, McNaught PJ, Laurent R. Prevalence and clinical features of lumbar zygapophysial joint pain: a study in an Australian population with chronic low back pain. Ann Rheum Dis 1995; 54:100–106.

34. Dreyfuss PH, Dreyer SJ, Herring SA. Contemporary concepts in spine care: lumbar zygapophyseal (facet) joint injections. Spine 1995; 20:2040–2047.

35. Kaplan M, Dreyfuss P, Halbrook B, Bogduk N. The ability of lumbar medial branch blocks to anaesthetise the zygapophysial joint: a physiologic challenge. Spine 1998; 23:1847–1852.

36. Bogduk N, McGuirk B. Medical management of acute and chronic low back pain. An evidence-based approach. Pain Research and Clinical Management, vol. 13. Amsterdam: Elsevier, 2002:187–196.

37. Geurts JWM, Lou L, Gauci CA, Newnhanm P, van Wijk MAW. Radiofrequency treatments in low back pain. Pain Pract 2002; 2:226–234.

38. Barnsley L, Lord S, Wallis B, Bogduk N. False positive rates of cervical zygapophysial joint blocks. Clin J Pain 1993; 9:124–130.

39. Schwarzer AC, Aprill CN, Derby R, Fortin J, Kine G, Bogduk N. The false-positive response rate of uncontrolled diagnostic blocks of the lumbar zygapophysial joints. Pain 1994; 58:195–200.

40. Dreyfuss P, Schwarzer AC, Lau P, Bogduk N. Specificity of lumbar medial branch and L5 dorsal ramus blocks. Spine 1997; 22:895–902.

41. Barnsley L, Lord S, Bogduk N. Comparative anaesthetic blocks in the diagnosis of zygapophysial joint pain. Pain 1993; 55:99–106.

42. Beaman DN, Graziano GP, Glover RA, Wojtys EM, Chang V. Substance P innervation of lumbar spine facet joints. Spine 1993; 18:1044–1049.

43. Lord SM, Barnsley L, Bogduk N. The utility of comparative local anaesthetic blocks versus placebo controlled blocks for the diagnosis of cervical zygapophysial joint pain. Clin J Pain 1995; 11:208–213.

44. International Spine Intervention Society. Lumbar medial branch blocks. In: Bogduk N, ed. Practice Guidelines for Spinal Diagnostic and Treatment Procedures. San Francisco: International Spine Intervention Society, 2004:47–65.

45. Manchikanti L, Pampati V, Fellows B, Bakhit CE. Prevalence of lumbar facet joint pain in chronic low back pain. Pain Phys 1999; 2:59–64.

46. Schofferman J, Kine G. Effectiveness of repeated radiofrequency neurotomy for lumbar facet pain. Spine 2004; 29:2471–2473.

47. Bogduk N. Clinical anatomy of the lumbar spine and sacrum, 4th ed. Amsterdam: Elsevier Churchill Livingstone, 2005:123–139.

48. Bogduk N, Wilson AS, Tynan W. The human lumbar dorsal rami. J Anat 1982; 134:383–397.

49. Bogduk N. The innervation of the lumbar spine. Spine 1983; 8:286–293.

50. Bogduk N. The lumbar mamillo-accessory ligament. Its anatomical and neurosurgical significance. Spine 1981; 6:162–167.

51. Lau P, Mercer S, Govind J, Bogduk N. The surgical anatomy of lumbar medial branch neurotomy. Pain Med 2004; 5:289–298.

52. Sanders M, Zuurmond WWA. Percutaneous intra-articular lumbar facet joint denervation in the treatment of low back pain: a comparison with percutaneous extra articular facet denervation. Pain Clin 1999; 11:329–325.

53. Hall JA. The role of radiofrequency facet denervation in chronic low back pain.hrrp://www.demsonline.org/jax-medicine/1998journals/october98/facetdenervation.htm.Accessed 09.05.05.

54. Kornick C, Kramarich S, Tim J, Sitzman T. Complications of lumbar facet radiofrequency denervation. Spine 2004; 29:1352–1354.

55. Pawl RP. Results in the treatment of low back syndrome from sensory neurolysis of lumbar facets (facet rhizotomy) by thermal coagulation. Proc Inst Med Chgo 1974; 30:150–151.

56. Lora J, Long DM. So-called facet denervation in the management of intractable back pain. Spine 1976; 1:121–126.

57. Deyo RA. Point of view. Spine 2001; 26:1417.

58. Carette S, Marcoux S, Truchon R, et al. A controlled trial of corticosteroid injections into facet joints for chronic low back pain. N Engl J Med 1991; 325:1002–1007.

59. Arner S, Lindblom U, Meyerson BA, Molander C. Prolonged relief of neuralgia after regional anaesthetic blocks: a call for further experimental and systematic clinical studies. Pain 1990; 43:287–297.

60. Butterworth JF, Strichartz G. Molecular mechanisms of local anaesthesia: a review. Anesthesiology 1990; 72:711–734.

61. Hollmann MW. Prolonged actions of short-acting drugs: local anaesthetics and chronic pain. (Editorial) Reg Anaesth Pain Med 2000; 25:337–339.

62. Niemisto L, Kalso E, Malmivaara A, Seitsalo S, Hurri H. Radiofrequency denervation for neck and back pain: a systematic review within the framework of the Cochrane Collaboration Back Review Group. Spine 2003; 28:1877–1888.

63. Geurts JW, van Wijk RM, Stolker RJ, Groen GJ. Efficacy of radiofrequency procedures for the treatment of spinal pain: a systematic review of Randomized clinical trials. Reg Anaesth Pain Med 2001; 26:394–400.

64. Cousins MJ, Walker S. Chronic pain: management strategies that work. Anaesth Analg 2001; 92(suppl 15–25):3S.

65. Deen HG, Fenton DS, Lamer TJ. Minimally invasive procedures for disorders of the lumbar spine. Mayo Clin Proc 2003; 78:1249–1256.

66. Concato J, Shah N, Horwitz RI. Randomized controlled trials, observational studies, and the hierarchy of research designs. N Engl J Med 2000; 342:1887–1992.

67. Benson K, hartz AJ. A comparison of observational studies and randomized controlled trials. N Engl J Med 2000; 342:1878–1886.

68. McCormack J, Greenhalgh T. Seeing what you want to see in randomized controlled trials: versions and perversions of UKPDS data. BMJ 2000; 320:1720–1723.

69. Rothwell PM. External validity of randomized controlled trials: "To whom do the results of this trial apply?" Lancet 2005; 365:82–93.

70. Chan AW, Altman DG. Epidemiology and reporting of randomized trials published in PubMed journals. Lancet 2005; 365:1159–1162.

71. Oxman A, Guyatt G. Summarizing the evidence. In: Guyatt G, Rennie D, eds. Users' Guides to the Medical Literature: A Manual for Evidence-Based Clinical Practice. Chicago: JAMA & Archives Journals, American Medical Association, AMA Press, 2002:553–608.

72. Furlan AD, Clarke J, Esmail R, Sinclair S, Irvin E, Bombardier C. A critical review of reviews on the treatment of chronic low back pain. Spine 2001; 26:E155–E162.

73. Gatchel RJ, McGeary D. Cochrane collaboration-based reviews of health care interventions: are they unequivocal and valid scientifically, or simply nihilistic? Spine J 2002; 2:315–319.

74. Hopayian K. The need for caution in interpreting high quality systematic reviews. BMJ 2001; 323:681–684.

30 | Intradiscal Heating

Richard Derby
Spinal Diagnostics and Treatment Center, Daly City, and Division of Physical Medicine and Rehabilitation, Stanford University Medical Center, Stanford, California, U.S.A.

Sang-Heon Lee and Yung Chen
Spinal Diagnostics and Treatment Center, Daly City, California, U.S.A.

INTRODUCTION

Treating axial and referred extremity pain is challenging, and until recently, the only micro-invasive treatments were nuclear decompressions using injected chymopapain or disc decompressions through small bore needles to remove or vaporize disc tissue (1–3). These procedures were designed and marketed as a treatment for radicular pain caused by disc herniations, but spinal fusions remained the standard treatment option for axial pain when conservative treatment failed. For many, however, a spinal fusion was not an attractive next option.

Thermocoagulation of the medial branches of the dorsal spinal nerve had long been an accepted method for treating zygapophyseal joint pain (4,5). In cases of disc injury where pain arises in part from the ingrowth and sensitization of nociceptive fibers within annular fissures, destroying these fibers by thermal destruction was first investigated by professor M. E. Sluijter. Sluijter (6) had long pioneered the use of radiofrequency nerve ablations for the treatment of chronic pain, and in the early 1990s, he treated a series of patients with chronic low back pain by inserting a radiofrequency needle into the disc center and heating the probe for 90 seconds at 70°C (7). His first clinical impressions were presented at the 6th International Congress Pain Clinic in Atlanta, Georgia (8), in 1994, and although his method did not ultimately survive a randomized controlled trial (RCT) (7), his technique was modified by others to include more posterior electrode placement and longer heating times. Using this modified technique, both Salinger and Derby presented two pilot studies, both claiming favorable outcomes in about two-thirds of the patients (9,10). The procedure, however, remained infrequently utilized until the pioneering work of two well-respected and published clinicians, Jeff and Joel Saal. Working with Hugh Sharkey and John Ashley at ORATEC Interventions, Inc., the team developed an innovative heating method using a resistive thermal coil threaded circumferentially around the disc nucleus and annulus to lie in close approximation to the posterior disc margin. This design, which was named intradiscal electrothermal treatment (IDET), offered much better access to the posterior annulus. Following the presentation of two independent prospective short-term outcome studies by Saal and Derby at the North American Spine Society (NASS) Thirteenth Annual Meeting, San Francisco, CA, 1998 (11), the procedure gained momentum. Several years later, Dr. Phil Finch, working with Tyco-Radionics, developed and introduced a radiofrequency heating catheter [intradiscal radiofrequency treatment (IDRT)], which was threaded across the posterior annulus (Tyco-Radionics discTrode) (12).

Developed as a method to reduce nociceptive input and modulate annular collagen, intradiscal heating has not gained universal acceptance, in part because, the mechanism by which heat reduces pain remains speculative. Although many mechanisms have been proposed, none have been proven. The various proposed mechanisms include alteration of spinal segment mechanics via collagen modification, thermal nociceptive fiber destruction, biochemical mediation of inflammation (13), stimulation of an outer annular healing response, cauterization of vascular ingrowth and induced healing of annular tears (14). The most commonly sited benefit of reducing the number or outer annular nociceptors was not substantiated in a sheep animal model (15). Shah et al. (14) reported histologic findings of denaturation, shrinkage, coalescence of annular collagen, and stromal disorganization following IDET using a standard protocol in a cadaver model. However, histologic and thermal data have suggested that collagen modification may not be the primary effect (16,17). Although temperatures sufficient to coagulate nociceptors may be achieved, temperatures sufficient to cause collagen contraction more than several millimeters beyond the catheter center have not been shown. In cadaver models, Lee et al. (17) showed no change in disc stability following IDET treatment, whereas Kleinstueck et al. (16) showed small decreases in the stability of flexion and rotation. Although the closure of annular fissures is one possible benefit of this approach, it has not been demonstrated experimentally. The general consensus of physicians who have performed repeat discograms following IDET is that radial tears are still present. Thus, it is unlikely that intradiscal heating using current protocols would cause either fissure closure or improved disc stability. On the other hand, it is unlikely that heating will cause destabilization and may help seal or promote the healing of the outer annular rim.

The therapeutic efficacy of intradiscal heating probably depends on the transfer of heat through the nucleus, annulus or both. Heat transfer was studied initially by Houpt (18), who showed that temperatures sufficient to ablate nociceptors could not be achieved at distances greater than 11 mm from the catheter, preventing adequate heating of the outer annulus. Troussier (19) also failed to show a substantial increase in posterior longitudinal ligament temperature using a radiofrequency probe placed in the nucleus. Comparing radiofrequency and electrothermal methods, Ashley and Saal (20) showed that a radiofrequency needle ineffectively heated tissue at distances greater than 1 mm, whereas an electroresistive catheter caused temperatures of 45°C in the outer annulus. Wright et al. (21) also achieved temperatures sufficient to coagulate nociceptors in the posterior annulus. In more recent work, Kleinstueck et al. (16) obtained maximum catheter temperatures of 90°C (~75°C in tissue) and temperatures of 50–60°C and 45°C at distances of ~6 mm and ~10 mm from the catheter, respectively. Although temperatures were similar to those achieved by Ashley and Saal (20), Kleinstueck et al. concluded that temperatures in the outer annulus were insufficient to ablate nociceptive fibers. However, Kleinstueck showed that even after 16 minutes of heating, a steady state had not been reached; thus, longer heating protocols could potentially achieve a toxic dose at distances up to 10 mm from the catheter (16). The placement of the heating element in the middle or outer annulus within 5–10 mm more readily achieves desired temperatures. The recently introduced Radionics Disc TRODE device (IDRT) was designed to pass the active element across the outer posterior annulus, permitting outer annular temperatures of 45–50°C within several minutes using radiofrequency-generated heat of about 70°C. Bono et al. (22) showed that a zone of potential denervation occurred at distances 12–14 mm from the catheter, with temperatures of 42°C achieved at distances up to 14 mm. Using an IDET catheter placed close to the area of pathology, Wright (21) measured mean outer annular temperatures of 43.9 ± 2.3°C and concluded that these temperatures are sufficient to coagulate nociceptors.

Although a catheter placed within 5 mm of the outer annulus may achieve temperatures toxic to nociceptors within outer and middle annular fibers, it is unclear if this mechanism correlates with the clinical recovery following IDET or IDRT. At issue is the duration of pain flare-up. Similar to medial branch neurotomies, one may expect several days to a week of flare-up owing to tissue trauma followed by clinical improvement. Few published studies (23) comment on the frequency and duration of postintradiscal heating flare-up. Derby et al. (23) showed that in a series of 32 patients, all reported flare-up lasting an average of five days. If patients having no flare or minimal (less than one week) flare achieved a significantly better outcome, these data would be consistent with the theory that intradiscal heating reduces pain by destroying nociceptor input.

Many patients have longer flare-ups and are prone to relapse. Heating tissue will cause a thermal injury and cell death. Similar to the proposed effect of hypertonic solutions, heat could potentially initiate a healing response. A recent study showed that although there was a loss of cell viability using live/dead staining after IDET treatment, IDET-treated discs maintained in cell-culture conditions demonstrated the ability to recover cell viability in the treated areas over two to four weeks (24). The authors found that the thermal modification of collagen following IDET treatment was demonstrated by histologic and scanning electron microscopic (SEM) changes in collagen morphology. The authors concluded that their findings were consistent with other studies showing that shoulder capsular tissues regain biomechanical integrity after thermal treatment.

If heating stimulates an outer annular healing response (14), one would expect an initial flare in pain owing to inflammation followed by a slow resolution of pain during healing of the outer annulus. Such a mechanism may account for the fragility of these patients to mechanical loading for one to three months following IDET. A potential benefit would result if pain originated partially from the ingrowth of nocioceptive fibers into the inner annular layers. In cases where the majority of disc pain results from abnormally high mechanical endplate loads (25), one would not expect heating to produce significant benefit. These difficult-to-identify cases could account for the modest outcome, despite stringent selection criteria. Although Derby et al. (23) have reported better outcomes in patients with low-pressure-sensitive discs during discography, the Pauza et al. study (26) did not confirm these findings.

In addition to the theoretical reduction in nocioceptive fibers, and the potential benefits of tissue regeneration, reduction of intradiscal pressure in younger and more hydrated discs could also contribute to improved outcomes. Using a recently introduced shorter electrothermal IDET catheter (SpineCATH Intradiscal catheter, Smith & Nephew®) the controlled intradiscal application of thermal energy on bovine disc material resulted in a 15% decrease in volume, 2% decrease in mass, and a 3% decrease in disc diameter (27). The authors postulated that this mechanism might provide an explanation for observed improvements in radicular symptoms in patients with lumbar herniated nucleus pulposus (HNP). In a similar study, Podhajsky et al. (27) found pressure reductions approximating to 30–50% in sheep nucleus pulposus following IDET treatment using a 1.5-cm electrothermal device (Decompression catheter, Smith & Nephew). The authors also found that the hydrophilic property of nucleus pulposus is temperature dependent, and that increasing the treatment temperature resulted in a decreasing ability for the nucleus to absorb water.

INDICATIONS

Proposed but unproven selection criteria include the following: unremitting low back pain or referred leg pain of at least six months' duration unimproved by aggressive nonoperative care; normal neurologic and negative straight leg raise (SLR) test; magnetic resonance imaging (MRI) negative for a neural compressive lesion; lack of satisfactory improvement with nonoperative care program and at least one epidural corticosteroid injection; <30% decrease in disc height; positive discography (generally ≥6/10 pain at ≤50 psi above opening pressure); no prior surgery; disc protrusion less than approximately 3 to 4 mm; absence of instability and moderate to severe stenosis; no inflammatory arthritis; no nonspinal conditions mimicking lumbar pain and no medical disorder precluding follow up (13,28,29).

CONSIDERATIONS FOR PREOPERATIVE PLANNING
Preoperative Imaging

Although a preoperative evaluation should include an MRI scan for the initial evaluation of structural pathology, standard MR techniques for the detection of annular tears are often unreliable (30). Abnormal MRI does not exclude significant changes in the peripheral structure of the intervertebral disc which can produce low back pain (31,32). The recently introduced dynamic lumbar spine MRI with axial loading may increase the sensitivity for the detection of annular tears (33), but a CT scan following discography remains the most accurate method for the detection of annular pathology (31,32,34).

Provocative Discography

Identifying symptomatic annular tears reliably is controversial, but discography is the criterion standard for identifying a painful internally disrupted intervertebral disc. In 1995, the NASS stated that CT-discography may be the only study capable of providing a diagnosis or permitting precise description of the internal anatomy of a disc and the integrity of disc substructures (35).

In contemporary practice, however, discography refers to provocation discography in which the most important component is the evaluation of pain reproduction caused by pressurizing the disc with contrast medium. Recently, Derby et al. introduced more precise methods and criteria for provocative discography using pressure-controlled techniques [e.g., reproducible visual analogue scale (VAS) pain ≥6/10 with ≤50-psi intradiscal pressure and <3.5-ml total volume] that may reduce the incidence of false-positive responses to an acceptable level (36,37). The recommended positive criteria for lumbar pressure-controlled manometric discography are as follows: *numeric rating scale of pain above 6/10, ≤50-psi intradiscal pressure above opening pressure, <3.5-ml total volume, and at least one negative control disc.*

In conjunction with the history, physical examination, MRI scan, and a CT scan following discogram, a positive response to provocative discography, will at a minimum, add confirming information that can be used to make a more informed judgment. However, a positive discogram cannot predict a favorable outcome (38).

SURGICAL TECHNIQUE
Intradiscal Electrothermal Treatment

The IDET procedure developed by Oratec (Oratec Interventions, Inc., Menlo Park, CA, U.S.A.) utilizes a navigable intradiscal catheter with a thermal resistive coil. The procedure can be performed under conscious sedation that typically includes 50–100 mg of Demerol or an equivalent dose of Fentanyl and 2–4 mg of Midazolam (Versed). Using a standard posterolateral discogram technique, a 30-cm catheter (SpineCATH Intradiscal Catheter or Decompression Catheter , Smith & Nephew) with a 5- or 1.5-cm active electrothermal tip is inserted through a 17-gauge introducer needle and advanced circuitously to the posterior annulus. Usually one catheter is enough, but in some cases, a bilateral deployment is required to cover the entire posterior annular wall (29).

The patient lies in a prone oblique position on a fluoroscopy table. Elevating the target side approximately 15° allows the fluoroscopy tube to remain in a more AP projection and reduce radiation scatter. If required, a folded towel or soft wedge may be placed under the patient's flank to prevent side bending of the lumbar spine. On the side selected for puncture, a wide area of the skin of the back is prepped and draped from the costal margin to the mid-buttock and from the midline to the flank.

A fluoroscopic examination confirms segmentation and determines the appropriate level for catheter placement. In the AP view, the fluoroscopy tube is rotated until the inferior vertebral endplate of the target interspace is parallel to the fluoroscopy beam. The fluoroscopic beam is axially rotated until the zygapophyseal joint space is located midway between the anterior and posterior vertebral margins. In this view, the insertion point is lateral to the lateral margin of the superior articular process (Fig. 1). The insertion point is marked on the skin. As the distance between the opposite superior articular processes increases at lower levels, the usual distance from the midline increases from about two to three fingerbreadths at the T12–L1 level to four to five fingerbreadths (~6 cm) at the L5–S1 level. Because of the iliac crest and increased interfacetal distance, at the L5–S1 level, the fluoroscopy tube is rotated only far enough to bring the zygapophyseal joint space approximately 25% of the distance between the anterior and posterior vertebral margins (Fig. 2).

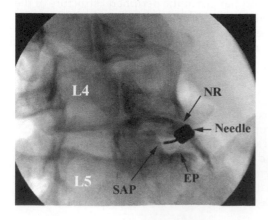

FIGURE 1 The introducer needle is usually advanced parallel to the fluoroscopic beam on the oblique fluoroscope view in which the zygapophyseal joint space is located midway between the anterior and posterior vertebral margins. In this view, the borders of the safe triangle include the nerve root for the superior tangential border, the vertebral endplate of the target disc for inferior border, and the lateral margin of the superior articular process for the medial side line.

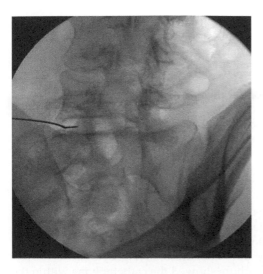

FIGURE 2 The oblique view of left L5–S1 level. Because of the iliac crest and increased interfacetal distance, at the L5–S1 level, the fluoroscopy tube is rotated only far enough to bring the zygapophyseal joint space, approximately 25% of the distance between the anterior and posterior vertebral margins.

Prior to needle placement, the skin, subcutaneous tissues, and deep muscular tissues along the needle trajectory are infiltrated with local anesthetic (1% lidocaine). To avoid potential neural injury, the needle should be directed into the safe triangle. The borders of the safe triangle include the nerve root for the superior tangential border, the vertebral end-plate of the target disc for inferior border, and the lateral margin of the superior articular process for the medial side line (Fig. 1).

One usually approaches the disc from the side opposite of the dominant pain. The modi-fied 17-G Tuohy needle is directed toward each disc under fluoroscopic guidance. To protect the discographer's hand from radiation exposure, forceps may be used to grasp the introducing needle. The introducer needle is advanced parallel to the fluoroscopic beam using an oblique fluoroscope view (Fig. 1).

A slight hockey-stick curve at the end of the introducer needle can improve navigation. If bony obstruction is encountered, the physician should confirm whether the needle has contacted the superior articular process or the vertebral body. If necessary, the needle may be slightly withdrawn and its trajectory modified. When the introducer needle contacts the disc margin, the ideal position in the AP projection is on a line drawn between the midpoints of the pedicles above and below (Fig. 3A). The introducer needle should not be advanced medial to the inner pedicle margins before contacting the intervertebral disc.

In the lateral view, the needle should contact the disc at the outer disc border between the posterior vertebral margins (Fig. 3B). When the needle contacts the disc, the position should be checked using AP and lateral views. Contact with the annulus fibrosus is characterized by the perception of firm but resilient resistance, and frequently, the patient experiences a momentary,

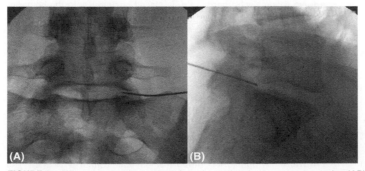

(A)   (B)

FIGURE 3 When the needle reaches the mid pedicle in the anteroposterior (AP) view, the position should be checked in the lateral views. The ideal position in the AP projection (**A**) is on a line drawn between the midpoints of the pedicles above and below. In the lateral view (**B**), the needle should contact the disc between the posterior vertebral margins.

sharp, or sudden aching sensation in the back or the buttock. There will be a sudden loss of resistance as the introducer needle enters the nucleoannular junction of the disc. The needle is then slightly advanced into the nuclear cavity of the disc and the position confirmed using AP and lateral imaging. After satisfactory needle placement, the needle bevel is turned to face posteriorly and the catheter is gently advanced to the opposite annulus with the preformed distal catheter curve facing posteriorly. One can monitor the passage of the catheter in either AP or lateral fluoroscopic view. When the catheter contacts the opposite annular wall, the tip will usually be directed toward the posterior lateral disc annulus (Fig. 4). The distance of the catheter from the outer annulus depends on the degree and location of the pre-existing annular disruption. Once the catheter crosses 4–5 mm of the opposite midline, it often turns back anteriorly (Fig. 5). Most of the active heating tip remains in the outer annulus on the opposite side, but in cases with a more extensive posterior annular disruption, the catheter will stay in the outer annulus as it crosses the midline (Fig. 6). The outer part of a portion of the catheter usually lies within 2 mm of the outer annulus (Figs. 7 and 8).

The catheter position is important (23,29). Ideally, the active length of the catheter should cross the "symptomatic" annular fissure and lie close enough (~5 mm) to the outer annulus to allow the spread of sufficient heat to both the outer and inner annulus (Fig. 8) (39).

Interestingly, the original Oratec company brochure showed the catheter lying within the nuclear–annular junction, and many of the original studies on inadequate spread of heat to the outer annular fibers were based on this catheter position. In clinical practice, however, the electrode tip inevitably ends up in the outer annular fibers. Although one may try multiple attempts and use a formed hooky stick bend on the outer catheter, ideal positioning 5 mm from the outer annulus is seldom achieved. Furthermore, frequent passage and multiple catheter removals could theoretically increase the risk of infection and often result in irrevocably damaging an expensive disposable device. In many cases, the catheter is in the outer annular fibers of the contralateral posterior lateral annulus and then passes more anterior (Fig. 5). The second bold

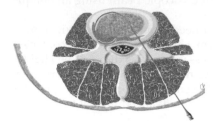

FIGURE 4 Using a standard posterolateral discogram technique, a decompression catheter (Smith & Nephew®) with a 1.5-cm active electrothermal tip is inserted through a 17-G introducer needle and advanced circuitously to the posterior annulus. Most of the active heating tip remains in the outer annulus on the opposite side. The very outer part of the catheter is usually within 2 mm of the outer annulus.

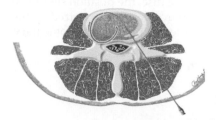

FIGURE 5 A SpineCATH Intradiscal Catheter (Smith & Nephew®), with a 5-cm active electrothermal tip, is placed circuitously to the posterior annulus and turns back anteriorly. The distance of the catheter from the outer annulus depends on the degree and location of the pre-existing annular disruption. Once the catheter crosses 4–5 mm of the opposite midline, it often turns back anteriorly.

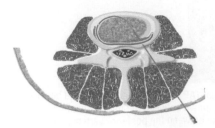

FIGURE 6 A SpineCATH Intradiscal Catheter (Smith & Nephew®) is placed circuitously in the outer posterior annulus. In cases with a more extensive posterior annular disruption, the catheter tip will stay in the outer annulus as it crosses the midline.

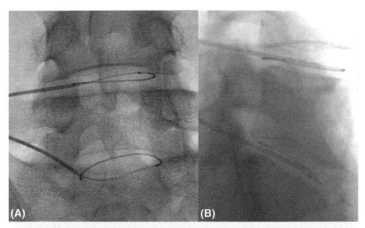

FIGURE 7 Fluoroscopy image of the intradiscal electrothermal treatment procedure. The intradiscal electrothermal catheter electrode (SpineCATH Intradiscal catheter, Smith & Nephew®) is placed within the L4/5 and L5/S1 discs.

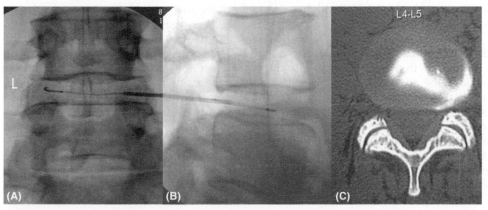

FIGURE 8 Fluoroscopy image of the intradiscal electrothermal treatment procedure. The shorter 1.5-cm eletrothermal wire (Decompression catheter, Smith & Nephew®) has been positioned within the torn outer posterior annulus of the L4/5 disc. After thermal heating, the patient was injected the fibrin sealant (Tisseel VH, Baxter Healthcare®) into the disc to help "seal" the painful torn annulus.

mark on the catheter must place beyond the introducer needle hub. Before heating, the position of the catheter should be confirmed and documented by AP and lateral view. The catheter should not be placed outside the annulus of the disc.

Heating Protocol. The original 5-cm active heating element catheter, introduced by Oratec, has the temperature electrode placed within the catheter and measured catheter temperatures that were on average 13°C higher than the adjacent disc tissue. The standard empirically derived protocol begins heating at 65°C with incremental changes of 1°C every 30 seconds to achieve a final temperature between 80° and 90°C. The final temperature was maintained for five minutes for a total treatment time of 13.5–16.5 minutes (40). Some advocated heating to higher temperatures but there was no standard method for determining the final temperatures. Analyzing study results using the 5-cm catheter, Derby et al. (37) could not show a correlation between higher temperatures and improved outcome at either eight months or 16 months postprocedure. In fact, when catheter positions were less than 5 mm from the outer annulus, higher thermal dosage was associated with longer flare-up durations postprocedure. The authors proposed an alternative protocol in which temperatures are incrementally increased to 80°C measured temperature, but the final temperature and duration were determined by the patient's pain response from baseline. Depending on the patient's pain tolerance and degree of sedation, incremental changes in temperature are stopped when the patient reports greater than 6–8/10 pain from their baseline pain. The temperature is then maintained for up to four minutes as long as the patient's back pain remain below 8/10 intensity.

The new shorter catheter (Decompression catheter, Smith & Nephew) uses a shorter 1.5-cm heating element which may help limit the destruction of normal disc annulus (Figs 4, 8). The temperature electrode is placed on the outside of the catheter, and therefore, measured temperatures reflect the adjacent tissue temperatures. The heating protocol still incrementally increases temperatures to 90°C and is then maintained for six minutes, but in effect, this temperature is 13 to 15°C higher than the 5-cm catheter. More heat reaches a shorter segment of the annulus, nucleus, or both, but because the catheter length is shorter, the total heat dose is probably less. Some practitioner's initial impressions suggest improved outcomes with shorter duration flare-ups and some feel that patients tolerate higher temperatures before complaining of excessive pain.

Intradiscal Radiofrequency Treatment

The approach to the intervertebral disc is similar to the earlier description, but rather than passing the introducer needle into the disc nucleus, the needle tip is directed into the outer posterior lateral annulus and the active electrode is advanced across the posterior annulus (Fig. 9). The device (discTRODE™ RF catheter, Radionics®) includes a sensing device that measures tissue resistance, and the higher resistance of the disc annulus can be detected with both sound and digital readings. By passing the needle tip slightly more posteriorly and medially in the disc annulus, an asymmetric opening in the needle tip would help direct the active electrode across the posterior disc annulus. The setup also includes a temperature-monitoring needle that can be placed into the outer posterior annulus and one can monitor the increase in the outer annular temperatures as the electrode is heated (Fig. 9A). A graduated temperature protocol beginning at 65°C is used but the final temperature is determined by measuring the temperatures in the contralateral annulus using the temperature-monitoring needle inserted into the contralateral outer annulus. When the temperature measured in the outer annulus by the temperature-monitoring needle reaches 45°C, the final temperature is maintained for four minutes. Although a seemingly more accurate method of determining the final temperature, the distance of the measuring electrode from the radiofrequency electrode is variable.

Postprocedure Care

After removing the catheter, an intradiscal antibiotic injection (e.g., 3- to 6-mg Cephalozin) combined with either local anesthetic or contrast media is typically injected through the introducer needle (23). The patient is monitored in the recovery room for one- to three-hours postprocedure

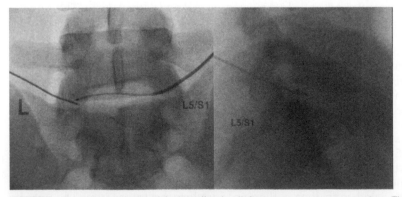

FIGURE 9 Fluoroscopy image of the intradiscal radiofrequency treatment procedure. The needle tip is directed into the outer posterior lateral annulus and the active tip is advanced across the posterior annulus. The setup also includes a needle with a temperature electrode that can be placed into the outer posterior annulus, and one can monitor the increase in outer annular temperatures as the electrode is heated.

and is discharged the same day (23). The patient is warned to expect a significant increase in his baseline pain and is told that the usual flare-up lasts two to seven days, but infrequently can last for an indefinite period of time. Patients are instructed to call if he or she experiences fever, chills, or severe (or delayed) onset of pain. Patients are contacted by telephone 48 to 96 hours after the procedure and are usually seen at a one-, three-, and six-month follow up (23,41).

Patients are typically braced for several weeks to several months after the procedure. During the initial several months, the outer annulus is rehealing and there is probably an increased risk of reinjury from excessive disc loading. Activities like walking and pool exercise are encouraged, but aggressive physical therapy is usually begun only after one- to two-months postprocedure (41). Most patients have reached maximal improvement by three months, but a minority may take three to six months (28,39,41,42). Several studies have documented stable and enduring pain relief in two-year follow ups (28,39,41,42).

COMPLICATIONS

Complications are infrequent. A retrospective study (13) reviewed the complications of 1675 IDET procedures performed at five different spine centers, and in addition, analyzed the data of 35,000 SpineCATH intradiscal catheters reported by the medical device reports (MDRs) of the United States Food and Drug Administration (FDA). A total of six nerve-root injuries were reported. All but one of the nerve-root injuries occurred during insertion of the introducer needle. Five of the six completely resolved and one case was resolving. No cases of discitis were reported. Six cases of post-IDET disc herniation were reported at the treated level two to 12 months after treatment. Four resolved with nonoperative care, and two required disc excision. Nineteen cases of catheter breakage were reported. All were associated with repeated catheter manipulation that resulted in kinking. In 16 cases, the catheter was uneventfully left within the disc. Eight cases of superficial skin burn at the needle puncture site were reported. One case of post-IDET bladder dysfunction was reported.

Although few, disc infections and neural injury can occur (43). Disc infections following intradiscal procedures have been most often described following lumbar discography and cervical discography. Causative organisms have been identified as *Staphylococcus aureus*, *Staphylococcus epidermis*, and *Escherichia coli* (44,45), suggesting inoculation with surface organisms or misadventure through internal organ perforation. Some authors consider discitis a rare complication of lumber discography (46–48), whereas others have found overall rates of 2.3% per patient and 1.3% per disc (49) or 0.1% per patient and 0.05% per disc (45). The incidence of discitis is higher for single, large-gauge needles and much lower for double-needle techniques (50). Animal studies have shown that intradiscal (51) and intravenous (49) antibiotics prevent discitis. The recommended regimen is 1 mg of Cefazolin per ml of contrast medium injected into the disc at the time of discography (51). However, many discographers use 3- to 6-mg Cephalozin (or an equivalent antibiotic) per ml of contrast. Even with prophylactic antibiotics, epidural abscess after discography has been reported (52,53). Stringent attention to aseptic technique is critical.

Striking a ventral ramus is a potential hazard. In a conscious patient, contact with the ventral ramus will be indicated by severe, sharp lancinating leg pain, which is an indication to withdraw and redirect the needle. Another potential complication is a subarachnoid puncture. If one closely monitors the lateral and AP fluoroscopic view, one should not pass the IDET introducer needle through the intervertebral foramen. In the AP view, the needle should not be seen passing medial to a line drawn between the medial edge of adjacent pedicles if the tip has not reached the posterior annulus in the lateral view. Subarachnoid needle placement is easily diagnosed, and although the patient would probably have a postprocedural headache, an epidural blood patch is an effective treatment. Whether a dural puncture increases the risk of heat injury to the cauda equine is unknown, but one might consider coming back another day instead of proceeding with intradiscal heating.

Passing a catheter through the outer annulus and into the epidural space is easily identified on a lateral fluoroscopic image. If this occurs, withdraw the catheter back into the disc and redirect. Heating an epidurally placed catheter should cause the patient to complain of the almost immediate onset of leg pain. Performing IDETs under general anesthesia is probably not a good idea. Ignoring complaints of excessive early pain onset or over-sedating a patient is also not preferred.

Procedural Risks

The IDET procedure is relatively benign but does carry risks beyond that expected with needle penetration of the disc. The risks inherent with discography or any percutaneous procedure directed into the intervertebral disc may also be associated with the IDET procedure. Intradiscal infection remains a concern; however, the use of preoperative IV antibiotics and postoperative prophylactic injections of antibiotics into the disc significantly reduce the risk of infection to less than 1/3000 cases (54). If the catheter penetrates the posterior annulus, it will lie in close proximity to the dura and spinal roots. In most cases, it is easy to determine if the catheter is outside the disc, but a catheter may navigate into a posterior disc protrusion and be seen posterior to the vertebral margin. Caution should be exercised if the catheter cannot be advanced to a more proximal position. Although transient increases in leg pain are not uncommon, prolonged increases in previous leg pain or occurrence of new leg pain is uncommon and has been documented in only a few reports. High temperatures in the epidural space adjacent to the disc may result from the occasional case when the catheter lies within a few millimeters of the traversing or exiting nerve root. Temperatures >45°C applied for an extended period of time might cause transient or prolonged leg pain. Endplate injury caused by heat is another possible complication, and although cadaver studies have not demonstrated significantly elevated endplate temperatures (55), it is difficult to determine the proximity of the catheter to the endplates with fluoroscopy, and in some instances, a portion of the catheter may contact an adjoining endplate.

Accelerated disc degeneration has been mentioned as a concern by some and as a goal by others. In the short term, however, there seems to be little change in the MRI reading pre- and post-IDET. Ho et al. (56) reported no change in the MRI scans of 72 patient at 12-months post-IDET.

OUTCOMES

Initial outcome studies following newly introduced treatment techniques, marketed and developed by device companies, often report overly optimistic results. Intradiscal electrothermal treatment was no exception. The initial prospective case series by the original developers, Saal et al., reported a positive response rate of 80%; Derby et al. initial studies reported positive-response rates of 73% when the catheter position was optimal and a 16.5% positive-response rate in patients with a fair catheter placement (23). Saal et al. (13,28) reported decreases in the SF-36 body pain of 59% to 78% and average decreases in VAS scores of 62% to 72%. Despite published results similar to the Saal's, Derby was earlier quoted in the Back Letter (57) as stating that about one-third of the patients were better, one-third were the same (a bit better), and one-third were worse (same or worse) following IDET. With the exception of the Karasek study (39), which included a convenience control group of patients denied insurance authorization who underwent a treatment protocol identical to patients receiving IDET, all early studies examined prospective cohorts without a control group. Depending on how one defined success, Karasek's series (39) showed as low as 23% or as high as 60% favorable results of the IDET group compared with the 5.9% favorable results of the control group. His patient selection included only patients with presumably healthier and better hydrated discs in which annular disruption was limited to two quadrants or less. The best reported outcome results were from Mauer et al. prospective series (58) that included only patients with an intact outer annulus. The outcomes were assessed by 10-point VAS pain scale, functional tolerance levels, and SF36 health survey questionnaire at baseline, three and six months. At six months, 94% of patients had a mean decrease of 4 points on VAS, the functional scale increased at an average of 75% and a highly significant increase in SF36 subscale scores were recorded at three and six months. In contrast to the studies performed by practitioners with a positive bias, less than stellar results were reported in two studies reported by surgeons (59,60). These two studies included a broad patient-selection criteria and both reported similar outcomes: one-third of the patients were significantly better, one-third slightly or questionably better, and one-third the same or worse (59,60).

Although initial IDET outcomes in well-selected patients were encouraging, selecting ideal candidates for a procedure designed to treat chronic low back pain is a complex problem. The cause of discogenic low back pain is not well understood, and probably varies from patient to patient and in any one patient from time to time. The patient's motivation to improve or report improvement is a confounding variable that is difficult to control and often contribute to reports of poor outcome. In addition, other sources of pain are often present and when one source is made better, others become worse. Even if we could precisely define the cause of a patient's pain, the potential benefit in heating annular tissue as a method of relieving low back pain remains speculative, and therefore, our ability to select optimal patients for intradiscal heating is limited. Despite these caveats, early studies indicated that maintained disc heights and limited annular disruption predicted better results. All studies required a positive response to provocative discography, and Derby et al. correlated improved outcomes in patients who reported concordant pain provocation during discography at low pressures and volumes (9). On the other hand, one prospective series (61) correlated poor results if patients were obese. The probability of post-IDET worsening of pain may be no greater than that observed in patients choosing not to undergo the procedure, and in fact, may be 6% to 20%, which is lower than the 30% of the sham control IDET group in the Pauza study (62). The number of patients undergoing surgery post-IDET varies, but probably averages between 10% and 15% at one year (39,59,61,63).

As IDET was promoted to treat discogenic low back pain, only one study compared the relief of extremity pain to relief of axial pain (64). Derby et al. noted that up to 84% of low back pain (LBP) patients who underwent IDET also presented with referred leg pain without radiculopathy (64). Their study showed that improvements in leg pain post-IDET procedure correlated well with improvements in back pain. Fifty-two percent of patients showed an improvement in leg pain with the mean improvement of 1.90/4 in the 5-point pain score.

Despite the difficulties in choosing ideal patients and despite varying initial outcome reports, IDET is one of the few interventional spinal procedures to have three randomized blinded controlled studies. The Pauza study (62) is a double-blind, placebo-controlled trial in carefully selected patients with single-level painful disc disruption identified with carefully performed pressure-controlled lumbar discography. The disc heights were maintained and protrusions, when present, were less than 20% of the disc height narrowing on lateral plain film radiographs (unclear). In addition, the patients had neither litigation nor compensation issues. The IDET procedures were performed by two separate clinicians, Kevin Pauza and John Pelosa, both of whom were experienced, technically proficient, and had positive clinical impressions regarding prior IDET outcomes. The catheters were navigated circumferentially to both the lateral and posterior annulus on both sides of the disc. Catheter insertions from both sides of the midline were performed, when necessary, to provide complete coverage of the outer annulus. After randomization, 37 were assigned to undergo IDET and 27 to sham treatment. Those undergoing a control procedure had a sham treatment in which the introducer needle was inserted to the lateral margin of the disc. Both groups exhibited significant improvements in pain scores and at six-month follow up, there was an average difference of 1.3 in VAS between the IDET and the control groups with a calculated p value of 0.045 (62). A similar pattern of improvement occurred in the bodily pain scores of the SF-36, but was not significantly different between the two groups ($p = 0.086$) (62).

Freeman et al. (15) performed a randomized double-blind controlled IDET efficacy study in which patients were selected on the basis of one- or two-level symptomatic disc degeneration with posterior or posterolateral annular tears as determined by provocative CT/discography. Patients were excluded if there was >50% loss of disc height or previous back surgery (15). The study did not demonstrate a significant benefit from IDET over placebo. No subject in either treatment group showed an improvement of >7 points in low back outcome score or specified domains of the SF-36.

Bogduk recently presented the IDET results of a controlled randomized study by Lau et al. (65) in patients with single-level painful disc disruption identified by a positive discogram using International Spinal Injection Society (ISIS) criteria. The study included six patients randomized to the control sham group, 11 patients randomized to the IDET group, and also included a benchmark group of patients who initially refused the requirements of enrollment randomization but had IDET performed after obtaining approval by their insurance company. Similar to the Pauza study, there was an average of 2.5 (7.0 to 4.5) decrease in the VA score at 12 months in the 11 patients in the controlled IDET group, and although the benchmark group showed less favorable outcome, there was no statistical difference in the groups, and the combined data from these two groups showed a statistical difference from initial VA score to the VA score at 12 months. Fifty percent of the randomized IDET cases achieved 50% or greater pain relief. The control IDET group, however, included six patients, and five of the six patients were somewhat better at three months. One control patient was pain free at three months and remained pain free at one-year follow up. Because of this one spontaneous recovery in the control group, the calculated number of patients needed to show a statistical difference between the active and sham group, which was approximately 100, and the study was stopped. Bogduk concluded that IDET was too weak a treatment to prove efficacy against a placebo conclusively without a large number of patients, but the results were probably not worse than any other of our treatments for this diagnosis.

Although there appears to be a modest improvement in pain compared with the natural history, the percentage of patients that would achieve various degrees of improvement is uncertain. The results of both Pauza et al. (62) and Lau et al. (65) are comparable with more recently reported outcomes in case series observational studies, and it appears that the number of treated patients needed for one to have 50% or more reduction in pain is between two and four with a pain reduction of about 2.5 on a 10-point VAS on an average. On the other hand, in both the Pauza and the Lau study, the number of patients in the randomized IDET group who reported worse pain at 12 months was less than 10% compared with the 30% of patients in Pauza's sham control group who reported increased VAS scores at follow up.

Return to work may be associated with both the percentage improvement in VAS and the VAS score after treatment (39). Karasek et al. (39) reported that for patients not previously working, achieving a VAS score of less than 3/10 predicted 75% of those who returned to work. The study also found that of all the patients achieving a VAS score improvement, at least 50% returned to work. However, no patients returned to work with less than 50% improvement (39).

Finally, technical variables influencing IDET outcome remain understudied. Derby et al. (66) evaluated the effect of heat intensity, heat duration, and the number of catheters on outcomes and pain flare-up following IDET in patients at a single level, with disc protrusion ≤2 mm and positive discogram with an annular tear. The results showed that in most cases, the catheters were within 2–5 mm of the outer annulus, and in those cases, higher temperatures and larger total heating doses increase the duration of postprocedure pain flare-ups and lead to less favorable outcomes at 8-month follow up (66). The author concluded that modifying the standard heating protocol downward depending on the amount of pain experienced by the patient during the incremental changes in temperature may reduce the duration of flare-up and would achieve similar or better results. Similar to these results, in a randomized trial using IDRT, Ercelen et al. did not find any difference in the six-month outcome following an intradiscal radiofrequency heating using a 120-second protocol versus a 360-second protocol (67).

FUTURE DIRECTIONS

Studies show that intradiscal heating causes thermal necrosis of tissue (2), and injury of the normal annulus caused by the long-heating elements could be a cause of prolonged flare-ups and unsatisfied outcome (40). The shorter 1.5-cm electrothermal devices might theoretically provide better outcomes with less-prolonged flare-ups (66). In contrast, under investigation is a new transdiscal radiofrequency treatment technique named transdiscal annuloplasty, which is designed to achieve a more uniform but significantly larger areas of heat spread. This device uses two separate electrode probes inserted from the right and left sides of the disc. The two probes are water cooled to reduce the heat adjacent to the electrodes and thus facilitating the spread of a lower heat across the posterior annulus. Pauza (68) showed that when the probes were inserted into the opposite posterior lateral disc annulus, the posterior annulus between the probes could reach a temperature of 60°C.

The addition of fibrin sealant could also help "seal" the annulus and prevent the leakage of inflammatory substances into the epidural space. During spinal surgery, fibrin sealant is used as an adjunct to hemostasis, wound healing, tissue adhesion, and to help seal dural leaks. Fibrin may enhance the repair process by acting as a biological glue, providing a scaffold for ingrowing fibroblasts, and stimulating cellular repare (4). Anecdotal reports by a few interventionalists have claimed improved outcome after the injection of fibrin sealant (Tisseel VH, Baxter Healthcare®) into painful annular tears (Fig. 5) (69).

SUMMARY

Intradiscal electrothermal treatment was one of the first micro-invasive devices designed specifically for treating discogenic low back pain (70). Both prospective and RCT studies have shown mostly consistent outcome results. As illustrated in a recent meta-analysis, the reviewers found on average, a clinically significant 2.7 improvement in back pain and a 17.7 improvement of the SF-36 bodily pain score when using the first-generation IDET catheter with a 5-cm active electrode (71). However, only about a third of the patients have dramatic pain relief (23). Most patients continue narcotics postprocedure and a few workers' compensation patients that were not working before the procedure return to work after an IDET procedure (61). Intradiscal heating does, however, provide a relatively benign next option for patients with chronic axial and referred extremity pain owing to one or two internally disrupted lumbar intervertebral discs. The unproven consensus is that disc heights should be relatively well maintained, internal disruption limited to two quadrants, and disc protrusions should not exceed 3–4 mm. The theoretical reason IDET might relieve discogenic pain remains speculative but the destruction of nociocepters or thermal modulation of collagen (27) could contribute to pain relief. In addition, heating the outer annulus may promote a healing response and repopulation of condrocytes might occur (27).

Diagnosing and treating discogenic low back and referred extremity pain is challenging. Many confounding variables make selection and outcome prediction difficult. Whether or not a newer generation of intradiscal heating methods and devices introduced in 2005 and beyond will improve future outcomes is speculative.

REFERENCES

1. The classic. Enzyme dissolution of the nucleus pulposus in humans. By Lyman W. Smith. 1964. Clin Orthop 1986; 206:4–9.
2. Chen YC, Lee SH, Chen D. Intradiscal pressure study of percutaneous disc decompression with nucleoplasty in human cadavers. Spine 2003; 28(7):661–665.
3. Andreula C, Muto M, Leonardi M. Interventional spinal procedures. Eur J Radiol 2004; 50(2): 112–119.
4. Dreyfuss P, Halbrook B, Pauza K, Joshi A, McLarty J, Bogduk N. Efficacy and validity of radiofrequency neurotomy for chronic lumbar zygapophysial joint pain. Spine 2000; 25(10):1270–1277.
5. Dreyfuss P, Baker R, Leclaire R, et al. Radiofrequency facet joint denervation in the treatment of low back pain: a placebo-controlled clinical trial to assess efficacy. Spine 2002; 27(5):556–557.
6. Sluijter ME. The use of radiofrequency lesions for pain relief in failed back patients. Int Disabil Stud 1988; 10(1):37–43.
7. Van Kleef M, Barendse G, Wilmink J, et al. Percutaneous intradiscal radiofrequency thermocoagulation in chronic non-specific low back pain. The Pain Clinic 1996; 9(3):259–268.
8. van Kleef M, Barendse GA, Dingemans WA, et al. Effects of producing a radiofrequency lesion adjacent to the dorsal root ganglion in patients with thoracic segmental pain. Clin J Pain 1995; 11(4):325–332.
9. Derby R, Eek B, Ryan D. Intradiscal electrothermal annuloplasty. Sci Newsletter Int Spinal Injection Soc 1998; 3(1).
10. Derby R, Eek B, Saal J. Intradiscal electrothermal coagulation by catheter. Paper presented at International Intradiscal Therapy Society 11th Annual Meeting, May 1998, San Antonio, TX.
11. Saal JA, Saal JS. A novel approach to painful derangement: collagen modulation with a thermal percutaneous navigable intradiscal catheter: a prospective trial. Paper presented at: NASS Thirteenth Meeting, October, 1998, San Francisco, CA.
12. Finch PM. The use of radiofrequency heat lesions in the treatment of lumbar discogenic pain. Pain Pract 2002; 2(3):235.

13. Saal JS, Saal JA. IDET related complications: a multi-center study of 1675 treated patients with a review of the FDA MDR data base. Paper presented at: International Spinal Injection Society 9th Annual Scientific Meeting, 2001.

14. Shah RV, Lutz GE, Lee J, Doty SB, Rodeo S. Intradiskal electrothermal therapy: a preliminary histologic study. Arch Phys Med Rehabil 2001; 82(9):1230–1237.

15. Freeman B, Fraser R, Cain C, Hall D. A randomized, double-blind controlled efficacy study: intradiscal electrothermal therapy (IDET) versus placebo. Paper presented at: International Society for the Study of the Lumbar Spine, 30th Annual Meeting, Vancouver, Canada, May 13–17, 2003.

16. Kleinstueck FS, Diederich CJ, Nau WH, et al. Acute biomechanical and histological effects of intradiscal electrothermal therapy on human lumbar discs. Spine 2001; 26(20):2198–2207.

17. Lee J, Lutz GE, Campbell D, Rodeo SA, Wright T. Stability of the lumbar spine after intradiscal electrothermal therapy. Arch Phys Med Rehabil 2001; 82(1):120–122.

18. Houpt JC, Conner ES, McFarland EW. Experimental study of temperature distributions and thermal transport during radiofrequency current therapy of the intervertebral disc [see comments]. Spine 1996; 21(15):1808–1812; discussion 1812–1803.

19. Troussier B, Lebas JF, Chirossel JP, et al. Percutaneous intradiscal radio-frequency thermocoagulation. A cadaveric study [see comments]. Spine 1995; 20(15):1713–1718.

20. Ashley J, Gharpuray V, Saal J. Temperature distribution in the intervertebral disc: a comparison of intranuclear radio-frequency needle to a novel heating catheter. Paper presented at Bioengineering Conference ASME, 1999.

21. Wright RE, et al. Precise in vivo measurement of peak intra-annular temperatures obtained during intradiscal electrothermal therapy. Paper presented at: 13th annual meeting IITS, June 8–10, 2000; Williamsburg, VA.

22. Bono CM, Garfin S, Iki K, Jalota A, Dawson K. Temperatures within the lumbar disc and end-plates during intradiscal electrothermal therapy: formulation of a predictive temperature map in relation to distance from the catheter. Paper presented at: ISIS 10th Annual Scientific Meeting, 2002, Austin, TX.

23. Derby REB, Chen Y, O' Neill C, Ryan D. Intradiscal electrothermal annuloplasty: a novel approach for treating chronic discogenic back pain. Neuromodulation 2000; 3(2):82–88.

24. Andersson G, Andrews N, Huckle J. Alteration of the collagen and cell viablity within the disc following intradiscal electrothermal therapy. Paper presented at: ISIS 12th Annual Scientific Meeting, 2004, Maui, Hawaii.

25. Adams MA, Dolan P, Hutton WC. Diurnal variations in the stresses on the lumbar spine. Spine 1987; 12(2):130–137.

26. Derby R. Outcome comparison between IDET, combined IDET nucleoplasty and biochemical injection treatment. Paper presented at: International Spinal Injectinon Society, 10th Annual Scientific Meeting, Austin, TX, September 7, 2002.

27. Podhajsky R, Belous A. The effects of temperature on Nucleus Pulposus; intervertebral pressure and hydrokinetics. Paper presented at: ISIS 12th Annual Scientific Meeting, 2004, Maui, Hawaii.

28. Saal JA, Saal JS. Intradiscal electrothermal treatment for chronic discogenic low back pain: prospective outcome study with a minimum 2-year follow-up. Spine 2002; 27(9):966–973; discussion 973–964.

29. Saal JA, Saal JS. Intradiscal electrothermal therapy for the treatment of chronic discogenic low back pain. Clin Sports Med 2002; 21(1):167–187.

30. Aprill C, Bogduk N. High-intensity zone: a diagnostic sign of painful lumbar disc on magnetic resonance imaging. Br J Radiol 1992; 65(773):361–369.

31. Osti OL, Vernon-Roberts B, Moore R, Fraser RD. Annular tears and disc degeneration in the lumbar spine. A post-mortem study of 135 discs. J Bone Joint Surg [Br]. 1992; 74(5):678–682.

32. Sachs BL, Vanharanta H, Spivey MA, et al. Dallas discogram description. A new classification of CT/discography in low-back disorders. Spine 1987; 12(3):287–294.

33. Saifuddin A, Braithwaite I, White J, Taylor BA, Renton P. The value of lumbar spine magnetic resonance imaging in the demonstration of anular tears. Spine 1998; 23(4):453–457.

34. Sachs BL, Spivey MA, Vanharanta H, et al. Techniques for lumbar discography and computed tomography/discography in clinical practice. Orthop Rev 1990; 19(9):775–778.

35. Guyer RD, Ohnmeiss DD. Lumbar discography. Position statement from the North American Spine Society Diagnostic and Therapeutic Committee [see comments]. Spine 1995; 20(18):2048–2059.

36. Derby R, Lee SH, Kim BJ, Chen Y, Aprill C, Bogduk N. Pressure-controlled lumbar discography in volunteers without low back symptoms (in press). Pain Med 2005.

37. Derby R, Lee SH, Chen Y. A prospective analysis of lumbar discography findings in select participants without low back symptoms. Paper presented at: North American Spine Society, 18th Annual Meeting, October 21–25, 2003; San Diego, CA.

38. Lau P, Mercer S, Govind J, Bogduk N. The surgical anatomy of lumbar medial branch neurotomy (facet denervation). Pain Med 2004; 5(3):289–298.

39. Karasek M, Bogduk N. Twelve-month follow-up of a controlled trial of intradiscal thermal anuloplasty for back pain due to internal disc disruption. Spine 2000; 25(20):2601–2607.

40. Kleinstueck FS, Diederich CJ, Nau WH, et al. Temperature and thermal dose distributions during intradiscal electrothermal therapy in the cadaveric lumbar spine. Spine 2003; 28(15):1700–1708.

41. Saal JA, Saal JS. Intradiscal electrothermal treatment for chronic discogenic low back pain: a prospective outcome study with minimum 1-year follow-up. Spine 2000; 25(20):2622–2627.

42. Bogduk N, Karasek M. Two-year follow-up of a controlled trial of intradiscal electrothermal anuloplasty for chronic low back pain resulting from internal disc disruption. Spine J 2002; 2(5): 343–350.

43. Thomas PS. Image-Guided Pain Management. Philadelphia: Lippincott-Raven Publishers, 1997.

44. Agre K, Wilson RR, Brim M, McDermott DJ. Chymodiactin postmarketing surveillance. Demographic and adverse experience data in 29,075 patients. Spine 1984; 9(5):479–485.

45. Guyer RD, Collier R, Stith WJ, et al. Discitis after discography. Spine 1988; 13(12):1352–1354.

46. Brodsky AE, Binder WF. Lumbar discography. Its value in diagnosis and treatment of lumbar disc lesions. Spine 1979; 4(2):110–120.

47. Simmons EH, Segil CM. An evaluation of discography in the localization of symptomatic levels in discogenic disease of the spine. Clin Orthop 1975; 108:57–69.

48. Wiley JJ, Macnab I, Wortzman G. Lumbar discography and its clinical applications. Can J Surg 1968; 11(3):280–289.

49. Fraser RD, Osti OL, Vernon-Roberts B. Iatrogenic discitis: the role of intravenous antibiotics in prevention and treatment. An experimental study. Spine 1989; 14(9):1025–1032.

50. Fraser RD, Osti OL, Vernon-Roberts B. Discitis after discography. J Bone Joint Surg [Br]. 1987; 69B(1):26–35.

51. Osti OL, Fraser RD, Vernon-Roberts B. Discitis after discography. The role of prophylactic antibiotics. J Bone Joint Surg [Br] 1990; 72(2):271–274.

52. Tsuji N, Igarashi S, Koyama T. Spinal epidural abscess—report of 5 cases. No Shinkei Geka 1987; 15(10):1079–1085.

53. Junila J, Niinimaki T, Tervonen O. Epidural abscess after lumbar discography. A case report. Spine 1997; 22(18):2191–2193.

54. Fraser RD. The North American Spine Society (NASS) on lumbar discography [letter; comment]. Spine 1996; 21(10):1274–1276.

55. Yetkinler DN, Nau WH, Brandt LL. Disc temperature measurements during nucleoplasty and IDET procedures. Paper presented at: 6th International Congress on Spinal Surgery, September 4–7, 2002; Ankara, Turkey.

56. Ho C, Kaiser J, Saal J. Does IDET cause advancement of disc degeneration? A one year MRI follow-up study of 72 patients. Paper presented at: 16th Annual Meeting North American Spine Society, October 31–November 3, 2001; Seattle, WA.

57. Two recent studies of thermal disc therapy. Back Lett 1999;14(8).

58. Maurer P, Squilante D, Dawson K. Is IDET effective treatment for discogenic low back pain? A prospective cohort outcome study (1–2 year follow-up) identifying successful patient selection criteria. Paper presented at: International Spinal Injection Society, 10th Annual Scientific Meeting, Austin, TX, September 7, 2002.

59. Davis TT, Delamarter RB, Sra P, Goldstein TB. The IDET procedure for chronic discogenic low back pain. Spine 2004; 29(7):752–756.

60. Spruit M, Jacobs WC. Pain and function after intradiscal electrothermal treatment (IDET) for symptomatic lumbar disc degeneration. Eur Spine J 2002; 11(6):589–593.

61. Webster BS, Verma S, Pransky GS. Outcomes of workers' compensation claimants with low back pain undergoing intradiscal electrothermal therapy. Spine 2004; 29(4):435–441.

62. Pauza KJ, Howell S, Dreyfuss P, Peloza JH, Dawson K, Bogduk N. A randomized, placebo-controlled trial of intradiscal electrothermal therapy for the treatment of discogenic low back pain. Spine J 2004; 4(1):27–35.

63. Lagattuta FB, Brady R, Hudoba P, Lai PH. Incidence of intervertebral fusion in patients treated with intradiscal electrothermotherapy. Paper presented at: American Association of Orthopedic Medicine Annual Meeting, May 4–6, 2000; Amelia Island, FL.

64. Derby R, Lee SH, Seo KS, Kazala K, Kim BJ, Kim MJ. Efficacy of IDET for relief of leg pain associated with discogenic low back pain. Pain Pract 2004; 4(4):281–285.

65. Lau P, Painter I, Govind J, Bailey B, Bogduk N. A controlled trial of IDET. Paper presented at: ISIS 12th Annual Scientific Meeting, 2004, Maui, Hawaii.

66. Derby R, Seo KS, Kazala K, Chen Y, Lee SH, Kim MJ. A factor analysis of lumbar intradiscal electrothermal annuloplasty (IDET) outcomes. Spine J 2005; 5(3):256–261; discussion 262.

67. Ercelen O, Bulutcu E, Oktenoglu T, et al. Radiofrequency lesioning using two different time modalities for the treatment of lumbar discogenic pain: a randomized trial. Spine 2003; 28(17):1922–1927.

68. Pauza K. Transdiscal anuloplasty: the first report cadaveric intervertebral disc temperature mapping. Paper presented at: ISIS 12th Annual Scientific Meeting, 2004, Maui, Hawaii.

69. Derby R, Kim BJ. Effect of short heating element IDET and fibrin injection on discogenic low back pain (in process). Arch Phys Med Rehabil 2005.

70. Djurasovic M, Glassman SD, Dimar JR, II, Johnson JR. Vertebral osteonecrosis associated with the use of intradiscal electrothermal therapy: a case report. Spine 2002; 27(13):E325–328.

71. Andersson G, Appleby D, Totta M. Meta analysis of the pain outcomes following treatment with intradiscal electrothermal therapy. Paper presented at: ISIS 12th Annual Scientific Meeting, 2004, Maui, Hawaii.

31 | Kyphoplasty for the Treatment of Osteoporotic Compression Fractures

Christopher M. Bono
Department of Orthopedic Surgery, Harvard Medical School, Brigham and Women's Hospital, Boston, Massachusetts, U.S.A.

James Sanfilippo
Department of Orthopedics, Thomas Jefferson University, Philadelphia, Pennsylvania, U.S.A.

Steven R. Garfin
Department of Orthopedic Surgery, University of California, San Diego Medical Center, San Diego, California, U.S.A.

INTRODUCTION

Approximately 28 million people in the United States have osteoporosis or clinically significant osteopenia. Osteoporosis is the leading underlying cause of fractures in the elderly and post-menopausal women. These fractures commonly involve the vertebral bodies, hip, and wrist. Annually, it has been estimated that there are 700,000 vertebral body compression fractures (VCFs) associated with osteoporosis (1), compared with 300,000 hip fractures and 250,000 wrist fractures. Of those, 700,000 fractures, about 50% will become clinically relevant. Vertebral body compression fractures alone account for approximately 150,000 hospital admissions yearly, each having an average length of stay of eight days and an average cost of $12,300 (2). Overall, the treatment of VCFs costs the U.S. healthcare system about $5-10 billion annually (3).

Osteoporosis is the result of an imbalance between bone resorption and bone production. Osteoporotic bone is histologically normal, though it has a lower number of trabeculae that result in a decreased amount of bone per unit volume (4). The most common method of diagnosis is by bone mineral density testing (BMD) by dual-energy X ray absorptiometry (DEXA) scan. With this test, osteoporosis has been defined by the World Health Organization as a BMD measuring less than 2.5 standard deviations below peak BMD of young, healthy individuals of the same sex. Once a fragility fracture has occurred, osteoporosis is considered severe.

Vertebral body compression fractures can lead to chronic back pain, pulmonary dysfunction, and compromise of the ability to perform activities of daily living. Despite these substantial effects, the vast majority of patients who are present with fragility fractures are unfortunately never started on an antiosteoporotic medication, (5,6) and often go on to develop subsequent compression fractures (7,8). This leads to an increased loss of vertebral body height, progressive thoracolumbar kyphosis, and potentially worsened pain, pulmonary compromise, early satiety, and functional disability (9). The impact of these complications is exaggerated in the affected elderly population that is often already compromised by other coexistent morbidities.

Nonoperative treatment of osteoporotic VCFs focuses on pain relief, physical rehabilitation, and initiation of an antiosteoporotic pharmacologic agent. Current pharmacologic agents include bisphosonates, selective estrogen-receptor modulators, and calcitonin (10,11). These function by blocking bone resorption and preventing bone loss. Recently, parathyroid hormone and its analogs have been used to stimulate bone formation and are the only effective pharmacologic means of increasing BMD (12). Fracture treatment can include bed rest, bracing, analgesics, and selective injections, all of which have met limited success (1). Admittedly, the most effective treatment is prophylaxis beginning in early adulthood, and includes exercise and adequate nutrition that maximize peak bone achieved (9).

Until recently, the options for surgical treatment of VCFs were limited. For a variety of reasons, open surgical procedures, such as instrumentation and fusion, are reserved for only the most severe cases of progressive deformity, pain, or neurological deficit. It is fraught with a variety of complications related to poor fixation and construct failure along with substantial surgical morbidity in the aged population.

Various techniques of less invasive surgery for fracture management have been developed over the last decade. Kyphoplasty and vertebroplasty are percutaneous techniques that have been introduced for the treatment of osteoporotic VCFs (13–17). Kyphoplasty is a technique that involves the insertion of an inflatable balloon tamp into the vertebral body to create a bone void and potentially restore height. Cement is then injected under low pressure into the void to provide longstanding mechanical stabilization. Many clinical studies have shown this to be a safe and effective method of treatment for symptomatic osteoporotic vertebral compression fractures (14–19).

INDICATIONS

Kyphoplasty is indicated for patients with painful osteoporotic thoracic and lumbar VCFs. Acute (less than six weeks), subacute (six weeks to three months), and chronic (greater than three months) fractures may be amenable to the procedure. The primary indication is pain relief, though a progressive kyphotic deformity related to collapsed fractures can also be an indication. In most cases, kyphoplasty is indicated after nonoperative methods have failed.

CONTRAINDICATIONS

Kyphoplasty is not indicated in the setting of a stable, well-healed, nonpainful fracture. More importantly, it is contraindicated in the presence of local infection, pre-existing spinal canal compromise, and some cases of vertebra plana, in which the pedicles are above the level of the vertebral body. Relative contraindications include middle-column involvement (i.e., burst fracture). However, there are some that feel kyphoplasty is safe, provided there is no neurologic deficit and no or minimal canal compromise. Uncontrolled or uncorrectable coagulopathies increase the risk for postoperative epidural hematomata, and should be considered a contraindication for percutaneous augmentation (20,21).

PREOPERATIVE PLANNING

Physical examination is a key component of preoperative planning prior to kyphoplasty. Back pain, particularly low back pain, in the elderly population, has a broad differential diagnosis, including spinal stenosis, facet-mediated pain, herniated discs, and degenerative disc disease. Therefore, it cannot be assumed that back pain is caused by a vertebral compression fracture detected on a radiograph. History and physical examination features that are supportive of a painful VCF are point tenderness with palpation of the spinous process of the vertebra in question, pain that is relieved by lying supine, and the lack of neurogenic claudicant-type lower extremity symptoms (21).

Appropriate imaging studies are essential in preoperative evaluation. Plain radiographs should include dedicated thoracic and/or lumbar radiographs, including AP and lateral views. Flexion and extension radiographs are needed prior to kyphoplasty; however, they should be obtained if there is a strong clinical suspicion for dynamic instability. Although their utility is yet to be clinically investigated, extension or supine films can be compared with flexion or standing films to assess fracture mobility as a possible predictor of kyphosis correction. This is particularly true for those patients with a nonhealed cleft within the vertebral body.

It is the authors' preference to obtain a magnetic resonance imaging (MRI) scan prior to surgery. It is useful in determining the acuity of the fracture. Acute or subacute fractures would demonstrate decreased signal within the vertebral bodies, signifying intraosseous edema, on T1-weighted images. T2-weighted images offer the greatest anatomicdetail and are useful for detecting fragment retropulsion and canal or foraminal stenosis. However, bone edema is less reliably detected. Short tau inversion recovery (STIR) sequences can be considered exaggerated

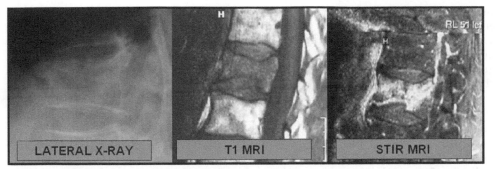

| LATERAL X-RAY | T1 MRI | STIR MRI |

FIGURE 1 Preoperative lateral radiograph and magnetic resonance imaging scans of an L1 osteoporotic compression fracture.

T2-weighted images in which signal from water (edema) is hyperintense (Fig. 1). Therefore, STIR images are the most sensitive method of determining fracture acuity based on an MRI (9,21). MRI is also helpful in differentiating between osteoporotic fracture and neoplastic or infectious processes, which may have a similar appearance on plain films.

If an MRI is contraindicated or cannot be obtained, a bone scan is an excellent alternative method for determining fracture acuity. Increased activity on bone scan signifies ongoing bone turnover, and indicates active fracture remodeling (9,21). Importantly, a bone scan can remain positive for up to 18 months after fracture, and thus, the relative intensity of uptake of radioactive dye of one level compared with another may be useful in determining the age of the fracture. In the authors' practice, a computed tomography (CT) is obtained in addition to the bone scan and plain films to characterize the fracture pattern and detect fragment retropulsion (21).

SURGICAL TECHNIQUE
Operative Setup

Kyphoplasty may be performed under local or general anesthesia. It is the authors' preference to use general anesthesia. If local anesthesia is used, patients can move themselves prone to a position of comfort on a radiolucent table prior to administration of intravenous sedation. In the authors' practice, the patient is sedated and intubated, and then carefully log-rolled into the prone position onto transverse chest and thigh rolls. This helps extend the thoracolumbar spine and aid in the reduction of the fracture. For middle and upper thoracic fractures, the position of the transverse chest roll is critical. If it is placed at the level of the fracture, it can exaggerate the kyphotic deformity, and therefore should be positioned proximal to the fracture whenever possible.

The use of an image intensifier (C-arm) is mandatory. Optimally, two C-rams are used to obtain simultaneous AP and lateral images (Fig. 2). The machines should be positioned prior to

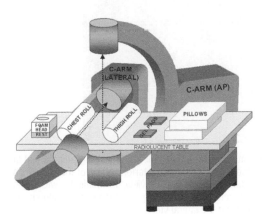

FIGURE 2 Operating room setup includes two C-arms to allow simultaneous anteroposterior and lateral views.

prepping and draping to ensure that adequate visualization of the operative area can be achieved. In some cases, the C-arm can be overrotated to obtain the "en face" view in lieu of the AP view. Angling the beam about 10° to 30° off the midline approximates the posterolateral to anteromedial orientation of the pedicle. This allows one to look "down the pipe" of the pedicle. In the authors' experience, it is most useful to confirm that the pedicle borders have not been violated after the placement of the Jamshidi needle. However, many surgeons find this view useful during needle placement as well.

After adequate radiographic visualization has been confirmed, the patient is then prepped and draped in the usual sterile fashion.

Entry into the Vertebral Body
Transpedicular Approach

For most lumbar and lower thoracic vertebrae, the transpedicular approach is preferred. In general, a pedicle diameter of at least 5 mm is required to adequately accommodate the kyphoplasty instrumentation. This can be assessed by measuring the transverse pedicle diameter on preoperative axial CT or MRI images. In most cases, both pedicles can be cannulated. The anatomic dangers of the transpedicular approach are the spinal cord or cauda equina medially, the nerve root inferiorly or superiorly, and the segmental vessel or visceral structures laterally.

Using both AP and lateral images, the injured vertebral level is identified. The skin is marked just lateral to the lateral border of the pedicle in the AP view. In the lateral view, the mark should allow for a path that passes within the mid-aspect of the pedicle.

A small nick incision is then made in the skin. A Jamshidi needle is inserted through this incision. The needle should be angled medially to achieve the proper trajectory within the pedicle. It is passed through the musculature until it comes into contact with the posterior aspect of the posterior elements. The optimal starting point is in the lateral aspect of the pedicle on AP view, and aligned with the pedicle on lateral view (Fig. 3). The needle is then advanced into the bone using AP and lateral imaging to ensure that the correct path is being followed.

It is essential to avoid breaching the cortices of the pedicle, as this can potentiate for cement leakage. As a guide, the tip of the needle should not pass medial to the medial border of the pedicle on AP view until the tip is seen to pass beyond the posterior cortex of the vertebral body on lateral view. If a breach of the medial pedicular cortex is suspected, the "en face" view can allow for better visualization of the needle within the pedicle.

Optimally, the Jamshidi needle should be angled medially toward the midline. With a superior endplate compression fracture, the needle can be directed toward the inferior half of the vertebral body. On the other hand, with compression of the inferior endplate, it can be directed toward the superior half of the body. This maximizes the amount of compactible

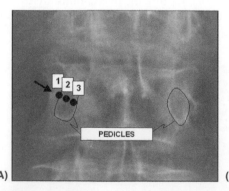 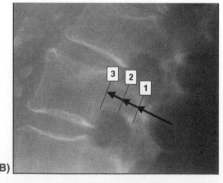

(A)   (B)

FIGURE 3 Landmarks for the transpedicular approach. On the anteroposterior (AP) view, the starting point is just at or lateral to the lateral border of the pedicle halo (**A**), which corresponds to the most posterior portion of the pedicle on the lateral view. When the needle tip is centered within the pedicle halo on the AP view, it should be within the mid-aspect of the pedicle on the lateral view (**B**). As the needle approaches the medial aspect of the pedicle halo on the AP view, it should be at the junction of the pedicle and vertebral body on the lateral view.

cancellous bone between the balloon and the injured endplate. If the vertebra is uniformly compressed, the needle can be oriented toward the middle of the body. Cranial-caudal position of the needle is best visualized on the lateral view.

Lateral Extrapedicular Approach

For thoracic levels with pedicles less than 5 mm (usually above T8), the lateral extrapedicular approach can be used. This approach considers the rib and pedicle together as an effective larger pedicle complex. As with the transpedicular approach, bilateral cannulation can be achieved with the extrapedicular approach. The anatomic structures in danger are the spinal cord medially (though at less risk than with the extrapedicular approach due to a more lateral entry portal), the segmental vessels and lungs laterally, and the nerve roots superiorly and inferiorly. Anterior penetration of the vertebral body can endanger the great vessels.

The skin incision should be more lateral than with the transpedicular approach to allow for a more medially angulated needle trajectory. The bony entry point with the Jamshidi needle is located just superior and just lateral to the pedicle halo, which usually correlates with the superolateral corner of the vertebral body image on the AP view (Fig. 4). Aiming toward the spinous process of the same level usually produces an ideal medial–lateral trajectory. On the lateral view, the needle should be aligned with the pedicle.

The needle is gradually and sequentially advanced into the bone. At no time should the needle tip cross the midline on AP view, which is highly suggestive of the violation of the spinal canal. Final needle positioning is similar to that of the transpedicular approach, which is the tip close to the junction of the vertebral body and the pedicle.

Posterolateral Approach

The posterolateral approach can be utilized for kyphoplasty of the L2–L5 vertebral bodies. The pedicle is not cannulated at any time; the needle enters the vertebral body through its posterolateral cortex using a trajectory that is similar to that used for discography. The incision is made 8- to 10-cm lateral to the midline, and the needle is angled 45° toward the midline. Entry and advancement should be visualized in the lateral view, making sure that the needle is anterior to the transverse process and the neural foramen. This positioning should avoid injury to the exiting nerve root within the psoas muscle. The posterolateral approach is a unilateral method of vertebral body entry; thus, the needle tip should arrive at or cross the midline in the AP view in order to ensure proper augmentation of the contralateral side.

Drilling and Insertion of the Balloon Tamp

Once proper placement of the Jamshidi needle is confirmed, the center stylet is removed. A guide pin is inserted through the Jamshidi cannula. Confirmation of the guide pin in the vertebral body on AP and lateral views is obtained, and the Jamshidi cannula is removed. A combination

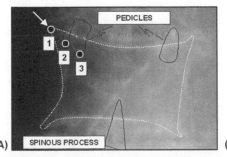 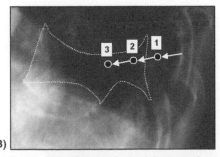

FIGURE 4 Landmarks for the lateral extrapedicular approach. The starting point is at the superolateral corner of the vertebral body on the anteroposterior (AP) view (**A**), and should be aligned with the trajectory of the pedicle on the lateral view. It is then advanced with a more exaggerated medial angulation than with the transpedicular approach, remaining lateral to the pedicle (**B**). Again, as the needle tip reaches the medial border of the pedicle on the AP view, it should be at or just past the junction of the pedicle and the vertebral body on the lateral view.

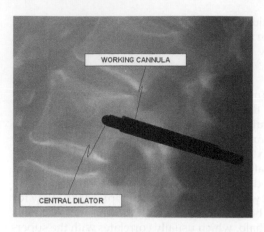

FIGURE 5   After guidewire exchange, the working cannula is inserted until the tip is just beyond the pedicle–vertebral body junction.

of dilator (center) and working cannula (outer) is then inserted over the guide pin (Fig. 5). Frequent lateral images should be obtained during this step to avoid inadvertent advancement of the guidewire through the anterior cortex of the vertebral body. Final placement of the cannula should be just beyond the junction of the pedicle and vertebral body in the lateral view.

The guide pin and central dilator are then removed, leaving the working cannula in position. If a biopsy is planned, it should be performed at this time. Otherwise, a finger-twist drill is inserted through the working cannula and carefully advanced to within a few millimeters of the anterior vertebral body cortex (Fig. 6). The drill is then removed, and the balloon tamp is inserted, with optimal positioning of the tamp within the mid-vertebral body on the lateral view. On the AP view, it is optimal to have the balloon tips converge upon the midline. Once the balloon tamp is in position, the guidewire (located within the lumen of the tamp, which increases its stiffness to facilitate insertion into the bone) is removed.

The balloon tamp is available with different sizes of balloons. In general, proximal thoracic vertebrae can accommodate a 10-mm balloon, whereas distal thoracic and lumbar vertebrae can accommodate a 15-mm balloon. A 20-mm balloon is also available, but is usually reserved for very large lumbar vertebrae. Balloon size should be determined preoperatively by measuring the radiographs or MRI. Also, the balloon is not a perfect sphere. It is cinched at the waist, creating an anterior and a posterior tamp, which can fill the body of the compressed vertebra more effectively, allowing for better reduction. There are radio-opaque markers on both sides of the balloon, allowing for better visualization with the image intensifiers.

The balloon tamp is then sequentially "inflated" with radio-opaque contrast dye under controlled pressure increments using a digital manometer. During inflation, frequent lateral and AP images should be monitored (Fig. 7). Optimally, the balloon should expand in a uniform manner, allowing it to elevate the depressed endplate. The balloon should not extend beyond

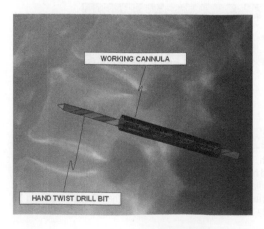

FIGURE 6   After the central dilator is removed, a hand-twist drill bit is carefully advanced to the anterior aspect of the vertebral body.

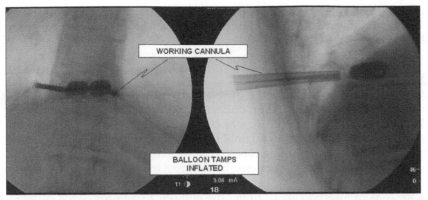

FIGURE 7 The balloon tamps are inflated simultaneously, frequently checking anteroposterior and lateral views to monitor expansion and detect any cortical breakout.

the borders of the vertebral body at any time. If this occurs, the balloon should be deflated and repositioned. Although superior, anterior, and lateral violation are more common, posterior breach can endanger the neurologic elements.

In many cases, the balloons do not inflate uniformly, as they follow the path of least resistance between the osteoporotic bone. Because of the three-dimensional deformations of the endplate, it is often difficult to determine if the balloon has violated this boundary. However, if the balloon appears to "flatten out" on either the AP or lateral view, it is most likely contained within the bone. The endpoints for balloon inflation are: (*i*) fracture reduction, (*ii*) uncorrectable cortical breakout, or (*iii*) approaching maximum safe pressure (400 psi).

Maximizing Fracture Reduction
Bone Curette
In some cases, the balloon tamp alone may not adequately achieve fracture reduction. In response to this, a bone curette has been developed that can be inserted straight, and once in position within the vertebral body, can deploy the tip into a 90° bend (Fig. 8A,B). Advancing and retracting this curette can be used to score the bone and potentially mobilize a fracture fragment. The curette is then removed and balloon tamp reduction is once again attempted.

Directional Balloon Tamp
As stated earlier, the balloon tamp follows the path of least resistance. Unfortunately, this path is not always optimal. If the tamp is expanding preferentially into an undesired region, such as

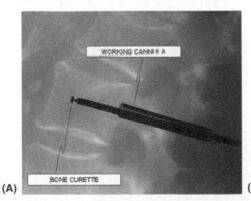
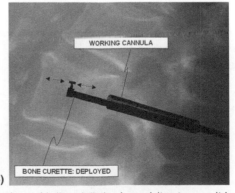

(A) (B)

FIGURE 8 A bone curette can be used to maximize reduction and balloon inflation in recalcitrant cases. It is inserted straight (**A**) and then deployed to achieve a 90° bend (**B**). It can then be advanced and retracted to mobilize bone fragments.

the uninjured vertebra, then one might consider the use of a directional balloon. This device enables inflation to be directed toward the injured endplate. The same care needs to be taken to avoid violation of the endplate.

Cement Insertion

Next, the balloon tamp is deflated and removed. A medium viscosity cement mixture of poly-methylmethacrylate (PMMA) and barium sulfate contrast is prepared. The cement mixture is used to fill several 1.5-cc bone filler devices (BFD), which are tubes and pushers that fit within the working cannula. The cement is allowed to set until the desired viscosity is reached, which is approximately the consistency of toothpaste. The BFDs are passed through the cannulae bilaterally into the vertebral body. Under continuous fluoroscopy, the pusher is used to fill the bone void.

The endpoints for cement insertion are (*i*) filling the anterior two-thirds of the vertebral body; (*ii*) filling of the posterior vertebral body; or (*iii*) any cement extravasation, particularly any posterior extravasation. Cement leakage through the body may occur with cement mixtures that are too fluid. If this occurs, cementing should stop, the cement should be given time to cure, and when the appropriate viscosity is obtained, injection should resume. In general, between 2 and 6 mm of cement can be used per side. Monitoring with fluoroscopy is a must to look for cement extrusion (Fig. 9). Fortunately, most cases of cement extrusion are clinically insignificant.

Final cement curing occurs in about five to 10 minutes. After this, the cannulae are twisted and removed. Final radiographs are taken to ensure proper cement placement, fracture reduction, and restoration of sagittal alignment. The patient should remain in the prone position for an additional five to 10 minutes to allow for final hardening of the cement in a reduced position.

POSTOPERATIVE CARE

As blood loss is minimal and pain relief is almost immediate, kyphoplasty can be performed as a same-day procedure. In the authors' practice, general anesthesia is usually used and an overnight stay is preferred. As PMMA cement is its strongest at the time of implantation, there is no indication for postoperative bed rest or bracing. Considering the various biomechanical data (22–25), the augmented vertebra is certainly stronger after cement augmentation than before it. Ideally, postoperative pain medications include oral narcotics for 24 to 48 hours, followed by acetaminophen or nonsteroidal anti-inflammatory drugs (NSAIDs). In reality, however, many of these patients take large dosages of narcotics, often including transdermal medications, which require a careful and gradual wean from dependency.

Because of the substantial deconditioning associated with osteoporotic VCFs, return to premorbid activity levels often requires physical and/or occupational therapy. This is

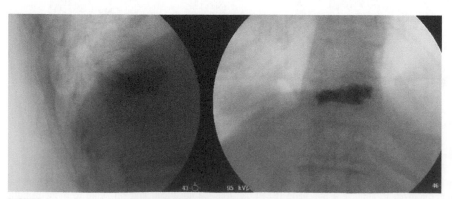

FIGURE 9   Cement is inserted to fill the void created.

dependent on the level of preprocedural disability and comorbidities of the patient (9,21). In addition to immediate postoperative radiographs, AP and lateral views should be obtained at one month postprocedure. Unless clinically indicated earlier, the authors also obtain radiographs at a one-year postoperative visit.

COMPLICATIONS

The overall complication rate following kyphoplasty is very low. In one study, clinically significant complications occurred in 1.2% of patients and 0.7% of fractures (14). Cement extrusion can occur in up to 9% of fractures (18). Fortunately, these are rarely associated with clinical sequelae.

Neurologic deficit following kyphoplasty rarely occurs (16,18,26). One study reported two cases of spinal cord injury. One patient developed partial paraplegia resulting from cement extrusion into the spinal canal. This was the result of improperly placed instruments. The other patient sustained a fracture at the junction of the pedicle and vertebral body during an extrapedicular approach. Subsequently, this patient developed an anterior-cord syndrome (16). In another large clinical series, no major neurologic injuries were noted (18).

The most common complication with kyphoplasty is transient pyrexia that may lead to short bout of fever. It is usually self-limited, resolving within three to four days. Pyrexia may be a result of the exothermic reaction of the PMMA curing, the pressure of the injection, or a inflammatory reaction (27). Other common complications include rib fractures from patient positioning and intraoperative hypotension from unreacted cement monomer. Epidural hematoma is a rare cause of neurologic deficit. As such, pharmacologic anticoagulation should not be started until four days after surgery (9,21).

OUTCOMES

The two major outcome measures after kyphoplasty are pain relief and restoration of vertebral body height. Most of the clinical studies published to date have been retrospective reviews. In a short-term follow up, Garfin et al. reported decreased pain in 90% of their patients (16). At an average 21-month follow up, Majd et al. found that 89% of their patients had significant improvement in pain and functional scores (19). In another report, Rhyne et al. demonstrated a mean seven-point improvement in visual analogue scale (VAS) pain score (28). In a small prospective study, Phillips et al. reported significant pain improvements within the first week after kyphoplasty (29). Coumans et al. also reported marked improvement in VAS and SF-36 scores (30).

The results of fracture reduction and vertebral body-height restoration have varied. Garfin et al. reported an average preprocedure anterior vertebral body height of 83% and a postprocedure height of 99% (16). Liebermann et al. showed an average of 50% restoration of vertebral body height in 70% of the levels treated (18). Majd et al. showed an average anterior-height restoration of 30% and an average middle-height restoration of 50% (19).

The amount of height restoration may be related to the time to kyphoplasty. Katzman et al. have reported a 57% restoration in fractures treated within two weeks (31).

Crandall et al. compared the results in acute (less than 10-week-old) and chronic (greater than four-month-old) fractures (32). They found that, although pain relief was equivalent, they were able to achieve a height restoration of 60% in the acute group but only of 26% in the chronic group. Also, Garfin et al. have shown that about 50% height restoration could be reliably achieved in fractures treated within three months (16).

There are currently no prospective randomized controlled studies comparing kyphoplasty with nonoperative management or to other methods of vertebral augmentation. In a recent nonrandomized prospective study, Kasperk et al. (33) compared kyphoplasty with nonoperative management in a group of patients with painful VCFs. The time of treatment was greater than one year. The kyphoplasty group showed statistically significant improvements in pain based on VAS scores and in vertebral body-height restoration. The control group showed no improvement in pain and demonstrated a loss of vertebral body height of 8% at final follow-up.

SUMMARY

As the population continues to live longer, osteoporosis and its related complications are projected to increase in frequency. Kyphoplasty has been shown to be a successful method of relieving pain and restoring some lost vertebral height with osteoporotic VCFs. Although PMMA appears to be an effective augmentation means, ongoing efforts to develop a resorbable bioactive cement have been made. With the optimal cement, surgeons may be more comfortable employing kyphoplasty for traumatic fractures in younger patients.

REFERENCES

1. Hanley E, Green NE, Spengler DM. An AOA critical issue: less invasive procedures in spine surgery. J Bone Joint Surg Am 2003; 85:956–961.
2. Riggs BL, Melton LJ. The worldwide problem of osteoporosis: insights afforded by epidemiology. Bone 1995; 17:505–511.
3. Botte MJ, D'Lima DD, Meunier MJ, et al. Specialty update: what's new in orthopaedic rehabilitation. J Bone Joint Surg Am 2001; 83:1920–1926.
4. Bono CM, Einhorn TA. Overview of osteoporosis: pathophysiology and determinants of bone strength. Eur Spine J 2003; 12(suppl):S90–96.
5. Freedman KB, Kaplan FS, Bilker WB, et al. Treatment of osteoporosis: are physicians missing an opportunity? J Bone Joint Surg Am 2000; 82-A:1063–1070.
6. Gardner MJ, Flik KR, Mooar P, et al. Improvement in the undertreatment of osteoporosis following hip fracture. J Bone Joint Surg Am 2002; 84-A:1342–1348.
7. Bono CM, Garfin SR. Multi-level thoracic and lumbar kyhphoplasty for rapidly progressing spinal osteoporosis in a patient with kyphoscoliosis. Adv Osteoporos Fracture Manag 2002; 1:98–102.
8. Ross PD, Huang C, Davis JW, et al. Vertebral dimension measurements improve prediction of vertebral fracture incidence. Bone 1995; 16:257–262.
9. Rao RD, Singrakhia MD. Current concepts review: painful osteoporotic vertebral fractures. J Bone Joint Surg Am 2003; 85:2010–2022.
10. Simon JA, Lewiecki EM, Smith ME, et al. Patient preference for once-weekly alendronate 70 mg versus once-daily alendronate 10 mg: a multicenter, randomized, open-label, crossover study. Clin Ther 2002; 24:1871–1886.
11. Maricic M, Adachi JD, Sarkar S, et al. Early effects of raloxifene on clinical vertebral fractures at 12 months in postmenopausal women with osteoporosis. Arch Intern Med 2002; 162:1140–1143.
12. Neer RM, Arnaud CD, Zanchetta JR, et al. Effect of parathyroid hormone (1-34) on fractures and bone mineral density in post-menopausal women with osteoporosis. N Engl J Med 2001; 344:1434–1441.
13. Gangi A, Dietemann JL, Mortazavi R, et al. CT-guided interventional procedures for pain management in the lumbosacral spine. Radiographics 1998; 18:621–633.
14. Garfin SR, Reilley MA. Minimally invasive treatment of osteoporotic vertebral body compression fractures. Spine J 2002; 2:76–80.
15. Garfin SR, Yuan H, Lieberman IH. Early outcomes in the minimally-invasive reductions and fixation of compression fractures. Proceedings of the NASS, 2000:184–185.
16. Garfin SR, Yuan HA, Reiley MA. New technologies in spine: kyphoplasty and vertebroplasty for the treatment of painful osteoporotic compression fractures. Spine 2001; 26:1511–1515.
17. Jarvik JG, Deyo RA. Vertebroplasty for osteoporotic compression fracture: effective treatment for a neglected disease. AJNR Am J Neuroradiol 2001; 22:594–595.
18. Lieberman IH, Dudeney S, Reinhardt MK, et al. Initial outcome and efficacy of "kyphoplasty" in the treatment of painful osteoporotic vertebral compression fractures. Spine 2001; 26:1631–1638.
19. Majd ME, Farley S, Holt RT. Preliminary outcomes and efficacy of the first 360 consecutive kyphoplasties for the treatment of painful osteoporotic vertebral compression fractures. Spine J 2005; 5: 244–255.
20. Gangi A, Kastler BA, Dietemann JL. Percutaneous vertebroplasty guided by a combination of CT and fluoroscopy. AJNR Am J Neuroradiol 1994; 15:83–86.
21. Spivak JM, Johnson MG. Perspectives on modern orthopaedics: percutaneous treatment of vertebral body pathology. J Am Acad Orthop Surg 2005; 13:6–17.
22. Belkoff SM, Mathis JM, Erbe EM, et al. Biomechanical evaluation of a new bone cement for use in vertebroplasty. Spine 2000; 25:1061–1064.
23. Tohmeh AG, Mathis JM, Fenton DC, et al. Biomechanical efficacy of unipedicular versus bipedicular vertebroplasty for the management of osteoporotic compression fractures. Spine 1999; 24: 1772–1776.
24. Belkoff SM, Mathis JM, Fenton DC, et al. An ex vivo biomechanical evaluation of an inflatable bone tamp used in the treatment of compression fracture. Spine 2001; 26:151–156.
25. Dean JR, Ison KT, Gishen P. The strengthening effect of percutaneous vertebroplasty. Clin Radiol 2000; 55:471–476.

26. Harrington KD. Major neurological complications following percutaneous vertebroplasty with poly-methylmethacrylate: a case report. J Bone Joint Surg 2001; 83A:1070–1073.
27. Cortet B, Cotten A, Boutry N, et al. Percutaneous vertebroplasty in patients with osteolytic metastases or multiple myeloma. Rev Rhum Engl Ed 1997; 64:177–183.
28. Rhyne A, III, Banit D, Laxer E, et al. Kyphoplasty: report of eighty-two thoracolumbar osteoporotic vertebral fractures. J Orthop Trauma 2004; 18:294–299.
29. Phillips FM, Ho E, Campbell-Hupp M, et al. Early radiographic and clinical results of balloon kyphoplasty for the treatment of osteoporotic vertebral compression fractures. Spine 2003; 28: 2260–2265; discussion 5–7.
30. Coumans JV, Reinhardt MK, Lieberman IH. Kyphoplasty for vertebral compression fractures: 1-year clinical outcomes from a prospective study. J Neurosurg 2003; 99:44–50.
31. Katzman SS. Operative treatment of osteoporotic vertebral body fractures: vertebroplasty versus kyphoplasty. Paper presentation 2003, American Academy of Orthopaedic Surgeons.
32. Crandall D, Slaughter D, Hankins PJ, et al. Acute versus chronic vertebral compression fractures treated with kyphoplasty: early results. Spine J 2004; 4:418–424.
33. Kasperk C, Hillmeier J, Noldge G, et al. Treatment of painful vertebral fractures by kyphoplasty in patients with primary osteoporosis: a prospective nonrandomized controlled study. J Bone Miner Res 2005; 20:604–612.

32 | Vertebroplasty for Osteoporotic Vertebral Compression Fractures

Fergus McKiernan
Center for Bone Diseases, Marshfield Clinic, Marshfield, Wisconsin, U.S.A.

Tom Faciszewski
Department of Orthopedic Spine Surgery, Marshfield Clinic, Marshfield, Wisconsin, U.S.A.

BRIEF INTRODUCTION AND HISTORY OF THE PROCEDURE

Vertebroplasty ordinarily refers to the percutaneous, intravertebral injection of polymethyl-methacrylate (PMMA) for vertebral stabilization and relief of pain. Galibert first described percutaneous vertebroplasty (PV) in 1987 in France as a minimally invasive treatment option for aggressive vertebral hemangiomas (1). The technique quickly found application to other infiltrative, metastatic, myelomatous, and metabolic vertebral pathology thereafter. Pioneering work by Jensen led to widespread use of PV in the United States to relieve pain from osteoporotic vertebral compression fractures (VCFs) refractory to nonoperative care (2). Osteoporosis is now the primary indication for PV worldwide.

Spine surgeons with experience in high-energy spine fractures should exercise caution in directly transferring that experience to the management of fragility fractures in frail, elderly patients with osteoporosis. Differences in classification schemes, biomechanics, and treatment principles in low-energy osteoporotic vertebral fracture are only becoming appreciated (3). This chapter limits its scope to conventional PV using PMMA for the management of painful thoracolumbar osteoporotic VCFs.

INDICATIONS

Percutaneous vertebroplasty is primarily indicated for the relief of pain of vertebral fracture origin (4). We consider PV appropriate when severe fracture pain has been substantially disruptive to activities of daily living or threatens functional independence in spite of at least one to two weeks of narcotic analgesia, bracing, domestic/institutional rest, nursing care, and physical assistance (5). Any specific threshold magnitude or duration of pain, degree of functional impairment or care paradigm is, in reality, largely subjective, untested, and lacks expert consensus. In some circumstances, PV performed immediately after fracture might be considered more "conservative" than initiating or continuing nonoperative management. Restorations of vertebral height or spinal alignment currently lack sufficient evidence to be considered sole indications for PV. In the authors' view, so-called "prophylactic" and "diagnostic" PV should not be performed.

PV is appropriate for both primary (e.g., postmenopausal, senescent) and secondary (e.g., glucocorticoid, endocrinopathologic) osteoporosis and may be considered in unusual causes of skeletal fragility such as osteogenesis imperfecta (6). Vertebroplasty of VCF resulting from high-energy trauma, in healthy bone and in young patients should be discouraged as any short-term benefit would not likely justify the permanent displacement of normally repaired and remodeled bone by PMMA. Furthermore, published PV outcomes would not apply to this patient population as (*i*) high-energy trauma results in other nonvertebral pain generators that would not benefit from PMMA fixation and (*ii*) augmentations under these circumstances would be subjected to greater biomechanical stresses for longer durations than those seen in the frail, elderly with osteoporosis. Medical contraindications to PV include uncorrected coagulopathy, unresolved systemic or local infection, and insufficient medical stability to endure the procedure. The anticoagulant/antiplatelet effects of coumadin, clopidogrel and, when possible, aspirin should have waned prior to PV. Other contraindications to PV include: (*i*) fracture severity when, in the absence of dynamic or latent mobility (see next), the degree of vertebral compression precludes safe augmentation, (*ii*) complex cortical disruption where venous, foraminal, or intraspinal PMMA leak appears unavoidable, (*iii*) myelopathy or neurologic deficit associated with VCF except possibly for dynamic radicular syndromes resulting from vertebral collapse in mobile VCFs. Fracture age is a surrogate for fracture healing and by itself is not an absolute contraindication to PV. Healed fractures should not be augmented.

Open surgical alternatives to PVA for fracture pain relief are rarely indicated, as they are associated with substantial morbidity and mortality. Neurologic deficit or severe deformity resulting from osteoporotic VCFs might justify open surgical intervention by operators experienced in spinal decompression and fixation in osteoporotic bone.

PREOPERATIVE PLANNING

Only about one-quarter of radiographically defined VCFs are recognized clinically (7). Of these, only about 40% are preceded by a specific "event" to which the patient can ascribe their VCF. Vertebral fracture pain is typically posterior and felt approximately at the anatomic level of the fracture but may wrap around the trunk or radiate caudally and be mistaken for pain emanating from more anterior, caudal, or visceral structures. Pain intensity is variable, may be transiently accompanied by paroxysms of halting muscle spasm, and is often intolerable during transitioning movements such as moving to and from the supine position. Patients are usually able to identify some position of comfort and can even be free of pain once that position is achieved. Surprisingly, approximately one-sixth reports standing or walking to be the position of maximum comfort (8). Therefore, VCF pain intensity and character range widely. Clinicians should be vigilant to consider osteoporotic VCF in any at-risk person presenting with back, flank, sacral, or abdominal pain.

This population has a high prevalence of medical and spinal comorbidities, particularly degenerative spinal stenosis and previous VCF (9). Careful characterizations of prefracture baseline back pain and physical function is critical for surgical planning and establishing postsurgical expectations. As fracture union matures (and after PV), pain associated with transitioning maneuvers diminishes. However, patients may also begin to report that their endurance for unsupported standing is limited to short periods of time by crescendo back aching, muscular fatiguing, and exhaustion. Acute VCF pain must be carefully distinguished from both prefracture baseline back pain and postfracture postural, fatiguing pain as neither of the latter will benefit from PV.

Findings on the physical exam are often nonspecific. The spinous process of the fractured vertebra may be painful with deep pressure but this is an insensitive indicator of the presence, absence, or level of fracture (10). Nevertheless thorough examination should search for unexpected synchronous vertebral, rib, pelvic, or hip fractures. When transition to the supine position (and subsequently to the seated position) is accompanied by severe pain or muscle spasm, or is forbidden by the patient, our experience predicts the presence of a dynamically mobile VCF and portends a favorable response to PV (1). Radicular signs and symptoms resulting from vertebral collapse and dynamic foraminal compromise are not necessarily contraindications to PV and may improve following stabilization when vertebral height restoration can be achieved. Myelopathic signs and symptoms are rare but should be considered contraindications to PV.

A comprehensive history and physical exam are mandatory. The examiner should be alert for less common causes of osteoporosis (e.g., hypercortisolism, hyperparathyroidism, hyperthyroidism). Early engagement of a metabolic bone disease specialist, geriatrician, or dedicated internist is recommended to assist with evaluation of the patient's skeletal fragility, preparation of the patient for PV, and management of the patient's osteoporosis postoperatively. Malignancy is always of concern in elderly patients with nontraumatic spine fractures and concern should be heightened when fractures occur cephalad to T5, have atypical radiographic features, or occur in the setting of significant constitutional symptoms or failing health. A complete blood count, comprehensive metabolic panel, erythrocyte sedimentation rate, serum and urine protein electrophoresis, and 25-hydroxy-vitamin D will detect most underlying infectious, metabolic, or malignant processes.

Plain radiography is usually the initial diagnostic imaging modality and bears important information for surgical planning and technique. Osteoporotic fracture classification schemes may be unfamiliar to some spine surgeons. Osteoporotic fracture morphology is characterized by configuration (crush, wedge, superior/inferior concave, biconcave) and degree of vertebral height reduction (anterior, middle, or posterior) as mild (20% to 25%), moderate (25% to 40%), severe (>40%), or vertebra plana (9). Additional important dimensions of the osteoporotic VCF include the presence of intravertebral clefts, dynamic mobility (Fig. 1A and 1B), and the integrity of the posterior cortical wall (3). Fracture age is usually based on the onset of pain ascribed to that VCF. An acute vertebral fracture is suggested by a change in configuration compared with recent radiographs or the presence of dynamic mobility. Remain vigilant when VCF is suspected clinically yet not detected radiographically because conformational changes of the fracturing vertebra typically lag days to weeks behind the clinical event. Osteoporotic VCFs typically occur in the context of diffuse skeletal demineralization. Isolated vertebral demineralization should raise concern for an infectious or neoplastic process. Ironically, a collapsed osteoporotic vertebra may appear denser as trabecular bone is compacted into a smaller space. Very dense compaction in nonmobile VCFs makes needle penetration surprisingly difficult and should prompt reconsideration of the need for PV.

There is increasing recognition that some osteoporotic VCFs change configuration under different loading conditions and in different body positions. This fracture property, termed "dynamic mobility," has been identified in as many as one-third of patients referred for vertebroplasty (11). In these patients, a preoperative supine cross-table lateral radiograph centered on the index vertebra will demonstrate an increase in fractured vertebral height compared with the height of the same vertebra on the standing lateral view (Fig. 1A and 1B). Care must be taken to exclude technical flaws (such as parallax and magnification errors) before concluding that a VCF is mobile. Dynamic mobility most frequently occurs at the thoraco-lumbar junction (T11–L1) and implies complete cortical and cancellous disruption. The radiographic correlate of this disruption is the intravertebral cleft (12). Large clefts occur most frequently beneath the superior endplate near the ventral margin of the vertebra. (Fig. 1C) Cleft margins appear increasingly sclerotic over time and intravertebral pseudarthrosis may result from persistent nonunion. Importantly, some osteoporotic VCFs demonstrate mobility only after maintenance of the supine position for 24 to 48 hours (Fig. 1C). Such "latent" mobility should be suspected in relatively recent, severe, thoracolumbar junction VCFs when dynamic mobility was anticipated but not appreciated. Dynamic mobility, latent mobility, and intravertebral clefts should be identified preoperatively because: (*i*) some severely compressed, but mobile, vertebrae might wrongfully be considered inoperable, (*ii*) failure to fill the entire cleft may result in persistent postoperative mobility and pain, and (*iii*) mobility can be harnessed intraoperatively for some vertebral height restoration.

Magnetic resonance imaging (MRI) is the single most useful imaging modality in the evaluation of osteoporotic VCF. MRI will identify intravertebral edema within hours of fracture, identify all involved fracture levels, define intravertebral clefts, and assist in the exclusion of pathologic fracture (Fig. 1D). High-intensity signal on T2-weighted or short-tau inversion recovery (STIR) sequences signify intraosseous edema. Involvement of the pedicle or posterior elements with signal abnormality or particularly the presence of soft tissue in the epidural or paraspinal space should alert the clinician to the possible presence of an underlying malignancy or infection. Computed tomography (CT) scanning with sagittal and coronal reconstruction is particularly helpful in assessing complex fracture patterns, visualizing the posterior cortical wall and when radicular syndromes demand precise visualization of the neuroforamen (Fig. 1C and 1E). Small sagittal and coronal intravertebral splits should alert the operator to potential pathways for PMMA flow. The size, shape, contours, and angular relationship of the pedicle to the vertebral body are best appreciated by MRI and/or CT and must be understood as they serve as the basis for subsequent needle trajectory.

Nuclear scintigraphic bone scanning is a sensitive, readily accessible, inexpensive means of detecting the locations and extent of fracture provided at least 48 to 72 hours have elapsed since the fracture event. Scintigraphic uptake can be nonspecific, however, and may persist up to two years after fracture thereby reducing diagnostic specificity. Multiple skeletal lesions may suggest metastasis. Single photon emission computed tomography (SPECT) scanning

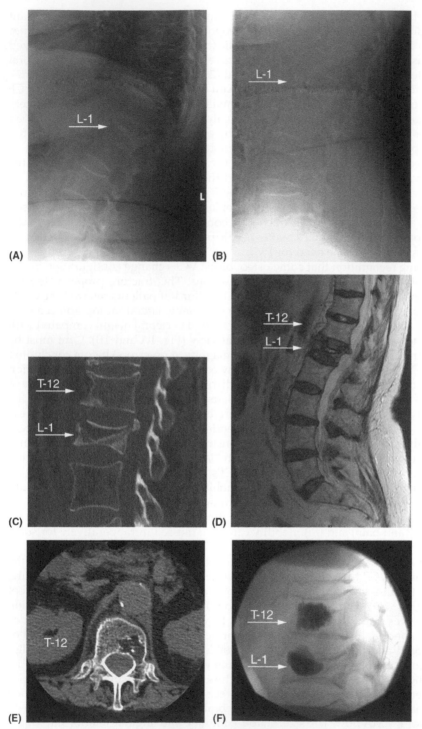

FIGURE 1 (**A**) Standing lateral radiograph reveals a severe, wedge L1 vertebral compression fracture (VCF). This degree of collapse precludes percutaneous vertebroplasty (PV). (**B**) Supine cross-table lateral radiograph demonstrates some dynamic mobility. An intravertebral cleft is seen as intravertebral gas. Even with some vertebral height restoration PV remains precarious. (**C**) After 24 hours in the supine position further vertebral height restoration ("latent" mobility) of L1 is demonstrated by computed tomography (CT). (**D**) Magnetic resonance (MR) shows the severe, edematous, clefted VCF with retropulsion. Note T12 superior endplate fracture. (**E**) Axial image demonstrates large posterior intra-vertebral defect within T12 further destabilizing the fracturing vertebra. (**F**) L1 with cleft fill pattern and T12 with trabe-cular fill pattern anteriorly. The patient had near complete relief of pain immediately postoperatively.

combined with nuclear scintigraphy more accurately localizes the anatomic site of radionuclide concentration and can, for instance, distinguish uptake in the posterior elements from uptake in the vertebral body when this distinction is necessary. Positron emission tomography (PET) scanning suggests malignancy when the standard uptake value (SUV) is greater than 2.5 in VCFs that are at least one month old. Low positive predictive value within the first postfracture month limits usefulness of PET scanning acutely (13). Both MRI and bone scans have the additional potential value of revealing synchronous, otherwise clinically unsuspected, fragility fractures in the pelvis and spine. Dual X ray absorptiometry (DXA) accurately determines the degree of skeletal fragility and is essential for subsequent osteoporosis management. In most cases, DXA can be postponed until after PV in order to limit painful maneuvering unless the degree of skeletal demineralization must be known preoperatively.

Percutaneous vertebroplasty may be undertaken after all anatomic dimensions and relationships are fully understood and needle access to the anterior vertebral body is judged to be safe.

SURGICAL TECHNIQUE

Percutaneous vertebroplasty can appear seductively straightforward but poor outcomes will plague the unwary. In appropriately selected patients, done well, vertebroplasty can provide relief of suffering that is profoundly gratifying (2,4,5,14).

PV may be performed in the interventional radiology suite, ambulatory surgery center, or hospital operating room. Secure venous access, emergency resuscitation equipment, continuous pulse oxymetry, blood pressure, and electrocardiogram (EKG) monitoring are mandatory. Universal precautions regarding handling of needles and sharps and strict aseptic technique are mandatory. General anesthesia, monitored anesthesia care, and local anesthesia are all acceptable modes of anesthesia. The mode of anesthesia should be individualized and determined by the patient's health and preference, the specifics of the vertebral fracture and augmentation goals, operator/anesthesiologist experience, and procedure location. Monitored anesthesia care using intravenous midazolam and fentanyl, or more recently, dexmedetomidine is the usual choice. We consider a general anesthetic (*i*) when better muscular relaxation is needed to facilitate vertebral height restoration when dynamic mobility permits and (*ii*) in patients with tenuous cardiopulmonary function to avoid risking a difficult, mid-procedure conversion to general anesthesia for more secure airway control. Preoperative intravenous antibiotic prophylaxis is recommended.

Extreme caution during transport, transfer, positioning, and dismounting should be exercised to prevent damage to fragile skin and bone. A radiolucent Jackson table allows positioning in extension and may facilitate the opportunity to harness dynamic mobility and effect height restoration. Patients are rolled to the prone position and all bony and neural prominences generously padded. Once the patient is securely positioned, the radiology staff should be prepared to image the index VCF. A well-informed, engaged, and proactive technical radiology staff is indispensable to successful PV. Protective eye and body wear are recommended as fluoroscopy can expose personnel to high levels of ionizing radiation. To minimize radiation exposure the gantries should be positioned so that radiation enters the patient from the side opposite the operator (lateral imaging) and from the floor [anterior–posterior (AP) imaging] (Fig. 2). Use continuous pulsed fluoroscopy with tight collimation while injecting PMMA or intermittent controlled fluoroscopy after delivery of small aliquots of PMMA. Avoid use of the magnification function and high-level fluoroscopy (2,15–17). Pregnancy should excuse women from the vertebroplasty suite to prevent harm from radiation scatter and PMMA vapors.

CT may provide better visualization for needle placement in high thoracic procedures but PMMA injection should always be performed fluoroscopically. Biplanar fluoroscopy allows for nearly instantaneous and simultaneous visualization of needle placement and PMMA flow. We recommend true lateral and AP imaging. Essential anatomic landmarks on lateral view are the anterior and posterior vertebral body borders, superior and inferior endplates, posterior aspect of the spinal canal, and the superior and inferior contours of the pedicles. Essential anatomic landmarks on AP view are the superior and inferior endplates, the lateral borders of the vertebral body, the spinous process, and the medial and lateral pedicle margins. These landmarks should

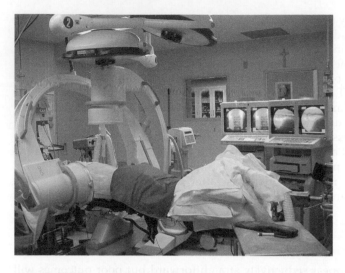

FIGURE 2 Typical vertebroplasty setup. Note position of C-arms relative to patient.

serve to rectify gantry angles. Some operators prefer the coned down pedicle view to the AP projection but this view may impair localization of the needle tip in relation to the midline. Inability to adequately identify all essential landmarks is sufficient reason to abort the procedure.

The pedicle margins in the AP view represent the waist; the narrowest portion of the pedicle. The pedicle waist is generally at the midpoint of the pedicle but its exact location may vary and its position must be confirmed on the lateral view. As the pedicle joins the vertebral body it flares and becomes trumpet-shaped. In general, thoracic pedicles flare less than lumbar pedicles. The position of the waist and the slope of pedicle flare are important determinants of needle trajectory. Successful needle placement is predicated on a thorough understanding of the pedicle–vertebral body relationship as gleaned from preoperative MRI and CT in two dimensions and the ability to conceptualize and engage this relationship in the third.

The center of the spinous process and the lateral and superior borders of both pedicles should be projected onto the skin of the patient's back and marked with a pen to serve as external reference points throughout the procedure (Fig. 3). The entry point for instrumentation is approximately 1 to 2 cm lateral to the intersection of a line drawn between both superior pedicle margins and the lateral margins of each pedicle. The precise entry point will vary depending on body habitus, vertebral anatomy, and the choice between transpedicular or extrapedicular approach. Once anatomic landmarks and imaging orientation are confirmed the patient is prepped and draped.

The vertebral body can be instrumented by either a transpedicular or an extrapedicular (trans-costovertebral, posterior–lateral) approach (2,4,15,16). In lumbar vertebral bodies

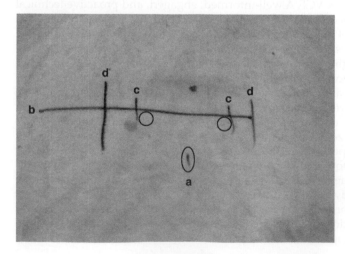

FIGURE 3 Vertebral landmarks projected onto the patient's back have been marked with a pen. (a) Spinous process, (b) tangent line drawn between superior pedicle margins, (c) lateral pedicle margins, and (d) approximate instrumentation entry point at intersection of lines (b) and (d).

(and at T12), larger pedicle size facilitates the transpedicular approach; however, satisfactory vertebral fill may require larger PMMA volumes and bilateral instrumentation. In the axial plane thoracic vertebral bodies are usually more conical/bullet shaped dorsal to ventral, their pedicles are narrower and positioned more cephalad than those of the lumbar spine. For these reasons, the parapedicular or trans-costovertebral approach is usually preferred for thoracic vertebrae. Smaller PMMA volumes are usually sufficient above T12 and these can often be delivered to the center of the vertebral body by unilateral instrumentation. Complex fracture patterns require individualized instrumentation strategies based on careful evaluation of preoperative and intraoperative imaging. For example, bipedicular instrumentation may be necessary when a severe biconcave deformity precludes navigation of the needle across the midline of the vertebral body.

Multiple proprietary vertebroplasty needle options are available (e.g., Stryker, Precision System®) and all are acceptable. Most are variations of the Jamshidi needle and are available with diamond or beveled (single or multiple) stylet tip options. A diamond tip stylet may reduce needle slippage on the cortical surface of the vertebra. An outer working cannula is available from some manufacturers as are various needle-handle options. After cortical penetration, some authors exchange the diamond tipped stylet for a single beveled stylet because they believe steering is improved using the latter. Needle length (10 or 15 cm) and gauge (11, 13, or 15 G) are determined by vertebral and patient anatomic factors. Innovations in needle technology have improved the ability to perform bone biopsy and facilitate re-entry into the vertebra by means of an outer working cannula (e.g., Oste-Mend, Stryker). Currently, operator preference and experience largely determines needle selection.

When appropriate, the skin is infiltrated with local anesthetic. Using the AP view, a 0.045-inch guide wire is passed through the skin and docked at the 10 o'clock and/or 2 o'clock positions on the left and right pedicle, respectively. A 1-cm cephalocaudal skin incision encompassing the docked guide wire(s) is made using a #10 scalpel blade (Fig. 4A). A vertebroplasty needle is then passed over the guide wire(s) and firmly docked into the vertebral cortex (Fig. 4B). The guide wire is removed, the needle trochar is replaced and, using a hand mallet, the needle is cautiously advanced in the predetermined trans- or extrapedicular trajectory (Fig. 4C). The little resistance

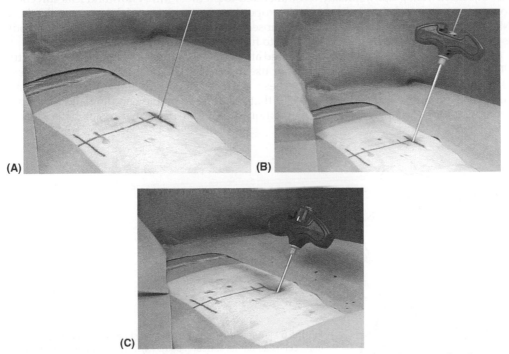

FIGURE 4   (**A**) Guide wire placed. (**B**) Needle advanced over guide wire. (**C**) Guide wire removed and trocar placed within needle.

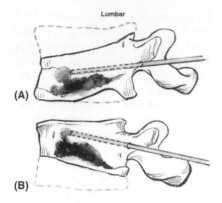

(A)

(B)

FIGURE 5 Lumbar vertebrae have larger pedicles in the cephalocaudal plane. (**A**) This superior wedge fracture requires a flat to caudal needle trajectory. (**B**) This inferior wedge fracture requires a cephalad needle trajectory.

offered by osteoporotic bone suddenly vanishes on entering an intravertebral cleft so that extreme care is necessary to prevent penetration of the anterior vertebral cortex or more ventral soft-tissue structures. In the transpedicular approach, the desired needle trajectory should form a near tangent with the medial trumpeted wall of the pedicle as it aims for the center of the vertebral body. The angle of needle trajectory will be determined by the location of the waist of the pedicle, the slope of pedicle flair as it joins the vertebral body, and the vertebral shape. The lateral view ensures appropriate needle trajectory in the cephalocaudal plane and monitors ventral needle penetration. The needle tip should not breach the medial pedicle shadow on the AP view until it has safely passed the posterior cortex of the vertebral body on the lateral view except when permitted by broadly flaring pedicles. When using the extrapedicular approach in thoracic vertebrae the 0.045-inch guide wires should be initially docked slightly cephalad and lateral to the 2 and 10 o' clock positions. The desired final needle depth is the anterior 20% to 30% of the vertebral body. Unlike pedicle screw instrumentation, the final needle position in the cephalocaudal plane will vary as this will be determined by the distorted configuration of the fractured vertebral body (Figs. 5 and 6). In bipedicular instrumentation, both needles should be placed prior to PMMA injection. Venography, initially recommended to predict PMMA flow and leak direction, has lost general support because the rheologic properties of contrast material do not predict those of PMMA and retained contrast may obscure subsequent PMMA visualization. If vertebral body biopsy is planned it should be performed prior to full needle penetration.

Historically, vertebroplasty was considered an "off-label" application for PMMA. Recently, the FDA has approved cements specifically for use in vertebral augmentation [e.g., Spineplex® (Stryker) and KyphX HV-R® (Kyphon)]. These cements consist of PMMA:barium sulfate mixtures in fixed ratios (approximately 70:30) that result in favorable handling and visualization characteristics. Mixing ratios, polymerization times, and performance characteristics of

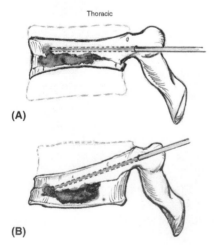

(A)

(B)

FIGURE 6 Thoracic vertebrae have smaller pedicles that are positioned more cephalad on the vertebral body. (**A**) This crush fracture requires a flat needle trajectory. (**B**) This superior wedge fracture requires a caudal needle trajectory starting from a more cephalad position.

non-FDA-approved PMMA products are unique and operators should thoroughly familiarize themselves with individual manufacturers' instructions. Modification of any PMMA product (e.g., by the addition of opacifying agents or antibiotics) alters their performance characteristics and creates a new, non-FDA-approved "device." Using FDA-approved PMMA products circumvents any potential medico-legal ramifications of "off-label" use.

Manual PMMA injection may be performed directly or remotely. Direct syringe-to-vertebroplasty needle injection using 1- or 3-cc PMMA-loaded plastic syringes affords the operator more direct tactile control of cement flow but at the risk of increased radiation exposure. Several proprietary devices (e.g., Parallax, Stryker) permit remote PMMA injection by interposing a delivery system between the operator and the vertebroplasty needle. Remote injection reduces radiation exposure but at the cost of dampened tactile control and increased resistance to flow within the delivery system.

The issue of cement viscosity has generated much rhetoric but supportive clinical science is scant. Conventional wisdom suggests that more viscous cement will result in fewer cement leaks. Optimal cement viscosity for injection is, in fact, unknown and may vary. Viscosity must be considered in view of the length and diameter of the delivery device, the rate of delivery, ambient temperature, intravertebral pressure, the configuration of the fracture, and the presence or absence of an intravertebral cleft. Some of these variables are operator-controlled while others can be anticipated but not directly controlled. We believe that resistance to injection is reduced and working times prolonged by combining somewhat less viscous PMMA with slower injection rates and we have reported low cement leak rates (5,11). Keeping PMMA monomer and polymer on ice prior to mixing will retard polymerization. Temperature differences between delivery tubing and vertebroplasty needle can result in rapid cement setting within the needle and result in a clogged needle.

Final cement fill volumes will depend on fracture level, morphology, severity, and fill pattern (Fig. 1F). In general, the minimum volume of cement sufficient to stabilize the vertebra (2- to 4-cc thoracic vertebrae, 4- to 8-cc lumbar vertebrae) is desired. Large sagittal, axial, or coronal intravertebral clefts become confluent reservoirs for PMMA and will require higher fill volumes (12). Clefts should be entered and completely filled to render the fracture nonmobile. Be cautious of smaller splits as they may fill preferentially and quickly wick PMMA into the disc or an extravertebral space. In the event of a small, innocent leak allow the PMMA to set, reposition the needle, and either cautiously resume injection or move to the contralateral side to complete the procedure. Vertebral filling should cease when, in the judgment of the operator, the biomechanically vulnerable segment (determined from preoperative imaging) has been filled, PMMA enters the dorsal one-third of the vertebra or a leak cannot be controlled. Spinning the needle prior to withdrawal usually amputates potential cement tails. We ordinarily limit augmentation to three vertebral levels during one procedure. Extreme care should be exercised during injection as PMMA is difficult to retrieve and a potential exothermal injury to contiguous tissue begins immediately.

At the completion of the procedure, the subcutaneous tissue and skin are closed with absorbable suture and the skin dressed. Patients should be kept supine for at least one hour following PV and actively monitored for potential adverse anesthetic, cardiopulmonary, and neurological events prior to dismissal. We keep some medically frail patients and those with high-risk augmentations (e.g., multilevel PV, large clefted VCFs) at rest longer or until their thoracolumbosacral orthosis (TLSO) are constructed when indicated.

COMPLICATIONS AND THEIR MANAGEMENT

Complications of PV are infrequent, generally avoidable, and usually relate to inaccurate needle placement or inattention to PMMA flow during injection. PMMA leak rates from osteoporotic VCFs range widely and reflect considerable ascertainment and reporting bias. Most contemporary operators report radiographic leak rates around 10% and symptomatic leak rates far less than 1% (5,15). Small asymptomatic PMMA leaks into the adjacent disc or paravertebral tissue, while undesirable, are probably harmless. Disc leaks may be anticipated by the presence of coronal and sagittal splits through the vertebral endplate seen on preoperative imaging. Increased subsequent adjacent VCF rate ascribed to PMMA disc leaks may have had more to do with the high PMMA fill volumes than the presence of cement within the disc (18). Paravertebral soft tissue leaks may occur through osteoporotic, pathologic, or iatrogenic cortical breach when PMMA filling volumes and rates exceed intravertebral (volume and pressure) capacity. Small paravertebral venous leaks are not uncommon. Vigilance during biplanar imaging is usually sufficient to stop injection and abort azygous or caval propagation so that clinical pulmonary embolism has been rare. Epidural venous leak can be avoided by terminating injection once PMMA reaches the junction of the mid- and posterior third of the vertebral body in the lateral position. Symptomatic foraminal venous leak may be problematic as the volume of PMMA necessary to compress the nerve root in the foramen is relatively small. The location and extent of PMMA leak will determine the presence and nature of any clinical symptoms. CT with 3D reconstructions will assist in the evaluation of a suspected symptomatic foraminal PMMA leak. Serious harm including spinal cord and nerve root injury, hematoma, hemothorax, PMMA pulmonary embolism, infection, and even death has been reported following PV (4). PMMA monomer cardiac toxicity, a concern during general orthopedic procedures, has not been problematic thus far during vertebroplasty.

Formal certification through sponsoring professional surgical and interventional radiology societies is highly recommended. Standards for the performance of PV have been published (19).

POSTOPERATIVE MANAGEMENT

Percutaneous vertebroplasty "fixes" a fractured vertebra but does not "fix" the patient with osteoporosis. Subsequent fracture risk in these patients is high and is increased further in the presence of more numerous and more severe VCFs, increased age, frailty, and falling (9). For this reason PV, a salvage procedure, should be embedded in a comprehensive osteoporosis management program (5). Patients must be provided with basic instruction in safe movements during essential activities of daily living such as dressing, toileting, and transferring either prior to PV or before returning home. Patients should be given explicit instructions regarding wound care. At the 7- to 10-day postoperative follow-up we routinely check a standing AP and lateral radiograph centered on the index vertebra, inspect the surgical site, initiate a more comprehensive rehabilitation program, and address the medical management of skeletal fragility (5). Physical therapy should emphasize fall risk reduction, safe body movements, and encourage a graduated, extension-based, core-strengthening program. Postoperative bracing using customized TLSO should be considered following biomechanically high-risk augmentations such as severe, dynamically mobile VCFs with large clefts at the thoracolumbar junction or multilevel augmentations. Identification and correction of hypovitaminosis D and dietary insufficiency for calcium, nearly ubiquitous in this population, will reduce falls and facilitate optimal skeletal responsiveness to drug therapy. Aggressive pharmacologic osteoporosis management may reduce subsequent VCF risk by 50% to 90%. In bisphosphonate-naive patients, anabolic therapy (Teriparatide, Forteo®) results in rapid mineralization, improved skeletal microarchetecture, and has the attractive, albeit unproven, potential for accelerated fracture repair.

OUTCOMES OF VERTEBROPLASTY

The quality of evidence pertaining to vertebral augmentation outcomes is variable (20). The level of evidence is limited to prospective case series (with or without concurrent observational groups), as no prospective, randomized, controlled trial has yet demonstrated superiority of PV over nonoperative care. In spite of these shortcomings, the available evidence uniformly demonstrates immediate, dramatic, and durable reduction in pain and improvement in quality of life following PV (5). Vertebral height restoration is possible during PV (11). In spite of much rhetoric, the clinical significance of the small restorations achieved thus far, by either augmentation method, remains to be determined. Subsequent vertebral fracture rate is an important conundrum that has not been fully resolved. The most recent literature suggests that subsequent VCF rate has declined and may reflect increasing surgical proficiency, smaller PMMA fill volumes, and implementation of aggressive osteoporosis-specific postoperative medical and physical therapy interventions. In the author's experience sustained pain relief, improved quality of life, and low subsequent VCF rate can be anticipated by combining PV with comprehensive osteoporosis aftercare (5).

PITFALLS AND BAILOUTS

Remember biopsy before injecting cement. In the absence of an access cannula clogged needles must be removed and the vertebra reinstrumented. Transpedicular instrumentation through very narrow pedicles may result in undesirable, lateralized needle tip position within the vertebral body. In such an instance, an extrapedicular approach must be chosen. The biomechanical implications of leaving a nonfractured vertebra between two augmented vertebrae or at the end of a long rigid biomechanical construct (e.g., ankylosing spondylitis, diffuse idiopathic skeletal hyperostosis, multilevel degenerative spondylosis with rigid osteophytosis) present a difficult conundrum. Thus far, we have resisted the impulse to augment the nonfractured vertebra. Finally, subsequent vertebral collapse on top of PMMA augmentation may result from incomplete filling or progression of the disease. Successful revision PV has been described (21).

SUMMARY/FUTURE DIRECTIONS

In carefully selected patients, PV safely and effectively relieves osteoporotic VCF pain when cautious patient handling, meticulous needle placement, and vigilance during PMMA injection are observed. It remains to be proven that PV is superior to nonoperative care for all patients. Optimal timing of PV and the effect of fracture level and morphology on outcome remain to be determined. The significance of vertebral height restoration and postural alignment is unknown and deserves serious study. Biomaterials and strategies that immediately restore vertebral strength and allow osseous reconstitution over time may replace PMMA in the future.

Synopsis

- PV safely and effectively relieves vertebral fracture pain.
- Operative strategy and success depends on familiarity with preoperative imaging and comprehensive understanding of fractured vertebral anatomy.
- Accurate needle placement and vigilance during PMMA injection will avert most pitfalls.
- PV should be embedded in a comprehensive osteoporosis management program.

REFERENCES

1. Galibert P, Deramond H, Rosat P, et al. Preliminary note on the treatment of vertebral hemangioma by percutaneous acrylic vertebroplasty. Neurochirugie 1987; 33:166–168 (French).
2. Jensen ME, Evans AJ, Mathis JM, et al. Percutaneous polymethylmethacrylate vertebroplasty in the treatment of osteoporotic vertebral compression fractures: technical aspects. Am J Neuroradiol 1997; 18:1897–1904.
3. Faciszewski T, McKiernan FE. Calling all vertebral fractures; Classification of vertebral compression fractures: a consensus for comparison of treatment and outcome. J Bone Miner Res 2002; 17:185–191.
4. Rao RD, Singrakhia MD. Painful osteoporotic vertebral fracture; pathogenesis, evaluation and roles of vertebroplasty and kyphoplasty in its management. J Bone Joint Surg Am 2003; 85-A:2010–2022.
5. McKiernan FE, Faciszewski T. Quality of life following percutaneous vertebroplasty. J Bone Joint Surg Am 2004; 86(12):2600–2606.
6. Rami PM, McGraw JK, Heatwole EV, et al. Percutaneous vertebroplasty in the treatment of vertebral body compression fracture secondary to osteogenesis imperfecta. Skeletal Radiol 2002; 31:162–165.
7. Fink HA, Milavetz DL, Palermo L, et al. For the Fracture Intervention Trial Research Group. What proportion of incident radiographic vertebral deformities is clinically diagnosed and vice versa? J Bone Miner Res 2005; 20:1216–1222.
8. Patel U, Skingle S, Campbell GA, et al. Clinical profile of acute vertebral compression fractures in osteoporosis. Br J Rheumatol 1991; 30:418–421.
9. http://www.surgeongeneral.gov/library/bonehealth/content.html, accessed July 2005.
10. Gaughen JR, Jensen ME, Schweickert PA, et al. Lack of preoperative spinous process tenderness does not affect clinical success of percutaneous vertebroplasty. J Vasc Interv Radiol 2002; 13:1135–1138.
11. McKiernan FE, Jensen R, Faciszewski T. The dynamic mobility of vertebral compression fractures. J Bone Miner Res 2003; 18:24–29.

McKiernan and Faciszewski

12. McKiernan FE, Faciszewski T. Intravertebral clefts in osteoporotic vertebral compression fractures 2003; 48:1414–1419.
13. Schmitz A, Risse JH, Textor J, et al. FDG-PET findings of vertebral compression fractures in osteoporosis: preliminary results. Osteoporos Int 2002; 13:755–761.
14. Evans AJ, Jensen ME, Kip KE, et al. Vertebral compression fractures: pain reduction and improvement in functional mobility after percutaneous polymethylmethacrylate vertebroplasty-retrospective report of 245 cases. Radiology 2003; 226:366–372.
15. Mathis JM, Wong W. Percutaneous vertebroplasty: technical considerations. J Vasc Interv Radiol 2003; 14:953–960.
16. Kallmes DF, Jensen ME. Percutaneous vertebroplasty. Radiology 2003; 229:27–36.
17. Kruger R, Faciszewski T. Radiation dose reduction to medical staff during vertebroplasty: a review of techniques and methods to mitigate occupational dose. Spine 2003; 28:1608–1613.
18. Lin EP, Ekholm S, Hiwatashi A, et al. Vertebroplasty: cement leakage into the disc increases the risk of new fracture of adjacent vertebral body. Am J Neuroradiol 2004; 25:175–180.
19. Barr JD, Mathis JM, Barr MS. Standard for the performance of percutaneous vertebroplasty. American College of Radiology Standards 2000–2001. Reston, VA: American College of Radiology, 2000: 441–448.
20. http://www.cms.hhs.gov/mcd/viewtechassess.asp?where=index&tid=25 and http://www.cms.hhs.gov/mcd/viewtechassess.asp?where=index&tid=26, accessed July 2005.
21. Gaughen JR, Jensen ME, Schweickert PA, et al. The therapeutic benefit of repeat percutaneous vertebroplasty at previously treated vertebral levels. Am J Neuroradiol 2002; 23:1657–1661.

33 | Vertebral Body Augmentation for Bone Tumor

Daisuke Togawa, Mark M. Kayanja, and Isador H. Lieberman
Cleveland Clinic Spine Institute, The Cleveland Clinic Foundation, Cleveland, Ohio, U.S.A.

A. Jay Khanna
Johns Hopkins Orthopedics, Good Samaritan Hospital, Baltimore, Maryland, U.S.A.

INTRODUCTION

The American Cancer Society estimated that 1.33 million patients were diagnosed with cancer in 2003 (1). Reportedly, metastases develops in two-thirds of cancer patients (2). The skeletal system is the third most common site of cancer metastasis behind the lung and liver (3). Cancer metastases are the most common skeletal tumors seen by orthopedists; the ratio of metastatic lesions to primary bone tumors is 25 to 1 (4,5). Delamarter et al. reported that only 29 of 1971 patients (1.5%) had primary neoplasms in a study of all cases of neoplastic disease (6). Although symptomatic, spinal cord involvement has been estimated to occur in 18,000 patients per year (7), 60% of all skeletal metastases (8) and 36% of vertebral lesions are asymptomatic (9) and discovered incidentally. The primary lesion remained unknown in 12.5% of the patients.

The spine is the most common site of metastatic skeletal involvement (10–16). Approximately 70% of spinal metastases occur in the thoracic spine, while the lumbar and cervical spine account for approximately 20% and 10% of the cases, respectively (17,18). Spinal metastatic disease can occur in the paraspinal regions, in the vertebrae, or in the epidural and subarachnoid spaces. Skeletal metastases are produced by almost all forms of malignant disease but are most often secondary to carcinomas of the breast, lung, prostate, kidneys, and less frequently thyroid and gastrointestinal carcinomas (7,9,13,19–28). Destruction of the vertebral body, often leading to vertebral body collapse, occurs in as many as 70% of the patients with multiple myeloma or metastatic cancer (29,30,64). Pain is the most common presenting symptom in up to 90% of the patients (29,30).

Recent advancements in the diagnosis and treatment of many types of cancers have prolonged and improved the quality of life for cancer patients. Unfortunately, the medical treatment itself can contribute to the already present osteolytic bone loss. If left untreated, vertebral body compression fractures can cause progressive kyphosis over multiple levels, cord compromise, or intractable pain. However, comorbid conditions and poor bone quality contribute to the difficulties of surgical intervention in this patient group. To alleviate these issues, percutaneous minimally invasive vertebral augmentation techniques have recently evolved that show promising results for this group of patients.

VERTEBROPLASTY
Indications and Technique

Percutaneous vertebroplasty is a minimally invasive technique commonly used to treat osteoporotic and osteolytic vertebral compression fractures. This technique was first performed by Galibert et al. and described in the French literature in 1987 (32). Typically, polymethylmethacrylate (PMMA) is injected into a compressed vertebral body under fluoroscopic guidance. The technique was used originally for the treatment of vertebral body hemangiomas, and then its use was gradually expanded to the treatment of pain associated with vertebral compression fractures with different pathologies. Vertebroplasty stabilizes a compression fracture but does not directly restore the vertebral body height.

The patient is positioned prone on the operating table. The procedure is performed under general anesthesia or intravenous sedation with local anesthesia. Contraindications to vertebroplasty are systemic pathology such as sepsis, prolonged bleeding times, or cardiopulmonary pathology, which would preclude the safe completion of the procedure. Other contraindications include neurological signs or symptoms, nonosteolytic infiltrative spinal metastases (e.g., prostate lesions), vertebral height collapse of more than 60%, vertebral bodies with deficient posterior cortices, or coagulopathy (33,34). Burst or vertebral plana fracture patterns are technically challenging and are relative contraindications.

Clinical Outcomes

From January 1985 to June 2005, 478 papers about vertebroplasty were published in peer-reviewed journals. Outcome data from over 1000 treated patients have been reported in several clinical series (35–51). Barr et al. reported complete pain relief in 50% of the patients with osteolytic fractures. Weill et al. reported a retrospective series of 37 patients who underwent 52 vertebroplasty procedures for spinal metastases (37). Seventy-three percent of patients had pain improvement. Cotton et al. also reported prospectively acquired data obtained in 37 patients who underwent 40 vertebroplasty procedures for osteolytic metastases (29 patients) and myeloma (eight patients). Partial or complete pain relief was observed after 36 (97%) of 37 procedures. Fourney et al. reported that complete pain relief or improvement occurred after 30 (86%) of 35 cases (52).

By virtue of the technique, vertebroplasty involves the injection of liquid PMMA into the closed space of a collapsed vertebral body. Although the incidence is low, the potential does exist for PMMA to extravasate into perivertebral veins, leading to pulmonary cement embolism (53–55). Several reports also describe that extravasation from the vertebral body could lead to cord compromise, necessitating emergent decompression (33,34,56–59).

KYPHOPLASTY
Indications and Technique

Kyphoplasty is a technique using an inflatable bone tamp to first create a cavity in the collapsed vertebral body in preparation for cement insertion. It has a number of potential advantages, including lower risk of cement extravasation and better restoration of vertebral body height (69,70,71). A biopsy needle is a convenient way to begin a kyphoplasty, following strategically placed 3-mm incisions and careful needle advancement, under multiplanar fluoroscopy. If a tissue diagnosis is needed, bone biopsy is recommended (63). A cannula is introduced into the vertebral body, via a transpedicular or extrapedicular route, followed by insertion of an inflatable bone tamp, which when inflated, reduces the compression fracture and restores the vertebral body toward its original height. This creates a cavity that is then filled with PMMA in a controlled fashion. Kyphoplasty offers several theoretical advantages over vertebroplasty including lower extravasation rates and greater height restoration (60–63,65–68,71).

Clinical Outcome
Metastatic Disease

Our ongoing study of kyphoplasty for the treatment of compression fractures resulting from spinal metastases has shown favorable preliminary results (72). We evaluated safety and efficacy of kyphoplasty in the first 21 patients over a three-year period for the treatment of spinal metastases (72). The mean age of the patients was 60.8 years (range: 40 to 88 years). The indication for the kyphoplasty procedure was painful osteolytic vertebral body compression fracture. Symptomatic levels were identified with plain radiographs and magnetic resonance imaging (MRI). The primary sources of the metastases included breast cancer (nine patients), lymphoma (four patients), lung cancer (three patients), and unknown location (five patients).

Postoperative evaluation showed that the procedure was well tolerated, with improvement in pain that resulted in early mobilization in all 21 patients. Preoperative and postoperative SF-36 data were available for 14 of the 21 patients, with a mean follow-up of 50 weeks (range: 3 to 206 weeks). Significant improvement (preoperative vs. postoperative scores, respectively)

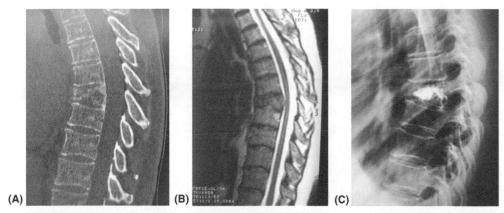

FIGURE 1   Breast cancer, 1 level osteolytic collapse, T. (**A**) Preoperative sagittal CT reconstruction. (**B**) Preoperative T2-weighted magnetic resonance image. (**C**) Postoperative lateral X ray.

was noted in the following areas: physical function, 20.9 to 33.5 ($P = 0.036$); vitality, 31.2 to 42.9 ($P = 0.012$); and social function, 37.5 to 66.1 ($P = 0.011$). No significant changes occurred in mental health (60.0 to 62.0), role-emotional (55.5 to 51.3), general health (52.1 to 46.0), bodily pain (31.6 to 39.0), and pain as measured by the Visual Analog Scale (6.5 to 3.9). All 21 patients tolerated the procedure well, and there were no substantial systemic complications. The fact that we found statistically significant improvement in only three SF-36 subscores may be because of the relatively small number of patients currently available. There was a trend toward decreased pain after kyphoplasty. It is important to note that our primary indication for the treatment of these patients was palliation and to avoid open conventional surgical procedures that could have had a negative impact on the general quality of life of these patients with multiple medical comorbidities and limited life expectancies. The fact that we were able to show a decrease in Visual Analog Scale pain scores from 6.5 to 3.9, although not statistically significant, suggests that there was a trend toward pain control (Fig. 1).

Multiple Myeloma

Dudeney et al. (73) have reported satisfactory results with kyphoplasty for osteolytic vertebral compression fractures secondary to multiple myeloma. We previously reported on kyphoplasty to treat 80 patients with multiple myeloma and associated vertebral body compression fractures (74). The mean age of our patients at the time of the procedure was 60.6 years (range: 35 to 85 years). Preoperative and postoperative SF-36 scores were available for 61 of 80 patients with a mean follow-up of 15.6 months (range: 2 to 59 months). No major complications related to the technique have been observed. Significant ($P < 0.05$) improvement in SF-36 scores (preoperative vs. postoperative, respectively) were observed for the following areas: bodily pain, 23.0 to 44.4 ($P < 0.001$); physical function, 25.5 to 36.6 ($P = 0.034$); vitality, 30.3 to 38.1 ($P = 0.039$); and social functioning, 35.4 to 67.5 ($P < 0.001$). Mental health scores showed an improvement of 60.3 to 66.2 ($P < 0.001$), whereas role-emotion and general health were essentially unchanged ($P = 0.086$ and $P = 0.054$, respectively). We believe these results suggest that kyphoplasty is efficacious in the treatment of vertebral body compression fractures secondary to multiple myeloma (Fig. 2).

FUTURE RESEARCH

Recently, Jang et al. reported the clinical efficacy of percutaneous vertebroplasty combined with radiotherapy in 28 patients with osteolytic metastatic spinal tumors (75). The use of these vertebral augmentation procedures in conjunction with radiation therapy is now being evaluated as a treatment for these malignancies both biomechanically and biologically. In addition, the access portals that permit the placement of working cannulas into the vertebral body for a vertebral augmentation procedure also can be used to instill chemotherapeutic agents or to perform brachytherapy-type procedures. It is still unclear what the exothermal effect of PMMA has on vertebral body tumor, and whether therapeutic agents can be mixed with filler materials.

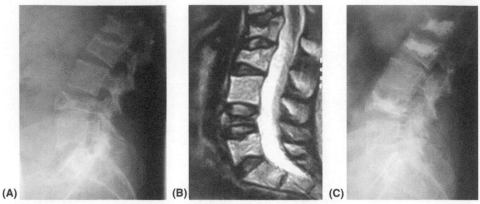

FIGURE 2   Multiple myeloma, 3 level osteolytic collapse. (**A**) Preoperative lateral X ray. (**B**) Preoperative T2-weighted magnetic resonance image. (**C**) Postoperative lateral X ray.

The safety and efficacy of this material containing both augmentation and chemotherapeutic components will need evaluation as to whether it fits the surgical procedure and whether it provides the necessary biological and biomechanical properties.

The next logical step beyond treatment of evident fractures is prophylactic augmentation. Prevention of osteolytic vertebral fractures with a combination of pharmacologics and timely reinforcement of at-risk vertebrae would be the goal. It is here that new osteoconductive synthetic composites will figure more prominently as an emerging alternative to cement (76).

CONCLUSIONS

Osteolytic vertebral body compression fractures pose a significant problem producing spinal deformity, pain, reduced pulmonary function, and morbidity, as well as overall increase in mortality in the elderly and those suffering from cancer. Traditional medical and surgical options in many cases prove inadequate. Percutaneous vertebral augmentation techniques such as vertebroplasty and kyphoplasty have proven to be beneficial in the treatment of these patients who are debilitated. The safety profile of vertebroplasty has been established, with most complications being minor or insignificant and resulting from the cement used in the procedure rather than the placement of the cannula. Kyphoplasty represents an alternative to vertebroplasty that may offer advantages in efficacy and safety. Our preliminary results with kyphoplasty for the treatment of vertebral compression fractures in patients with metastatic spinal malignancies and multiple myeloma suggest that the procedure is well-tolerated and efficacious. Although more data are needed to evaluate the use of kyphoplasty for the treatment of malignant compression fractures, the evidence is compelling that kyphoplasty can be used safely in the treatment of metastatic lesions of the vertebral body in patients who were previously considered poor surgical candidates because of limited life expectancies or the presence of other medical comorbidities. We now advocate early treatment of any osteolytic fractured vertebra and prophylactic treatment of any vertebra at risk of collapse. This concept should help avoid the structural and functional effects of progressive osteolytic spinal collapse.

REFERENCES

1. Cancer in America 2003. http://www.cancer.org/docroot/MED/content.
2. Shaw B, Mansfield FL, Borges L. One-stage posterolateral decompression and stabilization for primary and metastatic vertebral tumors in the thoracic and lumbar spine. J Neurosurg 1989; 70:405–410.
3. Boland PJ, Lane JM, Sundaresan N. Metastatic disease of the spine. Clin Orthop 1982; 169:95–102.
4. Francis KC, Hutter RV. Neoplasms of the spine in the aged. Clin Orthop 1963; 26:54–66.
5. Mirra JM. Bone Tumors: Clinical, Radiologic, and Pathologic Correlation. Philadelphia: Lea&Febiger, 1989:1495–1517.

6. Delamarter RB, Sachs BL, Thompson GH, et al. Primary neoplasms of the thoracic and lumbar spine. An analysis of 29 consecutive cases. Clin Orthop 1990; 256:87–100.
7. Black P. Spinal metastasis: current status and recommended guidelines for management. Neurosurgery 1979; 5:726–746.
8. Krishnamurthy GT, Tubis M, Hiss J, et al. Distribution pattern of metastatic bone disease. A need for total body skeletal image. JAMA 1977; 237:2504–2506.
9. Schaberg J, Gainor BJ. A profile of metastatic carcinoma of the spine. Spine 1985; 10:19–20.
10. Unni KK. Dahlin's Bone Tumors: General Aspects and Data on 11,087 Cases. 5th ed. Philadelphia, PA: Lippincott-Raven, 1996.
11. Gokaslan ZL. Spine surgery for cancer. Curr Opin Oncol 1996; 8:178–181.
12. Steinmets MP, Mekhail A, Benzel EC. Management of metastatic tumors of the spine: strategies and operative indications. Neurosurg Focus 2001; 11:Article 2.
13. Harrington KD. Metastatic disease of the spine. J Bone Joint Surg Am 1986; 68:1110–1115.
14. Berrettoni BA, Carter JR. Mechanisms of cancer metastasis to bone. J Bone Joint Surg Am 1986; 68:308–312.
15. Bhalla SK. Metastatic disease of the spine. Clin Orthop 1970; 73:52–60.
16. Johnston AD. Pathology of metastatic tumors in bone. Clin Orthop 1970; 73:8–32.
17. Barron KD, Hirano A, Araki S, et al. Experiences with metastatic neoplasms involving the spinal cord. Neurology 1959; 9:91–106.
18. Gerszten PC, Welch WC. Current surgical management of metastatic spinal disease. Oncology (Williston Park) 2000; 14:1013–1024, discussion 24, 29–30.
19. Clain A. Secondary malignant disease of bone. Br J Cancer 1965; 19:15–29.
20. Habermann ET, Sachs R, Stern RE, et al. The pathology and treatment of metastatic disease of the femur. Clin Orthop 1982; 169:70–82.
21. Milch RA, Changus GW. Response of bone to tumor invasion. Cancer 1956; 9:340–351.
22. Millburn L, Hibbs GG, Hendrickson FR. Treatment of spinal cord compression from metastatic carcinoma. Review of literature and presentation of a new method of treatment. Cancer 1968; 21:447–452.
23. Nottebaert M, Exner GU, von Hochstetter AR, et al. Metastatic bone disease from occult carcinoma: a profile. Int Orthop 1989; 13:119–123.
24. Adams M, Sonntag VK. Surgical treatment of metastatic cervical spine disease. Contemp Neurosurg 2001; 23:1–5.
25. Byrne TN. Spinal cord compression from epidural metastases. N Engl J Med 1992; 327:614–619.
26. Gilbert RW, Kim JH, Posner JB. Epidural spinal cord compression from metastatic tumor: diagnosis and treatment. Ann Neurol 1978; 3:40–51.
27. McLain RF, Weinstein JN. Tumors of the spine. Semin Spine Surg 1990; 2:157–180.
28. Wong DA, Fornasier VL, MacNab I. Spinal metastases: the obvious, the occult, and the impostors. Spine 1990; 15:1–4.
29. McLain RF, Weinstein JN. Tumors of the spine. In: The Spine. 4th ed. Herkowitz HN, Garfin SR, Balderston RA, Eismont FJ, Bell GR, Wiesel SW, eds. Philadelphia: W.B. Saunders Co, 1999: 1171–1206.
30. Sundaresan N, Krol G, Digiacinto G, et al. Metastatic Tumors of the Spine. In: Tumors of the Spine: Diagnosis and Clinical Management. Sundaresan N, Schmidek HH, Schiller AL, Rosenthal TD, eds. Chap. 29. Philadelphia: W.B. Saunders, 1990:279–304.
31. Lecouvet FE, Vande Berg BC, Maldague BE, et al. Vertebral compression fractures in multiple myeloma. Part I. Distribution and appearance at MR imaging. Radiology 1997; 204:195–199.
32. Galibert P, Deramond H, Rosat P, et al. Preliminary note on the treatment of vertebral angioma by percutaneous acrylic vertebroplasty. Neurochirurgie 1987; 33:166–168.
33. Bai B, Jazrawi LM, Kummer FJ, et al. The use of an injectable, biodegradable calcium phosphate bone substitute for the prophylactic augmentation of osteoporotic vertebrae and the management of vertebral compression fractures. Spine 1999; 24:1521–1526.
34. Cotten A, Boutry N, Cortet B, et al. Percutaneous vertebroplasty: state of the art. Radiographics 1998; 18:311–320, discussion 20–23.
35. Cotten A, Duquesnoy B. Vertebroplasty: current data and future potential. Rev Rhum Engl Ed 1997; 64:645–649.
36. Cortet B, Cotten A, Boutry N, et al. Percutaneous vertebroplasty in patients with osteolytic metastases or multiple myeloma. Rev Rhum Engl Ed 1997; 64:177–183.
37. Weill A, Chiras J, Simon JM, et al. Spinal metastases: indications for and results of percutaneous injection of acrylic surgical cement. Radiology 1996; 199:241–247.
38. Jensen ME, Evans AJ, Mathis JM, et al. Percutaneous polymethylmethacrylate vertebroplasty in the treatment of osteoporotic vertebral body compression fractures: technical aspects. Am J Neuroradiol 1997; 18:1897–1904.
39. Martin JB, Jean B, Sugiu K, et al. Vertebroplasty: clinical experience and follow-up results. Bone 1999; 25:S11–S15.
40. Deramond H, Depriester C, Galibert P, et al. Percutaneous vertebroplasty with polymethylmethacrylate. Technique, indications, and results. Radiol Clin N Am 1998; 36:533–546.

41. Evans AJ, Jensen ME, Kip KE, et al. Vertebral compression fractures: pain reduction and improvement in functional mobility after percutaneous polymethylmethacrylate vertebroplasty retrospective report of 245 cases. Radiology 2003; 226:366–372.

42. Cohen JE, Lylyk P, Ceratto R, et al. Percutaneous vertebroplasty: technique and results in 192 procedures. Neurol Res 2004; 26:41–49.

43. Cortet B, Cotten A, Boutry N, et al. Percutaneous vertebroplasty in the treatment of osteoporotic vertebral compression fractures: an open prospective study. J Rheumatol 1999; 26:2222–2228.

44. Cyteval C, Sarrabere MP, Roux JO, et al. Acute osteoporotic vertebral collapse: open study on percutaneous injection of acrylic surgical cement in 20 patients. Am J Roentgenol 1999; 173:1685–1690.

45. Maynard AS, Jensen ME, Schweickert PA, et al. Value of bone scan imaging in predicting pain relief from percutaneous vertebroplasty in osteoporotic vertebral fractures. Am J Neuroradiol 2000; 21:1807–1812.

46. Grados F, Depriester C, Cayrolle G, et al. Long-term observations of vertebral osteoporotic fractures treated by percutaneous vertebroplasty. Rheumatology (Oxf) 2000; 39:1410–1414.

47. Barr JD, Barr MS, Lemley TJ, et al. Percutaneous vertebroplasty for pain relief and spinal stabilization. Spine 2000; 25:923–928.

48. Kim AK, Jensen ME, Dion JE, et al. Unilateral transpedicular percutaneous vertebroplasty: initial experience. Radiology 2002; 222:737–741.

49. Kaufmann TJ, Jensen ME, Schweickert PA, et al. Age of fracture and clinical outcomes of percutaneous vertebroplasty. Am J Neuroradiol 2001; 22:1860–1863.

50. Heini PF, Walchli B, Berlemann U. Percutaneous transpedicular vertebroplasty with PMMA: operative technique and early results. A prospective study for the treatment of osteoporotic compression fractures. Eur Spine J 2000; 9:445–450.

51. Ryu KS, Park CK, Kim MC, et al. Dose-dependent epidural leakage of polymethylmethacrylate after percutaneous vertebroplasty in patients with osteoporotic vertebral compression fractures. J Neurosurg 2002; 96:56–61.

52. Fourney DR, Schomer DF, Nader R, et al. Percutaneous vertebroplasty and kyphoplasty for painful vertebral body fractures in cancer patients. J Neurosurg Spine 2003; 98:21–30.

53. Choe du H, Marom EM, Ahrar K, et al. Pulmonary embolism of polymethylmethacrylate during percutaneous vertebroplasty and kyphoplasty. Am J Roentgenol 2004; 183:1097–1102.

54. Jang JS, Lee SH, Jung SK. Pulmonary embolism of polymethylmethacrylate after percutaneous vertebroplasty: a report of three cases. Spine 2002; 27:E416–E418.

55. Yoo KY, Jeong SW, Yoon W, et al. Acute respiratory distress syndrome associated with pulmonary cement embolism following percutaneous vertebroplasty with polymethylmethacrylate. Spine 2004; 29:E294–E297.

56. Cotten A, Dewatre F, Cortet B, et al. Percutaneous vertebroplasty for osteolytic metastases and myeloma: effects of the percentage of lesion filling and the leakage of methylmethacrylate at clinical follow-up. Radiology 1996; 200:525–530.

57. Ratliff J, Nguyen T, Heiss J. Root and spinal cord compression from methylmethacrylate vertebroplasty. Spine 2001; 26:E300–E302.

58. Lee BJ, Lee SR, Yoo TY. Paraplegia as a complication of percutaneous vertebroplasty with polymethylmethacrylate: a case report. Spine 2002; 27:E419–E422.

59. Harrington KD. Major neurological complications following percutaneous vertebroplasty with polymethylmethacrylate: a case report. J Bone Joint Surg Am 2001; 83–A:1070–1073.

60. Kayanja MM, Togawa D, Lieberman IH. Biomechanical changes after the augmentation of experimental osteoporotic vertebral compression fractures in the cadaveric thoracic spine. Spine J 2005; 5:55–63.

61. Kayanja MM, Schlenk R, Togawa D, et al. The biomechanics of one, two and three levels of vertebral augmentation with polymethylmethacrylate in multilevel spinal segments. Spine 2006. In press.

62. Harrop JS, Prpa B, Reinhardt MK, et al. Primary and secondary osteoporosis' incidence of subsequent vertebral compression fractures after kyphoplasty. Spine 2004; 29:2120–2125.

63. Togawa D, Lieberman IH, Bauer TW, et al. Histological evaluation of biopsies obtained from vertebral compression fractures: unsuspected myeloma and osteomalacia. Spine 2005; 30:781–786.

64. Togawa D, Kovacic JJ, Bauer TW, et al. Radiographic and histologic findings of vertebral augmentation using polymethylmethacrylate in the primate spine—percutaneous vertebroplasty versus kyphoplasty. Spine 2006. In press.

65. Togawa D, Bauer TW, Lieberman IH, et al. Histologic evaluation of human vertebral bodies after vertebral augmentation with polymethylmethacrylate. Spine 2003; 28:1521–1527.

66. Kayanja MM, Ferrara LA, Lieberman IH. Distribution of anterior cortical shear strain after a thoracic wedge compression fracture. Spine J 2004; 4:76–87.

67. Coumans JV, Reinhardt MK, Lieberman IH. Kyphoplasty for vertebral compression fractures: 1-year clinical outcomes from a prospective study. J Neurosurg 2003; 99:44–50.

68. Lieberman IH, Dudeney S, Reinhardt MK, et al. Initial outcome and efficacy of "kyphoplasty" in the treatment of painful osteoporotic vertebral compression fractures. Spine 2001; 26:1631–1638.

69. Garfin SR, Yuan HA, Reiley MA. New technologies in spine: kyphoplasty and vertebroplasty for the treatment of painful osteoporotic compression fractures. Spine 2001; 26:1511–1515.

70. Ledlie JT, Renfro M. Balloon kyphoplasty: one-year outcomes in vertebral body height restoration, chronic pain, and activity levels. J Neurosurg 2003; 98:36–42.
71. Phillips FM, Ho E, Campbell-Hupp M, et al. Early radiographic and clinical results of balloon kyphoplasty for the treatment of osteoporotic vertebral compression fractures. Spine 2003; 28:2260–2265.
72. Khanna AJ, Reinhardt MK, Togawa D, et al. Functional outcomes of kyphoplasty for the treatment of spinal metastases. Abstract of papers, 72th annual meeting of American Academy of Orthopaedic Surgeons, Washington D.C., February 23–27, 2005.
73. Dudeney S, Lieberman IH, Reinhardt MK, et al. Kyphoplasty in the treatment of osteolytic vertebral compression fractures as a result of multiple myeloma. J Clin Oncol 2002; 20:2382–2387.
74. Khanna AJ, Reinhardt MK, Togawa D, et al. Clinical and functional outcomes of kyphoplasty for vertebral compression fractures. Spine J 2004; 4:S38–S39.
75. Jang JS, Lee SH. Efficacy of percutaneous vertebroplasty combined with radiotherapy in osteolytic metastatic spinal tumors. J Neurosurg Spine 2005; 2:243–248.
76. Lieberman IH, Togawa D, Kayanja MM. Vertebroplasty and kyphoplasty: filler materials. Spine J 2005; 5:S305–S316.

34 | Percutaneous Treatment of Vertebral Bone Cyst

Kathleen S. Beebe and Joseph Benevenia

Department of Orthopedics, University of Medicine and Dentistry of New Jersey, Newark, New Jersey, U.S.A.

INTRODUCTION

Percutaneous treatment of cystic bone lesions is most commonly performed for unicameral bone cysts (UBCs) and aneurysmal bone cyst (ABCs). Unlike ABCs, which commonly occur in the spine, UBCs of the spine are exceedingly rare. Thus, the focus of this chapter will be the percutaneous treatment of ABCs of the spine.

ABCs are benign, locally aggressive lesions that may be found primarily or secondary as part of a cystic component of another lesion. When encountered as a secondary lesion, they are most commonly associated with chondroblastoma, giant cell tumors, fibrous dysplasia, or nonossifying fibromas. The majority of the patients are under the age of 30. While the most common location of an ABC is around the knee, spine involvement is not uncommon, with the posterior elements being most frequently affected (1). Radiographically, the lesions are generally eccentric, lytic, and expansile (Figs. 1 and 2) (2). Computerized tomography (CT) and magnetic resonance imaging (MRI) may show septations and fluid-fluid levels (Figs. 3 and 4) (2); however, this is not pathognomonic for an ABC (3). Histologically, lesions should have cavernous blood-filled lakes (Fig. 5). The lesions can look radiographically and histologically similar to the more ominous telengectatic osteosarcoma. A lack of malignant cells on an adequate biopsy sample can exclude this malignant diagnosis.

Prior to any treatment, a biopsy of the lesion should be undertaken to confirm the diagnosis. This biopsy can be performed percutaneously with the caveat that fine-needle aspirates may be inconclusive. It often yields little tissue and only a nondiagnostic blood sample, necessitating a core tissue biopsy.

INDICATIONS

The indications and contraindications to percutaneous treatment of vertebral ABCs are not absolute. One must assess the risk and benefits of various forms of treatment for the cyst and the options must be weighed with most consideration given to the location of the lesion, spinal stability, and need for spinal mobility. The most definitive treatment is en bloc excision. While this reduces recurrence rates, it can be associated with unnecessary risks, such as physeal injury in children, and requires larger reconstructions. En bloc resection is more commonly employed in the treatment of the so-called expendable bones (such as the fibula). The most frequently utilized treatment for ABC is open curettage and bone grafting or cementation. This type of intralesional curettage carries with it a 20% to 30% recurrence rate and also poses a risk to the physis. Both procedures may be difficult depending on the location of the lesion. Lesions that are compressing vital structures as well as those that are causing instability are not well suited for percutaneous treatment for obvious reasons.

For lesions that are "inoperable" or those that have significant risk associated with surgical exposure and treatment, other treatment options need to be considered. External beam radiation therapy has been reported for the treatment of inaccessible lesions, but it carries the risk of radiation-induced osteonecrosis, sarcomas, growth disturbance, and myelopathy (4).

The use of percutaneous techniques for the treatment of vertebral bone cysts is a therapy that has received recent review. The advantages of percutaneous techniques include avoidance

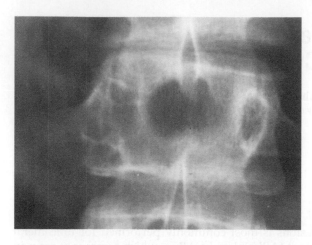

FIGURE 1 Anteroposterior radiograph of aneurysmal bone cyst. *Source*: From Ref. 2.

of the risk of open surgical incisions and the need for large reconstructions. In areas of vital neurovascular structures, this can be of utmost importance. In addition, recovery times, hospital stays, and cost may be lower.

Embolization of vessels that may feed the lesion has been suggested as a preoperative measure to reduce blood loss, as a salvage procedure for failed open surgical treatment, and as an alternative to operative intervention. There are two limiting factors associated with embolization. First, ABCs often lack large feeding vessels. Second, feeding vessels are often in close proximity or in association with major blood supplies to the spinal cord, which can risk postprocedural neurological deficit (4).

Sclerotherapy has been advocated as an alternative treatment option. Potential complications of using the sclerosing agent Ethibloc (Ethicon, Hamburg, Germany) include pulmonary embolism, local inflammation reaction (often associated with fever), and leakage of the agent that can occasionally lead to cutaneous fistulas or osteomyelitis (5). In addition, a fatality after embolization of the vertebrobasilar system following percutaneous injection of Ethibloc into an ABC has been reported (6).

Percutaneous treatment utilizing various agents has been advocated in the treatment of ABC. Injections of calcitonin and methylprednisolone into ABCs have been performed but most reports focus on more traditional sclerosing agents, such as Ethibloc (7,8).

Ethibloc is an emulsion of zein, alcohol, oleum papaveris, propylene glycol, and contrast medium. It has a high viscosity which allows for filling of a cyst. When placed in an aqueous medium, it thickens immediately to a chewing gum-like consistency. It then gradually hardens over a period of minutes. It promotes thrombus formation and induces local necrosis, inflammation, and fibrosis (9). In the treatment of lesions close to the spinal cord or nerve roots,

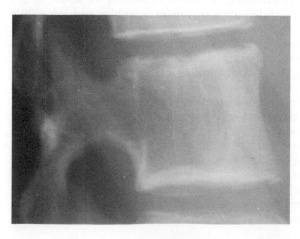

FIGURE 2 Lateral radiograph of aneurysmal bone cyst. *Source*: From Ref. 2.

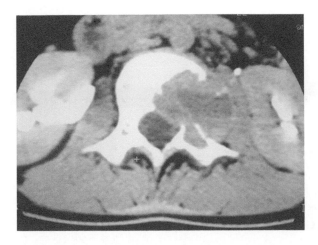

FIGURE 3 Axial computed tomography scan of aneurysmal bone cyst. *Source*: From Ref. 2.

inflammatory reactions can be dangerous and the use of histoacryl (cyanoacrylate) has been recommended for cranial or spinal ABC (4).

CONSIDERATIONS FOR PREOPERATIVE PLANNING

A thorough neurological exam should be performed prior to decisions about the type of treatment to be employed. Plain radiographs of the affected bone should be obtained. This will allow for both follow-up assessment of the response to treatment as well as correlation of findings with standard fluoroscopy. In addition, CT scanning should be performed to assess the intralesional matrix and bony architecture, with particular attention paid to areas of cortical thinning and expansion.

As mentioned before, MRI often demonstrates areas of fluid–fluid levels. Preoperative imaging not only assists with the technical aspects of the procedure but also in narrowing the differential diagnosis. In conjunction with appropriate radiographic imaging, a biopsy of the lesion should be performed to histologically confirm the diagnosis of an ABC before proceeding

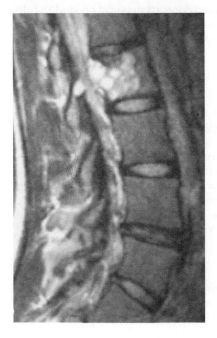

FIGURE 4 Sagittal magnetic resonance image of aneurysmal bone cyst. *Source*: From Ref. 2.

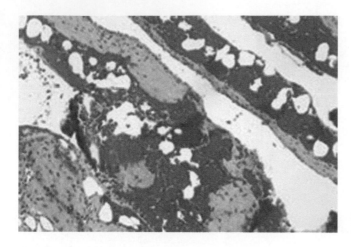

FIGURE 5 Histopathology of aneurysmal bone cyst.

with any treatment. In some cases, this is done by frozen section. In others, biopsy is preformed as an initial but separate procedure, with definitive treatment scheduled after permanent sections are reviewed.

SURGICAL TECHNIQUE

It is generally recommended that sclerotherapy be performed utilizing general anesthesia in the operating room or in the angiography suite. The technique for injection involves direct puncture of the cyst under CT or fluoroscopic guidance using a 14- to 18-gauge needle. Blood return should be noted and fluid may then be aspirated. Contrast medium is then injected into the lesion to demonstrate filling of the cyst. The volume of contrast material should be noted. If complete filling of the cyst does not occur, additional injection sites may be required. Incomplete filling may be the result of septations within the lesion. The venous drainage of the contrast material should also be assessed. It should be minimal. Without the ability to compress the venous drainage system, areas with marked venous drainage should not be injected, as this can risk embolization of the venous system (10). In areas around vital structures, histoacryl may be the sclerosing agent of choice. An amount equal to the injected contrast material needed to fully opacify the cyst should be utilized. This should be injected slowly with minimal pressure (11). Alternatively, injection with methylprednisolone acetate (80 to 125 mg) in conjunction with calcitonin (100 to 200 IU) may also be used (7,8).

COMPLICATIONS AND THEIR MANAGEMENT

Complications are generally related to the sclerosing agent that is utilized. Most complications have been reported with use of Ethibloc, although this agent is more typically used for ABCs in the extremities. Inflammatory reactions are common, although treatment of superficial (subcutaneous) lesions can lead to cutaneous fistulas. Inflammatory reactions can be managed with anti-inflammatories. While Ethibloc is still utilized in the treatment of extremity ABC, it is not recommended for use around the spine. The reports utilizing histoacryl note excellent response to the treatment occurred without major complications (4). In a review of the literature, no complications have been associated with the use of methylprednisolone or calcitonin injections, except for failure of the treatment to eliminate symptoms.

OUTCOMES

In a series of patients with lesions in the extremities and spine treated with sclerotherapy at one institution, excellent regression of the lesion (residual cyst less than 20%) was noted in 16 of the 17 cases. Complications in this series were minor and included local inflammatory reaction, small blistering, and insignificant leakage of sclerosing agent. No recurrences were noted (4). However, two of two patients with spinal lesions went on to have subsequent surgery despite radiographic regression of the lesion.

In contrast, Topouchian et al. (5) noted a high rate of complications (30%), which lead the authors to abandon this procedure at their institution. Despite this, 11 of their 15 patients had either partial or complete resolution of the lesion and did not require surgery. Three of the four patients who had cutaneous fistulas had superficial ABCs.

In the two case reports utilizing calcitonin and methylprednisolone, one patient demonstrated 95% resolution of the lucency on CT scan and a normal physical exam at follow-up (8). The other patient had resolution of the lesion noted by CT scan but had persistent pain and ultimately underwent a laminectomy for definitive treatment (7).

SUMMARY

In areas of the spine that are relatively inaccessible without instability or neurological compromise, sclerotherapy through percutaneous injection is an option to consider for ABCs. However, despite the high rate of partial or complete resolution of the lesion and low rate of reported complications, patients often go on to open surgery for more complete relief of their symptoms.

REFERENCES

1. Unni KK. Dahlin's Bone Tumors. Philadelphia, PA: Lippincott Raven Publishers, 1996.
2. Boriani S. DeIure F, Canpanacci L, et al. Aneurysmal bone cyst of the mobile spine. Spine 2001; 26(1):27–35.
3. Levesque J, Marx R, Bell RS, Wunder JS, Kandel R, White L. A Clinical Guide to Primary Bone Tumors. Baltimore, Maryland: Williams and Wilkins, 1998.
4. Dubois J, Chigot V, Grimard G, et al. Sclerotherapy in aneurysmal bone cyst in children: a review of 17 cases. Pediatr Radiol 2003; 33(6):365–372.
5. Topouchian V, Mazda K, Hamze B, et al. Aneurysmal bone cyst in children; complications of fibrosing agent injection. Radiology 2004; 232(2):522–526.
6. Peraud A, Drake M, Armstron D, et al. Fatal Ethibloc embolization of vertebrobasilar system following percutaneous injection into aneurysmal bone cyst of the second cervical vertebra. Am J Neuroradiol 2004; 25(6):1116–1120.
7. Rai AT, Collins JJ. Percutaneous treatment of pediatric aneurysmal bone cyst at c1: a minimally invasive alternative: a case report. Am J Neuroradiol 2005; 26(1):30–33.
8. Gladden ML, Gillingham BL, Hennrikus W, et al. Aneurysmal bone cyst of the first cervical vertebrae in a child treated with percutaneous intralesional injection of calcitonin and methylprednisolone. Spine 2000; 25(4):527–530.
9. Leclet H, Adamsbaum C. Interventional procedures in musculoskeletal radiology interventional techniques. Radiol Clin N Am 1998; 36(3):581–587.
10. Guibaud L, Herbreteau, Dubois J, et al. Aneurysmal bone cysts: percutaneous embolizations with an alcoholic solution of zein-series of 18 cases. Radiology 1998; 208(2):369–373.
11. deGauzy JS, Abid A, Accadbled F, et al. Percutaneous Ethibloc injection in the treatment of primary aneurysmal bone cyst. J Pediatr Orthop B 2005; 14(5):367–370.

SUMMARY

REFERENCES

35 | Spinous Process Distractive Devices for Lumbar Spinal Stenosis

Dimitriy Kondrashov, Ken Y. Hsu, and James F. Zucherman
Orthopedic Surgery, St. Mary's Spine Center, San Francisco, California, U.S.A.

INTRODUCTION

Lumbar spinal stenosis (LSS) had been first described in 1803 by Portal of France, who observed that narrowed spinal canals were associated with leg pain and atrophy (1). Our understanding of this condition was further enhanced by Verbiest, who described the anatomic changes of hypertrophic articular processes causing spinal canal stenosis (2). Subsequently, Kirkaldy-Willis described the three-joint complex and the pathologic changes found in degenerative spinal stenosis (3). Degenerative processes may start in one, two, or three joint complexes, including the disc anteriorly and the two facet joints posteriorly. With time, all three joints are involved. The degeneration of those joints also causes abnormal motion and abnormal stability, hence the term "mechanical low back pain." The abnormal motion may lead to osteophyte formation, as the body tends to stabilize the motion segment as seen elsewhere in the body [e.g., degenerative joint disease (DJD) of the hip, knee]. Ultimately the combination of disc protrusion, osteophyte formation, hypertrophy of facet joints and ligamentum flavum result in spinal stenosis, due to the lack of neural element space.

Approximately 1.2 million people in the United States have symptoms related to lumbar spinal stenosis and it is the leading preoperative diagnosis for adults older than 65 years who undergo spine surgery (4). The incidence of degenerative lumbar stenosis ranges from 1.7% to 8%. There does not appear to be gender predominance; however, degenerative spondylolisthesis associated with lumbar spinal stenosis is four times more common among women. Symptoms typically develop in the fifth or sixth decade of life in association with osteoarthritic changes in the lumbar spine. In 1996, almost 90,000 surgeries were performed for LSS (4). Symptoms are exacerbated by the upright posture and walking and include unilateral or bilateral radicular pain, sensory changes, leg muscle weakness and, more rarely, bowel and bladder dysfunction. Symptoms are typically improved or relieved with flexion of the lumbar spine, which increases the cross-sectional diameter of the spinal canal and neuroforamina.

Surgical decompression with or without fusion is the standard surgical treatment for the patients with significant LSS. While offering the potential to improve the quality of life for patients, it also has the potential for significant complications, especially when a fusion is performed. Postoperative complications may include the cardiovascular and pulmonary complications of general anesthesia, infection, iatrogenic instability, pseudarthrosis, hardware failure and the need for future surgery due to the development of disease at adjacent levels. A meta-analysis of the literature of spinal stenosis surgery by Turner et al. in 1992 showed the following complication rates for lumbar decompressive surgery: perioperative mortality (0.32%), dural tears (5.91%), deep infection (1.08%), superficial infection (2.3%), deep vein thrombosis (2.78%), and any complication (12.64%) (5).

Spacers placed between the lumbar spinous processes represent a promising surgical treatment alternative for a variety of spinal pathologies. Intuitively, they provide an unloading distractive force to the stenotic motion segment and have the potential to relieve the symptoms of neurogenic intermittent claudication (NIC) associated with spinal stenosis. The first-generation implant for nonrigid stabilization of lumbar spine was developed in 1986. It included a titanium interspinous blocker and an artificial Dacron ligament. The implant constituted "a floating system" without bony fixation to prevent any loosening. It achieved an increase in the rigidity of destabilized segments beyond normal values. Reportedly, those early implants were efficacious against low back pain (LBP) because of degenerative instability and free of major complications (6).

The second-generation implant was made of polyetheretherketone (PEEK) and named the Wallis implant. The proposed indications were: (*i*) following a discectomy for massive herniated nucleus pulposus (HNP) leading to substantial loss of disc material, (*ii*) following a second discectomy for a recurrent HNP, (*iii*) following a discectomy for herniation of a transitional disc with sacralized L5, (*iv*) disc degeneration next to a fusion, and (*v*) isolated Modic I lesion associated with chronic LBP (6). Those indications were mostly anecdotal and clinical trials are currently underway in Europe to determine its efficacy. Several other interspinous process decompression (IPD) devices have appeared in Europe and South America in the 1990s: Diam (Medtronic), Interspinous "U" (Fixano), X STOP (St. Francis Medical Technologies Inc., Alameda, California, U.S.A.) and Dynafix (GMReis) (Fig. 1). In general, there has been a paucity of peer-reviewed literature regarding those devices and the reported success as well as the indications for their use was predominantly anec-dotal. Some of those implants have been placed in the interspinous space to improve clinical out-comes following a primary surgical procedure, such as a microdiscectomy. Mariottini et al. from Italy have reported on 43 patients with lower extremity pain with back pain, treated by microsur-gical nerve root decompression and implantation of a soft intervertebral prosthesis (Diam) (7). Satisfying results were reported in 97% of cases at one- to five-year follow-up and the authors have concluded that the device was a reliable tool for curing LBP and sciatica. The study however lacks control subjects and it is unclear what the contribution of decompression relative to Diam is toward the symptomatic relief. With an increasing variety of these spacers being implanted, several varia-tions in the surgical technique to insert them have evolved. Some spacers require either the supra-spinous ligament or interspinous ligament to be significantly altered or removed before they can be inserted, and some spacers require the spinous processes themselves to be either modified or shaped. Several spacers are designed to function as stand alone devices while others incorporate an artificial ligament as an integral part of the design. The artificial ligament helps to maintain function that would otherwise be lost by sacrificing the ligaments, and it may also decrease the laxity of the motion segment, which could be an important component in treating certain patholo-gies such as degenerative disc disease. Placing the implant in the L5/S1 space represents a particu-lar challenge since the spinous process of the sacrum may not be prominent enough to support some spacers or to secure an artificial ligament. Variations in some of the current implant designs may therefore be necessary to address this level. Since the overwhelming majority of the LSS patients are elderly and are at high risk for osteoporosis, shaping the spinous processes or any bone removal reduces the bone strength and, in general, is best avoided in IPD procedures.

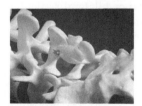

 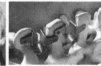

Fixano

DIAM

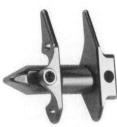 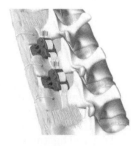

X STOP   Wallis

FIGURE 1 Modern interspinous devices.

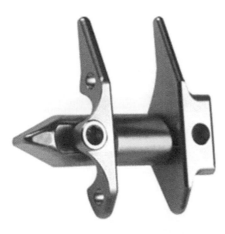

FIGURE 2 The X STOP device is available in both titanium and PEEK forms.

The first IPD device to be used in the United States for the treatment of patients with spinal stenosis was the X STOP device (Fig. 2), which is approved by the Food and Drug Administration (FDA). The X STOP (St. Francis Medical Technologies Inc., Alameda, California, U.S.A.) was developed specifically with the requirements of NIC patients in mind. We will describe in this chapter patient selection, current treatment options, the technique for performing IPD with the X STOP, as well as outcomes from clinical studies.

X STOP DESIGN RATIONALE

The X STOP was developed to fill the large void of treatment options between the safer, yet less effective conservative care, and the riskier, but more effective surgical decompression. The X STOP was designed specifically to limit the terminal extension movement at only the individual level(s) that provokes symptoms, while allowing unrestricted movement in all the other motion axes of the treated as well as untreated level(s). Because the implant was designed to be placed without removing any bony or soft tissues, the technique is minimally invasive and is usually performed with the patient under local anesthesia.

Several key design features allow for the straightforward implantation of the X STOP. The oval spacer separates the spinous processes and limits extension at the implanted level. The oval spacer helps distribute the load along the generally concave shape of the spinous processes and, by eliminating any sharp edges, reduces the likelihood of damaging the bone. The two lateral wings prevent migration anteriorly or laterally, and the supraspinous ligament, as well as the concave space between the spinous processes, prevents the implant from migrating posteriorly. The tapered tissue expander facilitates lateral insertion, allowing the supraspinous ligament to be preserved. Biomechanical studies have shown that the X STOP significantly prevents narrowing of the spinal canal and neural foramina, limits extension, and reduces intradiscal pressure and facet loading (8–10). In a magnetic resonance imaging (MRI) cadaver study, Richards et al. (8) reported that the X STOP increases the neural foramina area by 26% and the spinal canal area by 18% during extension (Fig. 3). In addition, foraminal width was increased by 41% and subarticular diameter by 50% in extension (8). In a kinematics cadaver study, terminal extension at the implant level was reduced by 62% following X STOP placement, while lateral bending and axial rotation range of motion were unchanged. In a cadaveric disc pressure study, Swanson et al. reported that the pressures in the posterior annulus and nucleus pulposus were reduced by 63% and 41% respectively during extension, and by 38% and 20% respectively in the neutral, standing position (Fig. 4) (9). Finally, Wiseman et al. performed a cadaveric facet loading study and reported that the mean facet force during extension decreased by 68% during extension (10). In each of those studies, the adjacent level measurements were not significantly changed from the intact specimen state. These preclinical studies indicate that the X STOP increases spinal canal and neural foramina space and also produces significant unloading of the disc and facets.

The requirement to maintain proper sagittal alignment and balance in patients receiving spinal implants is well understood. Lumbar fusion procedures that cause a flat back will

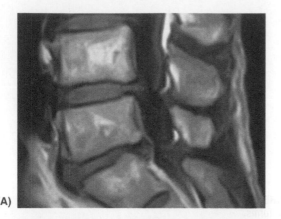

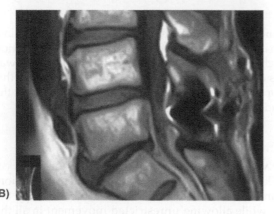

FIGURE 3 The increase in the neuroforaminal and the spinal canal area following rhe X STOP implantation. (**A**) Preoperative MRI of a patient with moderate spinal stenosis at L4–5 and retrolysthesis at L5–S1. (**B**) Postoperative MRI of the same patient s/p X STOP insertion at L4–5. The claudication symptoms have resolved.

overwhelmingly result in unacceptable clinical outcomes. Interspinous spacers are not fusion devices, but given their location posterior to the vertebral body and the axis of rotation, their possible impact on sagittal alignment is potentially significant. Three different radiological studies were therefore undertaken to measure any possible effect of the X STOP on sagittal

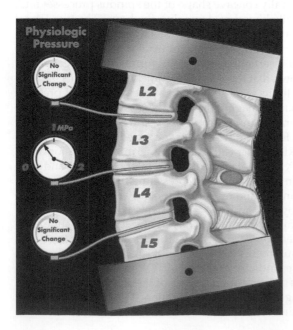

FIGURE 4 After the X STOP implantation into the cadaveric spines, the pressures in the posterior annulus and nucleus pulposus were reduced by 63% and 41%, respectively, during extension, and by 38% and 20%, respectively, in the neutral, standing position.

alignment. In the U.S. study, X-rays were taken at each follow-up visit for both X STOP and control patients and measurements were made of the lumbosacral angle (L1 to S1) and the intervertebral angle. At two-year follow-up, there were no significant differences in the mean scores between the two groups of patients (11). In the second study, preoperative X-rays from a subset of X STOP patients were digitally analyzed by digital metrics and compared to the standing films taken at two-year follow-up. In 23 patients with single level implants, the change in the intervertebral angle was only 0.5° (±2.0°) and the change in the lumbosacral angle was 0.1° (±3.8°). Similar values were recorded for 18 patients with double level implants. Interim data from an ongoing study by Dr. Douglas Wardlaw at the University of Aberdeen in Scotland have been recently presented, in which standing flexion/extension preoperative images were compared to postoperative images obtained in a positional MRI scanner. In addition to confirming in vivo the increases in the area of the foramen and canal that were measured in the preclinical in vitro cadaver study, results of this study confirm a change in angulation for both the lumbosacral angle and intervertebral angle of between 1° and 2°. These three studies confirm that the X STOP results in only minimal changes to sagittal alignment and this may be attributed at least in part to preserving the supraspinous ligament. This ligament is a substantial structure and its presence and the preservation of its original osseous insertion help prevent overdistraction of the segment. Its importance has been highlighted by several recent studies. The ultimate load and tensile strength of the interspinous/supraspinous ligament complex are 203 N and 1.2 Mpa, respectively (12). In another biomechanical study, the supraspinous/interspinous ligament complex was the largest contributor to resisting applied flexion moments in the porcine lumbar spine (13).

INDICATIONS

The ideal patient for the X STOP implantation has predominantly lower extremity complaints with or without LBP secondary to lumbar spinal stenosis at one or two levels. The clinical diagnosis of spinal stenosis should be confirmed with either MRI or computed tomography (CT) scan with or without a myelogram. The symptoms must be relieved with flexion. AS sitting places the lumbar spine in relative flexion, patients should be able to sit for about an hour without the pain. X STOP would be particularly indicated for the patients unable to undergo general anesthesia. The X STOP in its current design appears to be suitable for implantation at the L5/S1 levels in most patients, although in the clinical study conducted in the United States, patients with symptomatic stenosis at L5/S1 were excluded. In Europe, the X STOP is being successfully implanted at the L5/S1 level. Approximately one-third of patients in the United States have received implants at two levels, while triple levels procedures were not allowed in the U.S. study. As with L5/S1 procedures, triple level procedures are performed in Europe, but infrequently. Based on experience gained from more than 3000 X STOP procedures that have been performed worldwide, there appears to be a considerable amount of overlap in patients indicated for surgical decompression and patients indicated for the X STOP.

Patients with previous spinal surgery at the stenotic level are relatively contraindicated for the IPD. Theoretically those patients who have had prior microdiscectomy still have intact interspionous ligament and spinous processes and might me considered for the procedure. Grade 1 degenerative spondylolisthesis is not a contraindication for the X STOP. Patients with isthmic spondylolisthesis, however, are contraindicated. The presence of osteoporosis is not a contraindication. The presence of severe osteoporosis, as evidenced by a history of fragility fractures, may indicate insufficient bone quality to support the spacer and is a contraindication. Patients with grade 2 or higher degenerative spondylolysthesis, lateral lysthesis, or lumbar/thoracolumbar scoliosis with a Cobb angle greater than 25° are relatively contraindicated for the X STOP. Cauda equina syndrome is an absolute contraindication as these patients require emergent comprehensive surgical decompression.

SURGICAL TECHNIQUE

The patient is placed on a radiolucent table in a right lateral decubitus position and may be slightly sedated (Fig. 5). No general anesthesia is used. While patients can be treated in the prone position,

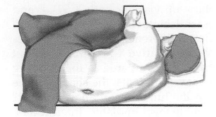

FIGURE 5 The patient is placed on a radiolucent table in a right lateral decubitus position and a midline 4 cm incision is made over the spinous processes of the stenotic level(s).

this may prevent them from completely flexing their spines during the procedure and could result in a less than optimal amount of distraction and an implant that is too small. The level to be treated is identified by fluoroscopy. After administration of a local anesthetic, a mid-sagittal incision of approximately 4 cm is made over the spinous processes of the stenotic level(s). This is carried down to the fascia which is split longitudinally 2 cm to the right and to the left of midline. It is of paramount importance to keep the supraspinous ligament intact. The paraspinal musculature is then elevated off the spinous processes and medial lamina bilaterally in the subperiosteal fashion using electrocautery and a Cobb elevator. Occasionally hypertrophied facets that block access to the interspinous space are partially trimmed with a rongeur to enable proper anterior placement of the implant. The spinal canal is not violated and neither laminotomy, nor laminectomy, nor foraminotomy is performed. Removal of any portion of the ligamentum flavum is unnecessary. A small curved dilator is inserted across the interspinous space abutting the posterior border of the facet joints at the most anterior margin of the interspinous space. After the correct level is verified by fluoroscopy, the small dilator is removed and a larger curved dilator is inserted (Fig. 6). The interspinous and supraspinous ligaments are left fully intact. After the larger dilator is removed, the sizing distractor is inserted. During the procedure, patients are able to assist by bringing their knees up against their chest and opening the interspinous space, which is distracted until the supraspinous ligament becomes taught. The correct implant size is indicated on the sizing instrument. The appropriately sized X STOP device is inserted between the spinous processes until being flushed to the right side of the spinous processes (Fig. 7). The screw hole for the universal wing on the left side is visualized and the universal wing screw is engaged (Fig. 8). The two wings are approximated towards the midline and the left sided universal wing screw is secured with a torque-limiting hexagonal screwdriver (Fig. 9). Anteroposterior (AP) and lateral fluoroscopy views are taken to verify the proper position. The incision is closed in the usual fashion. The drain is not routinely utilized. The use of a postoperative brace is unnecessary. The procedure is typically performed in less than an hour, and patients are discharged from the hospital within 24 hours.

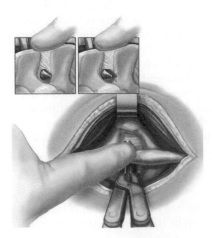

FIGURE 6 The interspinous space is sequentially dilated. The interspinous and supraspinous ligaments are left fully intact.

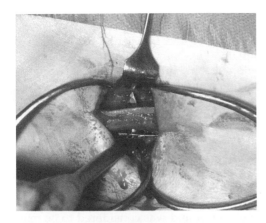

FIGURE 7 The appropriately sized X STOP device is inserted between the spinous processes until being flush with the right side of the spinous processes.

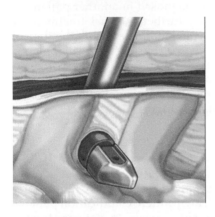

FIGURE 8 The screw hole for the universal wing on the left side is visualized and the universal wing screw is engaged.

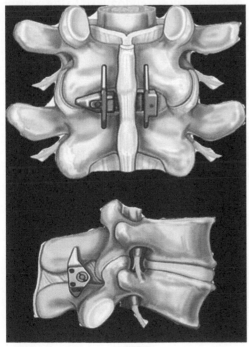

X STOP

FIGURE 9 The implanted X STOP device. Note the preservation of the supra-/ interspinous ligament complex.

COMPLICATIONS

Reported complications related to the IPD have been minor and transient. No procedures were converted to laminectomy during X STOP implantation. Four percent (4 out of 100) of the X STOP patients in the U.S. clinical study developed some minor operative site-related complications: one wound dehiscence, one seroma, one hematoma, and one report of incisional pain (11,14). There have been no reports of either vascular or neurological complications, which is anticipated since the laminae are left intact and the spinal canal and neuoforamina are not entered. Four percent (4 out of 100) of the patients developed device-related complications. One X STOP patient fell, causing the implant to dislodge, which was removed without any sequelae. A review of the patient's radiographs showed a very prominent facet that prevented the implant from being positioned properly. In retrospect, it could have been trimmed to allow more anterior placement of the X STOP. One patient reported worsening pain about one year after the procedure, which was determined to be possibly related to the implant. One implant was placed too posterior and was considered to be malpositioned. An asymptomatic spinous process fracture was diagnosed in another patient on routine six-month follow-up radiographs. This required no further medical treatment or surgical intervention and the patient's stenosis symptoms were eliminated from the time of the procedure onward despite the fracture. While unlikely, it is possible to fracture the spinous process during the surgical procedure, either by applying too much force to the sizing distractor, or by applying too much lateral force against the spinous process while attempting to insert the implant. Fracturing the spinous process would require the patient to be converted to laminectomy as the X STOP design completely relies on the support of the intact cephalad and caudad spinous processes.

X STOP OUTCOMES

A multicenter prospective, randomized controlled trial was performed in the United States comparing the outcomes of mild with moderate neurogenic intermittent claudication patients treated with the X STOP interspinous process decompression system to patients treated nonsurgically (11,14). There were 191 patients treated at nine centers. Eligible patients were randomized to either the X STOP group or the control group. Those randomized to the control group received at least one epidural steroid injection and had the option to receive nonsteroidal anti-inflammatory drugs (NSAIDs), analgesics, and physical therapy and additional injections as needed. Assessments were based on the Zurich Claudication Questionnaire (ZCQ), a validated, patient-completed outcomes measure specific to neurogenic claudication (15,16), as well as the SF-36.

   One hundred patients received the X STOP and 91 patients were treated nonoperatively. A total of 136 levels were implanted in 100 patients: 64 single levels and 36 double levels. One-level procedures took an average of 51 minutes and two-level—58 minutes. Blood loss was negligible: 40 ml for one-level procedures and 58 ml for two-level procedures. The most common level implanted was L4–L5 (89/136) and the second most common level was L3–L4 (43/136). The most common implant size was 12 mm. There were five X STOP sizes available during the trial, ranging from 6 mm to 14 mm. The procedure was performed under local anesthesia in 97 patients and under general in three patients. The length of stay was, on the average, less than 24 hours.

   At two-year follow-up, data from 93 of the 100 X STOP patients and 81 of the 91 control patients were available for analysis. The X STOP group had a significantly greater percentage of patients with an improvement in symptom severity domain of ZCQ than did the control group at each post-treatment visit. At two-year follow-up, 60% of the patients reported a clinically significant reduction in the severity of symptoms compared to the 18% of the controls. The X STOP group also had a significantly greater percentage of patients with an improvement in physical function domain of ZCQ than did the control group at each post-treatment visit. At the 24-month evaluation, 57% of the patients reported a clinically significant improvement in their physical function compared to 15% of the controls. At two-year follow-up, 73% of the patients were at least "somewhat satisfied" compared with 36% of the controls.

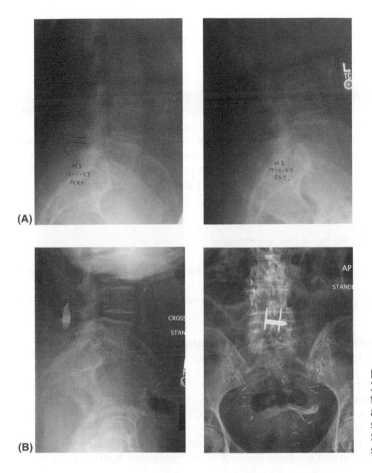

(A)

(B)

FIGURE 10 A case example from the X STOP pilot study with seven-year follow-up. (**A**) Preoperative X-rays of an 80-year-old patient with moderate spinal stenosis. (**B**) Seven years s/p X STOP implantation patient remains symtom-free.

Results of the SF-36 scores showed no significant differences in the pretreatment enrollment scores between the X STOP and control groups for any SF-36 domain. At all follow-up time points, the X STOP group scored significantly better than the control group in every physical domain.

It is not easy to interpret X STOP clinical results in the context of published outcomes of surgical treatment for stenosis, given the generally poor quality of that literature. To date, no randomized, prospective, multi-center study has been performed for either conservative treatment or a decompressive surgery in the treatment of LSS. The X STOP was clearly superior to nonoperative therapy in the randomized study conducted in the U.S. study, but it does not allow a direct comparison between the X STOP and laminectomy to be made.

During the course of the U.S. study, 24 patients in the control group underwent decompressive laminectomy for the relief of their stenosis symptoms and outcomes are available for 22 patients. At a mean follow-up time of 12.8 months outcomes for these patients were very similar to outcomes of the X STOP patients at two-year follow-up. Sixty-four percent had clinically significant improvement in symptom severity domain of ZCQ, 68% had clinically significantly improvement in physical function domain of ZCQ, and 60% were satisfied with the outcome of their treatment.

Of interest, 39 patients with grade I degenerative spondylolisthesis were treated in the U.S. study with the X STOP and 22 patients were treated nonoperatively. Using 15-point improvement over baseline scores in the ZCQ as the criterion of clinical success, 69% of the IPD patients had a successful outcome at two-year follow-up, compared with 9% of the control patients. The mean improvement score for the 39 X STOP patients was 26 points. There were no significant differences in the mean percentage of slip between X STOP and control patients at baseline or at two-year follow-up. The X STOP represents a significantly less invasive alternative therapy for these patients, resulting in very good clinical outcomes and most importantly, and no evidence that the implant results in any instability of the motion segment.

SUMMARY

IPD is a relatively new motion-preserving spinal procedure. There is a great deal yet to be learned regarding its possible application in a variety of degenerative spinal conditions. Thus far, X STOP is the only IPD device with the class I clinical data to support its efficacy. Similar to indirect fracture reduction techniques, the IPD utilizes ligamentotaxis to indirectly increase the foraminal and canal dimensions by reconstituting tension in the posterior ligamentous structures. Compared to most other developments in the motion-preservation field, such as disc arthroplasty, the apparent advantages of IPD compared with regular decompression include the following:

- No need for general anesthesia.
- Ease of application via the familiar posterior approach.
- Ease of revision.
- No opening of the spinal canal and, therefore, a minimal risk of injury to the neural elements.
- Being able to salvage with regular procedures (laminectomy alone or laminectomy with fusion).

The concerns regarding the procedure are mostly theoretical and extrapolated from other orthopedic disciplines, such as the total joint arthroplasty. They include the following:

- Wear debris generation owing to the implant and its clinical significance (should be minor because the articulation is bone-on-metal and unlikely to generate metal debris. In addition, any generated debris would not be likely to enter the spinal canal, since the canal is not violated during the X STOP placement).
- Longevity of the implants (a relatively minor concern because the metal is the strongest in compression, which is a predominant mode of loading of the implanted X STOP).

Future Developments

- Combining IPD with some degree of laminectomy/laminotomy at the same/adjacent levels (similar to the way some other IPD devices have been utilized).
- Performing IPD adjacent to a fusion or an artificial disc.
- Performing multilevel IPD (based on encouraging preliminary European results).
- Exploring the role of IPD in modulation of discogenic LBP (based on the reduction of intradiscal pressure observed with IPD application in the laboratory) and facet syndrome (based on the reduction of facet loading demonstrated in the laboratory).
- Investigating the role of IPD in patients with severe LSS and higher-grade degenerative slips.
- Performing a clinical randomized side-by-side comparison of IPD versus laminectomy.
- Perfecting the patient selection criteria for X STOP (symptomatic relief with standardized flexion-based test).
- Elucidating the role of bone densitometry prior to implantation to potentially include the subset of patients with severe osteoporosis.

In summary, X STOP interspinous process decompression is indicated for the elderly patients with one- or two-level mild-to-moderate lumbar spinal stenosis with predominantly lower extremity complaints which are relieved in flexion or sitting. X STOP outcomes have been demonstrated to be vastly superior to nonoperative therapy in the U.S. multicenter prospective randomized trial in LSS patients with mild-to-moderate symptoms. The patients with grade I degenerative spondylolysthesis seem to do at least as well after the X STOP implantation as the patients without the instability. The X STOP clinical outcomes are comparable to the results previously reported for patients who have undergone laminectomy.

Complications of IPD are relatively minor and uncommon. Placement of the X STOP device would not significantly complicate future laminectomy and/or fusion. Being a minimally invasive procedure, IPD helps avoid the major risks of laminectomy such as the risks of general anesthesia, direct neural injury, dural tears, and iatrogenic instability. In patients with grade I degenerative spondylolysthesis who are frequently treated with fusion, IPD also prevents the risks of pedicle screw placement and pseudarthrosis. Most importantly, being a motion-sparing device, X STOP does not increase the adjacent segment stresses and does not contribute to the adjacent segment degeneration and adjacent segment disease. X STOP and possibly other interspinous decompression devices will likely be a useful adjunct to the currently available surgical armamentarium for the successful treatment of spinal stenosis.

REFERENCES

1. Wiltse LL. History of spinal disorders. In: Frymoyer JW ed. Adult Spine. New York: Raven Press, 1991:33–55.
2. Verbiest H. A radicular syndrome from developmental narrowing of the lumbar vertebral canal. J Bone Joint Surg 1954; 36B:230–237.
3. Kirkaldy-Willis WH, Wedge JH, Yong-Hing K, Reilly J. Pathology and pathogenesis of lumbar spondylosis and stenosis. Spine 1978; 3:319–328.
4. Dartmouth Medical School. Center for the Evaluative Clinical Sciences. The quality of medical care in the United States: a report on the medicare program; the Dartmouth atlas of health care 1999 ed. Chicago, IL: AHA Press, 1999.
5. Turner JA, Ersek M, Herron L, Deyo R. Surgery for lumbar spinal stenosis. Attempted meta-analysis of the literature. Spine 1992; 17:1–8.
6. Senegas J. Mechanical supplementation by non-rigid fixation in degenerative intervertebral lumbar segments: the Wallis system. Eur Spine J 2002; 11 (suppl 2):S164–S169; epub 2002 June.
7. Mariottini A, et al. Preliminary results of a soft novel lumbar intervertebral prosthesis (DIAM) in the degenerative spinal pathology. Acta Neurochir 2005; 92 (suppl):129–131.
8. Richards JC, Majumdar S, Lindsey DP, Beaupre GS, Yerby SA. The treatment mechanism of an interspinous process implant for lumbar neurogenic intermittent claudication. Spine 2005; 30: 744–749.
9. Swanson KE, Lindsey DP, Hsu KY, Zucherman JF, Yerby SA. The effects of an interspinous implant on intervertebral disc pressures. Spine 2003; 28:26–32.
10. Wiseman CM, Lindsey DP, Fredrick AD, Yerby SA. The effect of an interspinous process implant on facet loading during extension. Spine 2005; 30:903–907.
11. Zucherman JF, et al. A multi-center, prospective, randomized trial evaluating the X STOP interspinous process decompression system for the treatment of neurogenic intermittent claudication. Spine 2005; 30:1351–1358.
12. Iida T, et al. Effects of aging and spinal degeneration on mechanical properties of lumbar supraspinous and interspinous ligaments. Spine 2002; 2(2):95–100.
13. Gillespie KA, Dickey JP. Biomechanical role of lumbar spine ligaments in flexion and extension: determination using a parallel linkage robot and a porcine model. Spine 2004; 29(11):1208–1216.
14. Zucherman JF, et al. A prospective randomized multi-center study for the treatment of lumbar spinal stenosis with the X STOP interspinous implant: 1-year results. Eur Spine J 2004; 13(1):22–31.
15. Stucki G, Daltroy L, Liang MH, Lipson SJ, Fossel AH, Katz JN. Measurement properties of a self-administered outcome measure in lumbar spinal stenosis. Spine 1996; 21:796–803.
16. Stucki G, Liang MH, Fossel AH, Katz JN. Relative responsiveness of condition-specific and generic health status measures in degenerative lumbar spinal stenosis. J Clin Epidemiol 1995; 48:1369–1378.
17. Atlas SJ, Keller RB, Robson D, Deyo RA, Singer DE. Surgical and nonsurgical management of lumbar spinal stenosis: four-year outcomes from the Maine lumbar spine study. Spine 2000; 25:556–562.
18. Cuckler JM, Bernini PA, Wiesel SW, Booth RE, Jr., Rothman RH, Pickens GT. The use of epidural steroids in the treatment of lumbar radicular pain. A prospective, randomized, double-blind study. J Bone Joint Surg Am 1985; 67:63–66.
19. Simotas AC. Nonoperative treatment for lumbar spinal stenosis. Clin Orthop 2001; 384:153–161.
20. Simotas AC, Dorey FJ, Hansraj KK, Cammisa F Jr. Nonoperative treatment for lumbar spinal stenosis. Clinical and outcome results and a 3-year survivorship analysis. Spine 2000; 25:197–203, discussions 4.
21. Gunzburg R, Keller TS, Szpalski M, Vandeputte K, Spratt KF. Clinical and psychofunctional measures of conservative decompression surgery for lumbar spinal stenosis: a prospective cohort study. Eur Spine J 2003; 12:197–204.
22. Katz JN, Stucki G, Lipson SJ, Fossel AH, Grobler LJ, Weinstein JN. Predictors of surgical outcome in degenerative lumbar spinal stenosis. Spine 1999; 24:2229–2233.
23. Benz RJ, Ibrahim ZG, Afshar P, Garfin SR. Predicting complications in elderly patients undergoing lumbar decompression. Clin Orthop 2001; 384:116–121.

24. Iguchi T, Kurihara A, Nakayama J, Sato K, Kurosaka M, Yamasaki K. Minimum 10-year outcome of decompressive laminectomy for degenerative lumbar spinal stenosis. Spine 2000; 25:1754–1759.
25. Khoo LT, Fessler RG. Microendoscopic decompressive laminotomy for the treatment of lumbar stenosis. Neurosurgery 2002; 51:146–154.
26. Postacchini F, Cinotti G, Perugia D, Gumina S. The surgical treatment of central lumbar stenosis. Multiple laminotomy compared with total laminectomy. J Bone Joint Surg Br 1993; 75:386–392.
27. Reindl R, Steffen T, Cohen L, Aebi M. Elective lumbar spinal decompression in the elderly: is it a high-risk operation? Can J Surg 2003; 46:43–46.

36 | Minimally Invasive Total Disc Replacement and Facet Joint Replacement

D. Greg Anderson and Chadi Tannoury
Department of Orthopedic Surgery, Thomas Jefferson University, Philadelphia, Pennsylvania, U.S.A.

INTRODUCTION

Low back pain is a very common condition affecting more than 80% of the population during the course of their lives. Fortunately, in most cases, symptom resolution is achieved with conservative management (1–3). The small percentage of patients continuing to experience chronic, disabling low back symptoms presents a challenge to modern medical systems. Experts often fail to agree on the exact cause or the best treatment for patients with severe degenerative low back pain, making the development of a well-accepted treatment algorithm difficult.

Low back pain surgery is performed most commonly at this time for symptoms related to degenerative disc disease. Patient selection for this type of surgery is critical to a successful clinical outcome and should include only motivated patients with localized disease (one or two spinal segments). Patients with psychological problems or secondary gain are generally poor candidates for surgery (4,5). The use of spinal surgery for patients with axial low back pain due to degenerative disease of the posterior element pathologies (i.e., zygapophseal joints) is not well-studied, but is thought to be a valid treatment option by some (6). Despite good patient selection, the published results of surgery for low back pain are generally less satisfactory than surgery for radicular symptoms. Among the reasons quoted for suboptimal results following spinal surgery for low back pain are poor patient selection, failure to understand the cause of the patient's symptoms and iatrogenic muscle, and soft-tissue injury from the surgical approach (7,8). In an attempt to decrease the morbidity of surgery, surgeons have developed less invasive treatment strategies for spinal pathology in recent years.

Although spinal arthrodesis has been the gold standard for surgical treatment of symptomatic degenerative disc disease for many years, the limitations of spinal fusion are well-known (9). Fusion leaves the motion segment in a nonphysiologic motionless state and may predispose to adjacent segment degeneration (10,11). In an effort to overcome the limitations of spinal fusion, motion-sparing surgical treatments have been designed and are in various stages of development. Although many of the motion-sparing solutions are not yet approved for use in the United States, enthusiasts predict that in time, motion-sparing spinal procedures will replace many of the fusion procedures that are currently performed. The spectrum of motion-sparing technology in development includes nucleus replacement, artificial disc replacement, posterior motion sparing implants, and facet joint replacement.

Generally speaking, motion sparing spinal implants have the potential to maintain quasi-physiologic spinal motion. It is hoped that the use of motion-sparing surgery rather than spinal fusion may reduce the incidence of adjacent segment degeneration, although none of the motion-sparing implants have enough follow-up data to support this hypothesis. It is the goal of this chapter to discuss how minimally invasive surgical techniques might be applied to the field of motion-sparing technology within the lumbar region of the spine.

MINIMALLY INVASIVE SPINAL SURGERY

Minimally invasive spinal surgery (MISS) is a family of surgical techniques that are aimed at reducing the iatrogenic damage to the soft tissues surrounding the spine during spinal surgery. The general principle of MISS is to work through smaller surgical incisions, using techniques to reduce muscle and soft-tissue injury when compared with traditional approaches to a particular spinal problem. To achieve these goals, special retractors, lighting systems, and magnification are often required. The theoretical benefits of a less invasive surgical approach include less postoperative pain, less blood loss, earlier recovery, and shorter hospital stay (12). Also, patients are generally more pleased with the cosmetic appearance of the incision following minimally invasive surgery compared with traditional surgery. The development of MISS began in the 1960s to 1970s with the advent of microdiscectomy for the treatment of herniated disc disease (13,14). Since that time, tubular retractor systems, fiberoptic lighting technology, spinal imaging, image guidance, and modern operative microscopes have become more readily available and have allowed progressively more sophisticated surgery to be performed through a less invasive approach.

Minimally invasive approaches have been described for all regions of the spine and essentially all categories of spinal pathology. However, the field of MISS is still in its infancy as only a fraction of the spine procedures performed worldwide use some form of MISS. Motion-sparing spinal technology is also in a relatively early state of development, with limited or no clinical experience available for many of the proposed motion-sparing implants. Therefore, only sparse data are currently available in the published literature combining minimally invasive surgical techniques for the implantation of motion-sparing spinal implants. However, there is a clear theoretical benefit in combining these two developing areas to achieve better clinical outcomes for patients with symptomatic lumbar spinal problems. In this chapter, we focus on three primary approaches that appear useful for motion-sparing implants including the anterior mini-open retroperitoneal approach, direct lateral approach, and Wiltse paramedian posterior approach. The current generation of motion-sparing implants appears to be amenable to the use one of these three approaches. As surgeons adopts minimally invasive techniques into their practice, it is important to be well-versed on these three "work-horse" approaches to the spine.

INDICATIONS AND LIMITATIONS

The exact indications for minimally invasive surgical approaches to lumbar spinal problems are still being defined. In general, patients are considered candidates for a less invasive surgical approach when the spinal condition is localized to a small region of the spine and the surgeon is familiar with the specific minimally invasive technique. Most minimally invasive techniques are more difficult in obese patients and those with prior spinal surgery. There is a well-defined learning curve to most minimally invasive techniques and thus the surgeon should begin with simple cases before tackling difficult procedures with a minimally invasive approach. In contrast, the indications for motion-sparing techniques are highly dependent on the specific technique and are still being defined in many cases. The best-studied motion-sparing technology to date has been artificial disc replacement.

Artificial Disc Replacement

Currently (2005), only one artificial disc prosthesis has received clearance from the U.S. Food and Drug Administration (FDA). It is indicated for severely symptomatic single-level degenerative disc disease at the L4–5 or L5–S1 segment. Contraindications for this implant include the presence of significant spinal canal pathology (e.g., stenosis), spinal instability (15–20), a history of prior spinal infection (21), significant osteoporosis/osteopenia (15,16,18,22,23), or symptomatic facet arthrosis (15–20,22–24). Also, patients with previous abdominal and/or retroperitoneal surgery are likely to be poor candidates for surgery due to the presence of adhesions in the retroperitoneal space that may prevent safe access to the anterior region of the spine (20).

The mini-open retroperitoneal approach is currently the most common approach used for implantation of artificial disc prostheses. This approach fulfills the goals of a minimally invasive approach because the muscle and soft-tissue injury related to this approach is generally minimal. Although this approach is simple to perform in theory, complications such as great vessel injury and vascular thrombosis are possible and therefore significant experience with retroperitoneal surgery is advisable when performing this approach for artificial disc replacement. At most U.S. centers, specialized exposure surgeons with experience in retroperitoneal vascular procedures perform the mini-retroperitoneal approaches when disc replacement surgery is being undertaken.

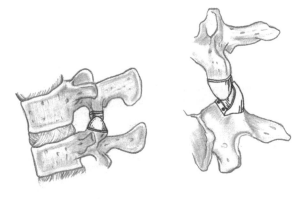

FIGURE 1 Schematic illustration of the artificial facet joints.

Posterior Motion-Sparing Procedures

The indications for posterior motion-sparing procedures including, pedicle-based tethers, interspinous process spacers, and facet joint replacement are not yet defined (Fig. 1). Posterior column pain generators such as the zygapophyseal facet joint have been more difficult to assess in the clinical setting. Facet joint injections with local anesthetic and/or steroid agents, as well as medial branch blocks have been used to diagnose and treat zygapophyseal joint pain. However, some studies suggest that these modalities are not reliable when defining the indications for surgical treatment (25,26).

Although the current indications for posterior motion-sparing techniques remains to be defined, it is in the posterior column of the lumbar spine that minimally invasive techniques might have their greatest utility. Tubular retractor access to the posterior spinal elements including the facet joint and spinal canal are well-established techniques that are already used in the field of spinal surgery. It seems that these approaches could easily be adapted to the implantation of posterior column minimally invasive implants if indeed these implants show adequate promise in the future.

Other technologies such as nucleus replacement and disc regeneration through tissue engineering are in development and appear to be ideally suited for a minimally invasive approach. Using either a lateral transpsoas portal or a posterolateral portal (outside the spinal canal), the disc can be accessed with minimal approach-related morbidity. Much additional work, however, remains to define the utility of these approaches before widespread clinical acceptance can occur.

PATIENT EVALUATION AND PHYSICAL EXAMINATION

The clinical evaluation must begin with a thorough history and physical examination of the patient. In addition to the general characteristics of the patient's symptoms and their prior medical history, the spinal surgeon must focus on a number of key points when considering a patient for surgery.

With artificial disc replacement, the surgeon should rule out a prior history of spinal infection or a prior retroperitoneal abdominal surgery. During the physical examination, the surgeon should evaluate the degree of obesity in the lower abdominal region and search for scars, which may indicate prior wounds or procedures that would impact the ability to achieve a safe anterior mini-retroperitoneal approach.

Preparation of the patient must include a frank discussion of the nature, risk, and benefits of the proposed operation. In addition, the patient should understand the symptoms that might respond to surgery and those that are unlikely to improve despite a technically successful surgery. The surgeon should also search for signs of psychological barriers that will impact the patient's ability to improve following surgery. Other preoperative issues to be explored include the use of narcotic pain medications or tobacco products. It has been our experience that patients generally do poorly if not weaned from narcotics medication prior to surgery and if they are not willing to quit smoking. Pending legal action or workman's compensation claims may decrease the odds of a clinically successful result from surgery. Optimal surgical candidates are highly motivated, well-educated, and take an active role in their recovery process (27,28).

PREOPERATIVE IMAGING

All patients should undergo imaging with plain radiographs to define the spinal alignment, disc space narrowing, and general bone quality. In addition, we use dynamic flexion/extension radiographs to define the degree of instability present over the spinal segments. Advanced imaging such as magnetic resonance imaging (MRI) and/or computed tomography (CT) myelography should be reviewed in all patients prior to surgery. CT myelography is usually obtained if a patient is unable to undergo an MRI or if additional information is required regarding the spinal canal or posterior elements.

When considering artificial disc surgery, the degree of disc collapse should be assessed along with the general quality of the bone. In cases where the bone quality is indeterminate, a DEXA study should be reviewed to rule out osteopenia, which might cause subsidence or dislodgement of the implant. The status of the facet joints should be evaluated on advance imaging studies to rule out significant facet arthrosis. Patients with advanced facet arthrosis may be better candidates for spinal fusion as opposed to an artificial disc procedure. Compression of the neural elements or spinal stenosis should also be ruled out. Although some disc protrusions may be addressed at the time of anterior discectomy prior to implantation of disc prosthesis, canal stenosis or sequestered disc fragments are not reliably addressed during a disc replacement procedure.

The surgeon should also evaluate the status of the surrounding lumbar discs on MRI. Severe disc space narrowing or endplate changes (Modic type 1 changes) indicate significant degeneration and may or may not be associated with lumbar symptoms. Discography may be used to elicit pain from the lumber discs. Although controversial, many surgeons believe that properly performed discography is useful to define the symptomatic level as a pain generator and to rule out pain at adjacent segments. Discography can also be helpful in defining patients who are poor candidates for surgical intervention on the basis of severe multilevel pain or a nonorganic response to the procedure.

In some cases, the vascular pattern (i.e., bifurcation of the aorta and vena cava) or the presence of vascular abnormalities can be defined on preoperative MRI. If significant concerns exist over the vascular anatomy in a particular case, arteriography or MR angiography may be useful. In revision anterior cases, placements of vascular and ureteral stents may be useful in identifying and protecting the major vessels and ureter during surgery.

Intraoperative imaging with a C-arm fluoroscopy unit is crucial to confirm correct placement of a disc replacement prostheses. We also find it useful to use the C-arm unit to define the optimal location of surgical incision prior to commencing the operation. By localizing the incisions directly over the surgical pathology, it is much easier to work efficiently through a small incision without compromising visualization. Although not widely used at the current time, imaging guidance technology may become more popular in the future to assist in alignment of disc replacement implants.

SURGICAL TECHNOLOGY FOR MINIMALLY INVASIVE MOTION-SPARING SURGERY

A variety of advancements have promoted the development of MISS. As a surgeon, it is useful to be familiar with the spectrum of technology that is used in MISS, although individual surgeon preferences differ according to the specific technologies employed. Some of the primary types of equipments that should be in the surgeons' armamentarium include the operative microscope, endoscopes, fiberoptic illumination systems, tubular retractors, and good quality portable fluoroscopy unit or image guidance equipment.

Patient Positioning, Spinal Access, and Operative Approach for Motion-Sparing Spinal Implants

The positioning and approach are dependent on the type of motion-sparing procedure that is being performed. In general, we prefer to use the Jackson table, because it is radiolucent and

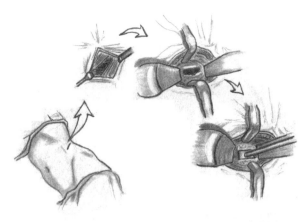

FIGURE 2 Schematic illustration of the mini-open lateral approach to the lumbar spine.

facilitates introperative imaging. In addition, the Jackson table facilitates safe positioning of most patients avoiding pressure in critical areas and can be used to reposition from supine to prone during the course of the surgery when needed.

Prior to the sterile preparation, the surgeon should ensure that the fluoroscopy unit can image the region of spine necessary for the planned procedure. The ideal location for the skin incision should also be marked at this time.

The operative approach depends on the procedure being performed. At the current time, most artificial disc surgery is performed through a mini-open retroperitoneal approach. The direct lateral approach is well suited to expose the L2–3, L3–4, and/or L4–5 levels and has been successfully used to perform nucleus pulposus replacement surgery (Fig. 2). Some are considering this approach for disc replacement surgery for the future, although the current generation of implants does not appear to be optimized for a direct lateral implantation.

In the posterior spine, the primary minimally invasive approach is the modified Wiltse paramedian approach. This approach provides excellent access to the spinal canal, posterolateral disc, facet joint, and intertransverse region of the spine. Specialized tubular retractor systems have improved spinal access via the Wiltse paramedian approach and are currently the standard for MISS in this area.

Specialized Spinal Minimally Invasive Spinal Retractors

A variety of specialized retractor systems have been designed for exposing the anterior aspect of the spine. Table-mounted frames that accommodate individual retractor blades are the most popular systems used for the anterior retroperitoneal approaches. Several manufactures provide systems with variable length blades that may be "snapped" onto the external frame and adjusted easily for optimal exposure of the anterior spine. Although first-generation artificial disc implants require bulky instruments for implantation, recent developments have improved the profile of the surgical instruments and may be used with more limited anterior incisions (Fig. 3) (19,29).

The lateral transpsoas approach may be performed with a table-mounted frame retractor system similar to the mini-open retroperitoneal approach or may be performed with expandable tubular retractors. The later approach can be performed through a smaller incision and is relatively simple to perform because no vascular mobilization is necessary to approach the disc spaces. Once the retroperitoneal space is identified, a guide wire can be inserted into the disc space. Working over the guide wire, the soft tissues of the retroperitoneal space can be opened with serial dilators, which are then "docked" to the spine. Finally, an expandable tubular retractor can be placed. By gently expanding the tubular retractor, excellent visualization of the lateral region of the disc can be achieved. During this approach, the surgeon depends on intraoperative fluoroscopy to assist with alignment of the retractor to the disc space.

In the posterior spine, tubular dilators and retractors are the standard for a limited exposure of the spine. Splitting rather than cutting the paraspinous muscles minimizes the

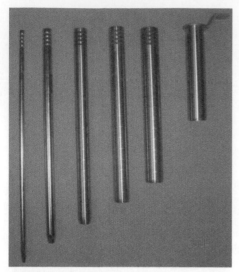

FIGURE 3 Serial tubular dilators and retractors are manufactured with variable lengths for optimal exposure of the spine.

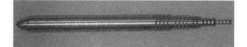

FIGURE 4 Use of sequential dilators allows serial dilation of the soft tissues and splitting of muscle fascicles rather than cutting or excising the muscle.

degree of soft-tissue injury secondary to the exposure (Fig. 4). A wide variety of tubular retractor systems are currently available, many of which can be expanded to improve the viewing area. Tubular retractors are generally secured to the operating table by an adjustable "arm" that helps to maintain the alignment and trajectory of the tubular retractor during surgery. This frees up the surgeon and assistant's hands for the operative procedure.

Perioperative Imaging/Image Guidance/Computer-Assisted Spinal Surgery

Compared with traditional open spinal surgery, minimally invasive spinal approaches are more dependent on the use of fluoroscopy. The portable C-arm fluoroscopy unit is the standard for intraoperative imaging. The type of unit is available in most operating rooms and is familiar and relatively simple to use. The surgeon must become familiar with the fluoroscopic anatomy of the spine to safely perform minimally invasive spinal techniques. Certain situation such as severe osteopenia or obesity can limit or prevent the surgeon from obtaining adequate images of the spinal anatomy on C-arm fluoroscopy. In these situations, an alternative approach (more traditional open approach with direct visualization of the spinal anatomy) may be required.

Prior to surgery, preoperative images should be carefully studied to identify the location of the spinal pathology relative to know spinal landmarks such as the pedicle. Because the minimally invasive spinal surgeon is able to visualize less of the spinal anatomy, it is important that all visual and tactile clues are used during surgery to identify relevant anatomy.

Image guidance technology, at least in theory, provides a means for the surgeon to improve the safety and efficiency of the spinal procedure by allowing real-time tracking of "virtual" surgical instruments on spinal images during the surgical procedures. Although a variety of different imaging strategies have been designed, most rely on fiducial markers attached to the spine and the surgical instruments which are "tracked" by a computer during the course of the surgery. This allows the surgeon to see the position of the instruments relative to fluoroscopic, tomographic, or reconstructed images of the spine. To identify spinal landmarks with the patient in the operative position, there is normally a step where the surgeon uses a pointer or an intraoperative image (fluoroscopy or isocentric fluoroscopy) to reference the spinal fiducials to the anatomy of the spine (30–34).

Image guidance generally lessens the need for fluoroscopy during the procedure and thus can reduce the exposure of the surgeon and surgical team to ionizing radiation (30). Image guidance also allows the surgeon to track instruments in the multiple views (anteroposterior and lateral) simultaneously, increasing the information available to the surgeon without requiring cumbersome shifts in C-arm position during the procedure.

The general adoption of image guidance technology in spinal surgery has been limited to date by the expense of the systems, complexity of the equipment, and added time necessary to perform the referencing procedure. However, as newer generations of image guidance technology become available, it is likely that the popularity and use of this technology will increase in spinal surgery.

Viewing Technologies

Precision optics and fiberoptic technology have produced excellent viewing options for limited access surgery (35,36). The specific viewing technology used is dependent on the experience and preference of the surgeon. Magnifying loops and a headlight remain a valid option for many spinal procedures, although the surgeon's focal length limits the size of the incision. Also, it is generally difficult for a surgeon and assistant to see down a small access portal simultaneously during surgery. In contrast, the operating microscope provides superior visualization of the spinal anatomy and reduces surgeon neck strain. In addition, it allows the surgeon and assistant to have equivalent views of the spine, despite the use of a small incision. The disadvantages of the operative microscope are its bulky size, as well as the relatively higher cost of the equipment, and the training required by the surgeon and staff to use the equipment properly. Endoscopy is also available and preferred by some. Endoscopy is able to visualize around corners better (use of 30° and 70° scopes) and is optimal in certain situations such as performing cervical surgery in the sitting position, where the microscope can be more difficult to use. However, depth perception with the endoscope is not as good as with the operative microscope and lens smudging remains a problem.

MINI-RETROPERITONEAL APPROACH FOR ARTIFICIAL DISC REPLACEMENT SURGERY

At the current time, the artificial disc is the primary motion-sparing technology available and approved by the FDA; although in the future it is likely that other motion-sparing options will become available. Therefore, the implantation of an artificial disc through a mini-retroperitoneal approach will be described in additional detail (37,38).

The patient is positioned in a supine position on a radiolucent table. We prefer to use an adjustable lumbar roll (a pump-style arterial line bag) in the lumbar spine, which can be adjusted during the procedure to increase or decrease the lordosis of the lumbar segments. Prior to the sterile prep, we use a C-arm to obtain a true anteroposterior view of the disc space and mark out the optimal location of the skin incision. By properly placing the incision, the need to extend the incision for exposure is eliminated. We prefer to use a pulse oximeter on the great toe of the side of the retroperitoneal approach to monitor the blood flow to the distal extremity during the procedure.

Following the sterile preparation and drape, a longitudinal incision approximately 5 to 6 cm in length is made and a mini-retroperitoneal approach is carried out (Fig. 5) We prefer to divide the linea alba between the two leaves of the rectus abdominus muscle to reduce the need to retract the rectus abdominus muscle for a true midline exposure of the spine. The preperitoneal space is identified and the peritoneal sac is bluntly swept toward the left (right retroperitoneal approach) for L5–S1 and to the right (left retroperitoneal approach for the L4–5 level). By employing the right retroperitoneal approach at the L5–S1 level, the left-sided retroperitoneal approach remains available without severe scarring should the patient require surgery at the L4–5 level in the future.

After blunt retraction of the peritoneal sac, the psoas muscle and vascular structures are identified. At the L5–S1 level, the middle sacral artery/vein is ligated and divided. At the L4–5 level, the ascending lumbar vein and the L4 segmental vessel are ligated and divided providing adequate exposure of the anterior aspect of the disc space. Great care is taken to bluntly sweep all pre-peritoneal tissues off the disc space particularly at the L5–S1 level to diminish the risk of retrograde ejaculation. Retractors are placed to protect the vascular structures and maintain a midline exposure of the spine.

The anatomic midline of the spine is then marked with a metallic screw and a true anteroposterior fluoroscopy image is obtained to confirm that the correct disc space has been exposed

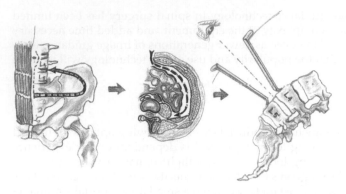

FIGURE 5 Schematic illustration of the anterior mini-retroperitoneal approach to the lumbar spine.

and that the midline is correctly identified. If needed, the midline marker is adjusted until it exactly marks the true midline of the vertebral segment.

Next, a thorough discectomy is performed with complete removal of the cartilaginous endplate, posterior anulus and lateral anulus to the margins of the vertebral body. The bony endplate is carefully maintained intact during the discectomy. Curettes are used to release any adherent anulus especially in the posterior and posterolateral corners of the disc. Occasionally brisk epidural bleeding is encountered posteriorly during the posterior release, which is controlled with a bipolar unit or packing with an appropriate hemostatic agent.

The disc space is then sized for the correct implant and alignment, fit, and lordosis of the segment are checked with anteroposterior and lateral fluoroscopy. After correct preparation of the disc space, the definitive implant is selected and placed. At the conclusion of the procedure, radiographic images are obtained to confirm good placement of the implant. The vascular and anatomic structures are inspected to ensure that there is no sign of injury and the surgical wound in closed in a standard fashion.

POSTEROPERATIVE MANAGEMENT

We examine the patient including distal pulses and neurologic examination as soon as possible following the conclusion of the procedure. The patient is encouraged to sit and flex as soon as possible after the procedure, but spinal extension is limited for the first six weeks after implantation. Generally, the patient is able to tolerate clear liquids on the night of the surgery and many patients are ready for discharge on the morning after surgery. We consider the use of an anticoagulation medication for the first three to four weeks following surgery to reduce the risk of a pelvis venous thrombus.

Normal activities are allowed as tolerated by the patient. Strenuous activities are deferred until the patient completes a comprehensive, supervised muscular rehabilitation program following surgery.

COMPLICATIONS

A variety of technical and medical complications are possible with disc replacement surgery. These include vascular injury, thrombosis or embolization (39–41), retrograde ejaculation (42,43), nerve root or cauda equine injury, injury to vital abdominal structures [e.g., ureter (44), bowel, or bladder], cerebrospinal fluid leakage, hernia formation, dislodgement or settling of the prosthesis, and prosthetic wear debris or osteolysis/loosening of the implant (45,46). Medical complications include infection (21), pelvic vein thrombosis, pulmonary embolism, cardiopulmonary compromise, stroke, and death. To reduce the risk of pelvic vein thrombus with pulmonary embolism anticoagulation may be warranted.

Learning Curve

It is important to remember that both MISS and disc arthroplasty represent complex procedures with significant learning curves. Therefore, the surgeon should plan appropriately for a learning curve as these techniques are adopted. During the early learning curve, longer operative times and possibly higher complication rates may be encountered.

OUTCOMES

Little has been published regarding the outcomes of minimally invasive total disc replacement procedures. In 1997, Mayer and Wiechert described a minimally invasive surgical approach to the anterior lumbar spine (29). In 2002, Mayer et al. reported using the minimally invasive anterior lumbar approach to implant series of artificial disc prostheses in the lumbar spine and noted satisfactory results in approximately 80% of the patients in the series. Complications occurred in 8.8% (three patients) of the patients but resolved in two or three patients (19).

SUMMARY

Minimally invasive spinal surgery is a developing and promising area of spinal surgery and can be adapted to a variety of motion-sparing spinal implants as these implants become available. The surgeon should become familiar with the current and rapidly changing technologies that facilitate this type of surgery. The mini-open retroperitoneal approach is currently the most commonly used approach for performing artificial disc implantation and is generally associated with little morbidity to the paraspinal muscular envelope. Although this approach is relatively straightforward, it is possible to encounter significant vein tears during the exposure and thus the surgeon performing this type of approach should be well versed in retroperitoneal abdominal surgery. Other approaches such as the direct lateral approach and modified Wiltse approach will likely play a role in the future as additional motional-sparing spinal implants become available.

Although patient recovery is generally quicker with minimally invasive approaches, the surgical technique for minimal access surgery is typically more technical than traditional open spinal surgery. Prospective studies are needed to compare minimally invasive spinal approaches with traditional approaches before definite statements regarding the efficacy of this developing field can be made.

REFERENCES

1. Mazanec DJ. Back pain: medical evaluation and therapy. Cleve Clin J Med 1995; 62(3):163–168.
2. Smeal WL, Tyburski M, Alleva J, et al. Conservative management of low back pain. Part I. Discogenic/radicular pain. Dis Mon 2004; 50(12):636–669.
3. Mannion AF, Muntener M, Taimela S, et al. A randomized clinical trial of three active therapies for chronic low back pain. Spine 1999; 24(23):2435–2448.
4. Anract P. Indications and limitations of surgery of common low back pain. Rev Prat 2000; 50(16):1793–1796.
5. Wipf JE, Deyo RA. Low back pain. Med Clin North Am 1995; 79(2):231–246.
6. Berven S, Tay BB, Colman W, et al. The lumbar zygapophyseal (facet) joints: a role in the pathogenesis of spinal pain syndromes and degenerative spondylolisthesis. Semin Neurol 2002; 22(2):187–196.
7. Schofferman J, Reynolds J, Herzog R, et al. Failed back surgery: etiology and diagnostic evaluation. Spine J 2003; 3(5):400–403.
8. Weatherley CR, Prickett CF, O'Brien JP. Discogenic pain persisting despite solid posterior fusion. J Bone Joint Surg Br 1986; 68(1):142–143.
9. Jaffray D, O'Brien JP. Isolated intervertebral disc resorption. A source of mechanical and inflammatory back pain? Spine 1986; 11(4):397–401.
10. Hilibrand AS, Carlson GD, Palumbo MA, et al. Radiculopathy and myelopathy at segments adjacent to the site of a previous anterior cervical arthrodesis. J Bone Joint Surg Am 1999; 81(4):519–528.
11. Goffin J, Casey A, Kehr P, et al. Preliminary clinical experience with the Bryan Cervical Disc Prosthesis. Neurosurgery 2002; 51(3):840–845. Discussion 845–847.
12. Jaikumar S, Kim DH, Kam AC. History of minimally invasive spine surgery. Neurosurgery 2002; 51(5 suppl):S1–14.
13. Williams RW. Lumbar disc disease. Microdiscectomy. Neurosurg Clin N Am 1993; 4(1):101–108.
14. Tong HC, Williams JC, Haig AJ, et al. Predicting outcomes of transforaminal epidural injections for sciatica. Spine J 2003; 3(6):430–434.
15. Zeegers WS, Bohnen LM, Laaper M, et al. Artificial disc replacement with the modular type SB Charite III: 2-year results in 50 prospectively studied patients. Eur Spine J 1999; 8(3):210–217.

16. Tropiano P, Huang RC, Girardi FP, et al. Lumbar disc replacement: preliminary results with ProDisc II after a minimum follow-up period of 1 year. J Spinal Disord Tech 2003; 16(4):362–368.

17. Zigler JE, Burd TA, Vialle EN, et al. Lumbar spine arthroplasty: early results using the ProDisc II: a prospective randomized trial of arthroplasty versus fusion. J Spinal Disord Tech 2003; 16(4):352–361.

18. Hochschuler SH, Ohnmeiss DD, Guyer RD, et al. Artificial disc: preliminary results of a prospective study in the United States. Eur Spine J 2002; 11(suppl 2):S106–110.

19. Mayer HM, Wiechert K, Korge A, et al. Minimally invasive total disc replacement: surgical technique and preliminary clinical results. Eur Spine J 2002; 11(suppl 2):S124–130.

20. Huang RC, Lim MR, Girardi FP, et al. The prevalence of contraindications to total disc replacement in a cohort of lumbar surgical patients. Spine 2004; 29(22):538–541.

21. Zheng Y, Lu WW, Zhu Q, et al. Variation in bone mineral density of the sacrum in young adults and its significance for sacral fixation. Spine 2000; 25(3):353–357.

22. Bertagnoli R, Kumar S. Indications for full prosthetic disc arthroplasty: a correlation of clinical outcome against a variety of indications. Eur Spine J 2002; 11(suppl 2):S131–136.

23. Lemaire JP, Skalli W, Lavaste F, et al. Intervertebral disc prosthesis. Results and prospects for the year 2000. Clin Orthop Relat Res 1997; (337):64–76.

24. Cinotti G, David T, Postacchini F. Results of disc prosthesis after a minimum follow-up period of 2 years. Spine 1996; 21(8):995–1000.

25. Moran R, O'Connell D, Walsh MG. The diagnostic value of facet joint injections. Spine 1988; 13(12): 1407–1410.

26. Axelsson P, Johnsson R, Stromqvist B, et al. Posterolateral lumbar fusion. Outcome of 71 consecutive operations after 4 (2-7) years. Acta Orthop Scand 1994; 65(3):309–314.

27. Parker LM, Murrell SE, Boden SD, et al. The outcome of posterolateral fusion in highly selected patients with discogenic low back pain. Spine 1996; 21(16):1909–1916. Discussion 1916–1917.

28. Moon MS. The outcome of posterolateral fusion in highly selected patients with discogenic low back pain. Spine 1997; 22(12):1419–1420.

29. Mayer HM, Wiechert K. Microsurgical anterior approaches to the lumbar spine for interbody fusion and total disc replacement. Neurosurgery 2002; 51(5 suppl):S159–165.

30. Mirza SK, Wiggins GC, Kuntz Ct, et al. Accuracy of thoracic vertebral body screw placement using standard fluoroscopy, fluoroscopic image guidance, and computed tomographic image guidance: a cadaver study. Spine 2003; 28(4):402–413.

31. Resnick DK. Prospective comparison of virtual fluoroscopy to fluoroscopy and plain radiographs for placement of lumbar pedicle screws. J Spinal Disord Tech 2003; 6(3):254–260.

32. Holly LT, Foley KT. Three-dimensional fluoroscopy-guided percutaneous thoracolumbar pedicle screw placement. Technical note. J Neurosurg 2003; 99(3suppl): 324–329.

33. Holly LT, Bloch O, Obasi C, et al. Frameless stereotaxy for anterior spinal procedures. J Neurosurg 2001; 95(2 suppl):196–201.

34. Foley KT, Simon DA, Rampersaud YR. Virtual fluoroscopy: computer-assisted fluoroscopic navigation. Spine 2001; 26(4):347–351.

35. Thongtrangan I, Le H, Park J, et al. Minimally invasive spinal surgery: a historical perspective. Neurosurg Focus 2004; 16(1):E13.

36. Egol KA. Minimally invasive orthopaedic trauma surgery: a review of the latest techniques. Bull Hosp Jt Dis 2004; 62(1-2):6–12.

37. Wolf O, Meier U. First experiences using microsurgical techniques for minimally invasive ventral interbody fusion of the lumbar spine (MINI-ALIF). Z Arztl Fortbild Qualitatssich 1999; 93(4):267–271.

38. Heniford BT, Matthews BD, Lieberman IH. Laparoscopic lumbar interbody spinal fusion. Surg Clin North Am 2000; 80(5):1487–1500.

39. McDonnell MF, Glassman SD, Dimar JR, et al. Perioperative complications of anterior procedures on the spine. J Bone Joint Surg Am 1996; 78(6):839–847.

40. Watkins R. Anterior lumbar interbody fusion surgical complications. Clin Orthop Relat Res 1992; (284):47–53.

41. Baker JK, Reardon PR, Reardon MJ, et al. Vascular injury in anterior lumbar surgery. Spine 1993; 18(15):2227–2230.

42. Flynn JC, Price CT. Sexual complications of anterior fusion of the lumbar spine. Spine 1984; 9(5):489–492.

43. Tiusanen H, Seitsalo S, Osterman K, et al. Retrograde ejaculation after anterior interbody lumbar fusion. Eur Spine J 1995; 4(6):339–342.

44. Isiklar ZU, Lindsey RW, Coburn M. Ureteral injury after anterior lumbar interbody fusion. A case report. Spine 1996; 21(20):2379–2382.

45. Patwardhan AG, Havey RM, Meade KP, et al. A follower load increases the load-carrying capacity of the lumbar spine in compression. Spine 1999; 24(10):1003–1009.

46. McAfee PC, Cunningham BW, Orbegoso CM, et al. Analysis of porous ingrowth in intervertebral disc prostheses: a nonhuman primate model. Spine 2003; 28(4):332–340.

37 | Percutaneous Nucleus Replacement Technology

Kern Singh
*Department of Orthopedic Surgery, Rush University Medical Center,
Chicago, Illinois, U.S.A.*

Alexander R. Vaccaro
*Department of Orthopedic Surgery and Neurosurgery, Thomas Jefferson University and
the Rothman Institute, Philadelphia, Pennsylvania, U.S.A.*

INTRODUCTION

Re-establishment of normal biomechanical properties in the diseased or degenerative disc continues to be a challenge in the field of spinal surgery. Since the 1950s, attempts have been made to develop and test models for restoration (1). Recent animal and human evidence suggests that the degenerative changes within the spinal unit begin in the nucleus (2,3). As such, the nucleus has become a focal point for recent developments in spinal replacement technology (4).

Anatomically, the nucleus is a gelatinous material with a cellular composition consisting of cells similar to pseudochondrocytes (5). The extracellular matrix is a unique combination of fluid-bathed collagens (types I and II), and proteoglycans, including chondroitin and keratin sulfate (6). The nucleus deforms or swells in response to changes in the hydraulic permeability of the endplates that is initiated by simple compressive loading (7,8). It has been theorized that changes in the diffusion of nutrients and water from the endplate alter the adaptive capabilities of the nucleus. Further changes in nuclear pressure may inhibit the ability of the endplate to nourish the avascular nucleus and annulus initiating a degenerative cascade (9–11).

Restoration of the nucleus with a prosthetic implant has undergone a gradual evolution in design and surgical approach modifications. The earliest attempts in replacing the nucleus were in conjunction with a discectomy for leg pain to maintain discal height and function, rather than as a functional alternative to spinal fusion (4,12–15). Fernstrom's attempt to preserve motion involved replacing the nucleus with stainless steel ball bearings while retaining the majority of the anulus fibrosis (16). At approximately the same time, Nachemson (17) injected silicon and Hamby and Glaser (1) injected PMMA into the disc space following a nuclearectomy. Issues regarding bone resorption, poor material containment, and questionable clinical results eventually led to the abandonment of earlier attempts in nuclear replacement (18).

Recent developments in nucleus replacement implants has paralleled the development of polymer and elastomer technology (18–20). The viscoelastic properties of these compounds hold theoretical promise for restoring the dynamic function of the nucleus under load. Based on these clinical advances, Ray and Schonmayr developed a hydrogel "pillow" or prosthetic nucleus device (PDN) composed of a dehydrated polyethylene, acrylonitrile/polyethylene, acrylamide covered by a woven polyethylene sack that allowed for free flow of fluid but remained constrained by an outer cover (21). Since 1996, over hundreds of patients have received the implants by means of an open annulotomy. Klara et al. reported marked improvements in disability assessment scores (Oswestry). However, these results were tempered by a continuing problem with extrusion and device migration (6%) with a 10% reoperation rate (21).

Recent advances in minimally invasive techniques may allow for access to the disc space via a limited annulotomy thereby decreasing the potential for device extrusion. Solid implant devices that have required an open annulotomy have been plagued with device migration and extrusion. Modifying the surgical approach from a posterior to posterolateral to anterior approach has decreased the incidence of device extrusion but has not eliminated it completely. Strategies to decrease implant migration have ranged from exploitation of expandable hydrogels that swell once inserted through a limited annulotomy to injectable polymers that are percutaneously injected into the nuclear defect or into a priory-placed balloon.

Percutaneous Insertion of a Nuclear Implant

An injectable biomaterial is ideal for restoration of the disc volume removed during a nuclear excision and for further prevention of disc height loss. Flowable materials may be injected percutaneously thereby interdigitating with irregular surgical defects and may, depending on the material used, physically bond to the adjacent tissue. Alternatively, flowable materials may be inserted into a percutaneously placed balloon to prevent any polymer extravasation through annular defects that may be present in a degenerative disc. Fluid pressurization of the intradiscal space may then allow for load transferring and sharing between the annulus and nucleus.

NuCore

An example of a percutaneously delivered nuclear implant is the NuCore™ (SpineWave Inc, Shelton, CT, U.S.A.) injectable polymer. Recent advances have been made allowing for the production of synthetically designed protein polymers consisting of repeated blocks of amino acid sequences. Block polymers are produced using a gene template-directed synthesis (22–24). Through the construction of synthetic genes, it is possible to specify the sequence of protein blocks many times greater than the limit of sequence control involved in chemical synthesis (22–24).

The protein polymer used in the NuCore™ injectable nucleus is a copolymer of silk fibrin and elastin, with two silk blocks and eight elastin blocks per polymer repeat (23,24). The protein polymer is synthesized using recombinant DNA techniques via an *Eschericia coli* strain K12. Using a technique of lysate precipitation, the cells are ruptured by homogenization and the protein polymer is purified (23,24). The identity and purity of the polymer is confirmed using amino acid composition, sequencing, mass spectroscopy, and other biochemical tests.

The NuCore™ material is comprised of a solution of the protein polymer and a polyfunctional cross-linking agent that closely resembles the properties of the human nucleus pulposus (Table 1).

Percutaneous Injection

The NuCore™ material is injected after mixing with a very low concentration of a diisocyanate-based cross-linking agent. The working time is approximately 90 seconds prior to the solution becoming a viscous gel. The gel time is approximately five minutes with the material reaching near final mechanical strength approximately 30 minutes following addition of the cross-linker (Figs. 1 and 2).

Safety

The NuCore™ material has been demonstrated to be noncytotoxic, nonirritating in several acute tests including cytotoxicity, sensitization (guinea pig), intracutaneous reactivity (rabbit), systemic toxicity (mouse), pyrogenicity, muscle implant evaluation, and genotoxicity testing. Chronic toxicity testing has also been conducted in a rat model, with material placed subcutaneously and evaluated at time points to one year and beyond, with no toxicity observed.

TABLE 1 A Comparison Between the NuCore™ Material and Normal Nucleus Mechanical Properties

Property	NuCore™ injectable nucleus	Natural nucleus
Protein content	19.4%	13.6–21.9%
Water content	79.1%	74–81%
pH	7.1	6.7–7.1
Complex shear modulus (G*)	26 kPa	7–21 kPa

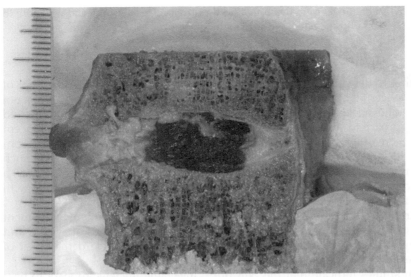

FIGURE 1 Sagittal image of NuCore™ material filling nuclear cavity. Note pigment used in cadaver studies to enhance visualization (Actual clinical product is nonpigmented).

Neurofunctional testing in a rat and intradiscal evaluation in a sheep model has also demonstrated no adverse tissue reactions.

Biomechanical Evaluation

Biomechanical cadaveric evaluation of the NuCore™ material after an annulotomy and partial nucleotomy demonstrated near-complete intradiscal height restoration. Specimens were also tested in six degrees of motion demonstrating no statistically significant difference between the NuCore™ material and the intact cadaver.

Additional testing of the cadaveric spinal units was performed to determine the NuCore™ material's ability to resist extrusive forces. Segments were tested in axial compression in both a neutral posture and in hyperflexion. In all cases, there was no extrusion prior to bony failure

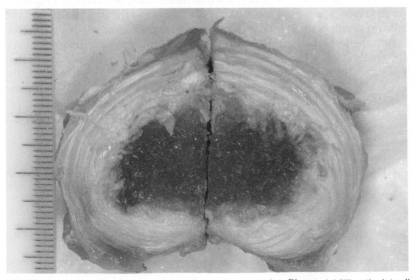

FIGURE 2 Axial image of the same specimen with the NuCore™ material filling the intradiscal space.

and/or endplate failure. Dynamic testing also revealed that the NuCore™ material was able to withstand cyclic loading (10 million cycles) with no signs of failure.

CONCLUSION

Surgeons are continuing to develop methods that allow the minimally invasive placement of nuclear replacement devices that prevent implant migration or extrusion. To date, this has not been successful with solid nuclear devices that remain the same size or expand with fluid adsorption. A novel approach to successful nuclear replacement strategies may be the concept of percutaneously delivered fluids that harden or cure in situ over a set time period and conform to the cavity in which they are applied. The deformation characteristics of hydrogels, such as silicone and polyurethanes, make this category of elastomers highly desirable. However, a problem with the percent monomer needed to obtain biomechanical strength comparable with a normal nucleus is a restriction because of its toxicity.

Future nucleus replacement designs must continue to focus on better patient assessment and profiling. Understanding the complex mechanisms between the outcomes of system and local degeneration will allow for the creation of prosthetic designs that retard the onset of degenerative disc disease.

Characterization studies indicate that the NuCore™ injectable nucleus appears to be a suitable alternative to replace the natural nucleus pulposus following a discectomy procedure. Extensive biomaterial characterization shows the NuCore™ material to be nontoxic and biocompatible. The mechanical properties of the NuCore™ material mimic those of the natural nucleus pulposus. Additional preclinical testing is underway in a variety of animal models, while laboratory testing has characterized the mechanical properties and durability of the material in spinal applications.

Other Percutaneous Nuclear Replacement Technologies

Also being developed for nucleus replacement or augmentation are injectable hydrogels. The Biodisc (Cryolife, Kennesaw, GA) is an injectable protein hydrogel device based on Cryolife's Bioglue surgical adhesive. The Biodisc material is injected into the disc space and begins to polymerize within 30 seconds, reaching pliable solid support state within two minutes. The polymerization process occurs with no appreciable exothermic reaction. The injectatable acts as a spacer with material properties similar to human nucleus pulposus. It restores disc height and motion. Early bench work fatigue testing at 10 million cycles reports 10% loss of disc height, which later recovers.

In summary, the restoration of nucleus function must demonstrate effectiveness in quality of life for those people disabled by acute or chronic back pain of discogenic origin. Methods of delivering these implants or polymers must be done in a nonmorbid fashion ensuring that the implant remains stable and functions appropriately. Percutaneous methods of implant delivery appear to be a promising method of ensuring implant stability especially with polymers that cure instantaneously and conform to the cavities into which they are introduced. Hopefully, further clinical studies of the NuCore™ injectable nucleus and other similar products for the treatment of early-stage degenerative disc disease may offer potential treatment options for this difficult clinical scenario.

REFERENCES

1. Hamby WB, Glaser HT. Replacement of spinal intervertebral discs with locally polymerizing methyl methacrylate: experimental study of effects upon tissues and report of a small clinical series. J Neurosurg 1959; 16:311–313.
2. Battie MC, Videman T, Parent E. Lumbar disc degeneration: epidemiology and genetic influences. Spine 2004; 29:2679–2690.
3. Holm S, Nachemson A. Nutrition of the intervertebral disc: acute effects of cigarette smoking. An experimental animal study. Ups J Med Sci 1988; 93:91–99.
4. Carl A, Ledet E, Yuan H, et al. New developments in nucleus pulposus replacement technology. Spine J 2004; 4:325S–329S.
5. Oegema TR Jr. Biochemistry of the intervertebral disc. Clin Sports Med 1993; 12:419–439.

6. Iatridis JC, Setton LA, Weidenbaum M, et al. Alterations in the mechanical behavior of the human lumbar nucleus pulposus with degeneration and aging. J Orthop Res 1997; 15:318–322.
7. Bao QB, McCullen GM, Higham PA, et al. The artificial disc: theory, design and materials. Biomaterials 1996; 17:1157–1167.
8. Iatridis JC, Weidenbaum M, Setton LA, et al. Is the nucleus pulposus a solid or a fluid? Mechanical behaviors of the nucleus pulposus of the human intervertebral disc. Spine 1996; 21:1174–1184.
9. Mwale F, Roughley P, Antoniou J. Distinction between the extracellular matrix of the nucleus pulposus and hyaline cartilage: a requisite for tissue engineering of intervertebral disc. Eur Cell Mater 2004; 8:58–64.
10. Niosi CA, Oxland TR. Degenerative mechanics of the lumbar spine. Spine J 2004; 4:202S–208S.
11. Sztrolovics R, Alini M, Roughley PJ, et al. Aggrecan degradation in human intervertebral disc and articular cartilage. Biochem J 1997; 326(Pt 1):235–241.
12. Ambrosio L, De Santis R, Nicolais L. Composite hydrogels for implants. Proc Inst Mech Eng [H] 1998; 212:93–99.
13. Bao QB, Yuan HA. New technologies in spine: nucleus replacement. Spine 2002; 27:1245–1247.
14. Sagi HC, Bao QB, Yuan HA. Nuclear replacement strategies. Orthop Clin N Am 2003; 34:263–267.
15. Sieber AN, Kostuik JP. Concepts in nuclear replacement. Spine J 2004; 4:322S–324S.
16. Fernstrom U. Arthroplasty with intercorporal endoprothesis in herniated disc and in painful disc. Acta Chir Scand Suppl 1966; 357:154–159.
17. Nachemson A. Lumbar intradiscal pressure. Experimental studies on post-mortem material. Acta Orthop Scand 1960; suppl 43:1–104.
18. Urbaniak JR, Bright DS, Hopkins JE. Replacement of intervertebral discs in chimpanzees by silicone-dacron implants: a preliminary report. J Biomed Mater Res 1973; 7:165–186.
19. Guyer RD, Ohnmeiss DD. Intervertebral disc prostheses. Spine 2003; 28:S15–S23.
20. Allen MJ, Schoonmaker JE, Bauer TW, et al. Preclinical evaluation of a poly(vinyl alcohol) hydrogel implant as a replacement for the nucleus pulposus. Spine 2004; 29:515–523.
21. Klara PM, Ray CD. Artificial nucleus replacement: clinical experience. Spine 2002; 27:1374–1377.
22. Edeland HG. Suggestions for a total elasto-dynamic intervertebral disc prosthesis. Biomater Med Devices Artif Organs 1981; 9:65–72.
23. Edeland HG. Some additional suggestions for an intervertebral disc prosthesis. J Biomed Eng 1985; 7:57–62.
24. Cappello J, Ferrari F. Microbial product of structural protein polymers. In: Plastics from Microbesed. Munich: Verlag, 1994.

38 | Percutaneous Posterior "Dynamic" Stabilization of the Lumbar Spine

Dilip K. Sengupta
Dartmouth-Hitchcock Medical Center, Lebanon, New Hampshire, U.S.A.

Harry N. Herkowitz
William Beaumont Hospital, Royal Oak, Michigan, U.S.A.

INTRODUCTION

Dynamic stabilization for the treatment of chronic low back pain is a relatively new concept. For the past few decades, fusion has been the mainstay of treatment via stabilization of a painful lumbar motion segment. With the addition of instrumentation, successful fusion rates have increased, but achieving successful clinical outcomes remained unpredictable. This has led to an increasing interest and enthusiasm in the use of nonfusion stabilization techniques during recent years. A large number of nonfusion devices have been recently introduced. Nonfusion devices may be broadly classified into two groups: prosthetic devices, which are applied after excision of an anatomical structure in the lumbar spine, and dynamic stabilization devices, which are applied to stabilize the spine without excision of any anatomical structure (Table 1).

OVERVIEW OF POSTERIOR DYNAMIC STABILIZATION DEVICES

The Graf artificial ligament, described by Henry Graf (1) in 1992, is one of the earliest dynamic stabilization devices and has formed the basis for many devices subsequently introduced. The system consists of a Dacron band (artificial ligament) that spans and axially compresses two or more pedicle screws together. This thereby locks the facet joints, which Graf thought to be the primary site of pain with spinal instability. Clinical experience with Graf ligament stabilization showed a high incidence of radicular symptoms secondary to either disc herniation or narrowing of the foramen (both presumably the result of undue axial compression). In addition, compressive forces along the posterior aspect of the disc may have led to more back pain (2). For these reasons, continued use of Graf ligament is limited to only a few centers in the Europe and Asia.

To prevent these harmful effects, subsequent dynamic stabilization designs incorporated a flexible rod system to connect the pedicle screws, which can maintain some degree of resistance to axial compression. The common proposed mechanism of action of all these devices is restriction of motion or flexibility of the unstable motion segment. However, with dynamic stabilization, preservation of motion is the aim, and the loss of flexibility is considered more of a side effect than the primary mechanism for pain relief.

This seeming paradox requires further explanation. It has been well-recognized that in degenerative diseases the range of motion of the lumbar spine is progressively decreased, rather than increased (3–5). Mulholland (6) hypothesized that the primary cause of pain in degenerative lumbar spine is an abnormal distribution of load and not an abnormally increased range of motion. More recently, Panjabi (7) described that clinical instability in lumbar spine is characterized by an abnormal quality of motion in the neutral zone (NZ), even when the total range of motion is in fact decreased. Summarizing these hypotheses, one of the authors, in a review article of the dynamic stabilization devices, described that the biomechanical goal of a dynamic stabilization device should be unloading the disc via load-sharing (8). This would, theoretically, prevent abnormal quality of motion with minimal restriction of range of motion (8). A suggested classification system of the currently available flexible rod systems for dynamic stabilization of the lumbar spine, based on their mechanism of action, is presented in Table 2.

TABLE 1   Classification of the Nonfusion Stabilization Devices

Disc prosthesis—Charite, Prodisc, Maverick, and the like.
Nuclear prosthesis—Ray PDNT, Mathys Spiral Coil, and the like.
Facet joint prosthesis—TOPS, TFAST, and the like.
Stabilization devices
   Spinous process distraction devices—X Stop, Wallis system, DIAM, and the like.
   Pedicle screw-based devices—Graf ligament, Dynesys, Dynamic Stabilization System II, and the like.

Abbreviations: TFAST, total facet arthroplasty systemT; TOPS, total posterior arthroplasty system.

One of the earliest flexible rod system introduced toward the end of last decade is Dynesys® (Zimmer Spine Inc., Warsaw, IN, U.S.A.) (Fig. 1) This is also the only example of a nonmetallic flexible rod. It consists of a polycarbonaturethane (Sulene-PCU) cylindrical spacer, held between the pedicle screws with an elastic ligament. The plastic cylinder applies a distraction force, unloading the facet joints, which is thought to be a cause of pain in the presence of a collapsed, degenerated disc. Biomechanical tests of Dynesys in cadaver spines show that the range of flexion is limited, apparently because the device holds the segment in nearly full flexion. The range of extension remains nearly normal, because the flexibility of the cylinder permits movement in this direction (9). No data are available in the literature regarding the degree of disc unloading with this device. Because of uneven restriction of flexibility of the motion segment, the device is exposed to higher forces at certain ranges of motion, and therefore the possibility of device failure remains a concern. On the other hand, it is known that the plastic cylinder softens at body temperature, as well as over time, which may lessen its efficacy in vivo while possibly protecting it somewhat against fatigue failure.

The Dynamic Stabilization System II (DSS-II) (Fig. 2) developed by one of the authors, is a flexible rod made of spring-grade titanium (10,11). It is connected to the lumbar spine through pedicle screws. The mechanism of action of this device is to produce distraction and lordosis, primarily to unload the disc, as well as the facet joints to relieve chronic, activity-related, mechanical low back pain. It is crucial that the device can apply an even unloading effect throughout the range of motion and avoid an uneven restriction of flexibility in order to prevent a device failure. The earlier design of this device consisted of a C-shaped spring, which appeared to unload the disc partially by load-sharing with the disc during flexion. However, it was found to be totally load-bearing during extension, leaving no load to be transmitted through the disc. This uneven unloading was presumed to be a characteristic that would predict device failure and the design was subsequently discarded. The second-generation device, the DSS-II, consists of a coil spring, which permits even unloading of the disc throughout the range of motion. The DSS-II has been used clinically.

The SoftFlex™ (Globus Medical Inc., Phoenixville, PA, U.S.A.) consists of a 6.5-mm titanium rod, made flexible by cutting out a spiral thread by one-and-a-half turns (540°) in its mid-section. The mechanism of action is also distraction and lordosis of the motion segment to unload the disc as well as the facet joints. The diameter of the rod is 6 mm, as it can be connected to a regular pedicle screw. The other advantage is that the same rod may contain a solid portion for fusion of one segment and a flexible portion for dynamic stabilization of the adjacent segment. The device has not been used clinically for dynamic stabilization as of the time of this writing (Fig. 3).

The Isobar® TTL (Scient'x USA Inc., Maitland, FL, U.S.A.) system incorporates a semirigid segment, consisting of disc springs, which can act as a shock-absorbing structure to axial load,

TABLE 2   Classification of Flexible Rod Stabilization Devices Based on their Mechanism of Action

Mechanism			Example
Stiffness	Distraction		Dynesys®
Stiffness	Distraction	Lordosis	Dynamic Stabilization System II
			SoftFlex™
Stiffness	Distraction	Axial shock absorption	Isobar® TTL
Selective stiffness of neutral zone motion			M-Brace™

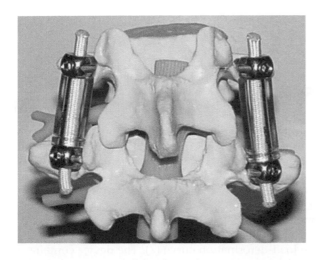

FIGURE 1 Dynesys® system consists of nonmetallic, flexible, cylindrical spacers, made of polycarbonaturethane (Sulene-PCU), held between the pedicle screws with a ligament.

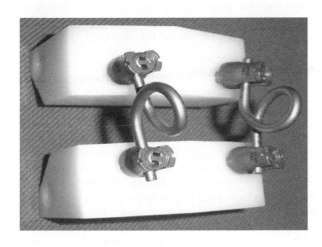

FIGURE 2 Dynamic Stabilization System II (DSS-II) system consists of alpha-shaped coils, made of 4-mm diameter spring-grade titanium rods.

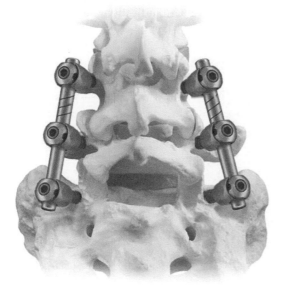

FIGURE 3 SoftFlex™ system consists of 6-mm diameter titanium rods, with spiral cuts, which makes it flexible.

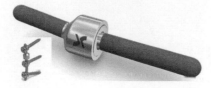

FIGURE 4 Isobar® TTL system consists of a flexible section between the 6-mm rods, made of disc springs, which offers not only lateral bending and rotational flexibility but also axial compressibility.

in addition to having lateral and rotational flexibility. The primary aim of this device was to reduce the rigidity of a fusion rod, in order to avoid stress shielding and to achieve a more solid fusion. However, this device may also be used for dynamic stabilization when no bone graft is used. No biomechanical data is available in the literature regarding its effect on flexibility or disc load in the lumbar spine. There is no published clinical data available regarding its application as a dynamic stabilization device (Fig. 4).

The M-Brace™ (Applied Spine Technologies, Inc. New haven, CT, U.S.A.) was originally designed by Panjabi, who has defined clinical instability of the lumbar spine as an abnormal quality of motion in the neutral zone of the load-deformation curve (7). The device contains a segment in the middle of a rod, which offers greater resistance to flexibility selectively in the neutral zone, but very little resistance toward the end zones. Therefore, the overall range of motion is minimally affected, and the load-deformation curve of a damaged spinal motion segment may be restored to that of an intact spine after application of this device (Fig. 5).

INDICATIONS FOR POSTERIOR DYNAMIC STABILIZATION

The indications and contraindications for posterior dynamic stabilizations are summarized in Table 3. The most important indication is disc degeneration with activity-related chronic mechanical low back pain, which fails to respond to conservative treatment. Typically, the patient describes worsening pain with activities of daily living and limitation of forward bending. More importantly, patients demonstrate a so-called instability catch characterized by sharp pain while getting up from forward bent posture. They may bend, twist or rotate the trunk, or support the body weight by putting hands on the knee and thigh, in order to avoid a painful arc while regaining the upright posture. When disc degeneration involves multiple segments, and the patient is relatively young, and a single painful disc cannot be localized, dynamic stabilization might be a better method of treatment (Fig. 6). Presence of facet degeneration is not a contraindication to posterior dynamic stabilization. It is preferable that the extent of disc degeneration is mild or moderate. More advanced disc degeneration with gross collapse of the disc space, and formation of large osteophytes may not respond to dynamic stabilization, and fusion may be a better alternative.

In the presence of concomitant radicular pain or neurogenic claudication, decompression and/or discectomy is the primary surgical goal. Posterior dynamic stabilization may be added

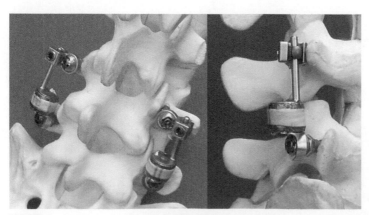

FIGURE 5 M-Brace consists of a flexible section, which offers selective resistance to the neutral zone motion but least resistance to the end-zone motion.

TABLE 3 Indications and Contraindications for Posterior Dynamic
Stabilization in the Lumbar Spine

Indications
Primary indications—in the treatment of instability
Disc degeneration with mechanical low back pain
Facet joint degeneration with mechanical low back pain
Degenerative spondylolisthesis
Salvage persistent pain after total disc replacement or nuclear replacement
Secondary indications—prevent instability
Adjacent segment to fusion
Following decompressive laminectomy for stenosis or listhesis
Relative Indications
Prevent instability following discectomy
Primary Total Joint Replacement—together with TDR
Contraindications
Advanced disc/facet degeneration with osteophytes
Degenerative spondylolisthesis exceeding grade I
Collapse of disc height exceeding 50%
Osteoporosis and similar metabolic bone disease
Infection

Abbreviation: TDR, total disc replacement.

to prevent instability and worsening back pain following decompression. Application of dynamic stabilization alone without decompression is unlikely to achieve clinical success (12,13). There is no data to justify addition of dynamic stabilization following simple discectomy for predominant radicular symptoms, unless the accompanying back pain itself would justify stabilization. The other important indication for dynamic stabilization is to salvage failure of other nonfusion stabilizations like nuclear replacement (Fig. 7) or total disc replacement (Fig. 8). In these cases, salvage with fusion may not be easy to achieve because of the presence of a prosthetic device between the vertebral bodies.

There is insufficient data in the literature to suggest which dynamic stabilization device would be more appropriate for a specific indication. Application of Dynesys is difficult through a minimally invasive approach, because the tensioner for the ligament requires exposure

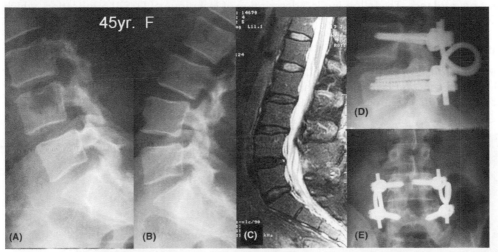

FIGURE 6 Case presentation: an ideal patient for minimally invasive dynamic stabilization. (**A,B**) This young female (45, F) presented with chronic, activity-related, mechanical low back pain, two years following discectomy at L4–5, and failed to respond to conservative treatment. (**C**) Magnetic resonance image showed multiple-level disc degeneration (L2 to S1), well-maintained disc heights, and high-intensity zone (HIZ) at L4–5 disc. Concordant pain response was reproduced only at the L4–5 segment. (**D,E**) She had complete resolution of symptoms after stabilization of the L4–5 segment with Dynamic Stabilization System II (DSS-II) system.

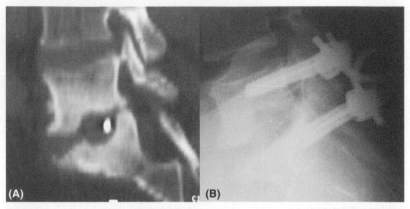

FIGURE 7   A case of failed PDN at L5–S1 segment, with persistent pain, but no extrusion of the implant, has been salvaged with Dynamic Stabilization System II (DSS-II) stabilization without fusion.

beyond the pedicle screw. Therefore, when minimally invasive isolated posterior dynamic stabilization is intended, any of the four other devices may be a better choice. On the other hand, for dynamic stabilization following open posterior decompression any of the devices, including Dynesys, may be used.

SURGICAL TECHNIQUE

In the absence of any indication for decompression, dynamic stabilization through a minimally invasive paraspinal approach is the method of choice. This can help prevent the so-called fusion disease, which more likely results from fibrosis of the paraspinal muscles damaged during exposure and retraction and possibly from damage to the facet joint capsule during pedicle screw insertion. When dynamic stabilization is applied following decompressive laminectomy, the pedicle screws may be inserted by the conventional technique. It is however important to remember not to disturb the facet joint capsule of both the stabilized segments as well as the adjacent segments. All the metallic flexible rods can be introduced by a minimally invasive posterior approach, with percutaneous insertion of the pedicle screws over guide pins under fluoroscopy guidance. The following is a description of technique of DSS-II application, which has been used clinically.

Patient Positioning

The patient is positioned prone on rolls to create ideal lumbar lordosis. This is checked by lateral fluoroscopy and is perhaps the most important step. It is possible to achieve further distraction, as well as lordosis during later stage of instrumentation.

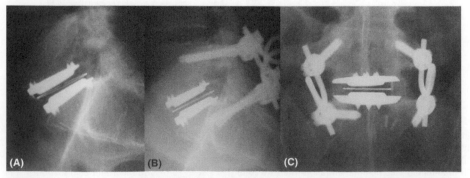

FIGURE 8   A case of failed Charite disc replacement at L5–S1 segment, with persistent back pain but no implant failure, was salvaged with Dynamic Stabilization System II (DSS-II) stabilization, without fusion.

Insertion of the Device

The pedicle screws are inserted by percutaneous technique using fluoroscopy, over guide pins and progressive dilators. Because of the lumbar lordosis, the trajectories of the pedicle screws of the same side converge to a small area on the surface of the skin. Pedicle screws on the same side may therefore be inserted through one 3-cm longitudinal skin incision. The tract between the two pedicle screws is created by splitting the erector spinae muscles with a dissector. Each screw head is connected to a slotted extension tube projecting outside the skin. Once satisfactory screw positioning is confirmed, the DSS spring is slid down the slot in the extension tubes of the pedicle screws to sit into the screw heads. The coil of the DSS-II device should be oriented in the sagittal plane before locking the nuts to the screw heads. Usually no distraction or compression is required, but when the disc height is collapsed to below 50%, distraction may be applied between the pedicle screws through the extension tubes. Because distraction is kyphogenic, if distraction is applied, it is important to ensure the lordosis of the segment. The average operative time for a single level is under 90 minutes and average blood loss is less than 50 cc. The postoperative morbidity is minimal and the patients can usually ambulate unsupported within a couple of hours after surgery and usually is discharged home the same day (Fig. 9).

COMPLICATIONS

The commonest perioperative complication is pedicle screw malposition. In a consecutive series of 83 cases, treated by stabilization with Dynesys with or without decompression, Stoll et al. (14) reported pedicle fracture (one case), screw misplacement (two cases), and screw loosening (eight cases). Schnake et al. (13) reported a similar (17%) incidence of screw loosening in a review of 26 cases of stabilization with Dynesys for degenerative spondylolisthesis.

Pedicle screw placement for dynamic stabilization is little more demanding than for fusion because of several reasons. First, the segment remains mobile, and therefore the pedicle screw needs to be inserted without damaging the facet joint capsule. This requires the starting point to be more lateral at the junction of the transverse process and the lateral aspect of the facet joint. Second, in fusion, the pedicle screws may be reinforced by cross-links, which is not possible in dynamic stabilization. Last, but most important, the pedicle screws for fusion has to provide stability only temporarily until fusion takes place, while for dynamic stabilization the pedicle screw needs to provide stability for an indefinite period. Should the pedicle screw appear to be loose, it may be replaced with a larger diameter screw, or a fusion should be performed instead of dynamic stabilization. Some advocate insertion of the pedicle screw at an earlier date, while bone growth around the pedicle screw threads may reinforce the screw–bone junction and application of the stabilization device at a second stage. No clinical experience with such a technique has been reported.

The other common pitfall is stabilization with inappropriate distraction and lordosis. Overdistraction may lead to undue stiffness and kyphosis of the segment. In contrast, underdistraction may not achieve adequate disc unloading. In a review of 50 cases with Dynesys stabilization, Rajaratnam et al. (15) reported better results in those cases where the standing lateral radiographs showed well-maintained lordosis, and less favorable results in cases with flat back or kyphosis. The appropriate degree of distraction should be estimated by the tactile feel of the tension between the pedicle screws, while observing the opening up of the disc space in fluoroscopy. The estimated degree of distraction force between the pedicle screws for adequate disc unloading is also dependent on patient positioning, and would be much different in the knee-chest position compared to prone position with hips and knees extended. For stabilization with DSS, we prefer to position the patient prone on a Jackson table with an appropriate degree of lordosis insured before instrumentation (16).

CLINICAL OUTCOMES

Long-term clinical results following posterior dynamic stabilization are only available for the Graf ligament. Grevitt et al. reported a two-year follow-up study on their first 50 cases with Graf ligament stabilization in 1994 (2). The majority of patients were young (mean age 41 years) with multiple segment degeneration and predominant back pain. They reported

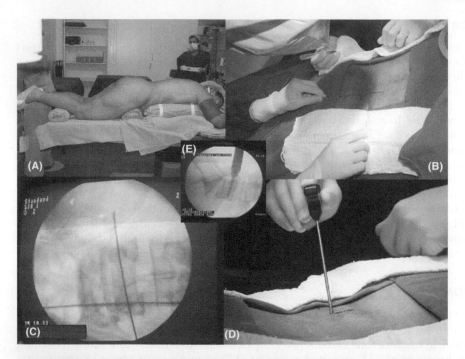

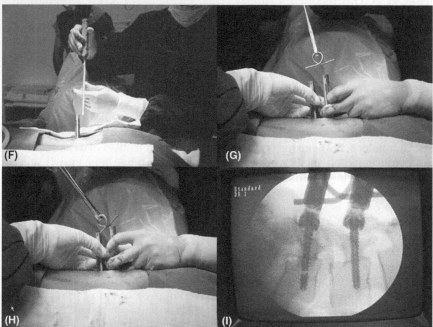

FIGURE 9 Technique for minimally invasive posterior dynamic stabilization, using Dynamic Stabilization System II (DSS-II) system and Pathfinder™ pedicle screw system (Abbott Spine Inc., Austin, TX, U.S.A.). (**A**) The patient is positioned prone, with restoration of adequate lumbar lordosis. (**B,C**) The pedicle screw is inserted percutaneously using fluoroscopy. K-wires are placed over the skin to identify the entry point centering over the pedicle. Because of the lordosis, usually, only a 5-cm incision is required for insertion of pedicle screws across one motion segment. (**D**) A guide pin is inserted into the pedicle, under anteroposterior and lateral fluoroscopy. Serial dilators and the cannulated tap are passed over the guide pin to prepare the track for insertion of the pedicle screw. (**E**) The cannulated pedicle screw with an attached slotted-cylindrical outrigger is inserted over the guide pin. (**F**) The second pedicle screw is inserted through the same skin incision. (**G–I**) The DSS-II coil spring is inserted, sliding it through the slots on the cylindrical outriggers, and sited into the screw heads under fluoroscopy guide. (**J**) The nuts are tightened making sure that the coil is maintained in the sagittal plane, and applying adequate distraction to restore the disc height and lordosis.

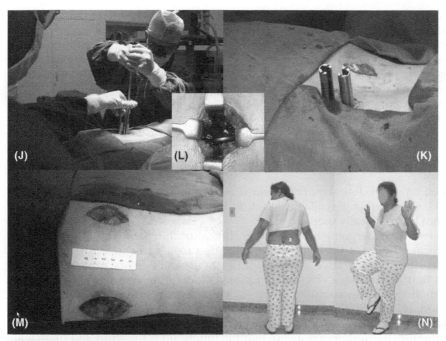

FIGURE 9 (*Continued*) (**K**) The procedure is repeated on the other side. (**L,M**) The coil of the DSS-II spring is buried well under the skin, and the skin incision rarely exceeds 5 cm on each side. (**N**) Because no muscle is cut or stripped off the bone, there is little postoperative pain, and the patients might be mobilized soon after the surgery.

excellent results in 72% and fair or poor in the remaining 28% cases. An independent review almost seven years later on the same group of patients showed excellent or good results maintained in 62% of the cases, and the authors concluded that the beneficial effects of Graf ligamentoplasty are sustained in the longer term in spite of the presence of an established degenerative process (17). In the original report by Grevitt et al., the commonest complication was new onset leg pain from narrowing of the neural foramen secondary to compression. Screw loosening was not particularly common, probably because of gradual stretching of the ligament within a few months following surgery, which relieves forces on the pedicle screws.

The first clinical experience with Dynesys was presented by the inventor of the system Dubois (14) in a review of 73 patients with mean of three years follow-up. The authors reported significant clinical improvement in terms of Oswestry Disability Index and functional scores, but no data were presented on the number or percentage of patients who had clinical improvement. The commonest indications were degenerative back pain with spinal stenosis and 67.5% of the patients had concomitant decompressive lumbar laminectomy. Device-related complications were reported in 11 cases (15%), all of which were related to pedicle screws. Pedicle screw loosening in the follow-up period was observed in seven cases (10%). The importance of this paper was that this was the first report of a multicenter clinical study with Dynesys, which reported clinical success comparable with fusion. However, a common criticism of this study was that it left unclear whether the clinical improvement was secondary to decompressive lumbar laminectomy or stabilization.

Clinical experience from authors not related to the development of Dynesys has been reported. Grob et al. (12), in a review of 31 cases with back pain as a result of degenerative instability, with a minimum of two years follow-up, reported a significant clinical improvement in half the cases (a lot 29%, some 21%, and a little 10%), and functional improvement in less than half the cases. Sixty-eight percent of cases would have the same operation again and 32% would not. It is important to note that clinical improvement was observed in only 39% of the cases who had Dynesys stabilization alone ($n = 18$), compared with 69% cases who had Dynesys following decompressive laminectomy ($n = 13$).

More recently, results of Dynesys stabilization for specific indications have been reported. Putzier et al. (18) reported that additional Dynesys stabilization ($n = 35$) following discectomy for disc herniation prevented progressive disc degeneration, compared with discectomy alone ($n = 49$) all of which showed progressive disc degeneration at a mean of 34 months follow-up. In another report, Schnake et al. (13) reported Dysesys stabilization following decompressive laminectomy for degenerative spondylolisthesis with spinal stenosis ($n = 26$ cases) with a minimum of two year follow-up. They found similar clinical improvement with this procedure compared with the results of decompression and fusion as published in the literature, but pointed out that the advantage of Dynesys was that no bone grafting was necessary. However, screw loosening was observed in 17% cases in the follow-up period. Currently, a Food and Drug Administration (FDA)-approved multicenter clinical IDE trial with Dynesys is in progress in the United States.

No published report of clinical outcome following dynamic stabilization with the DSS-II or The Isobar® TTL stabilization is available as yet. To the author's knowledge SoftFlex™ and M-Brace™ have not been clinically used as yet.

DSS-II is currently undergoing a prospective clinical trial in Sao Paulo, Brazil (16). To establish the clinical efficacy of the dynamic stabilization in the treatment of chronic low back pain as a result of degenerative disease with instability, the study protocol includes only those cases that do not have any leg symptoms, and do not require a concomitant decompression, or fusion in an adjacent segment. A preliminary report on 16 cases with DSS-II stabilization, with minimum one-year follow-up, showed excellent or good clinical outcome in 14 cases, and no incidence of implant failure or loosening. Although the initial results are encouraging, the authors are aware that the follow-up is too short and there were too few cases to make definitive conclusions concerning implant failure. Metallic flexible rods do not undergo creep or softening compared with the plastic cylinders. This prolongs the mechanical stabilization effect of the metallic devices, but also makes them more prone to fatigue failure.

SUMMARY

In the background of unhappy experience with fusion, dynamic stabilization has certainly created a new horizon in spine stabilization for degenerative back pain. In particular, minimally invasive posterior dynamic stabilization has the potential advantage of avoiding fusion disease. Like every other new spinal device, dynamic stabilization also has raised too much expectation, and consequently a large number of devices have been introduced in the clinical practice, often without adequate biomechanical or clinical studies. One of the greatest challenges of any dynamic stabilization device is that it has to balance the propensity for mechanical failure against the amount of motion preservation. Because of placebo effect, clinical efficacy will be difficult to establish. When the clinical studies involve multiple variables, like concomitant decompression or fusion or discectomy, it makes evaluation of the stabilization procedure nearly impossible. It is therefore pertinent that the device should have a careful biomechanical as well as clinical evaluation before considering its clinical use.

Fusion still remains the method of choice for advanced disc/facet degeneration and gross instability. However, multilevel disc degeneration, particularly in young patients, and adjacent segment degeneration following fusion are the so-called clinical targets of posterior dynamic stabilization. Before routine use can be recommended, it is crucial to demonstrate the clinical safety and efficacy of the device. In the age of spinal arthroplasty, additional indications may include salvage of a failed disc replacement or nuclear replacement.

Indications

A. *Primary indications*—in the treatment of instability
   1. Disc degeneration with mechanical low back pain
   2. Facet joint degeneration with mechanical low back pain
   3. Degenerative spondylolisthesis
   4. Salvage persistent pain after total disc replacement or nuclear replacement.

B. *Secondary indications*—prevent instability
1. Adjacent segment to fusion
2. Following decompressive laminectomy for stenosis or listhesis.
C. *Relative indications*
1. Prevent instability following discectomy
2. Primary total joint replacement—together with TDR.

Contraindications

1. Advanced disc/facet degeneration with osteophytes
2. Degenerative spondylolisthesis exceeding grade I
3. Collapse of disc height exceeding 50%
4. Osteoporosis and similar metabolic bone disease
5. Infection.

REFERENCES

1. Graf H. Lumbar instability. Surgical treatment without fusion. Rachis 1992; 412:123–137.
2. Grevitt MP, Gardner AD, Spilsbury J, et al. The Graf stabilisation system: early results in 50 patients. Eur Spine J 1995; 4(3):169–175; discussion 135.
3. Fujiwara A, Lim TH, An HS, et al. The effect of disc degeneration and facet joint osteoarthritis on the segmental flexibility of the lumbar spine. Spine 2000; 25(23):3036–3044.
4. Fujiwara A, Tamai K, An HS, et al. The relationship between disc degeneration, facet joint osteoarthritis, and stability of the degenerative lumbar spine. J Spinal Disord 2000; 13(5):444–450.
5. Frymoyer JW, Krag MH. Spinal stability and instability: definitions, classification, and general principles of management. In: Kahn A, ed. The Unstable Spine. New York: Grune & Stratton, 1986.
6. Mulholland RC, Sengupta DK. Rationale, principles and experimental evaluation of the concept of soft stabilization. Eur Spine J 2002; 11 (suppl 2):S198–205.
7. Panjabi MM. Clinical spinal instability and low back pain. J Electromyogr Kinesiol 2003; 13(4):371–379.
8. Sengupta DK. Dynamic stabilization devices in the treatment of low back pain. Orthop Clin N Am 2004; 35(1):43–56.
9. Schmoelz W, Huber JF, Nydegger T, Dipl I, Claes L, Wilke HJ. Dynamic stabilization of the lumbar spine and its effects on adjacent segments: an in vitro experiment. Spine 2003; 28 (suppl):418–423.
10. Sengupta DK, Mulholland RC. Fulcrum assisted soft stabilization system: a new concept in the surgical treatment of degenerative low back pain. Spine 2005; 30(9):1019–1029; discussion 1030.
11. Sengupta DK. Dynamic stabilization in the treatment of low back pain due to degenerative disorders. In: Herkowitz HN, ed. The Lumbar Spine. Vol. 1. 3rd ed. Philadelphia: LWW, 2004:373–383.
12. Grob D, Benini A, Junge A, Mannion AF. Clinical experience with the Dynesys semirigid fixation system for the lumbar spine: surgical and patient-oriented outcome in 50 cases after an average of 2 years. Spine 2005; 30(3):324–331.
13. Schnake KJ, Schaeren S, Jeanneret B. Dynamic stabilization in addition to decompression for lumbar spinal stenosis with degenerative spondylolisthesis. Spine 2006; 31(4):442–449.
14. Stoll TM, Dubois G, Schwarzenbach O. The dynamic neutralization system for the spine: a multi-center study of a novel non-fusion system. Eur Spine J 2002; 11 (suppl 2):S170–S178.
15. Rajaratnam SS, Selmon GPF, Mueller M, Shepperd JAN, Mulholland RC. Dynesis stabilization of the lumbo-sacral spine. Paper presented at Britspine, 2002; Birmingham, UK.
16. Pimenta L, Diaz R, K SD. DSS Minimally invasive posterior dynamic stabilization system. In: Fessler RG, ed. Dynamic Reconstruction of the Spine. New York: Thieme, 2006:323–329.
17. Gardner A, Pande KC. Graf ligamentoplasty: a 7-year follow-up. Eur Spine J 2002; 11 (suppl 2): S157–S163.
18. Putzier M, Schneider SV, Funk JF, Tohtz SW, Perka C. The surgical treatment of the lumbar disc prolapse: nucleotomy with additional transpedicular dynamic stabilization versus nucleotomy alone. Spine 2005; 30(5):E109–E114.

Index